Setting up Community Health and Development Programmes in Low and Middle Income Settings

T0201924

Setting up Community Health and Development Programmes in Low and Middle Income Settings

FOURTH EDITION

EDITED BY

Ted Lankester
Editor and lead author

Nathan Grills
Editor and author

With chapters by specialist authors
Editorial assistance from Eleanor Duncan

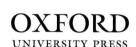

OXFORD
UNIVERSITY PRESS

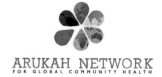

ARUKAH NETWORK
FOR GLOBAL COMMUNITY HEALTH

OXFORD
UNIVERSITY PRESS

Great Clarendon Street, Oxford, OX2 6DP,
United Kingdom

Oxford University Press is a department of the University of Oxford.
It furthers the University's objective of excellence in research, scholarship,
and education by publishing worldwide. Oxford is a registered trade mark of
Oxford University Press in the UK and in certain other countries

First Edition published in 1992
Second Edition published in 2000
Third Edition published in 2007
Fourth Edition published in 2019

Impression: 8

Published in the United States of America by Oxford University Press
198 Madison Avenue, New York, NY 10016, United States of America

British Library Cataloguing in Publication Data
Data available

Library of Congress Control Number: 2018962648

ISBN 978–0–19–880665–3

Printed and bound by
CPI Group (UK) Ltd, Croydon, CR0 4YY

READERS, PLEASE HELP US

Arukah Network believes and affirms that every community has the inherent gifts and skills needed to achieve health and wellbeing for its members, with appropriate support and accompaniment. Through our growing global network, and its *Clusters* of local people, we help to encourage these gifts and skills through intentional collaboration. *Clusters* demonstrate how this works in practice, thus enabling the network as a whole to increase and amplify its wisdom and expertise. *Communities* become better able to adopt life-changing improvements in their health and wellbeing, within their own cultures.

This book is designed to enable Arukah Network, and all others involved in health and development, to use evidence and examples of good practice to help communities develop and own their futures as effectively as possible. It also aims to help planners, academics and policy makers to grasp more fully the realities of field-based development.

This book is intended as a living resource in a fast-changing field. In community based health care we are always wanting to learn from each other. We are keen to hear from readers, whatever their background or experience, with comments, ideas, experiences, stories and examples relevant to any chapter of the book – or to any other health topic with a community based focus. Please contact us at team@arukahnetwork.org

Acknowledgements

When the first three editions of this book were first written starting in 1992, many friends and organisations gave support and encouragement, including SHARE, OPEN and TUSHAR projects, the Emmanuel Hospital Association, and Dr Kiran Martin of ASHA urban health programme.

With this edition Eleanor Duncan has carried out a full-scale editorial improvement and shortening of the complete text, and organised the references. She has given valuable editorial advice on most of the chapters. Dr Natalie Tan assisted her and contributed to the project in a variety of ways.

We have depended on the expert advice and careful review of each chapter by a worldwide variety of experts from universities, specialist agencies and the WHO. These include Andrew Tomkins, Nick Henwood, Krystle Lai, Henry Perry, Matt Reeve, Graham Carr, Tricia Greenhalgh, Priscilla Robinson, Helen Shawyer, Whitney Fry, Marko Kerac, Chris Morgan, Alison Morgan, Mark Pietroni, John Guillebaud, Giuliano Gargioni, Lana Syed, Veena O'Sullivan, Andi Eicher, Yael Velleman, Amulya Reddy, Kaaren Matthias, Kara Jenkinson, Jim Black, Stan Macaden, Anne- Marie Wilson, Nicole Bucher and Dan Munday.

Authors to Readers

We have written this book for two main audiences. The first is for those working in the field: programme managers, and practitioners from government and civil society involved in setting up or developing community health and development programmes, rural and urban. This book is also written for global health and other health care students, academics, policy makers and planners who wish to anchor their work into field-based situations. The link between valuable academic research and the impact of such research on the increased well being of vulnerable populations remains a thin line. Along with many others committed to the cause this book aims to broaden that line.

This is a radically revised fourth edition of a book Ted Lankester first wrote in 1992. In the 1980s, Ted became involved in working with colleagues to pilot ways of facilitating community based health care in remote areas where there was little effective coverage. The first edition started as his scribbled notes at the end of long days in the field. It finally saw the light of day as Ted and others broadened the scope of the book to include the experiences of many others. We are glad that despite its inadequacies the book has proved useful for many, seen several editions and reprints, a separate Indian edition and Hindi translation, and co-publication of the last edition by The Hesperian Foundation, California.

It is now 25 years since the first edition of this book was published. In addition to the topics covered in the previous editions there are many new and complex problems in promoting health at the community level. Each original chapter has been radically revised and updated with the latest evidence base along with stories, anecdotes and examples from wide ranging contexts. In addition Nathan Grills has joined as a Co-Editor and there are seven new chapters, two by Nathan, covering non-communicable diseases, mental health, disability, disaster reduction, domestic violence, palliative care and the use of Information and Communications Technology (ICT).

Although the context is very different to the 1990's, many of the core problems are similar. We remain exasperated that universal health coverage remains beyond the reach of so many. The Inverse Square Law still largely applies, which to paraphrase, states that those who most need health care are least likely to receive it.

If anything inequality and inequity in global health has grown with the increasing trend towards privatisation and corporatisation of healthcare.

As we study, lecture and travel, we see a gaping hole in global health – a giant jigsaw puzzle with the central pieces missing. This is the community – the community as an empowered group of individuals able to help plan, manage and increasingly "own" their health care, using inherent strengths, skills and abilities but in ways which also connect and integrate with government programmes This book is focussed on how communities, local health initiatives and trained health workers can help fill this gap and become the missing pieces of the jigsaw; how community members must be seen not simply as beneficiaries to whom we deliver a product – health care – but how they can be intimately involved in the solutions, as they learn to use their gifts and own their futures.

In the Bible we have an account of how Jesus used what was available – five loaves and two fish – to feed a crowd of 5000. Our hope and prayer is this: that those of us who are committed to universal health coverage and "turning off the tap of ill health" at higher levels will not be paralysed into inaction by the size of the task As the Chinese proverb states with brave simplicity: 'Many little things done in many little places by many little people will change the face of the world.'

Ted Lankester and Nathan Grills, 2019

Contents

Contributors

Smisha Agarwal Assistant Professor, Department of International Health, Johns Hopkins Bloomberg School of Public Health, Baltimore, Maryland, USA

Ian D Campbell Co-ordinator, Affirm Facilitation Associates, Woking, UK; Previously International Medical Advisor and Health Programme Consultant, Salvation Army, London, UK

Alison Rader Campbell Co-ordinator, Affirm Facilitation Associates, Woking, UK; Consultant Facilitator, Urban Health, Salvation Army, USA

Clement Chela Lecturer in Project Management Department of Public Health, University of Lusaka, Lusaka, Zambia

Julian Eaton Senior Advisor for Mental Health, CBM International, Bensheim, Germany; Co-Director, Centre for Global Mental Health, London School of Hygiene and Tropical Medicine, London, UK

Clare Goodhart Partner at Lensfield Medical Practice, Cambridge; WestCambs GP Specialty Training Programme Director; Honary Clinical Tutor at Cambridge University

Peter Grant Co-founder and Director (retired), Restored Relationships, Teddington, UK; Previously International Director, Tearfund, Teddington, UK

Nathan Grills Public Health Physician, Associate Professor of Global Health, Nossal Institute for Global Health, University of Melbourne, Melbourne, Australia

Joel Hafvenstein Executive Director, United Mission to Nepal, Kathmandu, Nepal; Previously Resilience Advisor, Tearfund, Teddington, UK. Co-Chair BOND Disaster Reduction Group, London, UK

Claire Thomas Salaried GP, Camberwell Green Practice President, VdGM European Young Family Doctors Movement, WONCA World Organisation of Family Doctors

Ted Lankester Founder and Co-Leader, Arukah Network (formerly CHGN); President Thrive Worldwide, Co-Founder, InterHealth Worldwide

Mhoira Leng Head of Palliative Care, Mulago Hospital and Makerere University, Kampala, Uganda; Medical Director, Cairdeas International Palliative Care Trust, Aberdeen, UK

Mandy Marshall Co-Founder and Director, Restored Relationships, Teddington, UK; Previously Advisor on Gender, Tearfund, Teddington, UK

Joshua Smith Research Analyst, Tearfund, Teddington, UK

Jubin Varghese Deputy Director, Disability Community Health and Development, Emmanuel Hospital Association, New Delhi, India

Trinity Zan Technical Advisor, Research Utilization, Global Health Population and Nutrition, FHI 360, Durham, North Carolina, USA

Abbreviations

ACT	Artemisinin combined therapy	**DMO**	District medical officer
AD	Auto-disable devices	**DOT**	Directly observed treatment
AFB	Acid-fast bacillus	**DOTS**	Directly observed treatment-short course
AIDS	Acquired immune deficiency syndrome	**DRC**	Democratic Republic of Congo
ARF	At-risk factor	**EC**	European Community
ARI	Acute respiratory infection	**ECHO**	European Community Humanitarian Office
ART	Antiretroviral therapy—sometimes known as HAART	**EDL**	Essential drugs list
ARVs	Antiretrovirals	**EPI**	Expanded programme on immunization
ASHAs	Accredited Social Health Activists	**EPMM**	Ending Preventable Maternal Mortality programme
BRAC	Bangladesh Rural Advancement Committee	**FBO**	Faith-based organization
CAG	Community action group	**FDC**	Fixed-dose combination
CB	Capacity building	**FGD**	Focus group discussion
CBD	Community-based distribution	**FGM/C**	Female genital mutilation/cutting
CBHC	Community-based health care	**FP**	Family planning
CBIOA	Census-based Impact Orientated Approach	**FPP**	Family planning provider
CCT	Conditional cash transfer scheme	**GADN**	Gender and Development Network
CEFM	Child, early, and forced marriage	**GAVI**	Global Alliance for Vaccines and Immunization
CHD	Community Health Development	**GVAP**	Global Vaccine Action Plan
CHGN	Community Health Global Network	**HBV**	Honour-based violence
CHP	Community health programme	**HCW**	Health care worker
CHW	Community health worker	**HFA**	Health For All
CMAM	Community-based management of acute malnutrition	**HIMS**	Health Information Management System
COPD	Chronic obstructive pulmonary disease	**HIV**	Human immunodeficiency virus
CPD	Continuing professional development	**HPV**	Human papillomavirus
CPR	Contraceptive prevalence rate	**HR**	Human resources
CPT	Co-trimoxazole preventive therapy	**HRC**	Home-based record card
CSO	Civil society organization	**HAS**	Health surveillance assistant
CSR	Corporate social responsibility	**HSV**	Herpes simplex virus
CTC	Community-based therapeutic care	**HW**	Health worker
DfiD	Department for International Development	**IAP**	Indian Academy of Pediatrics

iCCM	Integrated Community Case Management	**NID**	National immunization day
ICT	Information and Communication Technology	**NNT**	Neonatal tetanus
IDPs	Internally displaced people	**NPC**	Non-physician clinician
IMCI	Integrated Management of Childhood Illness	**NTD**	Neglected tropical disease
IMNCI	Integrated Management of Neonatal and Childhood Illness	**NTP**	National tuberculosis programme
IMPAC	Integrated Management of Pregnancy and Childbirth	**Ops**	Operations
		ORS	Oral rehydration salts/solution
INGO	International non-governmental organization	**ORT**	Oral rehydration therapy
		PA	Participatory appraisal
IPT	Isoniazid preventive therapy	**PHC**	Primary health care
IPTi	Intermittent preventive treatment in infants	**PLWH**	People living with HIV
IPTp	Intermittent preventive treatment in pregnancy	**PM&E**	Participatory monitoring and evaluation
		PPH	Postpartum haemorrhage
IRS	Insecticide residual spraying	**PPM**	Planned preventive maintenance
IUD	Intra-uterine device	**PPP**	Public-private partnership
JD	Job description	**QoL**	Quality of life
KAP	Knowledge, attitude, and practice	**RA**	Rural/Rapid appraisal
LAM	Lactational amenorrhea	**RBM**	Roll Back Malaria
LARC	Long-acting reversible contraception	**RDF**	Revolving drug fund
LLITN	Long-lasting insecticide-treated net	**RUTF**	Ready-to-use therapeutic food
LMIC	Low- to middle-income country	**SAM**	Severe acute malnutrition
M&E	Monitoring and evaluation	**SDG**	Sustainable development goal
MAM	Moderate acute malnutrition	**SHG**	Self-help group
MCH	Mother/child health	**SIA**	Supplementary immunization activities
MDGs	Millennium Development Goals	**SNID**	Sub-national immunization day
MDR-TB	Multidrug-resistant tuberculosis	**SP**	Sulfadoxine/pyrimethamine
MPW	Multipurpose health worker	**STI**	Sexually transmitted infection
MRSA	Methicillin-resistant Staphylococcus aureus	**TALC**	Teaching aids at low cost
MR	Measles-Rubella vaccine	**TB**	Tuberculosis
MSM	Men who have sex with men	**TBA**	Traditional birth attendant
MUAC	Mid-upper arm circumference	**TCA**	Tobacco control advocate
NCD	Non-communicable disease	**TFR**	Total fertility rate
NGO	Non-governmental organization	**THP**	Traditional health practitioner
		TOR	Terms of reference

TOT	Training of trainers	**VHC**	Village health committee
UHC	Universal Health Coverage	**VHT**	Village health team
UN	United Nations	**VIP**	Ventilated improved pit latrine
UNDP	United Nations Development Programme	**VVM**	Vaccine vial monitor
UNICEF	United Nations Children's Fund	**WASH**	Wash and sanitation programme
USAID	United States Agency for International Development	**WHO**	World Health Organization
VAWG	Violence against women and girls	**XDR-TB**	Extensively drug-resistant tuberculosis
VCT	Voluntary (HIV) counselling and testing		

SECTION 1
Community health principles

CHAPTER 1
Community-based health care
Setting the scene

Ted Lankester

What we need to know

This book is about community-based health care (CBHC). Its starting point is simple. Reliable and accessible health is rarely found among the poorest and most vulnerable members of our world. The facts are simple, and yet the reasons are complex.

A word of explanation about the word 'we' used throughout this book. "We" refer to all those who are in any way involved in working at community level, which includes community members and leaders, members of government and civil society organizations (CSOs), donors, academics, evaluators, and other stakeholders. Many people reading this book will be included by the term "we".

Before we look at the radical and effective ways in which communities themselves can be an answer to many of their health problems, we need to grasp the sheer scale of their needs and challenges, which are outlined next. These facts were accurate at the time of writing this book (2018).

Health problems: facts and statistics

Poverty and mortality

626 million people—about 8% of the world's population—live in absolute poverty, i.e. on less than 1.90 USD per day.[1] Each year, 303,000 women do not survive pregnancy or childbirth. The majority of these women die because they have no access to routine and emergency care.[2] Finally, each year, 5.5 million children—approximately 630 per hour—under the age of five years die. These deaths are largely due to preventable or easily treatable causes.[3]

Inequalities

A child born in Malawi can expect to live for only 47 years, while a child born in Japan could live for as long as 83 years—a thirty-six-year difference in life expectancy. In Afghanistan, Somalia, and Chad, the maternal mortality ratio is over 1000 out of 100,000 live births, while it is 21 for the European Region of the World Health Organization (WHO).[4]

Access to health care

Around half of the world's population lack access to full basic health care.[5] Additionally, 56 per cent of people living in rural areas worldwide do not have access to essential health-care services. In Africa 83 per cent of people in rural areas are not covered by essential health-care services.[6]

How CBHC can contribute to positive change

This book aims to show how CBHC can be one important part of the health system and part of the answer to responding to global health needs. For example, as the community takes initiatives, as health standards improve, and as other forms of development emerge, a new order starts to take shape. This is based on:

- *Justice*, where the rich are no longer tolerated in their exploitation of the poor, and the strong are less able to oppress the weak;
- *Equity*, where all have sufficient for their basic needs, and the differences between rich and poor are reduced;
- *Reconciliation* and *peace-making*, where individuals and community groups learn mutual respect and aim to resolve their differences;
- *Commonality of interest*, whereby as communities work towards common goals, conflict tends to lessen and divisive issues are more easily resolved.

In order for CBHC to reach any of these aspirations, it needs to be excellently managed and based on evidence and good practice. It must function as part of, or in the closest association with, national health systems.

This first chapter sets out to explain the unique features of CBHC, and how it links in with other forms of health care. It outlines the key role CBHC can play in helping to meet the major health challenges facing those in greatest need. We aim to address:

Where are we now?

Despite the figures shown above, we need to celebrate improvements that have been made. The good news is that the world has made real progress since the first edition of this book in 1991. The global under-five mortality rate has dropped from 93 deaths per 1,000 live

births in 1990 to 39 in 2017.[3] Life expectancy has risen worldwide in most countries.

However, progress has been uneven. In 2012, two-thirds of the reduction in under-five mortality rates had occurred in just five countries and thirteen countries have seen increases since 1990.[7]

Health gains are being lost in some of the poorest countries and communities, and a quote by Chen and colleagues from their 2004 study remains true in many of the most vulnerable communities: that 'after a century of the most spectacular health advances in human history, gains are being lost because of feeble health systems. On the front line we see overworked and overstressed health workers too few in numbers, losing the fight, with many collapsing under the strain'.[8]

It is not acceptable to tolerate this situation in a world where the richest and most favoured have excellent health care and life expectancies of more than 80 years, but where the poorest can only expect to live for around 50 years.[9] We therefore have an urgent duty to work and to advocate for a fairer deal for the poorest and most marginalized.

The source of our motivations to respond will vary, and often be inclusive of religious and humanitarian ideals. However, it will also help if we also recognize our mandate to improve the health and wellbeing of all the world's citizens. In 1948, the United Nations' Universal Declaration of Human Rights was ratified; Article 25 states that 'everyone has the right to a standard of living adequate for the health and well-being of himself and of his family, including food, clothing, housing and medical care and necessary social services ...'.[10] This book attempts to show how government, CSOs, and communities working together in strong and focused collaboration can improve global health through a wide range of tried and tested solutions. Chapter 3 helps to show how these are an essential part of health systems strengthening. In launching its 2008 World Health Report, *Primary Health Care—Now more than ever*, the WHO stated that 'Primary health care brings balance back to health care and *puts families and communities at the hub of the health system.* With an emphasis on local *ownership [it]... makes space for solutions created by communities, owned by them and sustained by them*' [italics added].[11]

Where have we come from?

Health care based in communities dates back to the dawn of human history. However, in the middle and second half of the twentieth century, specific models of CBHC started to emerge, with China's 'bare foot doctor' being an inspiring example. In 1946, the Constitution

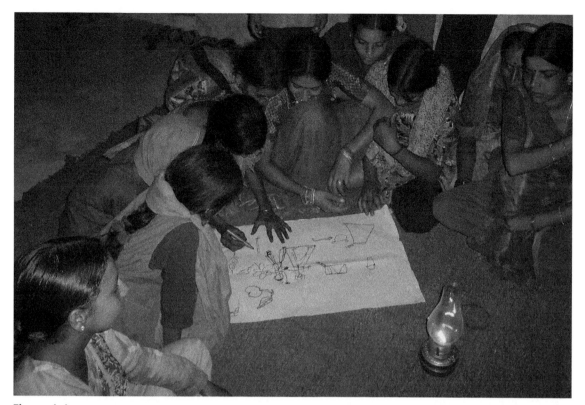

Figure 1.1 Community-based care is based on the excitement of learning together.

of the newly formed WHO defined health as (in what at the time was seen as a radical approach) 'a state of complete physical, mental and social well-being and not merely the absence of disease or infirmity'.[12]

However, we will take as our main starting point 1978, famous in primary health care circles as the year of the Alma-Ata Declaration.[13] There, under the joint leadership of WHO and UNICEF, Health Minsters and planners from 134 member states of the United Nations met at Alma-Ata in the then-Soviet Union (now Almaty, the former capital of Kazakhstan). They drew up a charter to bring basic health services within reach of every community and individual. Crucially, Target 5 of the Alma-Ata Declaration stated that a main social aim should be 'the attainment by all the people of the world of a level of health that will permit them to lead a socially and economically productive life. Primary health care is the key to attaining this target.' Out of this was coined a catchphrase of the time—'Health for All by the Year 2000'.

Alma-Ata inspired a number of effective and far-reaching programmes. Many of these continue today and have achieved spectacular results. For example,

the Comprehensive Rural Health Programme in Jamkhed, India (www.jamkhed.org) has improved the empowerment of women, helped communities to achieve economic independence in drought-ridden areas, and brought dramatic improvements in the health of women and children.[14]

However, the 1978 Declaration did not bring about the large-scale improvements that many had hoped for. Health for All (HFA) was a horizontal, comprehensive approach to health based on developing strong community-based partnerships, but it lacked the aims, expertise, and political will to be widely successful.

This caused a shift to a vertical approach concentrating on single topics or illnesses. These emerging vertical programmes were based on specific interventions, with health workers trained to deliver them. For example, UNICEF's Expanded Programme on Immunization (see Chapter 10) has been highly successful in vaccinating children against key diseases.

During the 1990s many other vertical programmes were added, including Roll Back Malaria, The Safe Motherhood Initiative, and what is now known as the End TB Strategy.

Table 1.1 shows the pros and cons of both a vertical and a horizontal approach. In summary, vertical approaches work well for tackling single, but often complex, health issues and diseases, but in so doing they are in danger of bypassing community action and ownership. They focus more on delivery than on empowerment. The result is that benefits may last only as long as the programme is funded. However, many programmes have also made spectacular gains—the virtual elimination of polio being an impressive example.

In the 1990s, WHO and UNICEF tried to bring the vertical and horizontal approaches together to meet the complex needs of children in an initiative known as Integrated Management of Childhood Illness (IMCI) (see Chapter 16).

In the year 2000, the Millennium Development Goals (MDGs) were introduced which, while valuable, were an incomplete set of focused objectives guiding many global health priorities. Some were reached, others were not. As of 2015, the MDGs were replaced by the Sustainable Development Goals (SDGs) running from 2015 to 2030, and which cover a far wider spectrum of planetary needs.

The SDGs include both the original priorities of Alma-Ata but now cover a far wider spectrum of illnesses. These goals acknowledge that health has a wide range of determinants, and that these need to be considered when thinking of community health. Accordingly, this edition of the book provides increased coverage of issues that determine human and planetary well-being. As we look ahead, CBHC has an ever-increasing role in meeting both the original and emerging needs.

As CBHC develops into the future we must still be guided by the revolutionary principles of Alma-Ata: equity, justice, health for all and community participation.

The Astana Declaration 2018 is an updated and expanded view of priorities and plans, written 40 years afterAlma Ata, which can be read in full at https://www.who.int/docs/default-source/primary-health/declaration/gcphc-declaration.pdf.

Major health challenges we face

The world is now going through what is known as a health transition. This means that we still have to deal with infectious diseases, malnutrition, and the classic diseases of poverty, high numbers of mothers dying in childbirth, and deaths of infants and children.

Table 1.1 Advantages and disadvantages of vertical and horizontal programmes

Vertical programmes

Advantages

Single topic or illness means programmes can more easily be expertly designed, managed, monitored, and delivered.

Priority illnesses can be effectively targeted.

Efficacy in implementing programmes dependent on evidence-based clinical guidelines, e.g. End TB Strategy.

Popular with donors.

Disadvantages

Often undermine community involvement.

Often bypass traditional healers.

Can impose western models of health care.

Often driven by donors and planners rather than by local priorities.

May be inefficient at community level as health workers are trained exclusively in one programme.

Often unsustainable when funding stops, or another health priority is considered more important.

Many health workers working at community level leave to join better-paid vertical programmes.

Horizontal programmes

Advantages

More opportunity for community partnership, design, and management.

Based on empowerment and behavioural change alongside delivery.

If well managed, more likely to be sustainable.

Less dependent on donors.

Emphasis given to strengthening health systems to address a wide range of problems.

Easier to focus on prevention as well as cure.

Community and family members can be involved as formal/informal health workers.

Interventions often technically simple.

Disadvantages

Less focus, which can be a problem if diseases are complex or a topic requires careful logistics and support.

Require good-quality, local management and leadership.

Often require more time, training, and patience to set up.

Need clear requirement for resources and supplies.

Funding is often harder to obtain.

But we also have ageing populations and non-communicable diseases (NCDs) as the leading causes of death, with associated disability, in most countries, plus the deadly effects of tobacco use, alcohol addiction, and substance abuse. These and other health priorities form the topics of many chapters in the second half of this book. Behind all these health needs are wider challenges. It is helpful to understand what some of these are from the CBHC viewpoint.

Lack of trained health workers

The world is short of 17.4 million trained health workers—doctors, nurses, midwives, and public health workers; by 2035 it will be 14.3 million short.[15]

There are many reasons for the shortage. Many countries lack the resources to train health care professionals or pay them adequately. As a result, many people leave for better paid jobs in cities or as private practitioners. Some join international organizations, NGOs, other CSOs, or vertical programmes that offer good salaries. Those more highly qualified are recruited by high-income countries who themselves need skilled workers. Additionally, in many low-income countries, health workers often have responsibilities at home caring for children and elderly relatives, many of whom are living longer and developing chronic illnesses.

Part of the solution to this problem, discussed in greater detail in Chapter 7 and subsequently, is suggested by the following quote at https://www.ncbi.nlm.nih.gov/pubmed/2621254:

With political will, however, governments can adopt more flexible approaches by planning CHW programmes within the context of overall health sector activities, rather than as a separate activity ... CHWs represent an important health resource whose potential in providing and extending a reasonable level of health care to undeserved populations must be fully tapped.[16]

Weak health systems and widespread corruption

Planning health services is vastly complex and involves not only specific health-related activities but also many other sectors such as agriculture, housing, water, sanitation, social services, and the environment. Resource-poor countries struggle in many of these areas.

Health systems are so weak in some places that plans cannot be implemented. In the neediest communities there are neither the systems nor the trained people for health care to happen at the local level. In many countries funds for national health systems are siphoned off at various levels through corrupt and illegal practices.

Health systems without a primary health care (community) basis

Where no national health system or insurance schemes exist, or there is little commitment to primary health care (PHC), the rich can usually still access good health care, but the poor are marginalized. This is evident in many countries, e.g. the United States and India. However, it is more helpful to look at examples where PHC does occur and brings good results. Where national governments are committed to PHC, huge gains can be made in reducing child deaths, deaths of mothers in childbirth, and increasing life expectancy.

How CBHC can help meet these challenges

The aim of CBHC is to ensure that in each rural and urban community, health programmes function effectively, prevention is given priority, that national health plans can be implemented, and that everyone has universal access to health care. Looking at this more specifically:

- CBHC goes a long way towards answering the need for more health workers—most of whom will be community members who can be effectively and economically trained (see Chapter 8).
- CBHC can strengthen health systems at a local level. This means programmes such as IMCI, vertical programmes, and other locally determined health initiatives can be implemented effectively with the full participation of the community (see Chapter 3).
- CBHC involves communities in planning and management so that even if specific programmes cease or donors withdraw funding, there will still be health systems in place at the community level.
- CBHC at its best draws in experience and best practice from around the globe, but also works in close co-operation with government health services and national plans.
- CBHC offers radical ways of meeting health needs, based on two powerful tools—empowerment and transformation. The meaning of these will emerge as we look at the distinctive features of a community-based approach in the next section.

Special features of a CBHC approach

CBHC emphasizes community

1. *CBHC encourages ownership by the community.*

The community participates, becomes a partner, and eventually shares ownership of the programme. CBHC aims to be a genuine partnership comprising health and development workers from government and CSOs as well as community members.

2. *CBHC responds to the needs of the community.*

CBHC starts with the local people; it helps them identify their needs, and works with them in finding answers.

3. *CBHC promotes self-reliance.*

CBHC aims to bring about healthy, self-reliant communities. People become armed with knowledge so they depend less on external sources of support.

4. *CBHC helps to encourage community life.*

CBHC encourages traditional practices unless they are actually harmful. New ideas are introduced with sensitivity. The aim of the health programme is always to build up confidence and dignity, and never to cause offence or humiliation.

5. *CBHC moves outwards to where the people live.*

Care, wherever possible, is based in the home and neighbourhood, not the clinic or hospital. It is decided according to the needs of the community, rather than the convenience of the doctor or health worker. Sick people are treated in their homes or as near to their homes as possible.

6. *CBHC moves forwards to the next generation.*

Children become a focal point of health activities. They are not simply targeted for improved health care but are involved in bringing it about. Healthy patterns of living absorbed by children today become the accepted practices of tomorrow (see Figure 1.2).

7. *CBHC helps to bring about behavioural change.*

Through the excitement of discovering new ideas and different practices that bring visible improvements, long-term changes in lifestyle start to occur and health begins to improve. CBHC is based at the local level and by its very nature behavioural change is a local process (see Chapter 4).

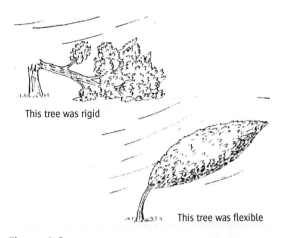

This tree was rigid

This tree was flexible

Figure 1.2 The flexibility of community-based health programmes enables them to respond to changing needs and situations.

8. *CBHC aims to include all community members.*

The poorest, neediest, and most at risk are given priority. Women are given equal status with men. The elderly and those living with disability are cared for. Members of the least-popular ethnic group, caste, or religion are equally valued. The rich and powerful are included where possible, but are never allowed to displace the poor or become too dominant. A person's need, rather than money or status, determines the type of health care received.

9. *CBHC aims to connect with all those committed to health and well-being.*

Health care professionals, community members, members of faith communities, and development workers are included and involved. Members of government and CSOs are welcomed and ideas mutually shared. CBHC is well placed to play a linking role between the community and various government services and other programmes (see Figure 1.3).

10. *CBHC encourages a style of leadership that is committed to caring and sharing rather than being top-down and dominant.*

CBHC emphasizes health

1. *CBHC is involved more in health care than in medical care.*

CBHC opposes 'PPNN'—a Pill for every Problem, a Needle for every Need. Instead, it emphasizes appropriate

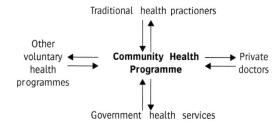

Figure 1.3 Community-based health programmes must work collaboratively wherever possible.

cure. Many health workers use excessive medicines and injections. CBHC aims to ensure that a rational list of essential, life-saving medicines is always available, affordable, and appropriately used (Figure 1.4).

2. *CBHC emphasizes health promotion and disease prevention.*

It aims to turn off 'the tap of ill health' and identify and reduce the higher-level causes and social determinants of ill health.

3. *CBHC follows a comprehensive, integrated, and holistic model of health care.*

It includes physical, mental, emotional, spiritual, and environmental health. Health is seen as an integral part

of social development. CBHC is committed to Planetary Health—'Healthier People on a Healthier Planet'.[17]

What CBHC is not

1. *CBHC is not in opposition to doctors, hospitals, and vertical programmes.*

Unless they disempower the community and impose inappropriate or short-lasting solutions, CBHC works in conjunction with these institutions. By concentrating on health care provided largely through trained community members it releases doctors and other senior health workers to use their training more effectively, and enables hospitals to use their facilities more efficiently.

2. *CBHC is not simply adding new structures on to old foundations.*

CBHC is not an extension of a hospital into the four walls of a community clinic. It is a restructuring of the health care system so that the people become partners with the providers. The place where illness occurs, the home and the community, also becomes the place where most health care takes place. Only when this fails is referral made to hospital or a health facility, i.e. health care takes place in homes, repairs take place in hospital.

3. *CBHC is not a second-rate health service for the poor.*

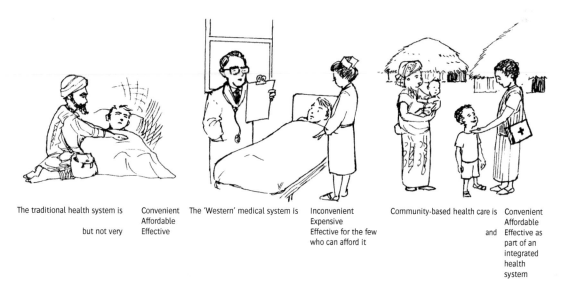

The traditional health system is Convenient Affordable but not very Effective

The 'Western' medical system is Inconvenient Expensive Effective for the few who can afford it

Community-based health care is Convenient Affordable and Effective as part of an integrated health system

Figure 1.4 Three models of health care.

CBHC is the key to an effective health system for all. But it must be correctly set up, excellently managed, and integrated into government health systems of which it is an essential part. The charter of the People's Health Assembly expands and explains many of these principles.[18]

CBHC: comparisons with other models

It is helpful to look at this according to three stages.

Stage 1: a traditional health model

Health care takes place in the community, according to the wishes and convenience of community members. Senior family members such as grandmothers are often seen as the traditional source of wisdom. In more serious situations, other traditional health workers are called in, and these are members of the community known to have specific skills or knowledge. Each community has its own traditional health practitioners. Examples include herbalists, shamans, priests, traditional midwives, and ayurvedic practitioners. Payment is made in cash or kind, usually at a level the patient can afford. This system has value when no better alternative exists, and when people's expectations remain low. Many remedies bring relief, and some are effective, such as in evidence-proved remedies from Chinese herbal medicine and Ayurveda (see Chapter 3). Today many rural societies still function largely on this system. Also, as health infrastructure collapses in failing states or in chronic complex emergencies, some communities are returning to this system.

Stage 2: a conventional hospital-based model

Health care takes place in the hospital or clinic largely at the convenience of the doctor, nurse, or other health practitioner. The health worker often has few links with the community. Hospital staff tend to direct and dominate the treatment of the patient. Often the cost of treatment is far beyond the reach of those most in need. Although often effective and acceptable to those able to pay for these services, this approach is commonly frightening, inconvenient, and unaffordable to the poor and marginalized. Many of the most excluded members of a community may never use it at all.

Stage 3: a modern primary health-care model

Health care returns to the community, with referral to clinic or hospital only when necessary.
PHC aims to ensure that good-quality care is available in the community, from a friendly provider, at an affordable cost. A referral system ensures that those who need clinic or hospital care are able to receive it. Prevention of ill health becomes the dominant theme:

Primary health care offers a way to organize the full range of health care, from households to hospitals, with prevention as important as cure, and with resources invested sensibly at each level of the health system. Primary health care increasingly looks like a smart way to get health development back on track ... In other words, primary health care becomes not only a system of appropriate prevention, cure, and care at community level, but a complete national health model for the way health services are provided.[19]

CBHC is at the heart of a PHC approach; often, the two terms are used interchangeably. Many countries, but not all, are committed to introducing and strengthening PHC as their preferred model, as advised by the WHO. But opposition to Universal Health Coverage (UHC) continues in some quarters. We need to understand the reasoning behind this opposition and advocate robustly for PHC as the system that most benefits the majority of citizens.

The role of civil society organizations (CSOs)

In many countries a wide range of CSOs are involved in health and development. These include a range and variety of which the following are the most commonly used; NGOs (non-governmental organizations), CBOs (community-based organizations), and FBOs (faith-based or faith-inspired organizations). Sometimes these collectively are known as the voluntary sector or the third sector.* This book uses the term CSO as it is probably the most inclusive.

CSOs have undoubtedly contributed a huge amount to the overall health care in many countries and to the most impoverished communities. But they also have their disadvantages, which include setting up alternative health care systems from the government rather than collaborating. Another disadvantage is that they may deliver a wide variety of services, which become unsustainable when the programme ends or the funding runs out. There are more details on the pros and cons of CSOs in Chapter 3.

Recently, the role of the faith-based sector is seen as increasingly important, particularly in sub-Saharan Africa.[20] More than 80 per cent of the world's population report having a religious faith, and most of this number reside in low- and middle-income countries.[21] This means that any failure to understand and respect local religious and cultural beliefs can add to the gap between the community and outsiders.

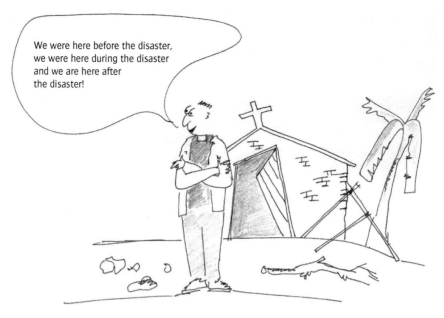

Figure 1.5 The church, mosque, or temple has a permanent presence.

In CBHC we should meet, respect, and encourage religious leaders who should be seen as allies in promoting healthy practices through their churches, temples, and mosques. But we must ensure they follow ethical, inclusive, and evidence-based practices (Figure 1.5).

When 'outsiders' come in to any community, whether government workers, members of CSOs, or any other organization we should bear in mind some of the following principles:

- Build trust and friendship.
- Recognize community skills and assets.
- Encourage community-led ideas and actions.
- Encourage maximum collaboration.
- Facilitate, encourage, and train.
- Never create dependence.
- Treat all community members with respect and dignity.
- Work towards sustainability.
- Amplify the voices of justice, compassion and equity.

What we need to do

Using CBHC to tackle poverty— the root cause of ill health

In his 1998 report on WHO activity, Jancloes stated that 'poverty is the main reason why babies are not vaccinated, clean water and sanitation are not provided, curative drugs and other treatments are not available, and mothers die in childbirth'.[22] We can interpret this statement to conclude that poverty is a root cause of ill health. Good and honest governance also plays a vital role, and communities can be taught how to hold local government and other health services accountable.

CBHC at its most effective tackles poverty head on. Through empowerment it helps communities to make the best use of existing resources, and generate new ones through other forms of community development, such as micro-enterprise. Through partnership, it enables communities to share their skills and resources, to everyone's benefit. Through connections with governments and other programmes, it helps to bring a wider range of resources to the community

The problem

Health workers soon come to realize that the diseases they see are usually symptoms of a much greater 'illness' that affects their communities. Health planners use the term 'social determinants of health' to describe these symptoms. A great deal of research and action is focused on trying to understand them.

Buse writes: "Those seeking to ensure health and wellbeing for all people at all ages should focus on the upstream determinants of sickness."

Even within the richest and poorest parts of cities the blight of poverty makes a huge difference. In the British city of Sunderland, life expectancy is 83 for a man from a wealthy neighbourhood, compared with 69 for a man from a deprived neighbourhood just a few kilometres away.[23]

Poverty is the main determinant of health. Most preventable illness in resource-poor areas and countries is a direct result of poverty. Poor people have little money, inadequate food and education, and little power; frequently, those who are wealthier have no concept of such deprivation, or that they partly may be the cause of it. The poor have a history of being exploited, quite often by those who own more land and have more money, including unethical corporations. Such exploitation is always found in association with poverty and both causes it and results from it.

Poverty does not usually disappear when a country becomes prosperous. Often the rich become richer still, and the poor make few gains; this divide continues to lead to greater inequity.

As those committed to CBHC, we must be aware of the forces that act against the poor and which lock them into lifestyles of poverty. We must understand and engage with other forms of development, such as adult literacy and children's education, both of which may reduce poverty and exploitation even more than the health programmes themselves. Figure 1.6 outlines some of the causes of poverty.

Each country, region, and community will have its own particular list of issues and prejudices that cause and embed poverty. Furthermore, human corruptibility multiplies the problems facing those who are the most marginalized and voiceless. For example:

- *greed* contributes to a wealthy minority at the expense of a poor majority;

- *dishonesty* may result in broken promises and pledges made to those depending on assurances of help or change; and

- *corruption* disproportionately affects the poor. Those unable to afford to bribes miss out on health care and, furthermore, funds allocated for the poor never reach them.

Our approach

In planning our response to poverty and exploitation we must consciously resist becoming discouraged or intimidated. Some of our actions will be directed at reducing poverty itself, especially if we are able to tackle some of the social determinants or work with others to encourage communities to follow enterprise-based approaches (including microfinance and income generation). We can also work indirectly by setting up systems to reduce the cost of providing services to community members

But first we must emphasize that the very concept of describing a community as 'poor' is in danger of betraying the existence of assets and abilities that are present in each individual, and which are richly present in all communities. For example, this author believes that, given the right nurture and encouragement, a community of 200 people or more is likely to possess a potential prime minister, a world-class actor, and an elite athlete.

There are some practical approaches we can follow when planning our programme:

1. *Understand the causes of poverty.*

Identifying the specific causes of poverty in the communities where we are working will help us to be more realistic in our planning.

2. *Understand we can do more together.*

While we can do very little as an individual, we can have a major impact when we work together with others, and when we form local, national, and global networks.

3. *Understand that CBHC is a multiplication process.*

The hospital-based approach treats illness but does little to prevent it. Someone has described it as trying to empty the ocean with a teaspoon. But a CBHC approach not only prevents illness, but by treating illness at an early stage greatly reduces the number of people who need to be referred to hospital. This approach reduces the health costs faced by the poor and by the country.

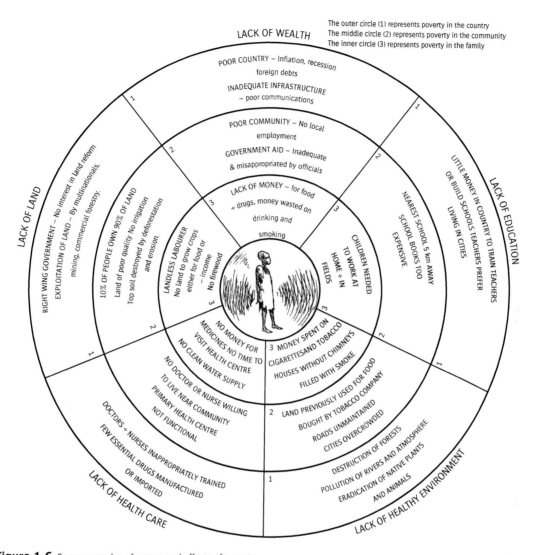

Figure 1.6 Some examples of causes and effects of poverty.

4. *Start with the skills that are present in the community.*

This is sometimes known as a strengths-based approach. Each community is rich in ideas, skills, and creative talent. These can be released, used, and directed, with far-reaching effects. Using skills from the community can lead to lower costs as more tasks are done by community members than are contracted to outsiders.

5. *Include community development in addition to health as soon as we are able.*

CBHC programmes need to be involved with government departments responsible for all areas of development that are essential for a community's health and well-being, e.g. agriculture and water. Tackling problems together is known as 'inter-sectorial collaboration', and will have a far greater effect on improving the health of our communities than through health interventions alone.

6. *Encourage people to claim their rights under the laws of the country.*

We can help community members to claim the services and supplies that are legally due to them. We can advocate for a rights-based approach. For more information on human rights and its value in promoting health, see details on the People's Health Movement in Further reading at the end of this chapter (see also Figure 1.7).

7. *Alter traditional patterns of life as little as possible unless they are actually harmful to health and well-being.*

This becomes increasingly difficult as 'globalization' brings the lure of riches, modernity, and glamour to those who can never attain them. Instead, income generation schemes, sports clubs, and other community initiatives can help to strengthen village communities and reduce unchosen or forced migration to cities.

8. *Resist injustice, and show solidarity where important humanitarian principles are involved.*

Advocacy plays an important part in CBHC and amplifying our collective voice is a key action we can take, and is mentioned in many sections of this book.

Sustainable Development Goals and Universal Health Coverage (UHC)

Two key frameworks—SDGs (see Figure 1.8) and Universal Health Coverage (UHC)—give us an internationally agreed reference point for advocacy. CBHC programmes specifically concentrate on the following SDGs but virtually all SDGs have an impact on health (numbers are as per Figure 1.8):

1. End poverty in all its forms everywhere.
2. End hunger, achieve food security and nutrition, and promote sustainable agriculture.
3. Ensure healthy lives and promote well-being for all at all ages.

5. Achieve gender equality and empower all women and girls.
6. Ensure availability and sustainable management of water and sanitation for all.
10. Reduce inequality within and among countries.

For a deeper explanation of the main SDGs relating to health,[24] interested readers are referred to http://sustainabledevelopment.un.org/focussdgs.html. In addition to working towards all the SDGs, we can also aim to help implement specific targets within Goal 3 (Figure 1.8):

3.1 by 2030 reduce the global maternal mortality ratio to less than 70 per 100,000 live births.

3.2 by 2030 end preventable deaths of newborns and under-five children.

3.3 by 2030 end the epidemics of AIDS, tuberculosis, malaria, and neglected tropical diseases, and combat hepatitis, water-borne diseases, and other communicable diseases.

3.4 by 2030 reduce by one-third premature mortality from NCDs through prevention and treatment, and promote mental health and well-being.[25]

We need to see UHC alongside the SDGs. The SDGs have been largely designed and promoted by the United Nations. UHC has been promoted more through the WHO. UHC has become one of the overarching themes of global health following the 'expiry' of the MDGs in 2015.

In UHC everyone has access to affordable health care as near to their homes as possible. The WHO definition of UHC[25] embodies three objectives:

1. Equity in access to health services—everyone who needs services should receive them, not just those who can afford them;

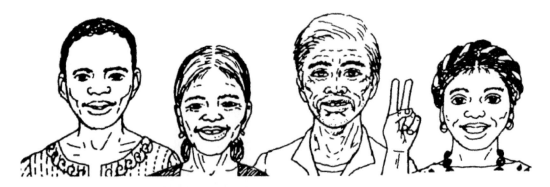

Figure 1.7 Working together in friendship and trust is one key to successful health programmes.

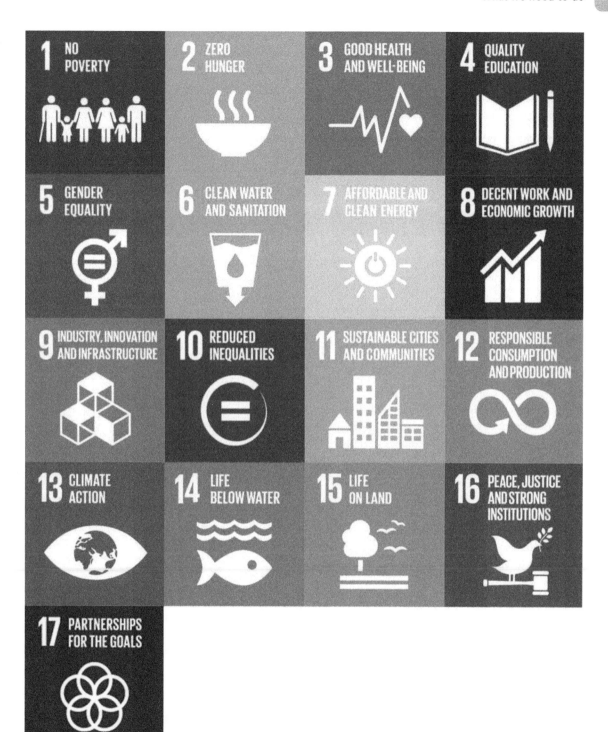

Figure 1.8 The Sustainable Development Goals.

2. The quality of health services should be good enough to improve the health of those receiving the services; and

3. People should be protected against financial risk, ensuring that the cost of using services does not put people at risk of financial harm.

Many global health planners and policy makers are encouraging countries to provide free access to health care because this leads to reduced death rates and fewer illnesses (i.e. to reduced mortality and lower morbidity).

However, in practice this is often impossible, given the lack of financial capacity in national health systems; additionally, at a local level, charging fees at an affordable rate can sometimes make the difference between the health programme continuing or closing down. This is discussed more in Chapter 12.

Setting up, strengthening, and scaling up programmes

Generally, there are three stages of health programmes that we may be involved with: Setting up, strengthening, and scaling up programmes. Each stage exists at both national and community levels. We will look at each from the viewpoint of CBHC.

Setting up refers to starting up new programmes where currently nothing effective exists. There are still large populations with no access to basic health care and in many areas, there are no effective programmes at community level. Examples include urban slums, poor and remote communities (especially in mountainous and desert areas), or rural areas where infrastructure is poor. Vulnerable and stigmatized communities may live alongside others who are relatively affluent. There are communities where conflict, disasters, or poor governance have undermined or overwhelmed health systems. In some countries, e.g. South Sudan, there are virtually no effective government health services.

Strengthening refers to working with existing programmes and building their capacity to increase their impact. This involves improving the knowledge and effectiveness of existing health workers, training new ones, improving systems, increasing quality, developing leadership skills, and enabling communities to use and trust their health services. It also involves including communities in planning and management strategies with government health services. (This book was almost given the added title 'strengthening' and most chapters will be helpful as programmes develop from their earliest stages.)

Scaling up, scaling out, or going to scale refers to making effective health programmes available on a wider scale

to increasing numbers of people. Although governments will need to take a lead in this, we can make major contributions in CBHC. For example:

- Ideas can spread between communities through word of mouth, leading to requests to extend existing health programmes.
- Health planners and practitioners can visit and learn from existing programmes to help in starting similar activities in their own areas.
- Governments can learn from effective CBHC approaches and implement them in other areas. For example, several states in India asked to learn from the model so successfully set up in Maharashtra by the Jamkhed Comprehensive Rural Health Programme (www.jamkhed.org), and the Uttarakhand Community Health Cluster (www.chgnuk.org).
- Scaling up needs to be higher on the priority list for community-based programmes than it has been in the past.

One effective way of scaling up is a social tool known as SALT, originally used in Zambia. This is a way of transferring knowledge, skills, and hope outwards in increasing circles from those communities originally involved in a health programme (see Chapter 2).

Long-term commitment or quick wins?

CBHC is almost by definition a long-term commitment. Empowerment and transformation are tools we use to encourage behavioural changes; these changes will lead to healthier communities but they often take many years. They can also be hard to measure. Communities may get discouraged when they don't see quick, clear, results, and they may start losing interest. This means we also need to ensure there are a few 'quick wins' which are more obvious to see and happen relatively fast. Put another way, we need to recognize and pick 'low-hanging fruit.'

Within the context of CBHC, Table 1.2 provides some examples of ideas that can bring about relatively quick and effective results.

New emerging challenges that CBHC can help to solve

Figure 1.9 gives the 2016 estimate of the ten leading causes of death. CBHC can help to prevent many of these a community level. Ischaemic heart disease is flagged up as the world's leading cause of death. For more details on this topic, see Chapter 22.

Table 1.2 Examples of some quick wins in the health sector

> Distribution of free, long-lasting, insecticide-treated bed nets to all children in malaria-endemic zones.
>
> Elimination or reduction of user fees for basic health services (providing financed by increased resources).
>
> Increased access to sexual and reproductive health including family planning and contraception information and services.
>
> Increased use of proven, effective drug combinations, e.g. for HIV/AIDS, TB, and malaria.

Source: data from Sachs, J.D. et al. The Millennium Project: a plan for meeting the Millenium Development Goals. *The Lancet*. 365(9456), 347-53. Copyright © 2005 Elsevier. This table is distributed under the terms of the Creative Commons Attribution Non- Commercial 4.0 International licence (CC-BY-NC), a copy of which is available at http://creativecommons.org/licenses/by-nc/4.0/.

Emerging/re-emerging diseases, and abuse

TB, HIV infection, dengue fever, chikungunya, Ebola, Zika, and others

In CBHC we may find ourselves at the front line of both helping to recognize and to treat various infections and conditions, e.g. Ebola in West Africa in 2014 and in

DRC in 2018/2019. Epidemiologists are concerned we are likely to see a disease which is both very dangerous and very infectious. In CBHC we can watch out for emerging diseases.

Neglected tropical diseases

Neglected tropical diseases (NTDs) include conditions like schistosomiasis and helminth (worm) infections. Tackling most of these types of problems needs a strong community basis. Approaches to NTDs have demonstrated how community-based distribution of effective medication can have a huge impact on large populations (see Chapter 11).

For example, in Nigeria, community health workers trained by Sightsavers have distributed a treatment for river blindness to nearly 5.5 million people. This approach has been replicated in over 15 African countries, resulting in the extension of the treatment to over 75 countries.[26]

Emerging antibiotic resistance

Antibiotic resistance is a topic likely to remain near the top of research and development in global health for the foreseeable future. In CBHC we have a twin duty both towards using appropriate treatment for community members and towards minimizing rapidly increasing

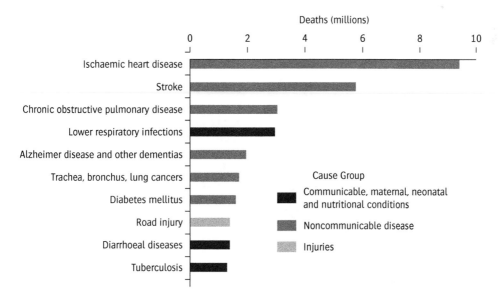

Figure 1.9 Top 10 global causes of death, 2016.

Reproduced with permission from Factsheet 2017: The top 10 causes of death. WHO. Copyright © WHO 2016. Available at: http://www.who.int/mediacentre/factsheets/fs310/en/. This image is distributed under the terms of the Creative Commons Attribution Non-Commercial 4.0 International licence (CC-BY-NC), a copy of which is available at http://creativecommons.org/licenses/by-nc/4.0/.

global resistance. We must ensure that antibiotics are used rationally, only when needed, and always according to careful protocols and group directions (see Chapter 11).

Non-communicable diseases

Not to be confused with NTDs, NCDs are now the leading cause of death worldwide. The recognition and maintenance treatment of many NCDs is best carried out at community level. This is an important new area for CBHC (for more information, see Chapter 22).

Mental health

Mental health is probably the most neglected area of health care worldwide and one that encompasses more human suffering than almost any other. It is estimated that four out of five people in the developing world who have mental health problems receive no treatment.[27] The field is wide open for new and effective community-based approaches to prevent, manage, and cure a majority of mental illness in the community setting[27–29] (see also Chapter 24).

Disability

The UN Convention on the Rights of Persons with Disabilities (UNCRPD) and the growth of the disability rights movement have resulted in a growing awarensss of the importance of disability in development programmes and of rights-based responses. The growing practice of community-based rehabilitation holds huge promise (see Chapter 23, Figure 1.10).

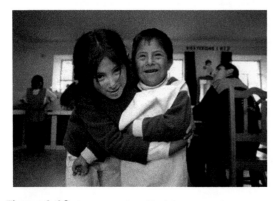

Figure 1.10 Community-based health care must be disability-inclusive. A picture from Peru.

Increase in drug abuse and alcohol and tobacco use

Tobacco is the leading cause of preventable death in the world. CBHC can work at community level to help reduce cigarette smoking and can add its voice to advocate against the tobacco industry, which is responsible for more deaths worldwide than all current wars and conflicts.[30]

Alcohol is estimated to cause nearly four per cent of deaths worldwide.[31] Reducing this at community and district level is a priority for community health programmes (see Chapter 22).

Physical and sexual abuse of women and children

Physical and sexual abuse affects communities worldwide—both urban and rural. Local community-based initiatives can strengthen family life and advocate against abusive practices, such as partner abuse, rape, and female genital mutilation (see Chapter 27).

Adolescent health

The WHO estimates there are 1.2 billion adolescents, i.e. young people between the ages of 12 and 19 years old, worldwide. Serious illness can start in these relatively healthy years, such as sexually transmitted infections, including HIV, and through unhealthy eating and living patterns. Depression, suicide, and violence are high, especially in urban areas.

CBHC can develop many ways of meeting the needs of adolescents. They can be actively included in health programmes and as members of health committees, youth, cultural, and sporting clubs. They can help to plan and implement solutions to problems faced by their peers, e.g. through becoming peer educators (see also Chapter 8).[32]

Obesity and unhealthy eating

These are becoming even more prevalent in low- and middle-income countries than in high-income countries. They especially occur in urban areas and in situations where the cheapest food available is often the least healthy, especially if there is also a lack of affordable or home-grown fruit and vegetables

CBHC programmes not only work through health promotion to encourage healthy eating, but also have an important role in research and advocacy for government legislation to regulate marketing, increase price of unhealthy foods, and increase access to healthy food.

Road crashes, drowning, and industrial injuries

Road crashes, drowning, and industrial injuries or so-called accidents, most largely preventable, are now one of the commonest causes of death worldwide. These disproportionately affect the young.

Increase in war, civil strife, natural disasters, terrorism, and fear

These situations can threaten years of development activity, in part because resources are diverted to support military aims. War and conflict also generate vast refugee problems. But refugees and internally displaced people (IDPs) can be educated in good health practices and trained as health workers. Modified forms of CBHC are highly effective in refugee situations and can help bridge the gap between disaster relief and long-term development.

Because natural disasters and human-generated conflicts affect an increasing number of communities, CBHC needs to help build the capacity of all communities to cope with those disasters most likely to affect them. Such disaster preparedness or risk mitigation empowers and unites communities to cope with an increasing number of problems themselves (see Chapter 25).

Recurrent periods of economic downturn

The burden of national debt, lack of employment, and rising costs of food always affect the poorest communities the most. CBHC can help find community-based solutions, such as micro-enterprise and co-operatives to reduce the impact of global recessions on communities.

Climate change

Climate change leads to global warming, rising sea levels, and unpredictable weather patterns, all of which affect the health of billions of people, often through less reliable rainfall or more frequent disasters such as flooding. The poor suffer disproportionately.[33]

For all these challenges, action will need to be taken by government at national and regional levels. But as problems expand so do the opportunities for CSOs. Our toolkit will remain the same—listening to communities, empowering them, and helping them to build capacity so they can respond with sustainable solutions into the future.[34]

Summary

Covering a wide range of topics, this chapter underlines a huge range of poorly met global health needs. CBHC is an important response to these problems. It is also a versatile approach which can address many current and emerging health and development challenges by using and enhancing the skills and assets of community members. It needs to be seen as an integral and connected part of emerging health systems, and as a key component of a PHC system.

Further reading

Balabanova D, McKee M, Mills A. *Good health at low cost 25 years on: What makes a successful health system.* London: London School of Hygiene & Tropical Medicine; 2011.

Chambers R. *Whose reality counts? Putting the first last.* London: ITDG Publishing; 1997. (A radical look at ways in which the needs and priorities of the poor can be understood, with the mapping of a future agenda.)

Commission on Social Determinants of Health. *Closing the gap in a generation: Health equity through action on the social determinants of health. Final Report of the Commission on Social Determinants of Health.* Geneva: World Health Organization; 2008.

Costello A., Managing the health effects of climate change. *The Lancet.* 2009; 373:1693–1733.

Global Health Watch. *Global Health Watch 3: An alternative world health report.* London: Zed Books; 2011. Available from: http://www.hst.org.za/sites/default/files/global%20health%20watch%203.pdf

Perlman D, Roy A (editors). *The practice of international health: A case-based orientation.* Oxford: Oxford University Press; 2009.

The Planetary Health Alliance. https://planetaryhealthalliance.org

The Lancet, 2018; 392 (10156): 1369–1486 [issue focussing on The Astana Declaration].

Rifkin S. Lessons from community participation in health programmes: A review of the post Alma-Ata experience. *International Health.* 2009; 1 (1): 31–3.

Rohde J, Wyon J (editors). *Community-based health care: Lessons from Bangladesh to Boston.* Cambridge, MA: Harvard School of Public Health; 2009. A wide-ranging book suitable especially for primary care and public health practitioners.

Siegel P, Checchi F, Colombo S, Paik E. Health-care needs of people affected by conflict: Future trends and changing frameworks. *The Lancet.* 2010; 375 (9711): 341–5.

World Health Organization. *Primary Health Care: Now more than ever.* World Health Report 2008. Geneva: World Health Organization; 2008. Available from: http://www.who.int/whr/2008/en/

References

1. The World Data Lab. *World Poverty Clock,* 2018. Available from: https://worldpoverty.io
2. World Health Organization. *Trends in maternal mortality: 1990 to 2015,* 2015. Available from: http://www.unfpa.org/sites/default/files/pub-pdf/9789241565141_eng.pdf
3. UNICEF. *Levels and trends in child mortality report,* 2018. Available from: http://www.un.org/en/development/desa/population/publications/mortality/child-mortality-report-2018.shtml
4. World Health Organization. *Fact file on health inequities,* 2011. Available from: http://www.who.int/sdhconference/background/news/facts/en/
5. World Health Organization and World Bank Group. *Tracking universal health coverage: Global monitoring report,* 2017. Available from: https://www.who.int/healthinfo/universal_health_coverage/report/2017/en/

6. International Labour Organization. *Global evidence on inequities in rural health protection: New data on rural deficits in health coverage for 174 countries*, 2015. Available from: http://www.social-protection.org/gimi/gess/RessourcePDF.action;jsessionid=wJJfYtqhFSsh6y2nwLdqQpgm5gy7hjK9QGZ4vBZ3z7hHKNWd6Tnx!-1211598784?ressource.ressourceId=51297

7. Morton, R. Offline: Positive and negative, *The Lancet*. 2012; 380 (9848): 1132.

8. Chen L, T Evans, S. Anand, JI Bufford, H Brown, M Choudhury, et al. Human resources for health: overcoming the crisis. *The Lancet*. 2004; 364 (9449): 1984–90.

9. World Health Organization. *World health statistics 2016: Monitoring health for the SDGs*, 2016. Available from: http://www.who.int/gho/publications/world_health_statistics/2016/en/

10. Universal Declaration of Human Rights, Resolution 217 A(III); UN Doc A/810 91, UN General Assembly, 1948.

11. World Health Organization. *World Health Report calls for return to primary health care approach.* (News release), 2008. Available from: http://www.who.int/mediacentre/news/releases/2008/pr38/en/

12. World Health Organization. *Constitution of WHO: Principles.* www.who.int/about/mission/en/

13. Declaration of Alma-Ata international conference on primary health care, Alma-Ata, USSR, 1978. Available from: http://www.who.int/publications/almaata_declaration_en.pdf.

14. Nossal Institute, University of Melbourne. *Course outline— Short course on primary health care in Jamkhed, India.* Available from: http://mdhs-study.unimelb.edu.au/short-courses/mspgh-short-courses/primary-health-care-in-jamkhed-india-nossal-institute/course-structure

15. World Health Organization. *Global strategy on human resources for health: Workforce 2030*, 2016. Available from: https://www.who.int/hrh/resources/pub_globstrathrh-2030/en/

16. Gilson, L, Walt, G, Heggenhougen, K, Owuor-Omondi, L, Perera, M, Ross, D, et al. National community health worker programs: how can they be strengthened? *Journal of Public Health Policy*. 1989; 10 (4): 518–32.

17. Whitmee, S, Haines A, Bayrer C, Boltz F, Capon AG, Ferreira B, et al. Safeguarding human health in the Anthropocene epoch: Report of The Rockefeller Foundation–Lancet Commission on planetary health. *The Lancet*, 2015; 386 (10007): 1973–2028.

18. First People's Health Assembly. *The People's Charter for Health*, 2000. Available from: http://www.phmovement.org/sites/www.phmovement.org/files/phm-pch-english.pdf

19. Chan M. Return to Alma-Ata. *The Lancet*. 2008; 372(9642): 865–6.

20. Olivier J, Tsimpo C, Gemignani R, Shojo M, Coulombe H, Dimmock F, et al. Understanding the roles of faith-based health-care providers in Africa: Review of the evidence with a focus on magnitude, reach, cost, and satisfaction. *The Lancet*. 2015; 386(10005): 1765–75.

21. Berkley Center for Religion, Peace and World Affairs. *Resources on faith, ethics, and public life.* Available from: http://berkleycenter.georgetown.edu/resources (Accessed May 26, 2014).

22. Jancloes M. The poorest first: WHO's activities to help the people in greatest need. *World Health Forum*. 1998; 19(2): 182–7.

23. Item No. 4: Overview of health and wellbeing in Sunderland 2011. Sunderland City Council. Available from: http://www.sunderland.gov.uk

24. United Nations. *The Sustainable Development Agenda.* Available from: http://www.un.org/sustainabledevelopment/development-agenda/ (Accessed 19th August 2017).

25. World Health Organization. *What is universal coverage?* Available from: http://www.who.int/health_financing/universal_coverage_definition/en/

26. Meredith SEO, Cross C, Amazigo UV. Empowering communities in combating river blindness and the role of NGOs: Case studies from Cameroon, Mali, Nigeria, and Uganda. *Health Research Policy and Systems*. 2012; 10 (16) [online]. Available from: http://www.health-policy-systems.com/content/10/1/16

27. World Health Organization. *Mental health atlas.* Geneva: WHO; 2014.

28. Roberts M. Mental health: Global effort sought. 2012; *BBC News*. Available from: http://www.bbc.co.uk/news/health-19883226

29. Patel V. *Where there is no psychiatrist.* London: Gaskell; 2003.

30. World Health Organization. Tobacco fact sheet, 2017. Available from: http://www.who.int/mediacentre/factsheets/fs339/en/index.html

31. Rehm J, Mathers C, Popova S, Thavorncharoensap M, Teerawattananon Y, Patra J. Global burden of disease and injury and economic cost attributable to alcohol use and alcohol-use disorders. *The Lancet*. 2009; 373 (9682): 2223–33

32. Patton G, Sawyer SM, Santelli JS, Ross DA, Afifi R, Allen NB, et al. Our future: A Lancet commission on adolescent health and wellbeing. *The Lancet*. 2016; 387 (10036): 2423–78.

33. World Bank. *Climate change complicates efforts to end poverty*, 2015. Available from: http://www.worldbank.org/en/news/feature/2015/02/06/climate-change-complicates-efforts-end-poverty

34. Sachs JD, McArthur JW. The Millennium Project: a plan for meeting the Millennium Development Goals. *The Lancet*. 2005; 365 (9456): 347–53.

CHAPTER 2
Working as partners with the community

Ted Lankester

Chapter 1 explained our main task, which is to work alongside communities, develop trust and friendship, and offer support, training, coaching, and connection when needed. Before discussing needs, we must listen and learn in order to appreciate the assets, gifts, and abilities of community members.

Whether we are working with government or civil society, in either case we will often be coming in as outsiders. Development models in the past (and often still) have been based largely on outsiders doing programmes *for communities*, owning the process, and then leaving with an unsustainable mixture of good ideas and muddled outcomes (Figure 2.1).

Worldwide, there is growing interest in financial and social enterprise. Community members with ideas, skills, and passion can help to lead the process of community development in ways that excite the community.

It is essential that communities own their own futures. Our task is to work alongside them in genuine partnerships to build their confidence and improve self-belief. At its best, a CBHC approach 'brings balance back to health care and puts families and communities at the hub of the health system. With an emphasis on local ownership it makes space for solutions created by communities, owned by them and sustained by them'.[1]

What we need to know

The subject of this chapter cannot be broken down into a formula that is guaranteed to work or a series of steps that must be followed. Rather, the ideas and suggestions in this chapter should be seen as guidelines and examples to stimulate the building of friendships and alliances on which our work largely depends.

Making contact with the community

We can't just walk into a community and start asking questions. We need time to build trust before rushing in with questions and suggestions. We can never bring

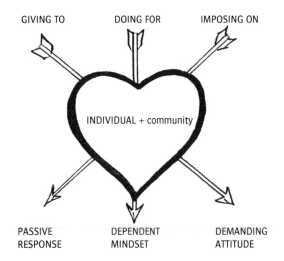

GIVING TO   DOING FOR   IMPOSING ON

INDIVIDUAL + community

PASSIVE   DEPENDENT   DEMANDING
RESPONSE   MINDSET   ATTITUDE

Figure 2.1 The effects of a top-down approach.

Reproduced courtesy of Ted Lankester. This image is distributed under the terms of the Creative Commons Attribution Non-Commercial 4.0 International licence (CC-BY-NC), a copy of which is available at http://creativecommons.org/licenses/by-nc/4.0/.

our own ideas and contributions unless the community learns to trust both us and our motives. Many vulnerable communities, after years of being exploited and disempowered, are wary of outsiders bearing clever-sounding promises.

Imagine you are a member of a community and a group of people visit you whom you have never met before, or even heard about. You might ask yourself who these people are, and if they can be trusted? Perhaps they are from a different ethnic group or a different part of the country. Are they foreigners or government officials with hidden agendas such as family planning. Could they be spies from another country? You may wonder if they are the same 'NGO' who visited before and then left, or another group of people who think they know more about the community than we do?

Quite often as a community you may wonder if this outsider is actually there to make money out of us, report on us, or abuse our women. Can't this outsider get a job anywhere else? Other community members may also be asking what can we get from working with these outsiders: handouts, money, a hospital, a resident doctor, tonics for the children, cigarettes, foreign goods, or guns.

It is only by getting to know the community that we will break down these suspicions. Only then will people from the community learn to trust us as we increasingly learn to appreciate both them and their culture.

As we make these first contacts we will often learn from the community some of the secrets of living,

relating, celebrating, or enduring hardship, which we, as health providers, may not have experienced. In making new friendships our own lives will often be enriched. Additionally, the community will come to realize that, although we may have some skills and experience which they haven't got, we come as ordinary people wishing to work with them.

The following twelve practical guidelines are always useful when we enter a new community:

1. Before visiting first learn about any customs we would be expected to follow.
2. On arrival meet the leaders and explain who we are.
3. Behave in an open and friendly manner and use the local greeting.
4. Dress appropriately and modestly, wearing the local style of clothes if possible.
5. Reduce the differences between ourselves and the community as much as possible, and take care not to show off expensive equipment.
6. Accept hospitality, and eat and drink with community members where possible.
7. Play and joke with the children, within the family context, and follow safeguarding principles.
8. Listen and learn, and don't ask too many questions until trust is established.
9. Don't make plans or promises that can't be kept.
10. Encourage good customs and practices, without being patronizing.
11. Avoid criticism both through our words and through our manner.
12. Don't take sides in any family, community, or political dispute.

The benefits of partnership

Community-based health care (CBHC) has come about because other models have often failed to bring basic health services to those who need them most. In many countries medical care follows a top-down model, is mainly curative, is dominated by health professionals and officials, and is frequently subsidized by donations from governments and outside agencies. People come to expect things to be given to them and done for them. Although in the process they may gain a degree of improved health, they often lose autonomy and self-belief (see Figure 2.1). In many situations this model of dependence is deeply ingrained and it will take time, patience, and mutual understanding to move into a new paradigm of development.

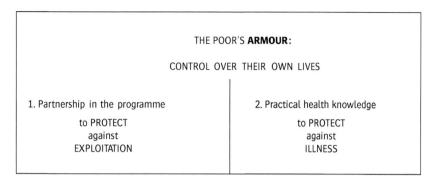

Figure 2.2 The Poor's Armour.

Our aim is to promote the health and well-being of the people, not just provide medical care for them.

1. Partnership helps to make a project sustainable.

If people themselves learn to change unhelpful health patterns for helpful ones, improved health will continue after the experts leave or the funding stops.

> Why, Tom—us people will go on livin' when all them people is gone.
>
> John Steinbeck, *The Grapes of Wrath*

2. Partnership helps to protect people from exploitation

Those with poor health, low income, or with little education are often exploited by others:

- Private practitioners may want them as patients—for a profit.
- Medicine stores may encourage them to buy inappropriate or excessive medicines (polypharmacy)—to make a profit
- The rich loan money—at high interest.
- Politicians make empty promises—for votes.

Partnership acts as a form of 'body armour' against these forces (Figure 2.2).

3. Partnership gives dignity to the poor.

As the benefits of partnership start to be visible, community members realize they no longer need others to do so many things for them. They come to see they can bring about change themselves and adopt healthier lifestyles, which means less medicine and fewer visits to the clinic. This new self-reliance gives a sense of worth to those who previously felt undervalued. Instead of being passive receivers, they become active participants.

For example, in one project in western India, newly selected female Community Health Workers (CHWs) covered their faces, looked down to the ground and said 'we are only useful for making bread and carrying water.' After a few months these same women, armed with practical health knowledge and new self-confidence, were teaching their communities and caring for health needs.[2]

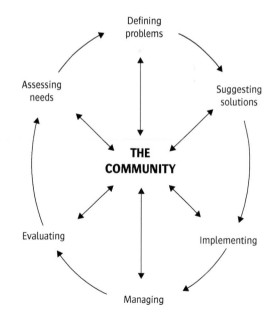

Figure 2.3 The community is central in all programme activities at the heart of the project circle.

4. Community members become effective health workers.

The skills, assets, and creative talents of the community become recognized and valued. Members realize that they themselves can play a major part in their own health care. CHWs can be selected, and trained, and in well-managed programmes, they often provide more appropriate primary care than outside health professionals: community members often understand local needs better than social workers.

> Outsiders can help, but insiders must do the job.
> Jimmy Yen, 1890–1990

5. Partnership acts as a multiplier.

When local people become excited by what they have achieved, they will want to spread the news to others. Imagine the ripple effect caused by throwing a stone into a pond. They themselves will become agents of change, taking new health patterns and new ideas to other communities. For example, A project in Delhi bought a mobile clinic van to extend health care for city slums into areas beyond where they had been working. Community health volunteers from the original programme area went along to encourage local people to participate, and took the lead in giving health teaching. Community partnership may seem slow at the start. Later this multiplier effect often causes a rapid increase in growth

6. Equipment is better looked after.

When people feel it is *their* clinic, *their* forestry plantation, or *their* water pump, they will take pride in looking after it.

7. Partnership helps to give stability at the grass roots.

At times of civil conflict and insecurity, community-based programmes will often continue because of their strength and self-reliance.

8. Partnership opens the eyes of the powerful.

Hierarchical systems isolate people at the top and prevent them from appreciating the wit, imagination, and skills of those at the bottom. Working in partnership enables people in authority to realize that poor people have many (intangible) assets.

Partnership as the foundation for all programme stages

Partnership moves us away from a dependency mindset, where community members are seen as beneficiaries

who are reliant on outside aid, and towards a situation where the community is central at all stages of the programme (Figure 2.3).

Factors that may obstruct partnership

Working with a community to improve their health and wellbeing is difficult, takes time and is complex. Being a facilitator requires social skills as challenging as a surgeon's technical skills. There are various problems that we are likely to face.

1. Blocks within the community

Many communities still expect a 'charity and donation' approach, partly because of inappropriate forms of aid programmes in the past. They will often expect us to do things for them and if we don't, they may lose interest. For example, an urban project in Nairobi had been providing services and handing out supplies to people in need for many years. It took this project great effort and patience to move from a donation approach to one in which local people were trained to be self-reliant. There was initial opposition to this change until people saw for themselves that there were greater benefits in this new way of working together.

2. Blocks from professionals

Health professionals often want to hold on to their knowledge, their skills, their income and their power. They may dislike or even oppose any system in which patients and people start learning about health or running a programme.

3. Blocks from government

Although governments increasingly support the concept of primary health care and community participation, they may give it only token attention. They will often have more urgent health priorities or very limited capacity, and they may have targets which are easier to meet by imposition rather than participation.

4. Blocks within programme managers

It is often much easier—and quicker—for outside programme managers and NGO country directors to run programmes according to their own priorities, timescales and donors' expectations. This can undermine their role as facilitators and in sharing management with the community.

What we need to do

Commitment to a partnership approach

We will never work in genuine partnership unless our own minds and attitudes are fully prepared. We need to be:

1. Committed to facilitating the community to own its own future.
2. Willing to recognize and mobilize the assets, skills and abilities of community members.
3. Willing to share knowledge, skills and connections whenever appropriate.
4. Prepared for delegation, mistakes and experimentation, and for the delays these may cause.
5. Ready to trust others and affirm them.
6. Willing to give credit to others. Our job is not to be heroes ourselves but to make heroes of others.

7. Willing to relinquish control.

Discover the importance of partnership

In order to actively start to develop partnership, we must prioritize plenty of contact time and dialogue between programme and community. By doing so, we will build trust through personal relationships and friendships. When trust is established, we can then work together on a specific activity, chosen by the community, which the programme can help to facilitate. Visiting a programme in which participation is active and effective can be inspirational. A visit may act as a stimulus both for the community we are starting to work with as well as for our programme team. One very effective way of doing this is to use the SALT method, initially pioneered by the Salvation Army (see Figure 2.4).

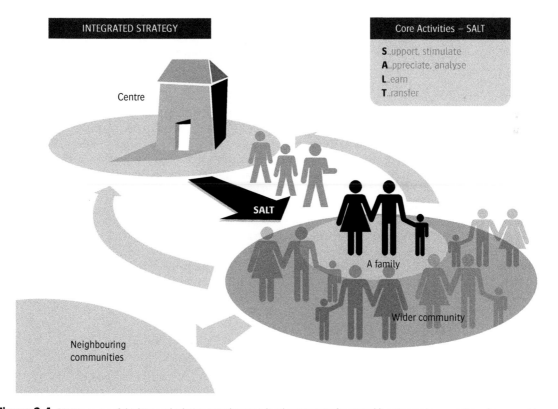

Figure 2.4 SALT is a way of thinking and relating ourselves to a local community for mutual learning and appreciation, change, and hope.

Choose a subject to work on together

Partnership does not happen at once and usually has to be described and modelled. Although our eventual aim is sharing the management of the programme, this happens in stages.

One effective way of starting this process is for the programme and the community to collaborate in choosing one activity where working together will clearly ensure success. When there are measurable and visible results from the initial activity, it becomes easier for other health priorities to be agreed together. If the activity is first suggested by the community, rather than by the programme staff, they will have ownership of it from the start.

The actual point in time when the first partnership activity begins may vary. It may be after we have completed Participatory Appraisal (PA, see Chapter 6) or after a more detailed community survey and joint planning exercise (Chapter 7). Or, it may occur earlier, perhaps if there is an obvious need after we first meet the community. In other situations, sometimes government plans may guide what activities we need to work on together.

An appropriate partnership activity will be a health priority strongly felt by the community, and that the community feels is obtainable. If the activity is too long or difficult people may lose interest. Finally, it should be something that is considered a 'quick win'. For example, a project in central India was able to work with the community in sinking tubewells, which not only brought drinking water to within the villages, but also rid communities of guinea worm. Everyone felt excited and wanted to work together on further activities. With this in mind, whatever activity is chosen, it must work and be enjoyable (Figure 2.5).

Some suggestions for starter subjects include community survey (Chapter 6),[3] a community immunization drive (Chapter 15), training CHWs (Chapter 8), a school deworming programme, or sinking a well (Chapter 21).

Learn how to set up community meetings

Setting up and facilitating community meetings are essential skills for team members to learn. If we are outsiders, it is essential we encourage community members to take on leadership tasks and for them (and us) to see our main role as trainers and coaches.

When planning ahead for meetings, elected or formal community leaders should be present if possible. Informal leaders may also attend such as teachers, religious leaders, or others who have genuine influence or a sense of community welfare.

The true leaders may be different again. They may be the community members who wield actual power because of their wealth, dominant personalities, or because of political or other connections. It is important to be aware of these aspects, as these people may try to dominate meetings or use them for their own personal ends.

In practice it is best for the community to decide, using their traditional forms of decision making, who should attend health and development meetings. However, we can try to ensure as much gender equality as possible and that no group is left out, e.g. adolescents, those living with disability, specific ethnic groups. One solution that often works well is for each household to send one representative. It is worth remembering that, in some societies, women will need their own separate meeting.

In harsh terrain, poor weather, or when communities are reluctant to come together we may need to think of creative ways to encourage people to attend. For example, Himalayan and other mountain programmes have distant and scattered villages. In one such programme, few villagers came to the meetings. Eventually, using a specific formula, a solution was found. A health film was shown at the beginning of the meeting to draw people in; a humorous one was shown at the end to encourage them to stay. In the middle, a useful debate was held about the health problems the village faced and how they might be solved.

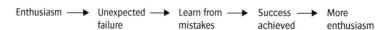

Figure 2.5 The value of enthusiasm.

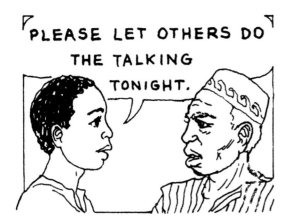

Figure 2.6 Please let others others do the talking tonight.

In planning a meeting, we should ensure that the location works for as many people as possible, and is acceptable, safe, and neutral. It is also important to make sure that the time of year and time of day is as convenient as possible. It is vital to avoid festivals, periods of major farming activity, and any planned days of strikes or civil protest. As with any meeting, we need to ensure that the meeting is the right length (tired people will soon fall asleep!), and that it doesn't try to address too many topics. Finally, it is important that it doesn't raise hopes that can't, or won't, be met.

Learn the skill of facilitating

Facilitation is a form of teaching and leading meetings where everyone learns together and reaches decisions under the skilled guidance of the facilitator. It is based on respect for the gifts and knowledge of each group member. Helping a group to identify problems and suggest solutions is usually an essential outcome of this approach.

Facilitation is one of the most important skills to learn in CBHC and community health development. It overlaps with the skills of chairing formal meetings but is more focused on drawing out ideas from everyone present. Some people have a natural ability to facilitate, but most have to learn how. One of our important roles is to train community members in facilitation so that they feel confident in leading meetings themselves.[4]

A facilitator will need to enable each group member to feel welcomed, relaxed, and sufficiently confident to share, and to explain the purpose of the meeting.

A facilitator will need to be well prepared in advance of the meeting, but remain flexible if the meeting doesn't go to plan. He or she must also help everyone to agree to some ground rules at the beginning, e.g. everyone is free to share, each opinion is respected, minority views are not dismissed, no interruptions or harsh comments allowed, no alcohol to be consumed. It is also vital for a facilitator to manage the expectations of those who have come to the meeting: often those attending at the start of a programme will expect some form of handout. Finally, if everyone agrees, he or she must ensure that someone is taking careful minutes, or records the meeting,

When facilitating, it is important to value each member's contribution, while also checking to make sure that everyone has understood what is being said. We must encourage all members, even those who seem shy, to take part as they feel comfortable. In many cultures, younger members, adolescents, and women may need encouragement to take part. Other important aspects of being a successful facilitator include the ability to:

- Communicate clearly.
- Encourage both appropriate humour and respect.
- Ensure dominant people do not 'hijack' the conversation (Figure 2.6).
- Steer the session in a useful direction.
- Keep to time, but don't be driven by the clock.
- Remain friendly and patient at all times.
- Learn to handle disagreement and conflict.
- Learn to cope with difficult questions.
- Summarize and draw together different ideas.
- Ensure the main findings and conclusions are recorded and shared.

It is also helpful to use 'energizers'—these are enjoyable activities that can be introduced at regular intervals to maintain interest.[5]

1. Playing 'mirrors': two people stand opposite each other—one does a certain action, the other mimics it. Then they swap roles.
2. Singing: someone starts up a local song and everyone joins in.
3. Stretching, running, and changing places: everyone gets up, stretches, runs, or walks around the circle once or twice, then takes up a different position.

Sometimes a helpful way to lead a discussion is by using the 'But Why?' approach:

'The child has an infected foot.'

'But why?'

'She stepped on a thorn.'

'But why?'

'She has no shoes.'

'But why?'

'Her father is a landless worker and cannot afford them.'

It can be helpful for those who lead meetings to meet together and practice facilitation skills as a role play.

Create a skills checklist

Ask yourself these questions each time you lead a small group discussion. It will help you to reflect on the development of your skills in facilitation.

- Did I use icebreakers or energizers to help people relax?
- Did I make sure everyone understood the questions and, if necessary reword, them?
- Was I comfortable with silence while people thought about the answers?
- How did I deal with someone who talked for a long time?
- Did I listen to everyone's responses?
- How did I encourage quiet people to join in?
- Did I make use of role play?
- How did I deal with someone who always answered the questions before anyone else had a chance?
- How did I encourage useful points to be discussed further?
- How did I cope when I didn't understand the answers?
- How did I cope when I felt people's views were unhelpful?
- How did I handle differences of opinion?

- Did I bring the discussion to a satisfactory conclusion?
- How could I do this better?

Generate enthusiasm

Just as vehicles run on fuel, so community development programmes run on enthusiasm (Figure 2.5).

To create enthusiasm:

- be friendly.
- encourage people's ideas.
- give support when things are difficult.
- celebrate successes.
- be fair in making decisions.
- avoid responding with blame or anger when things go wrong.

Involve many community members as early on as possible

It is important to involve community members in the programme as early as possible. We recommend three guidelines for involving others in the programme. These guidelines form the basis of what is known as 'task shifting'—a way to use skills and knowledge more efficiently, and bring encouragement to many people.

1. Don't do a job that someone *less* experienced can do just as well.
2. If there is a job that only you can do, teach someone *else* to do it as soon as possible.
3. The *least* qualified person to do a job *well* should do it.

Task shifting also ensures the skills pyramid is increasingly filled by community members (see Figure 2.7).

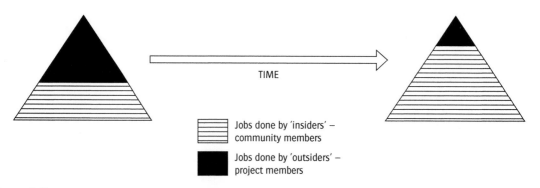

TIME

Jobs done by 'insiders' – community members

Jobs done by 'outsiders' – project members

Figure 2.7 The skills pyramid.

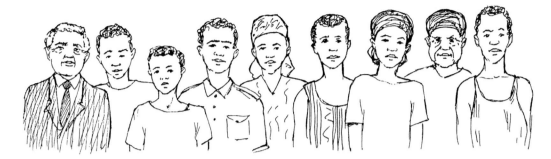

Figure 2.8 Village health committees must represent the whole community.

For example, when running a community clinic, we followed this sequence:

1. Community members were taught to register patients and to weigh babies,
2. With appropriate training, safeguards and government guidelines, community members helped dispense medicines.
3. CHWs saw patients under the guidance of a nurse or other qualified health worker.
4. The community largely took over the management of the health facility (an ideal task for a village health committee) and because of this, the community increasingly saw it as 'their clinic' (Figure 2.8).

Some helpful tips

Identify interests and abilities in community members

Suggest names of people who in your opinion have skills and abilities that could be used in the community and, if appropriate, train them and involve them. For example, in Sierra Leone, a team paid an unannounced visit to a remote rural community. Despite obvious health concerns and no access to health care, the conversation focused on what the community possessed in the way of abilities. In no time at all, a variety of skills became obvious. Who makes you laugh? Ah that's him over there. Which of you is the best actor? Oh, that's her. A range of skills and abilities in this community became apparent in under an hour.

Other important things to remember

Lead from the middle, not from the front.

Keep outside money, resources, and equipment to the minimum.

Be truthful and transparent.

Never make promises that cannot be kept, or raise expectations that cannot be met.

Show respect to everyone, even those who seem difficult to trust.

Never correct someone in front of their peers.

Demonstrate a kind and generous attitude.

Understand the power of affirmation.

Stop an activity if it is obviously not going to work.

Some pitfalls in developing community partnerships

Partnership in name only

Beware of activities that are only slanted towards the community, not based in the community. Such partnership is superficial rather than deep. Sometimes community members are keen to join a funded programme to help them on their own career path. They may, understandbly, hope that a good performance will be rewarded by a handout or new job opportunities.

Partnership is not maintained

We may originally aim for genuine community partnership, but when the health committee chairperson runs off with the funds, it is easy (and natural!) to want to change your mind! Even when problems arise, we must keep encouraging participation. Adverse or difficult situations can tempt us to retake control.

Partnership can cause divisions

Participation can release energy that works to start overcoming poverty. However, without any kind of monitoring or observation, that energy may get out of control or go in the wrong direction. For example, there may be those in the community who feel their needs are not being met, and they may become angry

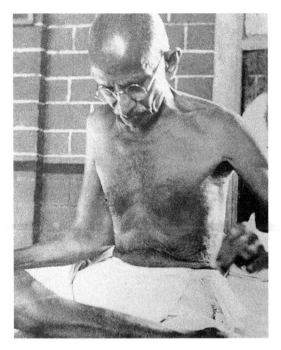

Figure 2.9 Mahatma Gandhi: a strong supporter of community involvement.

Reproduced courtesy of Camera Press. This image is distributed under the terms of the Creative Commons Attribution Non-Commercial 4.0 International licence (CC-BY-NC), a copy of which is available at http://creativecommons.org/licenses/by-nc/4.0/.

and violent towards programme members. Additionally, corrupt community leaders may try to exploit problems for personal gain. Finally, we must always be aware that some issues raised may be so strong that they can cause serious divisions within communities.

Build on existing groups

In order for partnership to succeed there need to be community organizations to underpin it. There may already be a variety of established community-based organizations (CBOs), including formal groupings, e.g. community elders, religious leaders, youth groups, or social action committees, or informal gatherings, e.g. women who meet regularly by the village well and share ideas about how to make their lives easier (Figure 2.9).

Additionally, there often will be a worshipping community based at a temple, mosque, or church. Some of these can be very effective and are often overlooked by government, NGOs, and other outsiders.

If an appropriate group already exists, we may be able to build on this group so that it forms the basis of a development committee or action group. However,

we must make sure it genuinely speaks for the whole community and that it is willing to engage with new ways of working.[6] Occasionally it will be easier to start from scratch.

Secrets of success for community groups include the following:

- Fair representation from within the community, ensuring women, adolescents, those living with disability or other marginalised or stigmatised groups are included wherever possible;
- Regular training;
- Effective, but not dominating, leadership;
- Trustworthiness in handling money and resources;
- Commitment to carrying out tasks agreed on;
- Achievable aims;
- Regular new challenges;
- Good governance arrangements and clearly understood purpose; and
- A way to gauge the group's effectiveness.

The following sections discuss three models we can partner with within the community.

Understand some models

Village Health Committees (VHCs)

This term is often used—not only in rural areas, but even in cities! The title Community Action Group is better, in that it helps the group to focus on goals and action. There are wide variations in functions of VHCs.

Usually a committee will start with one or two functions and learn to carry these out effectively. Later it can extend its activities. VHCs are often seen as helping manage health centres and health posts. But the horizon of the community should eventually move beyond seeing a health facility as the hub of their health system. Some common examples of health committee functions include CHW support, where members can help weigh children, keep records, and accompany the CHW on night calls where this is culturally appropriate. They can also support the CHW in the face of any criticisms. Note that women's groups can often have a more effective role, especially where CHWs are predominantly female; this is discussed further on.

Additionally, VHCs, if well-trained, can help organize the construction of a health post. They can be responsible for its upkeep and repairs. Furthermore, responsible VHC members can assist in clinics, where they can register patients, weigh children, and assist the health worker and the dispenser. They can also summon patients and organize patient flow.

Within the community they can remind people when clinic visits are due, e.g. for immunizations and antenatal care. Committee members can arrange publicity for immunization campaigns and help to gather children. They can assist with community and national immunization days by preparing the site and organizing people.

They can supervise the directly observed treatments (DOTs) for TB in the community (see Chapter 19). They may supervise treatment for hypertension or depression in less-educated communities until family members can take on this role, or the regular taking of antiretroviral therapy (ART) for people living with HIV/AIDS (see Chapter 20). Lastly, they can accompany sick patients to hospital. In all of these roles VHCs should follow any local rules on medical confidentiality. They need to work as friends of the community, not bosses (Figure 2.10).

If there is a need to organize a community survey, VHC members can visit homes beforehand to explain why the survey is being done. They can work with project members in carrying out the survey. They can explain results to the community after the survey is finished, and they can be involved in PA.

Public health activities are often high on the list of VHC responsibilities. Health committees can take responsibility for community hygiene, organize the digging of soakage pits and the construction and maintenance of latrines, water storage tanks, pumps and wells.

Additionally, VHCs can be contacts for government and outside agencies, and they can claim grants and benefits on behalf of the community. They can ensure government promises are carried out, and that the poor are treated fairly and receive any subsidies due. They can sometimes participate in research with academic institutes to show the evidence-based value of community activities. VHCs and programme leaders hold regular meetings for liaison, planning, and training.

How VHC members are chosen

If possible, the whole community should be involved, following the community's normal method of decision making. The process of selection is broadly similar to choosing CHWs (see Chapter 8). The committee should not be chosen only by or from the rich and powerful (see Figure 2.8), and the committee should be large enough to represent the main social groups in the community and small enough to unite and get things done. Six to

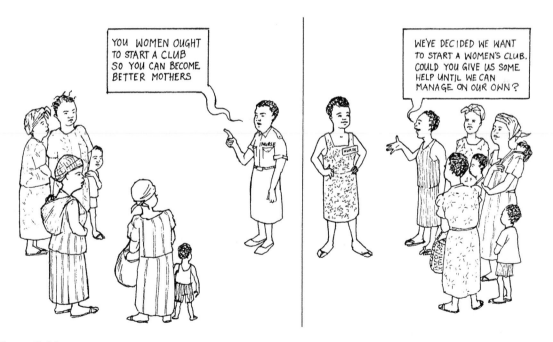

Figure 2.10 Women's groups are more likely to succeed when the people themselves want to start them.

twelve members is ideal. Smaller 'sub-groups' can be appointed in addition.

In a VHC each main group in the community should be represented including women, adolescents, the landless, the low-caste, and members of any minority ethnic group. Teachers and religious leaders can be useful members. In very small communities each household can send one member. It is vital that every health committee, no matter how small, includes women, and at least one member of the poorest subgroup of the community.

How many people should the VHC represent?

The size of the community represented by a VHC varies a great deal. Usually each geographical community such as a village, a plantation, or a defined area in a city slum has its own committee. However, this is not always possible. When villages are very small or scattered, either two or more villages can join together, providing they are close enough, or health committees can be set up for each health centre rather than for each village.

In city slums or large towns an appropriate area needs to be defined. This could be a street or a cluster of dwellings. Some slums, especially illegal settlements, are small enough for a single committee. In mixed slum communities we must see that all groups are represented.

Generally, it is hard for a VHC to represent more than 1000 people. A much smaller number is preferable.

When to select the VHC

There are three possible times that a VHC can be selected.

1. At the start of the project.

Although this is a common practice, members may find it hard to grasp the functions of the committee and what role they can play.

2. After a period of six to twelve months.

By this time those with a genuine interest in health will be known both by the programme and by the community.

3. Before a special activity.

For example, at the building of a health post or the improving of a water supply, members have a goal to aim for and are more likely to work effectively.

Training VHC members

VHCs need thorough and regular training. This should include learning the ways of functioning together as a group, with an emphasis on team-building and leadership skills. It is also important to be able to form

and maintain good governance structures, as well as to understand roles and responsibilities. Finally, many members may require specific task-related training.

How VHCs develop

An African health leader has described four stages through which VHCs often pass.

Stage 1

Members are busy working out their own relationships and seeing which individual or which group is likely to gain control.

Stage 2

Members test out the benefits to which they are entitled. Common ones include lifts in project vehicles, free medicines, or priority in clinics.

During this stage members seem very interested in project activities, but mainly because of the privileges they hope to obtain.

Stage 3

VHC members start requesting special things for the community. Common examples of these types of requests include a resident doctor, a hospital or a new vehicle. They may also demand handouts supposedly for the poor. Through these demands, members may hope to increase their own standing in the community. If demands are unsuccessful, some members may lose interest.

Stage 4

Those remaining VHC members start working with the project and serving the community with genuine commitment.

Put another way, most teams go through the four stages of 'Forming', 'Storming', 'Norming' and 'Performing'.

VHC benefits and challenges

In some projects VHCs have proved successful, and in others they have been disappointing. Researchers have looked at a wide range of health facility committees to see how effective they are.[7] Because their situations are so different it is hard to be clear about what works and what doesn't. However, there is evidence that if well set up, trained and monitored, these committees can have a useful function.

Benefits of VHCs are based on the fact that their members are chosen by the community and live in the community. They have authority to carry out health-related activities. They can also liaise closely, or be integrated with, local or district health services, where they can be a voice for the community.

However, VHCs can sometimes run into problems. Often, members join for mixed reasons, e.g. personal prestige, perks, and privileges, rather than from an interest in the health and development of their community. Additionally, the VHC may be slow and bureaucratic; in these cases, members may lose interest and the VHC may ultimately fail unless they regularly have new challenges and activities to maintain interest. Ideally, the new challenges and activities are suggested by the committee itself. Most importantly, the VHC may become politicized. Those with political ambitions may dominate, and divisions in the community may be reflected in the committee. This is a particular risk in urban slums, areas with social unrest, or in the run-up to elections.

All these problems can be lessened by the careful choice and training of VHC members. VHCs are often most successful when they take responsibility for broader community development as well as for health.

Women's groups

Groups or clubs have one main advantage over committees: people join them out of genuine interest, rather than to gain privileges. Women's groups specifically have another main advantage in that women are usually more interested in the welfare of their family than in personal gain. Women acting together can be highly effective in community development, and they

can help to overturn harmful community practices or resist exploitation from outside (Figure 2.11).

Each programme and community should set up its own guidelines. Some will encourage any woman who lives in the community to attend. Others will suggest that each household sends one female member. It is important, however, that membership is inclusive, embracing all ages, all social groups or castes, people with disabilities, and those with non-infectious physical or mental illness. Furthermore, it is important that men are also involved in development activities. Encouraging men's support and interest should be a priority for any women's group.

A group should only be started if sufficient women are interested and ideally if the community is willing to give it support. If women initially lack interest or confidence to form a group, programme staff can explain the value of starting a club. Usually at an early stage, group members with leadership gifts will emerge and can be endorsed as leaders by the rest of the group. If no leader is immediately forthcoming, a CHW can take on this role.

Club members may appreciate having one healthcare worker who can work with them, and act as their mentor. Such a person will need to be sensitive, enthusiastic, and willing to let others lead.

The group should have a facilitator, whose tasks might include encouraging interested women to call a first meeting, helping women bring ideas and suggestions, and nurturing leadership skills in others.

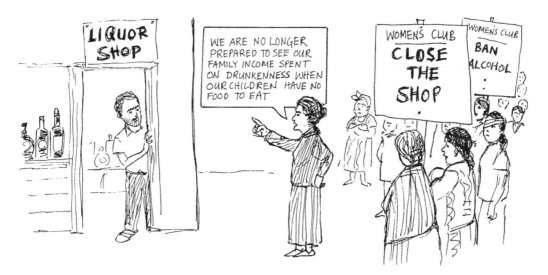

Figure 2.11 Women's clubs can act as effective pressure groups to overcome social evils.

Additionally, they may teach group members about practical health matters and assist group members to seek loans, or pursue justice issues relevant to the community. Finally, a facilitator will help to set up a simple governance system with an understanding of roles and responsibilities. Suggestions for initial meetings include sharing a common religious observance after making sure it is acceptable to all who are present, or discussing a topic of current interest, asking 'but why?' and 'so then what?'.

Health-related activities for women's groups

Worldwide, women's groups carry out a huge variety of activities. Usually they start with one or two activities that prove successful and enjoyable. Some valuable research has now shown that women's groups can reduce mortality associated with pregnancy and childbirth if they follow some basic guidelines.[8] The use of women's groups in one study showed that more than one-third of deaths in pregnant women and over one-fifth of death in newborns could be prevented.

Here are some of the secrets for success:

- Careful training of the women's groups (known as participatory learning) in relevant topics.
- Home visits to counsel mothers, provide newborn care and make referral easier.
- Interactive learning that involves identifying problems during pregnancy, at delivery and after delivery.
- Working out practical ways for women to identify problems, deal with these at home and refer when necessary.

Women's groups are ideal for giving practical support and encouragement to the CHW.

In addition to engaging in the health topics tackled by VHCs, women's groups often take special interest in the health needs and feeding of children, immunization, preventing diarrhoea and teaching about methods of rehydration, women's health problems, family planning and child spacing, taking of ART and home care of those with AIDS and of orphaned children, supervising TB DOT treatment, setting up home care programmes for the people living with disability, housebound or those with terminal illnesses, and promoting personal hygiene.

Social activities for women's groups

Examples might include running a crèche for young children so mothers can work in the fields or earn a living in the city. Additionally, women's groups can help to organize festivals or cultural activities. Starting a sewing circle might lead on to economic activities (see below).

Educational activities for women's groups

Women's groups can arrange literacy classes or non-formal education for children or adults. The group may have a member who is an effective teacher. Alternatively, a group member could be sent on a training course and then do the teaching herself.

Economic activities for women's groups

These activities should not be started too soon. Group members should first establish trust among themselves and gain experience in group activities. Possibilities include:

1. Starting a special savings fund into which each member pays a monthly amount. Funds could be used for:

- emergency grants to any member in special need, e.g. following a death in the family.
- an item of equipment that could be used by the club or hired out to others.

   For example, one group in Maharashtra, India, bought tents and musical instruments used for weddings. These were then available for the families of group members and hired out to others for a profit.

- Giving repayable loans to members.

   These could be used for useful items that the family could not otherwise afford. Examples might include a sewing machine, farm animals, or improved seeds or fertilisers.

2. Income generation and community banking.

For example, Project Hope encourages groups of about 25 women to take out loans from a village health bank to start small businesses. Health promotion is given priority whenever the bank meets.[9]

Agricultural activities for women's groups

Women's groups can teach members to start kitchen gardens. Vegetables grown by women in kitchen gardens are likely to be used as a food crop for the family, benefiting children.

Social action

Once a group is well established, women can work together in solidarity against social problems. For example, women can make a united stand in the community to discourage husbands/partners and community members from abusing alcohol and drugs. They can also work together to save the environment. A few years ago, women in the Himalayas banded together to prevent contractors cutting down trees and ruining the soil. When axemen appeared, they hugged the trees and when lorries arrived, they lay down in the road. Another example, the Murihi Project in Kenya, is a group started by church members, mainly women, who wanted to clean up the environment, reduce dependence on charcoal, which depletes the nearby forests, and generate income. They weave baskets of recycled plastic, make cooking briquettes from renewable resources, and grow trees.

A simple constitution

At the start, members can simply meet together, and no formal leadership is needed. Later, the group may wish to appoint a secretary, a president, and a treasurer. Eventually, the group may wish to draw up a written constitution, establish governance procedures, and become registered— sometimes in an association with neighbouring women's groups. A small yearly membership fee can be paid by each member to cover costs.

Common problems faced by women's groups

Frequently, men oppose women's groups, often out of jealousy and suspicion. The remedies for this are to include and inform partners. Once men understand that activities are likely to benefit the family and pose no threat to their own role position, the problem is often reduced. In rural communities, members of young farmers' clubs can work in association with women's groups.

Group members may expect great things to happen quickly. When they don't, interest drops and women stop coming. The remedy is to start small with modest expectations and the understanding that progress takes time. It is helpful to choose engaging starter projects with relatively quick outcomes. Fun, celebration, and arranging community events help boost motivation.

Finally, there is always a risk of opposing views within the group, or members taking sides or forming factions. Rifts like this can threaten the success of the group. Therefore, from the beginning, everyone must know and agree that learning to work together is the main purpose of the group. The facilitator may be able to suggest a fair way of solving any serious dispute. Success for women's groups, as for all community organizations, depends upon effective, fair leadership.

Children's clubs

Children's clubs can give children a key role in the community programmes.[10] For example, in Auguri, Nigeria, a group of 10–16-year-olds belonging to a child's rights club identified and targeted the low rates of immunization. Based on their work, in the geographic area they covered, around 328 children were immunized each month over an eight-month period compared to only eight children per month before the club started.

Clusters

The Arukah Network (formerly the Community Health Global Network) is setting up clusters which are proving very effective in helping to bring a wide range of community members into strong local collaborations.

In most communities worldwide, there are a variety of players such as government services, religious centres, faith-based organizations, social entrepreneurs, CHWs, NGOs, and village elders. Often these groups compete rather than co-operate. Clusters aim to bring groups together in order to bring long-term collaboration and sustained outcomes.

At the beginning, an Arukah facilitator visits and explains the purpose of the cluster, and invites a wide variety of groups to meet for a cluster launch, which may take one to two days. During this launch an atmosphere of trust, friendship, and transparency is encouraged as the basis for future co-operation. Community priorities are discussed and agreed upon and ways forward mapped out. Arukah has found this to be a 'winning formula' in a number of places. It has drawn up guidelines including tips for success and pitfalls to avoid.

In the Uttarakhand cluster in north India, over fifty groups now meet together regularly. The cluster is able to have a far greater impact than groups working alone. It has been asked to run specific programmes by the government, including disability, tobacco control, non-communicable diseases, child health, and disaster relief during monsoon floods. It has also been asked to train District Medical Officers.

The Cluster model has proved a 'win-win' for member organizations, government, and community members. For more details on Arukah Network's cluster model interested readers are referred to http://www.arukahnetwork.org.

Summary

Current development models are largely moving away from the donor/beneficiary model towards partnership with communities to help community members manage their programmes and own their futures. Partnership protects people against exploitation, creates interdependence, and enables communities to identify problems and devise solutions.

Partnership should be the basis of all programme activities. Skills as facilitators and leaders are needed to ensure abilities and skills in the community as widely as possible. For partnership to succeed, health team members must have clear aims and helpful attitudes, and give the community good training.

Partnership is helped by setting up health committees, women's groups, or similar community organizations. The relatively new cluster model being pioneered by the Arukah Network and others shows great promise.

Further reading

Arole M, Arole R. Jamkhed: the evolution of a world training center. In: Taylor-Ide D, Taylor CE, editors. *Just and lasting change: When communities own their futures.* Baltimore: The Johns Hopkins University Press; 2002.

Asset Based Community Development Institute (ABCD). Publications available to download. http://www.abcdinstitute.org/publications/downloadable

Babul F. *Child-to-Child: A review of the literature (1995–2007).* London: Child-to-Child Trust; 2007. Available from: http://www.childtochild.org.uk/wp-content/uploads/2014/08/CtC-Literature-Review-Final-2007.pdf

Bailey D, Hawes H, Bonati G. *Child-to-Child: A resource book.* London: Child-to-Child Trust; 2007.

Maphogoro S, Stutter E. *The Community is my university: A voice from the grass roots on rural health and development.* Amsterdam: Koninklijk Instituut Voor de Tropen; 2003.

Tearfund. *Child Participation: Roots 7.* Teddington: Tearfund; 2004. Available from: www.tearfund.org/tilz

Tearfund. *Partnering with the Local Church: Roots 11.* Teddington: Tearfund; 2007. Available from: http://tilz.tearfund.org/en/resources/publications/roots/

Werner D, Sanders D. *Questioning the solution: The politics of primary health care and child survival.* Palo Alto, CA: HealthWrights; 1997.

References

1. World Health Organization. *World Health Report 2008: Primary health care: Now more than ever.* Geneva: World Health Organization; 2008. Available from; http://www.who.int/whr/2008/whr08_en.pdf

2. Arole M, Arole A. *Jamkhed: A comprehensive rural health project.* London: Macmillan; 1994.

3. Rifkin S, Pridmore P. *Partners in planning.* London: Macmillan; 2001.

4. Tearfund. *Facilitation skills workbook.* Teddington: Tearfund; 2000. Available from: www.tearfund.org/tilz

5. International HIV/AIDS Alliance. *100 Ways to energize groups: Games to use in workshops, meetings and the community. A facilitator's guide to participatory workshops with NGOs/CBOs responding to HIV/AIDS.* Brighton: International HIV/AIDS Alliance; 2003. Available to download from: http://www.aidsalliance.org/assets/000/001/052/ene0502_Energiser_guide_eng_original.pdf?1413808298

6. Carter I. *Building the capacity of local groups, mobilizing the community.* Teddington: Tearfund; 2001. Available from: https://learn.tearfund.org/~/media/files/tilz/publications/pillars/english/pillars_building_capacity_e.pdf

7. McCoy DC, Hall JA, Ridge M. A systematic review of the literature for evidence on health facility committees in low- and middle-income countries. *Health Policy and Planning.* 2012; 27 (6): 449–66.

8. Badas E. *Good practice guide: Community mobilisation through women's groups to improve the health of mothers and babies.* London: ADAS/Ekjut/Women and Children First (UK)/UCL; 2011. Available from: https://www.k4health.org/sites/default/files/Good%20Practice%20Guide.pdf

9. Project Hope. Available at: www.projecthope.org

10. Hanbury C, editor. *Children for health: Children as partners in health promotion.* London: Macmillan; 2005.

CHAPTER 3
Community health as part of the health system

Ted Lankester

This chapter considers how community-based health care (CBHC) relates to and strengthens the national health system. It looks at the variety of linkages that CBHC needs to establish with a wide variety of players, which include:

For the sake of simplicity in this chapter, the term civil society organization (CSO) is used. It includes non-governmental organizations (NGOs and INGOs), community-based organizations (CBOs), faith-based or faith-inspired organizations (FBOs), and the voluntary or 'third' sector.

Working with government

This section is designed to help organizations that are not officially part of government to work effectively in a co-operative spirit with government departments. It is also useful for those in government to understand principles that are important for CSOs.

What is government?

As far as health programmes are concerned, the main government health services are run by the Ministry of Health, which has various levels. The central level is where nationwide health policy and planning takes place. State, provincial, and regional levels or sub-regional levels adapt and carry out national health policy according to the area's needs. At the district level (or similar name), the district medical officer (DMO) organizes and carries out all aspects of health care in the district. The district is seen increasingly as the key component of a health service—large enough to manage health care and small enough to support services at local level. Many countries, e.g. Uganda, also have sub-districts, sometimes called counties, with deputy medical officers. Sometimes FBOs are responsible for district or sub-district hospitals or other health services, especially in Sub-Saharan Africa. Finally, the local level includes the primary health centre, which would normally include a few in-patient beds and facilities for skilled delivery, and smaller health posts or dispensaries (NB: terms vary from country to country). Health committees and a cadre of community health workers (CHWs), attached either to government or to CSO, may be linked in at primary or district level.

In addition to the Ministry of Health, other ministries or departments have an influence on health such as agriculture, forestry and environment; energy and renewable resources; social welfare departments; human resources; education; urban or rural development; and water.

Who provides health care more effectively—government or CSO?

It is important to understand that the government of the country is, or should be, primarily responsible for overall health services and health systems, including public health and preventative and curative care. In many resource-poor areas these services may be under severe strain and health systems may sometimes be absent altogether. Often CSOs can work alongside and enhance coverage, but it is important all these activities are done in association with the government wherever possible. It is still helpful to look at the respective roles and strengths of government on the one hand, and CSOs on the other (Figure 3.1).

Activities often done best by government include:

- Planning national, regional, and district health policy, often guided by the World Health Organization (WHO), UNICEF, and other official bodies.
- Funding nationwide health care (although other sources are increasingly necessary, but are usually channelled through government).
- Establishing primary, secondary, and tertiary health care—primary health centres, district, and regional hospitals.

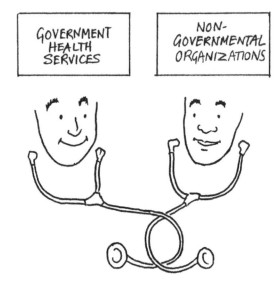

Figure 3.1 An essential partnership for the most effective care in most countries of the world.

Reproduced courtesy of David Gifford. This image is distributed under the terms of the Creative Commons Attribution Non-Commercial 4.0 International licence (CC-BY-NC), a copy of which is available at http://creativecommons.org/licenses/by-nc/4.0/.

- Oversight of training for doctors, nurses, and other senior health professionals.
- Co-coordinating nationwide programmes, e.g. End TB Strategy, Roll Back Malaria, Integrated Management of Childhood Illness (IMCI).
- Regulating the activities of other health care providers, both individuals and organizations.
- Collecting routine data on disease prevalence, patterns of diseases and on management of these condition.
- Scaling-up effective methods and ideas (often pioneered by CSOs at local or district level) that need government and legislative powers to be rolled out nationally. These are all tasks that require both high expenditure and nationwide planning to be effective.

Activities often done better by CSOs include:

- Helping primary care health to be operational in underserved areas.
- Encouraging the full participation of the community.
- Training, teaching and motivating health workers and community members.
- Advocacy for health-related rights and benefits entitled under the constitution, and more widely, including relevant human rights.
- Meeting local needs with flexible, appropriate programmes.
- Working in remote or difficult areas, with neglected, vulnerable, or isolated groups.
- Integrating primary health care and development activities at local level.
- Establishing urban health care; working among the urban poor will become an increasing focus for CSOs.

These are tasks that spring from the strengths of the CSO—enthusiasm, flexibility, community involvement and manageable size.

How can government and CSOs work together?

Working relationships between government and CSOs usually follow one of three models.

1. CSO and government set up a joint programme.

The CSO works closely with the government, and carries out a specific programme or task that government services are not providing. In some areas of Nepal, the government concentrates on providing curative services at local level leaving the CSO to train community health workers. In another example, in China, international

CSOs partner with government health services in many poor or remote communities.

Programmes are discussed with each level of the health service. Often the main tasks carried out by the CSO include training and helping to improve health care at grass roots level. There can be drawbacks in this approach—it may be hard to define who does what and which organization is responsible for which part of the programme. A great deal of time is taken in planning and meeting. The CSO may be restricted and unable to make best use of its enthusiasm and flexibility.

2. CSO sets up a programme on its own terms.

In this model the CSO takes a lead role in some or all of the health care at primary or district level or for specific wider health priorities. This approach is widely used in South Sudan in the absence of government services in many areas. However, wherever possible the CSO must liaise with and be accountable to government and integrate with national programmes, such as immunization and TB control.

CSOs can sometimes be competitive and lacking in respect. A DMO told the author on a recent post-Ebola visit to Sierra Leone, 'It's nice that you came to see me to share your ideas. Most NGOs don't even bother to knock on our door—they just get on with their own programmes'.

If a CSO programme proves effective, the government may help to fund it, learn from it or copy it, using its approach in other parts of the country. The Nigerian Lardin Gabas project made effective use of storytelling for health education. The government adopted its ideas and methods elsewhere.

3. Government delegates or contracts out primary and (sometimes) secondary health care to the CSO for local or district-wide implementation.

This is an exciting opportunity for CSOs (Figure 3.2). Here are three examples: In many areas of the Democratic Republic of Congo, hospital beds are provided by church-related institutions. In India, the charity ASHA providing health care among the urban poor of Delhi is responsible to government for providing CHW training, urban health clinics, and other development activities. A third example is the Arukah Network Clusters in Uttarakhand, India which undertake a variety of tasks and services on behalf of government (see Chapter 2).[1]

We are likely to see more health services being provided by CSOs in the future, especially where programmes co-operate and negotiate with government on a group basis.

Practical guidelines for working with government

Build personal relationships

Building relationships is of value in itself and not something we do simply in order to obtain goods and services from those in authority. One way of building relationships, in addition to arranging meetings and meals, is to invite government officials to attend or speak at special events.

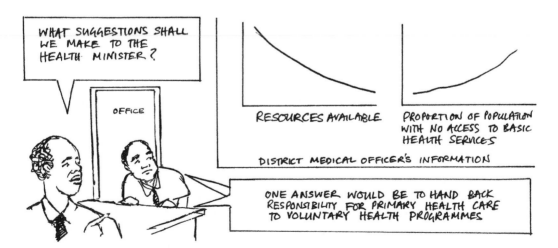

Figure 3.2 An example of value in government and NGO working together.

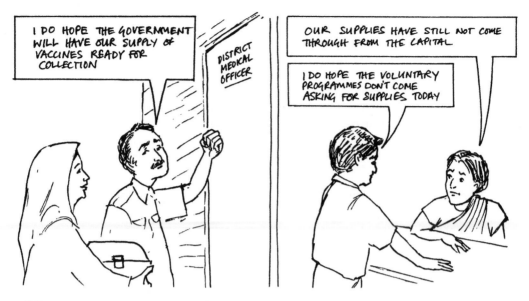

Figure 3.3 A common example of government and NGO needing to co-operate.

Reproduced courtesy of David Gifford. This image is distributed under the terms of the Creative Commons Attribution Non-Commercial 4.0 International licence (CC-BY-NC), a copy of which is available at http://creativecommons.org/licenses/by-nc/4.0/.

In some countries this approach can be complex. From our viewpoint, strategic people include the DMO and the DMO's equivalent, deputy, or any officer responsible for liaising with CSOs. District medical staff are transferred continually. We need to keep on friendly working terms with all those we deal with regularly, ranging from the DMO to the junior staff who, for example, sign out vaccines or provide supplies (Figure 3.3).

We can make strategic use of any school, community, and family links between health team and community members and government officials. For example, we may find the DMO and a member of the village health committee were at school together or played on the same football team. This approach is known as homophily and is valuable, providing it is used appropriately. However, we need to avoid nepotism, i.e. inappropriate favours given to those with family connections.

Discuss plans for the programme

Programme plans should be discussed with the most senior appropriate government officer. This may be at state, regional, or district level. If this person is found to lack interest, we should persevere, e.g. invite them to be a guest of honour or speaker at a community function, which helps government to understand what a community initiative can achieve. Alternatively, we may need to search out another senior government officer who is supportive of our work. When starting

a programme, we may need advice and ideas from the DMO, both about the location and the type of programme we should carry out. As the programme develops, we should inform the DMO of any important changes of plan or expansion into new areas. If we have been planning with a government officer other than the DMO we should ensure the DMO is kept informed.

We are likely to be involved in one or more national programmes co-ordinated by the government, such as the End TB Strategy or countrywide programmes on Neglected Tropical Diseases (NTDs, see Chapter 16). In these situations, we need to cultivate close and ongoing links with the government and to follow national adaptations and recording systems. It is worth remembering that in many areas hit by serious poverty, natural disasters, or civil conflict, there will be a breakdown in government health care. We will need to keep well informed, and balance our commitment to the poor with requests or restraints from government, sometimes adopting an advocacy role.

Send regular reports, returns, and information

We should send in any statistics or reports requested by government (Figure 3.4). This will include immunization figures (Chapter 15), reporting on TB control (Chapter 19), aspects of the IMCI (Chapter 16), or any other activity that is part of a national health strategy. If our returns are regular, accurate and show good coverage, this will help our standing with the government.

```
┌─────────────────────────────────────────────────────────────┐
│                        REPORT FORM                          │
│                                                             │
│              Monthly report for ....................         │
│                                  (month)                    │
│                                                             │
│  Weighing group (hamlet) .............. Village ............ District ......... │
│                                                             │
│  Date of weighing............ Field Worker ............ Number of kaders helping ........ │
│                                                             │
│  Total hamlet population .......... in .......... families  │
│                                                             │
│                                                             │
│  1. Total children under 36 months old      ............    │
│                                                             │
│  2. Total children with weight charts        ............    │
│                                                             │
│  3. Total newly entered this month           ............    │
│                                                             │
│  4. Total with increased weight this month   ............    │
│                                                             │
│  5. Total with no increase in weight         ............    │
│                                                             │
│  6. Total weighed with last month weight unknown            │
│       (therefore, do not know if weight increased)  ....... │
│                                                             │
│  7. Total weighed this month                 ............    │
│                                                             │
│                                                             │
│       Participation score        = # 2/1                    │
│       Activity score             = #7/2                     │
│       Growth score               =#4/(7 − (3 + 6) )         │
│       Overall score              = # 4/1                     │
│                                                             │
│       Use of supplies this month:                           │
│         Weight charts            ...............             │
│         Oralyte packets          ...............             │
│         Vitamin A high-dose capsules  ...........           │
│         Iron folate tablets      ...............             │
└─────────────────────────────────────────────────────────────┘
```

Figure 3.4 A report form from Indonesia for sending monthly statistics to the government.

Define areas of responsibility

In joint programmes with government we must ensure that the exact responsibilities of CSOs and government are clearly defined. If the government has given us responsibility for part of the programme, we should make sure that it also gives us the authority to carry it out, and that the community knows we have been given this responsibility.

Help that may be obtained from the government

Drugs and supplies

The government often provides free or subsidized supplies. These may include TB drugs for registered programmes, antiretroviral drugs for HIV, family planning supplies, Vitamin A and zinc supplements, iron and folic acid, delivery kits for midwives, long-acting insecticide impregnated mosquito nets, materials for water and sanitation programmes, and vaccines whose use is part of the national programme. These can usually be obtained via the DMO or District Hospital. We should use government supplies whenever possible, but remember that they may be not be dependable and there may be excessive paperwork.

Financial grants

These may be available from the government, usually for a specific purpose. However, they may be late or never arrive (meaning we should not be dependent on them) and they may have strict conditions attached. If possible, we should obtain grants for general purposes, not specific ones, so that the programme can decide on the most appropriate way of using the money. Some countries are so poor that no funds may be available at all. Alternative non-governmental sources may be available such as multilaterals, bilaterals, The Global Fund, etc.

Working with funders and donors

There is more information on this important topic in Chapters 5 and 12. This section looks at ways to work effectively with organizations, donors, or individuals who support our organization.

Questions asked by programmes

From time to time we may wonder:

- Why are the donor's forms so long and complex?
- Do we *have* to complete a logframe?
- Why does it take so long for funds to reach us?
- Why does the agency send representatives to question us and request evaluation? Why don't they send representatives to give us ideas, information, and encouragement?

It helps to answer these questions if we understand the problems faced by agencies (Figure 3.5).

Problems faced by donor agencies

Many agencies, especially those that are less well-resourced or have been hit by economic recession are under pressure, especially as demands on their funds are constantly rising. We should remember that:

1. Many agencies are dependent on their own supporters, who in turn will expect reassurance that their money is well spent, and want information including stories and photographs. The more of these supporters receive, the more money they will give to the agency.
2. The agency may have insufficient funds to meet all the requests, often because a major disaster has just occurred, or because disaster relief takes priority.
3. There are problems in communication because forms may be incomplete or wrongly completed. In some countries postal delays prevent letters, proposals or

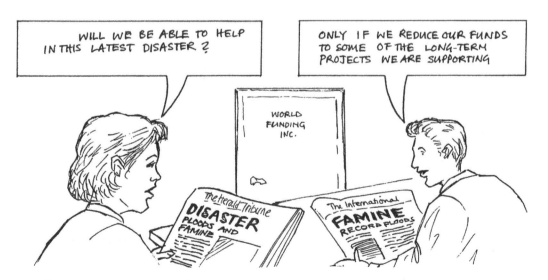

Figure 3.5 A common dilemma facing funding agencies.

financial support from arriving. Sometimes unreliable electricity supplies and Internet connections make email contact difficult.

4. Donor fatigue is where individual donors and donor agencies get overwhelmed by the number of requests made of them. There is a seeming endless list of needs and appeals for financial assistance.

Ways in which programmes can work with funders and donors

- Send reports and budgets accurately and on time. If programmes don't do this they will soon lose the confidence of donors even if they are doing a good job.
- Keep costs as low as possible.
- Reply promptly to letters, emails and other communications.
- Inform the agency of any major changes of plan.
- Welcome visitors from the agency.
- Send additional reports, short stories, and photos as appropriate
- Thank any donors promptly with two or three paragraphs of relevant and interesting information. This helps and pleases donors.

If two or more agencies are supporting a programme, then the area of support and contribution of each should be carefully defined and recorded. Finally, we should remember that most funding agencies want to work in partnership with us. Usually they are genuinely interested in what we are doing. Consultants and visitors who come and see our field work are often experts who have previously worked in similar programmes.

Avoid being donor driven

We must remember that the gifts and abilities present in our community are a crucial part of development. With training and encouragement, they can lead to start-ups and enterprises—both financial and social. This new wave of self-belief is growing in many countries and will hopefully lead to communities (and countries) becoming less dependent on donors and international aid. Our programmes must tap into this refreshing spirit of enterprise and self- belief which the millennial generation increasingly demonstrates.

We may, of course, still need funds for our programmes. Increasingly, funding is more available for clearly defined programmes and capital costs, but less often for running costs. If we participate in vertical programmes such as the End TB Strategy or Roll Back Malaria, some of our running costs may be met. But in practice we need

funds to set up our programme systems, pay salaries, and spend time building community relationships, planning, and training. These are often harder to find. But if we have worked out both needs and goals with the community and designed an effective proposal which includes administrative funds, we are more likely to make a good case. This is important because we want at all costs to avoid being donor-driven. At its worst this can undermine our programme, as we chase funds to carry out the latest government programme or donor fashion in the hope that our programme will survive. Instead, we should start with our strengths and passions. Donors prefer funding passion to funding fund-chasers.

Understand partnership and capacity building

Foreign governments and donor agencies, are increasingly guided in making funding available by these two principles:

1. Partnership.

An agency and its field partner share aims and objectives, work for mutual benefit and learn from each other. An 'us together' approach replaces a 'we and them' attitude. Partnership needs to be learned by both sides. It involves regular contact, the building of trust, a direct, open approach and long-term commitment. Everyone benefits, not least the communities we are serving. Collaboration is also seen as an essential part of the future. Many networks, such as Arukah Network, are increasingly committed to this principle.

2. Capacity building.

The supporting agency helps build the field partner's knowledge, capability and administrative systems. In turn, this enables the field partner to become increasingly self-sufficient and non-dependent. Capacity building includes training (especially in management and leadership skills, e.g. through coaching), making links, and connections between groups with their own respective strengths.

If we are looking for an outside donor we should ask about their attitude to capacity building and partnerships. Capacity building works best when the field partner is involved in determining those areas where they need their capacity to be built.

Working with other CSOs

We should aim to work as closely as possible with other voluntary programmes present in our area. These will include development projects tackling the root causes of ill health through forestry, agriculture, literacy, poverty reduction, and education (see Figure 3.6). Many, but not all, of these will be non-governmental. They may include businesses with ethical policies, academic institutes, and government departments. One entity that is present almost everywhere is a community of *faith and worship*, whether based in a church, mosque, temple, or other place of sanctity. Many health and development programmes have been slow in working with FBOs and local places of worship. More often than not the leaders of these faith communities have a strong desire to serve their community. We should seek opportunities to build relationships with priests, imams, and other religious leaders, offer training on health-related topics, and integrate them into our programmes.

Two pieces of research have highlighted the importance of this. Research commissioned by the WHO discovered that between forty and seventy per cent of health care services in Sub-Saharan Africa are provided by FBOs.[2] Additionally, a World Bank study showed that the poor trust faith-based and religious leaders more than the secular institutions that tended to partner with the World Bank.[3]

Those of us from the global north need to remember that the secularist worldview often goes against the culture of communities in the global south for whom the spiritual is an integral part of their individual, family, and community life.[4]

One excellent example of an international organization that partners with local church-based entities worldwide is Tearfund. One programme they have pioneered is a development training programme and model known as Umoja. This is proving of great value in many communities in Africa, Asia, and Latin America.[5]

Although our aim is to co-operate as much as possible we must also carefully assess any group with whom we wish to develop special links. In practice we will usually only wish to work closely with organizations that follow a community empowerment model and prioritize care according to need, rather than giving special favours to those with a particular ethnic or religious background. We also wish to work with those which base their activities on evidence, good practice, transparency and accountability.

If, however, another CSO seems to share our values and goals we can:

1. Co-operate or collaborate.

Collaboration might include visiting each other's programmes, training each other's staff, sharing expensive equipment, setting up a combined system for ordering and drugs, and sharing leisure activities. Another is the mutual visiting of programmes using a SALT approach (see Chapter 2). There is always opportunity for intentional linking between programmes, government, FBOs, and other health players in the surrounding area (Figure 3.6).

2. Define programme areas.

If there is genuine overlap between programmes, it will be necessary to define clearly where each programme should work and what each programme should do.

3. Join any voluntary health organization that encourages programmes to work together and share activities.

For example, in India the Voluntary Health Association of India does this effectively with many state groups. In Africa many countries have national Christian or Church Health Associations.[6]

4. Become a member of a national or international network.

Increased contact with other, larger organizations will enable us to learn, share information, and work together. There are an growing number of these, including HIFA, VISION 2020, Arukah Network, and the People's Health Movement.

Working with the private sector

It is worth considering these three inter-related factors:

1. An increasing amount of wealth is owned by the private sector, both by successful national companies and by multinational corporations.

2. The financial needs of health and development programmes are growing rapidly.

3. The governments of many developing countries are seriously short of money, meaning they struggle to finance health care. This makes a link between the wealthy private sector and the needy development sector an obvious one to explore.

Many openings arise from company-supported Corporate Social Responsibility programmes (CSRs) started by businesses who wish to contribute, or be seen to contribute, to the common good. In addition, some of the wealthiest individuals in the world have set up philanthropic organizations, trusts, and foundations targeting global health.

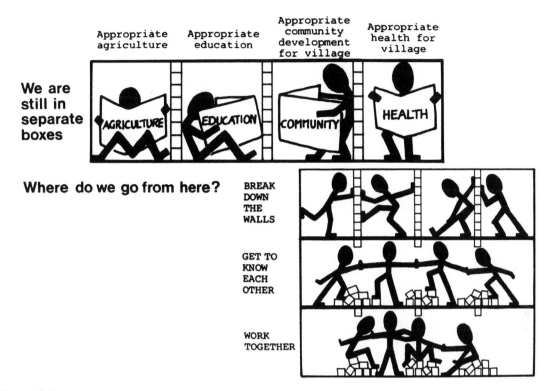

Figure 3.6 We must get rid of 'silos'.

There are, of course, some drawbacks. There are dangers and disadvantages we need to be aware of, particularly the difference in values. Often the motivating factor in the corporate sector is profit and expansion, but in the humanitarian sector, service, care and compassion.

We need to follow some basic principles:

- Define clearly the needs of the programme in terms of funding, resources, drug supply and other inputs.
- Understand clearly what any public or private company is willing to provide, whether money, supplies or services.
- Work out a way in which both programme and company can benefit from the partnership.
- Ensure that the company does not drive or set the health programme's agenda, either through persuasion, aggressive advertising or illegal incentives.
- Make no links with any company that has unethical policies or products. Obvious examples include tobacco or weapons, unregulated baby milk substitutes, or anything that pollutes or damages the environment.
- Set up a careful agreement for a limited period and then review it.

Some examples of co-operation

- A pharmaceutical company that donates or subsidizes an essential medicine needed on a wide scale. This could include antimalarials, deworming treatment, TB drugs and antiretroviral medicines. Some very effective collaborations have involved international pharmaceutical companies donating free treatment for a number of NTDs such as schistosomiasis (bilharzia) and onchocerciasis (river blindness).
- A locally based company might sponsor a training programme.
- A bank might help to set up a co-operative.
- Businesses sympathetic to the programme may give regular or one-off grants.

Working with doctors and private practitioners

This section discusses working with doctors and qualified practitioners who have undertaken some formal medical training, although this may be less than the normal MBBS or MD or equivalent. Some will work in government service and some in the voluntary sector, but many will work as full- or part-time private practitioners. Many government doctors also have private practices.

Some characteristics of doctors

Doctors often approach community health according to similar patterns. These comments are not criticisms but an outline of doctor's strengths and weakness in engaging with community health.

1. There is a tendency for doctors to be more interested in treatment and cure than in prevention.

They generally prefer working in hospitals or their own offices. They often put an emphasis on investigations and laboratory testing which are expensive. Money and status may be important to them.

2. They may have less interest in primary or community-based health.

They may believe it will not use their skills and training to the full. They usually prefer working in towns or cities rather than in remote rural areas.

3. They may show interest in the health programmes we set up.

This may happen for a variety of reasons—perhaps out of social concern, or out of fear that successful health prevention will reduce their patient numbers. However surgeons in particular have a key role in caring for patients referred in by the community.

4. Many doctors, especially if hospital-based, are very busy.

Understandably, doctors tend to be reactive to situations, e.g. curing illness, rather than proactive, e.g. preventing illness, or looking for 'up-stream' causes (see Chapter 1).

With this in mind, it is worth considering that doctors who specialise in public health will often have priorities more in line with CBHC.

How best to collaborate with doctors in our programme area

On the one hand, we will want to collaborate and work alongside existing health facilities and other health providers in our area. On the other, we will also need to guide community members against being treated inappropriately with unnecessary and expensive medicines and injections. Getting this balance right will need diplomacy and persistence. Here are some ideas that may help:

- Build personal relationships with other doctors and practitioners.
- Explain who we are and what we are doing.

Make it clear that our main aim is not primarily to treat patients, but to prevent illness and improve the health of the community.

1. Never publicly criticize or speak out against other doctors or their practices.

Even if we strongly disapprove of the way a colleague is treating a patient, we should be slow to criticize either in public or to one of the doctor's patients. If the case is serious we should see the practitioner ourselves.

2. Provide health education to local doctors.

Most doctors have little chance for continuing medical education. From the day they qualify, most will receive information largely from the representatives of pharmaceutical companies promoting their products. We can, therefore, invite doctors to our staff training days, run local health courses or seminars, loan health books or journals, and welcome them to use the programme library or access on-line resources.

3. Include practitioners in our health programme.

For example, a doctor working in or near our programme area may, with some training and orientation, became a part-time member of the health team.

The doctor's role in Community Health Programmes (CHPs)

This section discusses various roles that qualified doctors can take on within a CHP. Although it is a tradition that when a doctor goes to a clinic or health centre he/she sees the patients, this is can be unhelpful in a community health setting. It undermines any other health workers who have been trained to do this (Figure 3.7). It also goes against the whole principle of task shifting (see Chapter 1). Instead, doctors should only see patients who need specialist diagnosis, care or treatment, referred to them by other health workers.

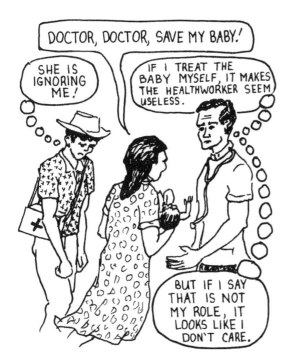

Figure 3.7 A practical field programme.

Teacher and Trainer

The doctor's aim should be to pass on relevant skills and knowledge so that other health workers quickly learn to diagnose, treat and prevent common diseases.

Planner and strategist

Doctors have an important function in identifying health priorities, and helping to draw up plans and strategies. But they should do this alongside the community, who themselves will identify problems and solutions. It is easy for programmes to become 'doctor-driven' unless any doctor in a leadership role fully understands the CBHC approach.

A liaison role

Doctors are usually best placed to liaise with government officials, medical officers and programme directors of other health care programmes. This is especially important when we are involved with national programmes such as Stop TB or IMCI.

Compiler of a Model List of Essential Medicines

Because a doctor's training emphasizes the use of medicines to cure illness, any list of essential medicines a doctor draws up will need to be discussed with others. For example, a nurse experienced in CBHC or a medical assistant can advise whether the list is too long; the director or finance officer whether it is too expensive (see Chapter 11).

Adviser

Doctors can advise on all health-related topics, including clinical care, the use of medicines, immunisation schedules, clean water, latrines, and the setting up of clinics and programmes for mothers and children.

Programme Director

In practice, doctors are often the directors of community health programmes (CHPs), but there are three good reasons why leadership should be either shared or handed over to others.

1. Doctors usually understand CBHC only if they have been strongly exposed to primary health care models or have been 'converted' to a CBHC model of care, distinct from a hospital-based approach.

Nurses, on the other hand, often make appropriate CHP leaders, provided that doctors support them in strategic and advisory roles. In practice, doctors are often unwilling to work under the leadership of a nurse, as in many areas of the world nurses, wrongly, have lower social status.

2. Doctors and other health professionals are rarely trained in programme management.

Thus they may make poor managers unless they have natural gifts or get additional training. Generally programmes should employ managers after the startup phase of any programme, even though doctors will normally retain some form of leadership role. Often staff members with special aptitude can be trained and mentored into management roles.

3. Doctors often base success on patient numbers.

Because they tend to evaluate the effectiveness of a health programme by how many patients are brought to the hospital, they may not understand that, in contrast, the aim of the community health programme is usually to reduce the number of people going to hospital.

Working with traditional health practitioners (THPs)

What are THPs?

Most patients in the poorest parts of the world, and especially in rural areas, first seek advice from THPs. In many areas of Africa, up to eighty per cent of people visit THPs. In areas with better health services, increasing numbers of patients first consult scientifically trained (allopathic) health workers. Where health services are declining or becoming too expensive, people are returning to THPs for their main source of health care. THPs include a huge range of people. Some follow long-established, traditional, medical systems, such as Ayurvedic, Unani, and Siddha practitioners in south Asia, traditional Chinese medicine, and Inyangas (herbalists) in South Africa. What nearly all have in common is a deep understanding and strong connection with the communities they serve. Although many remedies they use are unproven and some are dangerous, many medicines used today were originally derived from herbs and traditional medicines. This includes artemisinin, now the most effective treatment for malaria, which has been used for centuries in China and is extracted from the plant *Artemisia annua*. Most countries have networks of THPs, ranging from those who are ethical, established, and registered to those with little or no training or who use dubious or dangerous practices.

The WHO has set up guidelines on the use of traditional and complementary medicine (T&CM).[7] They have identified three ways in which traditional medicine can be more effectively used, in view of its huge and growing size:

1. Build the knowledge base that will inform national policies on their use and potential.
2. Strengthen their quality, safety, and use by more careful regulation and training of practitioners.
3. Promote universal health coverage by integrating T&CM into health care services and into appropriate self-health care.

The varied knowledge and practices of THPs mean that we can never have one universal way of working with them. We must develop a strategy for our own situation.

Guidelines for working with THPs

1. Gather information about THPs working in the programme area.

Some of this information will come through meeting THPs in the community, e.g. as part of a participatory appraisal (see Chapter 6) and from working alongside community members. We can find out:

- if they follow any particular systems?
- what sorts of treatment do they use?
- which members of the community consult them?
- what types of ailment do they treat?
- how much do they charge?
- are they paid in money or in kind?
- do people perceive that their treatments are effective?
- are they respected?
- do they use any dangerous or harmful practices?
- what is their attitude to allopathic medicine?

Once we have answers to some or all of these questions, we can decide how to work with THPs.

2. Devise a model for working with THPs.

We should remember that whatever services our programme provides, many patients will continue to visit THPs, especially for the treatment of pain, epilepsy and symptoms of chronic disease. In practice, we will probably work with some types of THP, but may decide that others use approaches or have belief systems that would conflict with the programme. Programmes quite commonly work with traditional birth attendants (TBAs) or established practitioners of traditional systems, such as Ayurveda. For any group of THPs we have three options:

a. Incorporate THPs into our health programme.

This will work only if we develop a strong level of personal trust, if THPs share a broadly similar value system, and if they are prepared to work in close partnership with us and undergo further training.

b. Co-operate with THPs in specific areas of health care.

In this model THPs will continue with many of their traditional activities but, through the training we offer, help to promote better health practices in the community. For example, in Malawi, THPs within the Queen Elizabeth Hospital catchment area in Blantyre were successfully given briefing sessions on the symptoms of TB, and provided with referral slips so they could refer on patients with chronic cough for sputum testing.

c. Decide against any formal links with THPs, if values and approach seem too far apart, or if their approach results in harm to patients.

Regardless of which option seems best for the project, before developing a permanent model we should run a small pilot scheme first.

3. Set up THP training.

Having chosen which THPs to work with and how, we then need to design training programmes. Our training must be based on trust, a sharing of information, establishing common areas of understanding, correcting harmful beliefs, and affirming helpful ones. THPs probably learn best through apprenticeship, and by observation and discussion, rather than formal training.

4. Find ways in which THPs are able to benefit CBHC.

While many programmes use THPs, some fail to make best use of them. Where they have been involved in health programmes, their contributions have often been valuable. THPS can do these tasks:

- Providing important information about health needs in the community, or their referral area
- Working as CHWs or alongside them.

- Encouraging improvements in hygiene and nutrition practices.
- Be advocates for improved sanitation, including latrines.
- Promoting breastfeeding and use of oral rehydration solution (ORS).
- Working alongside trained TBAs or skilled attendants in the care of pregnant women and newborns.
- Working as observers in TB DOTs programmes.
- Cooperate with the programme in the prevention and treatment of Sexually Transmitted Infection, TB, and HIV/AIDS.
- Become involved in home care programmes.
- Involvement with community-based mental health services.[8]
- Monitor programmes involving THPs.

We will need to monitor occurrences of harmful or dangerous practices such as dissuading patients from using ARVs to control HIV, or medicines to cure TB. We will also need to keep track of actual or perceived benefit felt by the programme, the THP, and the community.

Working with hospitals

Some CHPs are attached to a base hospital, and others are independent. Whichever arrangement is used, one principle is essential: hospitals and CHPs must work in partnership (Figure 3.8). Hospitals provide a whole range of backup services for the primary health care level.

There are usually three levels in a national health system. Sometimes a level may be divided into subdivisions and the levels may have different names depending on the country.

1. Primary level.

This includes CHWs working in the community, dispensaries, health posts, subcentres and primary health centres.

2. Secondary level.

The district, first referral or 'base' hospital gives backing to the primary level, and takes referrals from it. It has inpatient beds, can usually perform routine surgery, caesarean sections and a range of investigations.

3. Tertiary level.

Well-equipped regional hospitals perform major surgery and complex investigations, and offer a range of specialist care. They take referrals from the secondary level.

When this system works correctly (see Figure 3.9), it is good for patients, health workers and the economy. It is good for *patients* because they receive primary care near their home, saving them time, money and worry. It is good for *health workers* because they see patients appropriate to their level of training and have job satisfaction. It is good for the *economy* because the majority of patients are seen by CHWs rather than highly trained, well-paid doctors.

The model described in this section is the primary health care model recommended by the WHO and others as the most effective and equitable system, following many of the principles of the Alma Ata Declaration of 1978 (see Chapter 1).

How health services often work in practice

Breakdown of health services

In many parts of the world health services are severely short of funds. Staff may be absent or demoralized. Equipment may have broken down and drug supplies

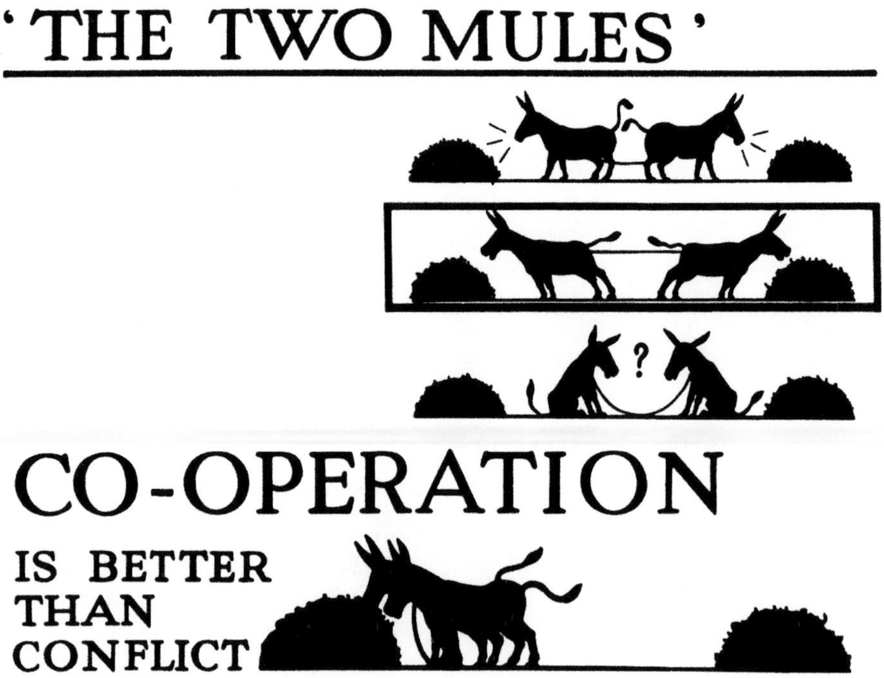

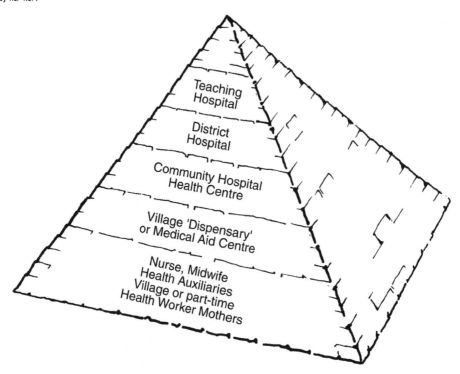

Figure 3.8 Everyone benefits when hospitals and primary health programmes work together.

Figure 3.9 The Health Pyramid. Patients should normally enter at the lowest level and only move upwards by referral.

may have run out. Some levels of the health system may have ceased to function. CBHC has to work within whatever structure is available, drawing support where it can but being self-sufficient when necessary.

Non-existent referral systems

Owing to poor quality health services, many people bypass the primary levels of the health service and go to the secondary or tertiary levels for their health problems. In particular, the wealthy and powerful like seeing smart doctors in smart hospitals even for minor ailments. This has unfortunate results:

- The rich get over-treated, so setting an inappropriate pattern, which others start to follow.
- The poor are undertreated, or not treated at all, as there is little capacity to handle serious problems referred from the primary level.
- Health workers are unfulfilled: doctors spend time seeing patients with minor problems, and so become

bored; CHWs and middle-level workers are bypassed except by the very poor, and so become discouraged.
- Costs increase as more hospitals are built.

The correct role of the hospital

Acting as a referral centre

Most patients will be referred in from the primary health centre. Acutely ill patients in the community nearby may be referred directly by CHWs and bypass the primary health centre. A few patients will be self-referred (Figure 3.11). Patients requiring referral to hospital will include emergencies, those needing surgery, caesarean section, or assisted delivery, and those needing more complex investigations (either as outpatients or inpatients). In acting as a referral centre the hospital will have three important tasks:

1. It will receive patients, trying where possible to admit any patient referred from the primary level especially if coming in from a long distance.

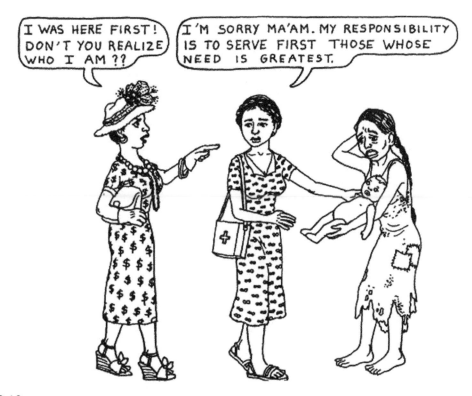

Figure 3.10 A question for health care in the twenty-first century: 'Will this health worker submit to the demands of the rich or respond to the needs of the poor?'

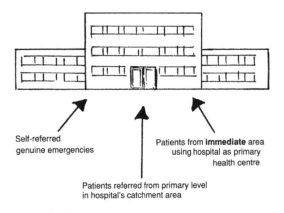

Figure 3.11 The correct use of a referral hospital.

2. It will care for patients in the ward, where staff should be taught to give dignity and special care for the poorest and sickest. Often in practice staff respect the rich and push the poor aside (Figure 3.10).

3. It will discharge patients back to the community, first contacting the primary health centre team to arrange a suitable time and means of transport. A doctor or nurse will write a discharge summary.

The time immediately after discharge is often difficult for patients. They may not know what should happen next or what treatment they should be taking. To help them, base hospitals and the Community Health team must communicate well.

Acting as a teaching centre

In some programmes, teaching of the health team, including the CHWs, is done in the hospital, and in others it is done mainly in the community with occasional visits to the hospital. Patients will usually pay more attention to what the hospital says than to what the community health team says. Therefore, it is important that both give the same message and that the hospital supports the teaching of the CHWs.

Backing up with supplies, equipment and management

The hospital may be the simplest place to obtain medicines, vaccines and equipment. It may arrange to sterilize instruments. It may have more expensive items that CHPs can borrow or use, such as teaching aids or vehicles. The hospital may do the CHP's accounting, prepare statistics, or help produce the annual report. It may have salary structures and management systems

that can be adapted. It may have a photocopier and a more functional Internet.

Discouraging self-referrals while providing a neighbourhood primary health programme

The role of the hospital is to treat serious cases referred from the primary level, not to act as a primary health centre for anyone who walks in. The hospital should discourage patients from attending unless they have a referral letter or are a genuine emergency. However, the hospital can set up a primary health programme or centre with appropriate staff for people who live in communities very near the hospital. They can carry out community health activities like a regular CHP, selecting and training CHWs and referring internally (see Figure 3.11).

How hospitals and CHPs relate to each other

There are several different models of how this can happen.

1. CHP under hospital management

This is the traditional arrangement. The hospital is established and decides to start a CHP. The government may now be promoting the use of CHWs and the hospital may seem the obvious place for them to be based for training and support. Increasingly, more doctors and health workers are seeing the importance of prevention.

2. CHP separate from hospital

When the CHP is separate from the hospital, there may be no fixed hospital for referral. In this situation, the CHP is truly on its own and dependent on its own resources, planning, and expertise. Patients needing referral will be sent to different practitioners, clinics or hospitals, with whom piecemeal arrangements are made. Many urban projects follow this model.

Where there are fixed hospital(s) for referral, the programme remains separate but builds special contacts with one or two hospitals as referral centres. This pattern has much to commend it and if well set up, it enables a programme to be independent yet have access to hospitals for referral.

3. CHP served by hospital

This radical pattern, though rare, is probably the best. The hospital is part of the CHP and its main aim is providing referral and support services. Staff move freely between hospital and community, patients feel welcomed in the hospital, and those in need are treated with understanding.

An excellent example of this approach is the Comprehensive Rural Health Programme in Jamkhed, India (www.jamkhed.org). In practice, some rural hospitals past and present have started with this vision but the demand for curative services became overwhelming, the hospital became the profitable arm of the programme, and the vision was lost.

Practical solutions for good CHP–hospital relations

Problems can also arise when CHPs are managed by hospitals. Poor co-operation can result in or stem from misunderstandings or even rivalry between the hospital and the CHP. Additionally, poor care can be given to the poorest patients. Hospital staff often prefer looking after the rich who can pay for services, rather than the slum-dweller or villager who can't pay and doesn't understand. Finally, priority is often given to the hospital. As the hospital is seen as the most important service, when shortages of money or staff occur, it is the CHP that suffers.

The secret of a successful partnership is the development of a friendly working relationship between the primary and the secondary level—between the CHP and the hospital (See Figure 3.12). We should make this a definite goal in our programme. There are several keys to good CHP–hospital relations and one leads from the other:

- Mutual understanding of each other's role.

CHP members need to spend time in the hospital, understand how it works, and getting to know its staff. It is essential that hospital staff spend time in the community, understand the way of life, and share in identifying problems and solutions.

- Mutual respect.

As each branch of the health team understands the other, so mutual respect grows, which in turn leads to:

- Interdependence where everyone benefits, and the poor receive appropriate treatment.

This partnership between primary and secondary levels will not happen on its own. Staff continually change and everyone is busy. One or two people in the hospital and CHP must champion this process. Special times for celebrating national events, anniversaries, birthdays and successes can be fun occasions and build friendships, as can sporting activities like football and volleyball matches.

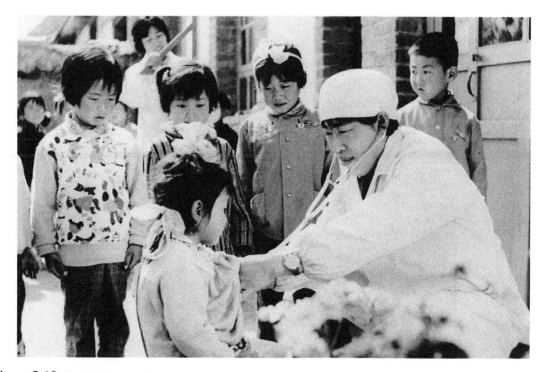

Figure 3.12 Close links between hospital doctors and primary health services in China benefit all members of the community.

Summary

CHPs must be seen as an integral part of a national health care system. They need to establish a wide range of connections and useful collaborations. They should learn to co-operate with government in a well-defined partnership, each recognizing the strengths and roles of the other. They must co-operate with donors and funders and provide necessary information promptly. They should work with other CSOs in the programme area, providing their values and goals are similar. They should be open to alliances with the private sector, for example, through corporate social responsibility (CSR) programmes and philanthropic organizations, providing that the CHP's values are safeguarded. CHPs will use and relate to doctors in a variety of ways. They should consider carefully how to work in co-operation with any private practitioners or THPs in the programme area. Finally, CHPs should integrate with other levels of the health service, including referral hospitals, so that each tier carries out the jobs for which it was designed. This results in increased job satisfaction for health workers, provides more effective services for patients, and greatly reduces costs. Underlying all co-operation is the building of friendship and trust between the health programme and colleagues in government, neighbouring programmes, and hospitals.

Further reading

Carter I. *Building the capacity of local groups: A pillars guide*. Teddington: Tearfund; 2001. Available from: www.tearfund.org/tilz.

Busia K, Kasilo OMJ. Collaboration between traditional health practitioners and conventional health practitioners: Some country experiences. *WHO African Health Monitor*. 2010; 13. Available from: www.aho.afro.who.int/en/ahm/issue/13/reports/collaboration-between-traditional-health-practitioners-and-conventional-health

Amonoo-Lartson G, Lovell IH, Rankin J. *District health care*. 2nd ed. London: Macmillan; 1996. Out of print. May be available second-hand or on-line through library services.

World Health Organization. *Legal status of traditional medicine and complementary/alternative medicine: A worldwide review*. Geneva: World Health Organization; 2001. Available from: http://apps.who.int/medicinedocs/en/d/Jh2943e/4.38.html

Hoff W. *Traditional practitioners as primary health care workers*. Geneva: World Health Organization; 1995. Available from: http://apps.who.int/medicinedocs/pdf/h2941e/h2941e.pdf

World Health Organization. *Traditional medicine strategy 2014–2023*. Geneva: World Health Organization; 2013. Available from: http://www.who.int/medicines/publications/traditional/trm_strategy14_23/en/ In addition the WHO website links to regional research publications about plant-based traditional medicines in specific countries.

References

1. Arukah Network for Global Community Health. Available from: https://www.arukahnetwork.org/uttarakhand

2. The World Health Organization. *Faith-based organizations play a major role in HIV/AIDS care and treatment in sub-Saharan Africa*. Geneva: World Health Organization; 2007. Available from: http://www.who.int/mediacentre/news/notes/2007/np05/en/index.html

3. Narayan D. Voice of the Poor. In: Belshaw D, Calderisi R, Sugden C, editors. *Faith in development: Partnership between the World Bank and the churches of Africa*. Oxford: Regnum Books/The World Bank; 2001. p. 39–50. Narayan D, Patel R, Schafft K, Rademacher A, Koch-Schulte S. *Voices of the poor: Can anyone hear us?* Oxford: Oxford University Press; 2000.

4. Grills N. The paradox of multilateral organizations engaging with faith-based organizations. *Global Governance*. 2009; 15 (4): 505–20.

5. Tearfund. *Umoja*. Available from: http://tilz.tearfund.org/en/themes/church/umoja/

6. Africa Christian Health Associations Platform. Available from: http://africachap.org/en/

7. World Health Organization. *Traditional medicine strategy 2014–2023*. Geneva: World Health Organization; 2014. Available from: http://apps.who.int/iris/bitstream/10665/92455/1/9789241506090_eng.pdf?ua=1

8. Alem A, Jacobssen L, Hanlon C. Community-based mental health care in Africa: Mental health workers' views. *World Psychiatry*. 2008; 7 (1): 54–7.

9. Campbell-Hall V, Petersen I, Bhana A, Mjadu S, Hosegood V, Flisher A, et al. Collaboration between traditional practitioners and primary health care staff in South Africa: Developing a workable partnership for community mental health services. *Transcultural Psychiatry*. 2010; 47 (4): 610–28.

CHAPTER 4
Health teaching and behavioural change

Ted Lankester

What we need to know

At the outset of setting up any programme, we need to remind ourselves that communities and their individual members make their choices based on the understanding and knowledge they possess. Community members are more expert about their own situations than any outsider, even if sometimes their health information is incomplete or incorrect.

After some training most health and development workers are able to give good health teaching (Figure 4.1). But in community-based health care (CBHC), teaching is not our primary aim. Our purpose to accompany the community so as to help bring about improved wellbeing and new patterns of healthy living. For this to happen there first needs to be a transformation in the attitudes of the health team, starting with the programme leaders.

Transformation means a radical and permanent change from one set of attitudes and behaviours to another. We need to exchange the negative ways in which we see ourselves and others with positive and affirming attitudes that encompass everyone.

We must also recognize any cynical, unhelpful attitude that we start to develop at an early stage before it causes discouragement to ourselves and those around us. For example, we may feel superior to the people we are working with because we are better educated, come from a city, or belong to a different tribe or caste. Conversely, for a variety of reasons we may feel inferior and need to learn to appreciate our own gifts.

We may blame community members for their ignorance and unhealthy habits, or we may think less of others because they are poor. This is especially true if we have never been poor ourselves or if we have overcome poverty but become arrogant in the process of doing so.

A health team that trusts, affirms, and believes the best about the community it works with will naturally encourage and empower that community. Self-esteem and self-belief will grow. But while it is easy to talk about the need for transformation, it can be difficult to bring about. How can we transform our attitudes?

Transforming our attitudes

We must begin by realizing and accepting that it takes time to change. Changing attitudes is a long-term process, like learning a new skill: it takes practice. In the early stages of a programme, we are often more open

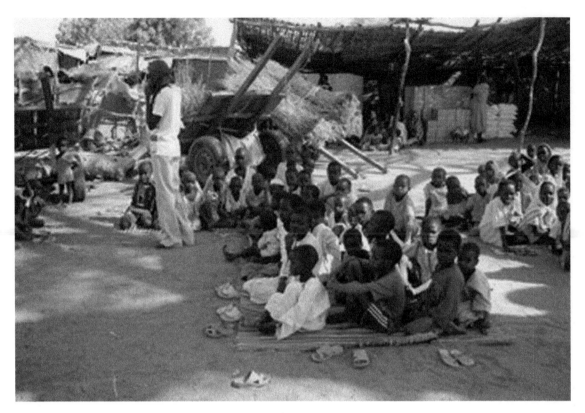

Figure 4.1 Health teaching in practice.
Reproduced courtesy of Tearfund. This image is distributed under the terms of the Creative Commons Attribution Non-Commercial 4.0 International licence (CC-BY-NC), a copy of which is available at http://creativecommons.org/licenses/by-nc/4.0/.

to change, so new attitudes can start to take root in ourselves and in those around us.

Spiritual pilgrimage

This is often underplayed, but relevant for the eighty six per cent of the world population that claims to have a religious faith. All of us in the health programme, as well as community members and those coming from outside, may be able to draw strength and guidance from prayer, meditation, self-awareness, or the examples of spiritual teachers. Our day may start this way in a common observance.

Jesus told us to love our neighbour as we love ourselves (Matt. 22:39). Therefore, in addition to loving our neighbours we also need to learn to love and appreciate ourselves—who we are and what we can become—in an attitude of humility. Then, this love of ourselves becomes the measure and encouragement for loving others. Jesus goes further: he encourages us to love our enemies, those whom we may not naturally like, or with whom we don't agree. The Quran teaches

'And walk not on the earth with conceit and arrogance' (*Sura* 17, v. 37).

Live with those we serve

For a period of time each project member, including those in leadership, should ideally live within the community and experience the hardships—and joys—of community life. This will help us to understand and appreciate the community's lifestyle, thinking and behaviour. Then we will be less likely to make judgments and more likely to show respect. Finally, we can ask ourselves two questions to discern if we are judging instead of accepting:

• What would these community members have achieved if they had been given my opportunities?

• What would I have achieved if I had suffered their disadvantages?

Sometimes it is worth carrying out an 'attitude brainstorm'. To do this, the team meets together and everyone shares ideas about helpful and unhelpful attitudes they have seen in themselves and in others. Someone lists these in two columns on a flipchart. As people come to recognize helpful and unhelpful attitudes within the context of a supportive group, it helps the process of transformation. Later on, there can be a review session and members can share their experiences and ways in which their attitudes have changed. One golden rule: no one is criticized or humiliated for anything personal they share.

Visit 'model' programmes and use role models

Sometimes there will be health programmes where we can observe the process of transformation or see the results of it. By living for a time in a new environment we will be more open than usual to new ideas, attitudes and practices.

We can also follow the example of role models. Often attitudes are caught, not taught. Each person in the team is encouraged to think of one or two friends or community or national figures whose values they admire. For many of us, the dignified unselfishness of the villager or the single mother bringing up a family successfully in an urban slum is its own inspiration.

Use role play

Role play can be an effective way of identifying the natural attitudes we possess, and learning how to change them. For example, we can role play the way we would naturally react to an uneducated community member who repeatedly fails to grasp our health teaching. Then, after group discussion, we repeat the role play using a different, more affirmative approach.

Health teaching and behavioural change

Our ultimate aim is to turn off the tap of ill health in the communities we work alongside (Figure 4.2). This comes about through a permanent behaviour change, which prevents many illnesses from occurring and enables community members to treat many more at an early stage before they become serious.

This is a complex and very important subject in CBHC, and there are several ways to approach this. This section provides two examples: the Stages of Change model,[1] which can help us understand the process of behavioural change. The second is a four-stage approach to bringing about change, found to be useful by a group of programmes with which the author is associated. These stages can apply to an individual,

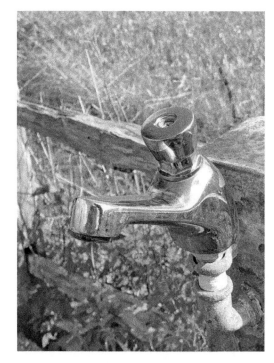

Figure 4.2 Turning off the tap of ill health.

family, neighbourhood, or entire community. We will call these Model 1 and Model 2, but they overlap at various points.

Models of behaviour change

Model 1: stages of change

There are five stages in this model:

1. Precontemplation (Not Ready)
2. Contemplation (Getting Ready)
3. Preparation (Ready)
4. Action
5. Maintenance

Precontemplation

People in this stage do not intend to act in the foreseeable future, i.e. the next six months. Health professionals may consider such people and communities as resistant or unmotivated. In practice, the community may not see how the planned change can benefit them.

Contemplation (getting ready)

People in this stage intend to change within the next six months. They are aware of not only the good reasons for changing, but are also aware of the downsides. This weighing up of costs and benefits can keep people at the contemplation stage for long periods of time. Outsiders may feel these people are either unable to make up their minds, or are procrastinating or stalling. In practice, they instead may need further guidance in understanding how the change can bring them real, tangible benefits.

Preparation (ready)

People in the preparation stage intend to act soon—usually within the next month. Typically, they have already taken some significant action in the past year. These individuals have a plan of action, e.g. pregnant women who agree to attend antenatal classes and have a facility-based delivery.

Action

Those in the action stage have made specific changes in their lifestyle within the past six months. Health professionals may feel encouraged that their programmes are working, but, in practice, this may be only one part of the change process, albeit an important one. For example, a reduction in cigarettes smoked or switching to low-tar cigarettes may seem like useful action especially across a whole community, but only total cessation will bring full benefits.

Maintenance

This final stage is where people have changed their lifestyles and are working to prevent relapse. During the maintenance stage, people become less tempted to relapse and grow increasingly more confident about maintaining their new behaviour. Based on current evidence, maintenance lasts from six months to five years. For example, US research showed that after 12 months of continuous abstinence from tobacco, forty-three per cent of individuals returned to regular smoking. After five years of continuous abstinence, the risk of relapse dropped to seven per cent.

Model 2: progress through four practical stages

The second model is a more traditional approach. It guides us against the wishful thinking that health teaching in itself will bring about change. It won't. Teaching about health is only one part of a behaviour change process.

Health teaching

Health information alone does not bring change, but health teaching is often where we need to start. It is often most effective when it addresses a topical, important need that community members have.

Many staff in busy health programmes and hospitals spend their time curing illness in health centres and outpatient departments. They give health education only if there is time left over. This approach will never improve a community's health.

However, things can start to change when we prioritize health teaching—probably the most important of all community health activities. It should take place on all appropriate occasions, e.g. not only in clinics, but also in schools and whenever community members and health workers come together. Teaching needs to be interesting, fun, and involve the active participation of learners. Later sections in this chapter look at ways we can do this.

Health awareness

The purpose of health teaching is not simply to impart knowledge about health. Even if people know more, knowledge does not always guarantee action. A community may have health knowledge, but not be healthy; people may have heard endless health talks, but maintained their harmful habits. Our main aim, therefore, is not simply to teach, but to create awareness of how making changes in health behaviour can lead to healthier lives, less illness, fewer work-days lost and less expense. For example, a mother may know she should wash her hands before preparing food, but does not do so. Because she is not aware how this would make a difference in her particular situation, she is unmotivated to change.

Motivation

Community members who have been made *aware* of a particular problem see the importance of doing something about it. In other words, they become motivated to make changes because they realize that making these changes will be to their advantage (Figure 4.3).

Behavioural change

Once a person or community feels motivated to embrace a new way of thinking and acting, they will start the crucial phase of behavioural change. Without this last stage all the health teaching in the world makes little impact. This community (or individual) is now able to say: 'We know, we understand, we are motivated, we will change our behaviour'. Some people call this moving a community to an 'Ah, Yes!' moment.

For example, consider a tobacco control programme. An unaware community buys and smokes cigarettes, and young people start smoking as a matter of course. As the community increases its awareness about the health

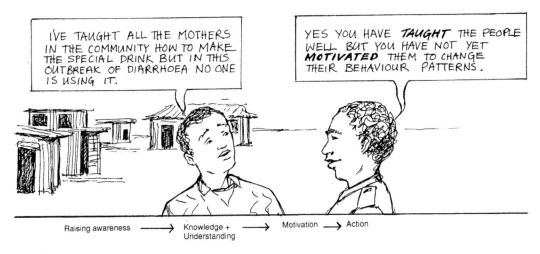

Figure 4.3 A process of raising awareness.

risks and expense of smoking, its greater understanding of the issue may lead to fewer people adopting the habit. A motivated community starts to see the value of stopping buying and smoking cigarettes. Individuals will make the decision to stop smoking, and share with others their experience of quitting.

Behaviour change then starts to spread as people learn from each other. A community whose behaviour has really changed may then encourage other communities they know, e.g. an Arukah Network Cluster (see Chapter 2), to start their own programme of tobacco control, or they may join an advocacy group to prevent companies from selling cigarettes in or near their community.

It is important to note that a vital part of this stage is *sustaining* the behavioural change. Even in highly motivated community members, changes in health behaviour need to be continually reinforced or people will return to their old ways. For example, it is relatively easy to teach people about the value of hand washing to reduce the amount of diarrhoea in the family. For a few days they will follow what seems a sensible practice. But it is difficult for them to sustain this over a period of time unless it is reinforced until it becomes a firm habit.

One way of doing this is to use an 'emotional driver' such as disgust, or the concept of being 'uncool'. For example: 'It's disgusting to think you would prepare food for your family without washing your hands first', or 'It now seems so uncool to sit down to eat without everyone washing their hands'.

What we need to do

Choosing an appropriate subject

Health teaching should start with one or two concerns already important to the community, and grow from there. Often such concerns come up in discussions with the community or become clear from the participatory appraisal (PA) or the community diagnosis (see Chapter 6).

Creating awareness about a felt need is usually quite easy. People already understand the problem, and they are now ready for solutions. Creating awareness about a real but unfelt need takes longer. For example, when dealing with moderate malnutrition in children, although the health team knows that children who are underweight on the growth chart are at greater risk from childhood illnesses, these children may look normal and healthy to members of the community.

Choosing an appropriate method

There are many ways of teaching and creating awareness. We should learn to use one or two effectively, rather than trying to master them all. Any method chosen needs to be:

1. Appropriate to the local culture.

For example, storytelling or singing may be part of the local tradition. If so, we can use these in our teaching. We should avoid methods that are strange to our community, cause offence, or send the wrong message. We must make sure that any teaching, without compromising any important health messages, is in line with religious or social customs. Colours and symbols may have particular meanings in a community, and using the local language or dialect will help a community feel ownership at an early stage.

However, we should be prepared for unintended results. For example, after watching a TV programme on how to prepare for healthy childbirth, instead of queuing up for the next antenatal clinic, members of the community were found consulting local moneylenders about raising credit to buy their own TV set!

2. Appropriate to the subject we are teaching.

For example, teaching how to overcome drunkenness can be shown very effectively through drama or puppets. Teaching is enjoyable, the audience feels involved, and the message is clear. The drama can be paused at key moments, and the audience asked to suggest what should happen next.

3. Appropriate to the level of education.

For example, health professionals may be used to learning from lectures and PowerPoint presentations, but community members will become bored and turn off. Role play, health games, or other action-based learning are more appropriate for those with less education or difficulty in reading and writing. Also, the processes of the PA can be valuable (see Chapter 6).

4. Appropriate to the gifts of the people.

In CBHC we should always be recognizing and using the gifts, talents, and skills present within the community. There are likely to be people who are natural actors, singers, storytellers, and entertainers. Use these gifts wherever people are willing.

5. Appropriate to the resources of the programme and community.

For example, some programmes find using films helpful. In the author's experience this works well, even in remote areas, providing that the community and health programme work together on this. Team tasks can include checking the resources, spare parts, fuel, and expertise for using and maintaining projectors.

We should always work with the community and learn from them the methods that they know work best in their community. One good example comes from a group living in the Congolese forest for whom song and dance are ways to relax and celebrate. By writing their own words and expressing them through dance rhythms, the prevention and treatment of diarrhoea took a big leap forward.

Preparing to teach

Teaching and creating awareness will only be successful if we are well organized beforehand. We will need to prepare: teachers, materials, equipment, and the community itself.

Teaching and facilitation

Some people are gifted teachers and facilitators and others find it difficult to engage an audience. Most health team members and community health workers can learn to teach adequately if they have some guidance and encouragement. This may be through observing good practice or attending a teaching course. It could be through group or individual coaching. When it comes to specific skills needed, e.g. using flashcards, puppet shows, PowerPoint on computers, team members should practise their skills in the classroom together before trying them out on the community. Training of Trainers courses (TOTs) can be very helpful.

Materials needed

Teaching materials need to be chosen and prepared with care. See if it is possible to adopt and adapt materials already used in the community or in neighbouring programmes. Be aware when choosing to use flipcharts, flashcards, or pictures as visual aids that many rural people are 'pictorially illiterate'—they may not understand a picture's message even if it seems obvious to us (Figure 4.5).

Visual aids and other forms of health education are best prepared by local people. Alternatively, field-test them with a small community group before use, encouraging them to comment freely and incorporating their suggestions into the final version. Ask questions like: What does this picture show? What do you like or dislike? What would you do to make this easier to understand?

Any special equipment such as projectors, generators, or even props for a drama need to be assembled and checked carefully beforehand. Make sure that everything is there and works. Make a checklist of everything needed and use

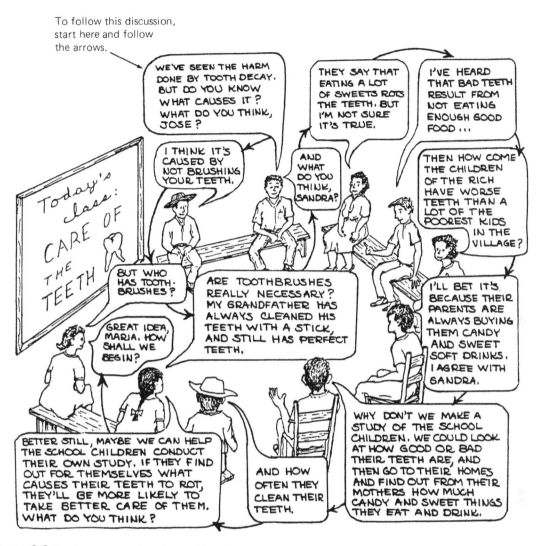

Figure 4.4 Creating awareness through group discussion.

it before setting out. As more sophisticated equipment becomes available at community level it becomes even more important to try it out first. For example, flashcards can now be shown through iPads and similar devices, but the user will need to be confident in using this technology in front of small groups.

The community setting

We should aim to plan all health teaching activities with the community, encouraging them to choose subjects, organize the programme, and invite as many people as possible to attend. Plenty of time and money has been wasted by the arrival of well-prepared health teams to distant communities who were unaware of when and why the health team was coming. Check places and times with mobile phones ahead of time

Methods of raising health awareness

Group discussions

Any form of community meeting when people come together to share ideas, problems and solutions is a valuable way of raising awareness about key issues (Figure 4.4). This can be done by a facilitator following the guidelines in Chapter 2.

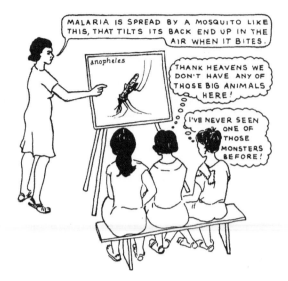

Figure 4.5 Make sure that people understand your pictures.

Reproduced from Hesperian Health Guides, www.hesperian.org. Copyright © 2017 Hesperian Health Guides. This image is distributed under the terms of the Creative Commons Attribution Non-Commercial 4.0 International licence (CC-BY-NC), a copy of which is available at http://creativecommons.org/licenses/by-nc/4.0/.

Personal advice at the point of need

This takes place whenever a community member and health worker get together. The setting may be a clinic or a home, a village path, a city street, or during a community survey. People listen and learn most effectively when they have a problem and want to find an answer.[2] For example, a mother meets the Village Health Worker on the path. She is worried about her child, now dehydrated from two days of diarrhoea. She listens and responds to a health worker who talks to her about the problem and how she can use rehydration solution to help the child now and prevent this from happening again.

She is more likely to adopt the new health behaviour when she hears about it in the context of a critical need than in a health talk when her children are well and she has no concerns. This factor is described in the Health Belief Model,[3] which predicts the likelihood of people taking action on health.

Practical guidelines here include:

1. Use opportunities to teach at the point of need.
2. Congratulate the person on any good health practice, and build on that success.
3. Use simple, non-medical language, and check understanding.
4. Ask the person to repeat back the main point you explained.

5. When working in a clinic, leave the door open, so other family members can 'learn by overhearing', providing this does not break locally accepted views on confidentiality.
6. Teach by repetition. A good example of this is the use of 'Health drills' (see Chapter 13).

Flashcards

Flashcards are cards with pictures, symbols, or words on the front, and often there is a message or explanation for the teacher on the back as a prompt for what to say about each card. They are a good way of unfolding a story with a health message. Although they have been used for many years, flashcards are still a valuable, interesting, and portable teaching aid, especially in community settings. They can also be used on electronic devices for smaller groups such as a family or a group of CHWs.

Before using flashcards make sure that the message is topical for the audience. For example, in a mother and child health clinic, show cards on issues relevant to mothers and children. Also make sure that any pictures and script are easily understood. It is best to use illustrations, ideas, and words familiar to people. Lastly, always make sure that the cards are in the right order. Check them through and practise telling the story with them beforehand.

While using flashcards, ensure you know the subject well and speak with confidence. It is equally important to involve the audience. Ask questions, make jokes, and refer to recent events in the community, such as a death from diarrhoea, an injury from drunkenness, or a measles epidemic.

After using the flashcards, develop a discussion. Invite someone from the audience to retell the story or show the flashcards themselves. Finally, make sure to stop before the people become bored, tired, too hot, or too cold.

Flipcharts

Flipcharts consist of several large sheets of good quality paper fastened together and bound with strong tape at the top of a board. After one sheet is filled, it can be flipped over. Flip charts can also be prepared beforehand with any information to share with the audience. Flipcharts are very useful for recording ideas in brainstorming sessions and guiding group discussions. They become even more useful if used by someone gifted at drawing cartoons. They can be photographed and these images can also be used on mobile phones.

Flannel boards (flannelgraphs, cloth boards)

A flannel board consists of two parts: a board covered in rough cloth or flannel and mounted in a frame; and cut-outs of people and objects with a rough backing such as sandpaper. Cut-outs can be moved about to develop a health message. Ready-made flannel boards with story ideas can be bought. Better still, the project and community can make their own. Before using a flannel board, good health stories must be prepared and practised using the cut-outs. Digital format flannel boards are also possible.

Stories and songs

Stories and songs are excellent ways of teaching health, especially in communities where storytelling and singing are part of the culture. They are popular because they use people, places, and events that are familiar and often much loved by the community. Health teachings can be woven into traditional stories or folk epics, or new stories can be created using familiar characters and settings.

A few practical guidelines for using stories or songs include:

1. Select or write a story/song that tells an important health message. Better still, help a community member to write a story.
2. Tell the story to everyone gathered.
3. Divide people into small groups of four to six and get them to retell the story in their group.
4. Encourage groups to act out the story as a drama, now or on another occasion.
5. Weave an actual community event into the story— either a bad one as a warning, a good one as an example, or an amusing one to help people remember.
6. Discuss issues raised by the story.
7. Songs remind people of important health messages and can be learned quickly by others. Set them to catchy or popular tunes.

Encourage local people, such as CHWs, to make up their own words. Write a special song to mark an important event and ideally draw in a local musician. Organize a competition between individuals or groups for the best health song, and arrange a cultural evening to hear and judge them. For example, in the Prem Jyoti community health programme in Bihar, north India, singing is an important part of the culture. Some people are still illiterate in this area, and the village health workers and community, guided by the health team, have written nearly 30 songs (many set to popular tunes) to illustrate ways to lead a healthier life. Also, in northern Mozambique a band called Massukos has set health messages to music. A musician called Santos wrote a song called *Wash Your Hands*, which quickly became a hit. The non-profit organization Estamos used the song to promote the installation of water pumps to bring clean water and Ecosan toilets.[4]

Role play

This is a simple form of drama where two people take on the roles of other people and act them out. One of the main values of role play is to help those actually performing it to know how it feels to be the people they portray.

Practical guidelines for role play include:

1. Make sure the members of the group already know and trust each other.
2. Choose simple subjects and divide people into twos or threes. If groups of three are used, members take turns to observe the two doing the role play, make comments, and then later feed back ideas to the class.
3. Give simple guidelines to each couple and a few minutes for them to plan.
4. Allow each pair five to ten minutes.
5. Discuss together at the end, drawing attention to the attitudes (both good and bad) acted out.

Role play is often enjoyed most by more outgoing people. Some people may need encouragement to overcome their shyness. Don't force people to take part if they don't wish. Role plays are often most effective among groups who already know each other.

Skill sharing

Health and development depend on learning new skills. We may have a particular skill we can teach others or we may wish to learn a new skill from someone else in the group.

Drama

Drama is one of the best ways to teach. It is enjoyable and engaging. People can relate to the characters and the things being said. Furthermore, drama is an especially good way of creating awareness and motivating communities. Theatre does not require the audience to be literate or well informed, and it appeals to all ages. Drama and theatre can be fun and hold people's attention. Most importantly, it appeals to our thoughts, ideas, emotions, and wills, and it challenges us to change our behaviours (Figure 4.6).

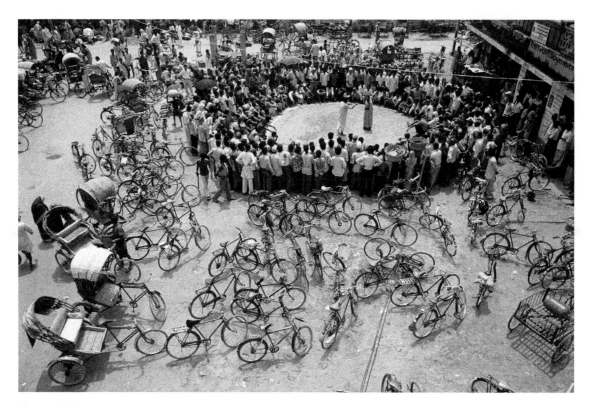

Figure 4.6 Theatre provides a creative way to both engage with and learn from a local community.

Reproduced courtesy of Anders Thormann. This image is distributed under the terms of the Creative Commons Attribution Non-Commercial 4.0 International licence (CC-BY-NC), a copy of which is available at http://creativecommons.org/licenses/by-nc/4.0/.

Short, simple dramas can be used in many situations, such as CHW teaching lessons, community meetings, marketplaces, school health lessons, or CHW box-giving ceremonies (Chapter 8). Longer dramas can be used during festivals or at special meetings. The Rampa Fund in Kyrgyzstan, Central Asia produced an interactive street theatre programme that promoted local culture and healthy lifestyles. We can find out if anything similar occurs in our country or region.

It is important to note that producing a drama takes a lot of time and energy. A drama production should only be undertaken if we have the resources, including team or community members with initiative, gifts and enthusiasm. Creating a drama is worthwhile when there is a major issue that the community needs to understand and when the drama can be used on a number of occasions (see Box 4.1).

Steps for a successful production must also include doing your research beforehand to guarantee a positive outcome. After all your hard work,

- Take care that nothing is being said or done in your organization's name that could affect your reputation.

- Make time to train the actors and people who produce and direct the play so they do this as well as possible: poor performances undermine the message (Figure 4.7).

- Make sure to get the facts right, and that any health information or message is based on good evidence.

- Ensure that the play is not too long or complicated and highlights one or two simple messages.

For example, *Theatre for a Change* works in several African countries using drama to raise awareness about HIV, sexual exploitation, and gender rights. It concentrates on these issues in ways that are carefully tuned to the cultures of the communities where they work (http://www.tfacafrica.com).

Puppets

Puppets, like drama, are enjoyable and involve the audience. They can say almost anything without offending people. They are useful in sex education. See Box 4.2 for how to use puppets.

Box 4.1 Things to consider when producing a drama

1. Choose an appropriate theme.
2. Prepare and practise using a script if necessary, but leave space for improvisation.
3. Start by using health team members as main characters and anyone in the community keen to take part.
4. Choose a site that has enough space for actors and audience.
5. Make sure the audience can see properly. Hang lights to shine on players.
6. Make sure the audience can hear properly. Actors must face the audiences and speak out. Before starting, ask someone to sit at the back to check the play can be heard easily.
7. Use only simple props and costumes. For example, dress a rich man in a T-shirt marked with a dollar sign, a poor man in rags, a crook can carry a toy gun, and a health worker a stethoscope round the neck. Consider making masks to represent some well-known character, animal, or emotion.
8. Write explanations and scene descriptions on a piece of cardboard. Hold this up between acts to explain what is going on and where the action is taking place, or use a narrator.
9. Mix the serious with the funny. For example: After an important statement, everyone can nod and look wise. After a wrong idea is given, other actors can boo or hiss depending on what is appropriate in that community.
10. Include songs with a health message and teach them to the audience.
11. Develop a discussion after the drama is over, to consider the issues raised or to plan community action.
12. Plan to repeat the play or perform it in another community if it proves popular.
13. Avoid causing offence to any community members, even unintentionally. A drama that compares a wise sister who cares well for her baby and a foolish one who doesn't may teach a useful lesson, but cause the minority of people who identify with the foolish mother to lose face and leave discouraged.

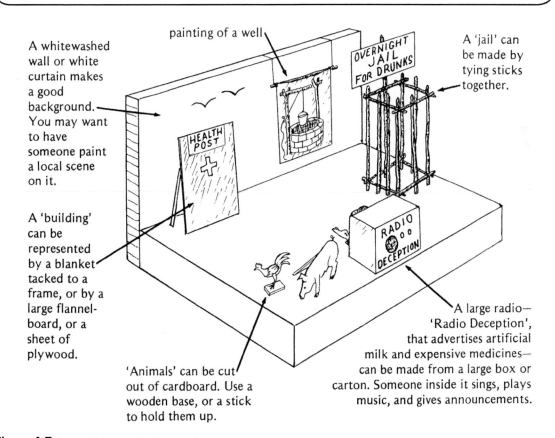

A whitewashed wall or white curtain makes a good background. You may want to have someone paint a local scene on it.

A 'building' can be represented by a blanket tacked to a frame, or by a large flannel-board, or a sheet of plywood.

painting of a well

OVERNIGHT JAIL FOR DRUNKS

A 'jail' can be made by tying sticks together.

HEALTH POST

RADIO DECEPTION

'Animals' can be cut out of cardboard. Use a wooden base, or a stick to hold them up.

A large radio— 'Radio Deception', that advertises artificial milk and expensive medicines— can be made from a large box or carton. Someone inside it sings, plays music, and gives announcements.

Figure 4.7 Props add a sense of reality to a play.

Box 4.2 **Practical guidelines for using puppets**

1. Construct some puppets. These can be made out of papier mâché. Alternatively, stick or glove puppets can be made.
2. Arrange a puppet workshop. Call in someone with experience to lead a teaching session when team or community members can learn how to make and use puppets.
3. Prepare and practise a story outline leaving plenty of scope for adding in funny or topical lines.
4. Erect a screen at the right height. This can be a cloth stretched between two poles. The screen should completely hide the people holding the puppets.
5. Puppets should face the audience, open their mouths, nod their heads, and move when they speak.
6. A different voice should be used for each puppet.
7. Puppets should have exaggerated actions and characteristics, for example, laughs should be loud, tempers should be bad, noses should be long.
8. Avoid silences.
9. Puppets can ask questions to the audience and encourage them to join in. They can lead a discussion afterwards.

Health teaching using live examples

People themselves can act as very effective visual aids, providing they and their family feel comfortable with this. When giving a talk on malnutrition, perhaps use as a live example a child now well-nourished, but known to have been seriously malnourished in the past. This approach is an example of what is known as 'Positive Deviance'.[5] Or, when giving an anatomy lesson, use a young man on which to draw the outlines of organs such as heart, lungs, and liver. This will be of greater interest than simply using a chalkboard. Cured TB patients can be trained to give brief health talks in the clinic. By explaining how they struggled but succeeded in taking medicine regularly, how they continued to support their family, and how their illness was cured, they can have great impact. Such talks can also be given by people living with HIV/AIDS who have taken antiretroviral therapy (ART). Again, this is all the more effective if people remember the person's state of health before treatment.

Still images (slides, digital photographs)

Using stills is a good way to teach and create interest, if the equipment is available. People enjoy seeing photos, especially of people and places they recognize (Figure 4.8).

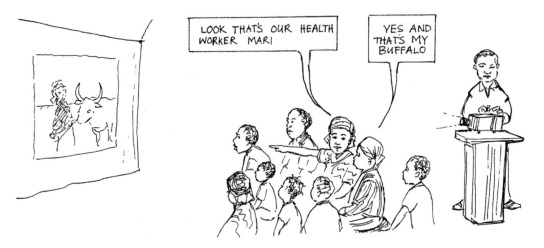

Figure 4.8 Photo sequences taken 'on location' always arouse great interest.

Collect together good quality, digital photos, preferably those which have been taken locally, perhaps by community members, or which show images of familiar places and people. To do this:

- Ask for volunteers with an interest and skill in photography.
- Decide together on the title(s) of the slide sequence to be made. Suitable subjects might be 'Immunize your Child'; 'What happens in a Maternal and Child Health Clinic'; or 'A Day in the Life of a Community Health Worker.'
- List the subjects and situations for which photographs are needed.
- Make sure that local people will be comfortable having pictures taken of them which may be shown publicly or end up on social media

Encourage the photographers to take action shots and close-ups in the project area. Each photo should be of a specific subject or make a particular point: they need to be good quality. Once you have the photos that you can use:

- Link photos into a teaching sequence. Aim to put about 30 slides together.
- Photos can be uploaded onto software and shown using a data projector.
- Show the sequence to the audience, using each slide as a discussion starter.

For example, we could ask:

- What does this picture show?
- What is the picture trying to teach us?
- How could we do this in our community?

Before the presentation we should practise showing the sequence, and make sure the data projector and other equipment is correctly linked up and working. If we are using an unfamiliar location, we should visit the meeting place beforehand, work out how the equipment will be set up, and ensure there is a dependable power supply.

If used wrongly, photo sequences become sleepy entertainment. If used correctly, they can arouse interest and motivation. Their success depends on the skill of the teacher, the quality of the pictures, and how much people are involved in discussion.

CD-ROMS, the Internet, and mobile phones (SMS)

The use of CD-ROMS continues to be valuable in areas with poor Internet connection, but at the time of writing, these are likely to be replaced by other technologies. Many relevant teaching materials are available and can be used individually or in small groups. Where equipment is available and connections reliable, fast enough and affordable the use of the Internet is increasingly valuable. Mobile phones can receive text messages on health or be used with apps. Their use is rapidly increasing and is almost limitless. Linking people together in shared learning and specialist topics is a valuable way of maintaining interest and stimulating creative ideas. Facebook, Google Groups, and WhatsApp are current widely used examples. Health wikis are increasingly used, e.g. by the Hesperian Foundation. Also, be aware of relevant webinars and podcasts. Chapter 26 on the use of ICT (IT) in health and development has further information on how ICT can be used in health teaching and raising awareness.

Moving images (films, "streaming" DVDs, YouTube and video)

Greater numbers of people are watching a wide range of health information on ever increasing platforms and technologies. Find out what is available locally or nationally. When choosing films, or other means of pick short, appropriate films with a clear health message or similar. Before going to a wider group, considering giving a trial showing to a selected audience to make sure the message is important, relevant, easy to understand, and unlikely to cause offence. Films on small screens can only be seen effectively by a limited number of people, so when showing the film, make sure everyone can see and hear clearly. Importantly, ensure that the film is in the correct format for your equipment, with good quality image and sound (this is not the time for bootleg copies!). Check all the equipment is in working order before starting.

Before the film begins, introduce the programme and indicate the key things to look for. After it ends, summarize the key points and open up discussion on the issues raised. Films are best shown where people naturally gather, such as the village meeting hall, a bar, or room attached to a place of worship.

Lastly, if try making a film or video using a camcorder or mobile phone. Call in skilled outsiders to help.

Radio and television

Many TV and radio programmes reflect unhealthy values and consumerist lifestyles, but with care and pre-planning we can still use the media for health education. In some countries, radio soap operas are proving very popular and effective. For example, *Urunana* has been a popular radio programme broadcast in Rwanda, which also reaches neighbouring countries. *Urunana* has a well-written and entertaining storyline and includes valuable health lessons, such as education about HIV/AIDS.[6] Similar programmes have also been produced in South Africa, Somalia, Afghanistan and Cambodia.

Health education by radio is more effective when combined with entertainment. Some people use the words inform, entertain and inspire as marks of successful teaching. The use of short animations, ideally with musical background known to the community, is becoming popular. BBC Media Action is involved in developing innovative use of radio and television in a variety of subjects including health.[7] When considering using radio or television as a teaching aid, use these practical guidelines to ensure success:

1. Publicize the times of relevant health-related TV or radio programmes.
2. Encourage people to watch or listen in groups.
3. Arrange discussions on issues raised afterwards.
4. Participate by:

   - writing to the producer with ideas and questions;
   - sending in a health story or song;
   - entering health competitions.

Other forms of health teaching

- Calendars.

The community can design these, writing in appropriate health texts and making illustrations. They can sell them locally to make a small profit.

- Printed leaflets and handbills.

These should be short, well laid out, illustrated, and easy to read. Comic strips can be used. Leaflets are reminders to people of something they have been taught, e.g. how to make home-made oral rehydration solution (ORS).

- Lecturing and using PowerPoint.

These are useful for more educated audiences. Maximum time is one hour, of which only 20–30 minutes should be lecture and the rest interactive. Using PowerPoint well needs training and experience. Some excellent material on avoiding 'death by PowerPoint' is available online.

- Chalkboards (blackboards) and whiteboards.

These are useful for summarizing what is being taught, or recording contributions from learners, perhaps in the form of a diagram.

- Health quizzes and health games.

A variety of games can be used or devised by the team or community. This can be an enjoyable way to revise or to test knowledge.

- Brains trusts.

An expert panel answers questions. Questions are submitted before but can also be asked 'from the floor'.

- Books, journals, and websites.

Consider setting up a simple project library with suitable books and articles arranged according to levels of difficulty and subject matter. Make a list of relevant health and development websites available for anyone with Internet access.

- Visits to seminars, conferences, and other projects.

Arrange for programme members, CHWs, or community leaders to attend appropriate seminars. Arrange visits to other projects to generate new ideas. Consider using SALT methodology (see Chapter 2). Finally, we can devise our own methods of teaching. Perhaps some of the best ways are yet to be discovered.

Evaluating progress

We need to know if our health teaching is effective. Some simple ways of finding out include simply talking with the community. We will soon get ideas and suggestions about ways to improve. Or, instead of face-to-face inquiries, make a questionnaire. This is useful for evaluating CHW teaching or at the end of special courses for health workers. A questionnaire can ask which sessions or subjects were considered most interesting and important, and which forms of teaching were most enjoyable or helpful. Ask participants to grade their answers using a scale from best to worst. Ask for suggestions about how to improve teaching. Anonymous questionnaires may be more reliable. Other ideas to gauge progress include assessing progress within the community, or setting an examination; however, remember that a test may show how much people have understood and remember, but not whether knowledge is being put into practice.

In reality, the best way of evaluating our teaching will be the participation, enthusiasm, and progress of the health team and the community. Good teaching eventually leads to good statistics. For more suggestions on monitoring and evaluation, see Chapter 9.

Summary

Our aim is to create awareness and teach effectively so that individuals and communities develop healthier lifestyles and learn how to prevent illness within their homes and neighbourhoods. Before being able to do this effectively our own attitudes need to undergo transformation. This process can happen more quickly if we spend time living in the community. We also need to learn the art of reflection and to draw strength from spirituality.

We must understand that the sequence that begins with health teaching leads on to health awareness, motivation, and the behavioural change leading to healthier lifestyles.

Before carrying out health activities, both team and community members need to be well prepared. Communities should be helped to understand one or two major health issues at a time, using methods that are appropriate to their culture, and the subject being taught. Many methods are available but the most effective ones actively involve the community. These include group discussions, storytelling, song, drama and puppets. The use of radio, TV, films, videos, the Internet, SMS technology, apps, CD-ROMs and social media play an ever-growing role in effective health teaching.

Feedback on the success of health education programmes can be obtained through discussions with the community and by questionnaire. The real mark of success is a healthier, happier and more productive community.

Further reading and resources

Abba F. *Teaching for better learning: A guide for teachers of primary health care staff.* 2nd ed. Geneva: World Health Organization; 1992.

Clarke S, Blackman R, Carter I. *Facilitation skills workbook.* Teddington: Tearfund; 2004. Available from: http://tilz.tearfund.org/~/media/Files/TILZ/Fac_skills_English/Facilitation__E.pdf

Ellis K. Stop and Think—An Educational Puppet Show. 2008, PDF downloadable free from TALC.

Hope A, Timmel S. *Training for transformation.* Zimbabwe: Mambo Press; 1999.

Hubley J. *Communicating health.* London: Macmillan; 2004.

Kukulska-Hulme A, Trailer J. *Mobile learning: A handbook for educators and trainers.* New York: Routledge; 2005.

Linney B. *Pictures, people and power: People-centred visual aids for development.* New York: Macmillan; 1995.

Maphorogo S, Sutter E. *The Community is my university: A voice from the grass roots on rural health and development* [CD Rom]. Amsterdam: KIT; 2009. Free for use in developing countries from TALC.

Medicine and creativity. *The Lancet.* 2006; 368 (Special Issue). Contains essays about use of song and theatre in health.

Prentki T, Lacy C. Using Theatre in Development. *Footsteps.* 2004; 58. Available from: http://tilz.tearfund.org

Rohr-Rouendaal P. *Where there is no artist: Development drawings and how to use them.* 2nd ed. Rugby: IT Publications; 2007. https://artworkbypetra.com/where-there-is-no-artist/

Shaw J, Robertson C. *Participatory video: A practical approach to using video creatively in group development work.* London: Routledge; 1997.

Werner D, Bower B. *Helping health workers learn.* Berkeley, CA: Hesperian Foundation; 1982.
A classic that each programme should have a copy of.

Useful websites

Source: International online resource centre on disability and inclusion www.asksource.info

Pinterest: For ideas on making visual aids, flannel boards, etc. https://in.pinterest.com/

References

1. Prochaska JO, DiClemente CC. Stages and processes of self-change of smoking: Toward an integrative model of change. *Journal of Consulting and Clinical Psychology.* 1983; 51(3): 390–5.
2. Rosenstock IM. Why people use health services. *Milbank Memorial Fund Quarterly.* 1966; 44 (3): 1107–8.
3. Glanz K, Rimer BK, Viswanath K. *Health behavior and health education: Theory, research, and practice.* 4th ed. San Francisco: Jossey-Bass; 2008.
4. McAfee M, reporter. Mozambique: Guitar Hero [television broadcast]. *Frontline/World.* Berkeley, CA: Public Broadcasting Service; 2008 May 27. Available from: http://www.pbs.org/frontlineworld/stories/mozambique704/
5. Positive Deviance Initiative. *Background.* Available from: https://positivedeviance.org/background/
6. Umutesi D. Urunana soap opera script writer talks about the value of drama in Rwanda's society. *New Times* [online]. 2012 May 24. Available from: http://www.newtimes.co.rw/section/article/2012-05-24/102546/
7. BBC Media Action. *Transforming lives through media.* London: BBC. Available from: http://www.bbc.co.uk/mediaaction/what-we-do/health.

CHAPTER 5
Initial tasks

Ted Lankester

What we need to know

Our ideal is for the community, the government and civil society organizations (CSO) to work together in close collaboration, remembering that the community should increasingly lead this process and own their future. Different communities will be at widely different stages in their development. Some may need to learn leadership skills and programme management almost from scratch, while others, through existing good health leadership, may already be far advanced. Some may have functioning health systems and health centres, while others virtually no access to health care.

Although we always want to encourage the self-sufficiency of communities, there are times of emergency or insecurity when outside aid and relief is needed to prevent a community or area from disintegrating as the problems they are facing are too large to cope with alone. For more details on this topic, see Chapters 25 and 27.

When we work in community development, especially in very resource-poor settings, we will often find that not all community members put health at the top of their priority list. For example, if decision makers are young and male, they are likely to see electricity supply, better roads, or employment opportunities as more pressing needs than health. Health is often deemed a greater need for women, especially those with children. As health workers we must remember the 'social determinants' of health—issues which cause

ill health and which need to be dealt with upstream. Providing curative health care alone will not lead to healthier communities.

In the setting up community-based health care (CBHC), we face different scenarios. Some projects will involve setting up health services from scratch 'beyond where the road ends', and others will involve developing health services from an existing hospital or health centre. Sometimes we will simply need to strengthen what already exists. There may be good services in one area, but there may be a need to scale up or scale out services to underserved areas, perhaps via new health posts or a mobile clinic. Or, we may simply need to concentrate on health training that focuses on community health workers (CHWs) and women's groups.

Whether our own role is as a member of the community, government, or CSO, we need to become effective leaders and facilitators and be efficient and well organized. This chapter explains the first steps to take, and looks at six starter topics. It highlights some of the key areas to consider, and signposts resources from which all projects can learn. It is worth noting that some of these steps are complex, especially obtaining funds. Chapter 10, Managing Personnel and Finance, covers other areas of programme management and can be read alongside this chapter.

Choosing a community

We may be leading a CSO programme and able to choose for ourselves where to work, and are often responding to a specific need for which the community has requested our help. Increasingly, we will be working alongside government health services and responding to their requests. Community-based health programmes operate in a wide range of contexts. Many are rural but an increasing number are meeting the more complex needs of urban slums. For effective collaboration we need to answer these questions:

1. Has the community, or the government, requested outside help?

If the answer is no, we should be asking why we want to start at all. If for various reasons we still believe this is the right thing to do we will need to build relationships with community members, until they reach a point where they welcome our involvement. We should remember that an apparent interest shown by a community in outside help may be because they see it as a source of funds. We need to explain our approach clearly from the outset.

2. Do community leaders show a genuine interest in working with us?

This is especially important in urban areas where leaders are sometimes more subject to corruption, or more suspicious of those wishing to work in their communities. It is important for the success of a programme that community leaders want to work alongside it (see Figure 5.1). For example, do community leaders have:

• readiness to trust, and work with, members of the community?
• concern for people's welfare, especially the most vulnerable?
• a reputation for honesty?
• their community's respect and confidence?
• Does the community seem united?

Almost all communities have splits and divisions. If these are serious, follow racial or tribal lines or are very long-standing, it is hard to establish a good partnership. However, working towards common health goals can sometimes bring reconciliation and encourage unity.

4. What scope is there for our potential role?
   • Is there serious ill health?
   • Do the people generally seem healthy or sick?
   • Do many children die before the age of five?
   • Is there year-round clean water?
   • Is there much disability or blindness (not always obvious)?

One way to determine the answers to these questions is through using a Participatory Appraisal (PA) (see Chapter 6).

5. Are existing health services adequate?

Is universal health coverage present? If so, are people genuinely able to access health services as needed? Is this the case for the poorest members of the community—and for the people living with disability? We may find that government services exist but are underused; that private doctors are present but charge exorbitant rates; that other health programmes or hospitals exist but offer only curative services.

6. Have we sufficient resources?
   • Have we the personnel, expertise and resources to help this community develop the services it needs or 'plug the gaps'?
   • Can we help the community with their felt needs?
   • Can we help the community tackle root causes of ill health, such as contaminated water, lack of food, alcohol abuse, poverty, and exploitation?
   • Is there an existing referral system, for problems we cannot handle ourselves? If not, can we help set one up?

7. Is the target area a suitable size?

If it is too small, rapid health improvements may occur, but the project may not be cost-effective. Focusing on too small an area may cause jealousy and misunderstanding with other nearby communities. If it is too large, we may become swamped with urgent problems and be unable to help the people bring about lasting health improvements. At the start of a project we should usually confine our work to an area within a single health district, and not spread ourselves too thin unless we bring a very specific skill or focus that is needed over a wider area.

8. Does the government approve the programme plans?

If our programme is not already working closely with the government, we should contact the district medical officer (DMO) or equivalent to find out:

• if the government is already doing community-based work in the area.
• if we are following national or district health priorities.
• if the DMO approves of our plans, feels able to work in partnership with us or is willing to draw up a written agreement.

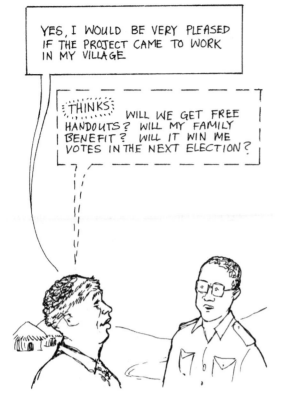

Figure 5.1 Different expectations.

Reproduced courtesy of David Gifford. This image is distributed under the terms of the Creative Commons Attribution Non-Commercial 4.0 International licence (CC-BY-NC), a copy of which is available at http://creativecommons.org/licenses/by-nc/4.0/.

Governments in the most resource-poor countries are usually unable to provide adequate services at community level, owing to weak health systems and insufficient staff. When governments and CSOs work in a co-operative spirit and share their plans in line with mutual targets and government health plans, co-operation can work very well. If a CSO gains a good reputation the government may 'contract out' aspects of primary health care to the CSO, or ask for help to extend an existing programme.

In one example, a health programme in Sichuan, western China, where a non-governmental organization (NGO) has been partnering with government health services, was so effective in training village doctors and helping to set up community-based projects in townships, that the NGO was asked by the state government to work with them to cover the entire prefecture (district).

In another example, the World Health Organization (WHO) has estimated that between 30 and 70 per cent

of health care infrastructure in Africa is owned by faith-based organizations.[1] With churches and other religious organizations often being the dominant CSO, there is huge potential for more partnerships between such groups and government health services.

Lastly, the Arukah Network (previously known as Community Health Global Network) has brought together nearly 50 separate health-related programmes in the state of Uttarakhand, North India. By working together and registering as a society, the government and other donors have been willing and able to contract out a variety of health services to the 'Uttarakhand Cluster'. These have included tobacco control, disaster responses, disability programmes, and the training of CHWs.

Having decided with a community to work together, we must then decide whether this should cover all the people in the target area, or just the neediest groups within it. As a general rule, it is better to work with the entire population but give special attention to the poorest members and those with the greatest health needs.

There are a few exceptions:

- Where there is an obvious group that is deprived or different, such as refugees, nomads, or the landless.
- Where we have particular skills such as in water and sanitation (WASH) programmes,[2] or in the community treatment of non-communicable diseases (see Chapter 22), or those suffering from specific illnesses, e.g. neglected tropical diseases.
- With certain health problems such as tuberculosis (TB), HIV/AIDS, mental health problems, substance abuse, or addiction, there may be value in more specific targeting. Equally, it may be good practice deliberately to mainstream them into integrated community-based health programmes.

Appointing health team members

In the start-up phase, community-based health teams will comprise different levels of staff, from CHWs, who are usually members of the local community, to senior leadership including a nurse and administrator, and often a doctor. Of course, there will be wide variation between programmes.

Who should be appointed?

Here are some qualities needed in health team members:

1. A genuine interest in the community

Those who want to work on the project should not merely be interested in financial gain or prestige. Field workers will often work long hours. Those with a genuine interest in the project are more likely to continue in the project if they possess vision for the work.

2. A willingness to learn

It is better to include team members who realize they have a lot to learn, rather than those who believe they are experts already. Often those who have previously worked in formal curative settings, e.g. hospitals, will need careful retraining for the very different world of community health.

3. A readiness to take on any job

Health team members must be ready to take on any activity, ranging from clinical work or teaching to more menial tasks. They must be ready to take initiative. For example: many health programmes have drivers whose sole responsibility is to drive and maintain the vehicle in good working order. But they often have several free hours in the day. During this time, they could learn basic health skills and join in with clinic or teaching activities between journeys.

4. Respect and appreciation of poor or stigmatized community members

Many religious teachers have taught special love for the poor. Many of the best health workers are happy to be known as friends of the poor.

5. A willingness to work as part of a team

Being a team player is important in community health. In practice this means an attitude which values working with colleagues from different parts of the country or from different backgrounds. It means being slow to anger, and quick to forgive—or apologize. Inappropriate words or behaviour in front of community members or public disagreements can set back the programme. Unresolved anger against a colleague can harm team relationships.

6. Adequate health for the job in hand

While the programme should have an inclusive attitude to mental and physical disability (see Chapter 23), strong physical and mental health is important for some jobs. However, those with poorer health or those on long-term treatment, e.g. for HIV, psychological health problems or diabetes, must never be excluded or stigmatized. The key question is one of occupational health as to whether the applicant is fit enough to carry out the tasks required, and if not, whether adjustments acceptable to the programme can make their involvement possible.

7. A balanced team

Health teams will need a balance of those who have gifts in vision, ideas, and networking (the ideas people), those able to find common ground and solve disputes (the smoothers), and those who are methodical and able to complete tasks efficiently (the finishers). Each type of person will need to recognize and respect the other's gifts and different approaches (see Chapter 10).

Qualifications

In CBHC, character and personality are as important as qualifications. Many community health skills are best learned on the job.

For junior health workers, basic education up to the standard school-leaving age, plus enthusiasm, is a good profile to look for. Learning on the job and via appropriate training courses is often more appropriate than formal professional training, although team members may wish to gain more formal education, for example, on day release or online courses. Health workers increasingly need documentation of any training, qualifications and continuing professional development (CPD).

Programmes also need professionally trained staff:

- A doctor or medical advisor who can act as facilitator, trainer, and part-time clinician. Doctors will need a good understanding of a community health approach. Otherwise they may slant or even 'hijack' a project back to a curative model.
- A 'non-physician clinician' (NPC), such as a nurse or medical assistant, often makes the best team leader or director of a smaller programme.
- An operations (Ops) manager or administrator is essential to co-ordinate tasks and manage finance for all but the smallest programmes. Expertise in financial emanagement is a crucial skill.

The ultimate success of a programme is largely determined by how well it is led and managed.

Managers will need personal talent and training appropriate for the programme. They will be managing people as well as supplies, so their style must be democratic and inclusive.

Where to recruit suitable people

Some possible places to recruit people for the project include:

- *The local community*: in CBHC most junior team members are drawn from the local community. We should look out for appropriate people to nurture and train.

- *Networks*: through networks of friends and contacts suitable workers may be found from a wider area.
- *Training schools and institutions*
- *Voluntary health associations or religious bodies*
- *Transfers from hospitals, sister projects, or government programmes*: this must only take place after careful evaluation of their skills and approach.
- *Through advertisements in papers and journals*: this approach often attracts inappropriate people and, understandably, may result in applications from people mainly interested in simply finding a job.

There is one danger area worth mentioning—'poaching' good staff from nearby community health programmes should be avoided. Instead, we should aim to develop relationships *with* other programmes based on mutual respect, and co-operation (see the section 'clusters' in Chapter 2). In the Uttarakhand Cluster, transfers of staff between the 50-member programmes require a no-objection letter from the programme head before the transfer can be completed. Competition between different CSOs has become a stumbling block and an absurdity that should be replaced by more sensible and collaborative ways of working.

Another emerging problem is the serious shortage of health workers in many developing countries. One common reason is that health workers, especially doctors and nurses, are recruited to work in higher paid jobs abroad, in cities, or in well-funded aid agencies or 'vertical' programmes (see Chapter 1). This is making it harder to find appropriately qualified staff who are willing to work for the lower salaries that a voluntary programme can afford. We must therefore be committed to the principle of 'task shifting'; see Chapter 1, which explains how the least qualified member of a team that can carry out a task effectively should do it.

Selecting team members

We need to make sure we are recruiting team members based on good human resources (HR) principles that are both fair and legal;[3, 4] see also Chapter 10. There are three useful ways of recruiting, which often work well in community-based settings.

Personal recommendation

Recommendations should be from reliable, unbiased sources, ideally from those who know the programme's aims and values.

Interview

Sometimes people who are inappropriate for the job may perform well at interview. Conversely, excellent workers may not do themselves justice out of nervousness.

Trial period

Trial periods can be very useful. It may be worthwhile inviting applicants to spend a few days in the community. Some programmes spend time informally with applicants to test their suitability in field situations, but this 'test run' needs to be made clear to applicants and done according to national legal practice. Guarantee from the start that applicants understand the nature of the trial period and will accept any decision about whether they are employed.

Situations that require caution

Employing relatives

Existing team members may ask if their relatives can be employed in the programme. This is not usually a good plan, unless there are objective ways of checking out their suitability. Sometimes such relatives may have failed to find other jobs. Often two or more members of one family in a programme may exert undue influence and cause division in the team (see Figure 5.2).

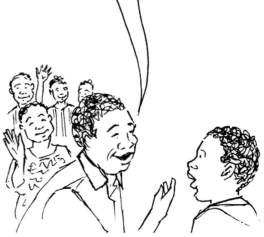

Figure 5.2 A commonly found conflict of interest at community level.

Overloading with members of one tribe, caste, or district

Too much similarity or homogeneity between team members can cause suspicion among the community. This can be especially true if most team members are from outside the programme area.

Unmarried and unpartnered women

Any young unpartnered women in the team will need safe working and living conditions. In some countries it is not appropriate or legal to employ them. In other countries, they will need to work or live in a group setting or in the company of older married women, according to local culture and security considerations.

Employment laws

It is important to ensure that all Human Resource (HR) policies, including recruitment, are in line with the laws of the country where the project is based.

Understanding the project cycle

At an early stage in setting up a programme it is helpful for us to understand the concept of the project cycle. Firstly, this enables us to be methodical in our thinking and secondly, many donors tend to follow this pattern and will expect us to be aware of it and follow it. Looking at Figure 5.3 and, starting at the top, we can first identify the problems, assets, and solutions on which the health team and the community can work together. This is done largely by a needs assessment such as the PA or the community survey (see Chapter 6). We then need to plan the programme (see Chapter 7), which leads to a design that is best set out in a logical framework. Next,

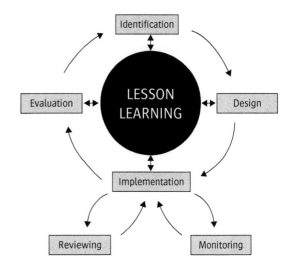

Figure 5.3 The project cycle.

we need to implement the project; various chapters in this book describe ways to do this.

At regular intervals we will need to monitor and review our progress (see Chapter 9). As the programme develops, we must continuously evaluate and reflect on any changes that are needed, and ways to make these changes.

See also Figure 2.5 in Chapter 2, which provides a similar perspective, but more from the community's point of view.

What we need to do

Obtaining funds

This section is about initial tasks, which includes obtaining initial funds (Chapter 12 looks at long-term funding and sustainability in more detail). But from the beginning of the project, we must be fully aware that improving the long-term health and well-being of a community requires sustainable sources of money or subsidy. This does not automatically mean that it needs funding from outside the country. Indeed, the assumption that outsiders can fund programmes far into the future is rarely true and is disempowering to the

community and undermines its ability to become more self-reliant. It is important first to attempt to procure means of obtaining income sources from within the community and from within the country.

Obtaining funds is a good example of where the community itself needs to be involved at the very beginning. Community members need to understand that it is at least partly their responsibility. From an early stage we need to ensure that community members play their part in locating funds from within their own country or region, and learn to write successful proposals (both of which may require a great deal of training and self-belief). Additionally, there may be entrepreneurs within the community whose business skills can make a valuable contribution to the project. In any discussion between government and programme, sustainability must be high on the agenda. The developing world is full of abandoned programmes and people with shattered hopes. More often than not, all parties involved in a project assume they will be able to find outside funding sources far into the future; usually, they don't.

Before making promises to the community and raising their hopes, it is vital to plan ahead and work out approximately how much funding is needed for at least the first three years. Of course, this can only be approximate as plans are likely to change as we respond to the community's needs, or current government priorities. While Chapter 10 looks at financial management in more detail, and Chapter 12 on sustainability addresses how we can ensure that programmes can continue in the long term, this section looks both at how we can obtain seed funding to make a start, and discusses some broad principles. In obtaining funds, we first need to choose sources whose funding criteria are most in line with our programme. Second, we need to follow the best sequence in applying for these funds.

Choosing the funding source(s)

Before writing off to foreign donors, we should first identify sources of funds within the community. Only after these options are exhausted do we then move outwards to wider possibilities (Figure 5.4).

Sources within the community itself

Currently there is a strong movement against charging user fees. It is seen as going against the concept of universal health coverage and resulting in the poorest members of the community being unable to afford health care. However, there are many who do not agree with this conclusion and believe that it is possible to design a fair and workable model that protects the poorest. The section 'Ways to increase programme resources' in Chapter 12 gives some examples of how user fees can partially fund health programmes.

Community-based health insurance schemes can be an alternative to or work alongside user fees. Experience shows that charging nothing makes community members undervalue the services and medicines they receive; if a medicine is cheap or free it may be regarded as useless, past its expiry date, or 'dumped' by a foreign project or government. Worse still, it may seem like a bribe to encourage people to adopt some political or religious point of view. However, some countries have abolished user fees and we need to be aware of the laws and the viewpoint in the region where we are working. In practice, modest user fees from patients can make a small but useful contribution.

The base hospital

If the project is run by a hospital, some funds may be available. For example, if the hospital has a high reputation, funds may flow in from private patients. Sometimes, joint applications can be made for a combination of community- and facility-based services. In practice most, but not all, hospitals are seriously short of funds and have little to give towards community health care (see Chapter 12).

Local organizations and those in nearby cities

Try any appropriate sources—churches, temples, mosques, co-operatives, Rotary and Lions clubs, charities, local business associations, the 'generous rich'. Many international companies have adopted the practice of corporate social responsibility (CSR) and by building relationships with appropriate companies, funds may occasionally be made available, sometimes on a recurring basis.

Additionally, creative thinking can come up with successful solutions. For example, a project on the east coast of Africa, hoping to improve the health of communities through local income generation and improvements to the environment needed seed funding to get started. Before writing to sources outside the country they approached local tourist hotels in the area, explained the programme, and by doing so, secured sufficient donations to enable the project to begin.

The government—district, state, or national

Funds are often available, especially for programmes working in collaboration with the government. Although such sources may not always be dependable, they are worth pursuing. In addition, certain supplies are often available which reduce programme costs. These include vaccines, insecticide-treated bed nets, TB medicines, and antiretroviral therapy (ART). In many of the poorest countries, government health services may have few general funds but they may have more specific funding from international programmes.

Non-governmental organizations and faith-based organizations

There are a very large number of these mid-level agencies. Personal connection, rather than 'blind' proposal writing, is nearly always the best approach. Well-known examples include Save the Children International, World Vision, Tearfund, Christian Aid, Water Aid, Bread for the World, Lutheran Federation, Mennonite Central Committee, the Aga Khan Foundation, Oxfam, and Project Hope.

International sources

The majority of international donors have country-based or regional offices and these are usually where funds are distributed. It is usually unsuccessful to request funding from the country of origin except through personal connections and contacts. In practice when a community health programme is starting out, there is little chance they will have the capacity to engage multilateral or bilateral donors.

Multilateral aid agencies

These are usually part of the United Nations, including the United Nations Development Programme (UNDP), the WHO, the United Nations Children's Fund (UNICEF), the World Bank, and others.

Bilateral aid

Most governments of so-called donor countries have aid agencies. Examples are the United States Agency for International Development (USAID) (the largest), the UK's DfID, or Global Affairs Canada. Governments tend to focus on particular countries or regions, often for historical or political reasons, and will have country or regional offices in those places that handle funding

applications. Significant sums may be available but normally a national of that country needs to be connected with the project.

The European Community (EC) has its own agency, the European Community Humanitarian Office (ECHO), which funds certain types of projects.

Other international funding agencies

The Global Fund was established in 2002 to fight AIDS, tuberculosis, and malaria, and is a non-profit international financing organization that makes grants to local organizations. The Bill and Melinda Gates Foundation is a private trust that funds the work of selected partner organizations. Even though we may have our own specific community-based priorities, these sometimes overlap with and are eligible for some of these largely vertical funding sources.

Before applying for foreign funds, i.e. those sourced from outside our country in different currencies, we will almost certainly need special agreements with the government to receive foreign contributions. In addition, there are other possible disadvantages:

● Dependence

If foreign funds are available, community members may expect handouts and well-paid jobs to be available for them. They may be less ready to contribute their own time, money, and resources if they see foreign programme vehicles or receive foreign medicines (Figure 5.5).

Wise Funding Inc.
Bigtown
Anystate, USA
30 March 2008

Dear Project Leader

Thank you for the funding application which you sent on behalf of your organization, "Cure all People" (CAP).

Although we do have funding available it is our policy only to release this if we have an assurance that all local and national sources have been tried first. We also require outline plans of how your project plans to become sustainable when outside funding stops ...

Figure 5.4 A priority in seeking outside funding.

Dependency, suspicion, separation from people as foreign funding increases

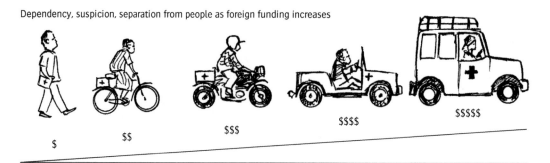

Figure 5.5 An effect of increasing foreign funding.

- Suspicion

In some countries, rumours may spread that foreigners attached to projects may be involved in illegal activities or as undercover agents.

- Reporting requirements

Some international funding agencies, e.g. USAID, have very stringent reporting requirements that are time consuming to comply with, and this should be borne in mind when applying for funding.

- Lack of sustainability and the danger of being donor driven.

Foreign funds are usually only available for a limited time frame. The priorities of donors continually change, so programmes that are started through one donor often need to seek further funding from elsewhere. This sequence of seeking donors and adapting the health programme to fulfil their requirements can be exhausting for the health team and confusing for the community. The programme may end up being donor–driven, which may result in "project creep" or in a change to the intrinsic mission statement of the original project.

In CBHC we need to think very carefully about when, how, or even whether we apply for international funds (see Figure 5.5; see also Chapter 12).

Applying for funds

Always remember that applying for and receiving funding takes time. We must start applying as soon as our plans begin to take shape. In the case of government or foreign funds, it may take six to twelve months or longer before funds are actually received (see Figure 5.6). In the case of smaller trusts or less-formal funding sources, e.g.

faith-based groups or charitable organizations known to us, this can be quicker, but amounts will usually be smaller.

There are some further helpful ideas in Chapter 3 that expound on the need to co-operate and build relationships with those who share their resources with our programme.

There are stages in applying for funds that must be followed carefully. If we bypass them and send in a full project proposal to an agency without prior warning it is almost bound to be rejected as an unsolicited request for funds. We need to bring a potential donor on side in a carefully considered sequence.

1. *Personal contacts*: We can follow up any personal contacts with the agency or with its staff, its trustees, or through mutual acquaintances. This can work well with smaller trusts and foundations but is unlikely to be acceptable to a larger donor except to gain information as to how best to take the proposal forwards.

2. *Letter of enquiry*: This states in just a few paragraphs what we are doing and why we wish to approach this donor. It asks what further contact would be acceptable if the agency wishes to consider supporting

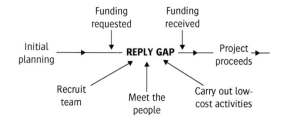

Figure 5.6 Reply Gap.

the project. A good outcome would be for the donor to agree to a face-to-face meeting; alternatively, they might suggest we complete a full project proposal or send more information through a concept note.

3. *Concept note*: This gives basic concise information needed by a donor in one to three pages. It can include in summary form some of the items required in more detail in project proposal forms.

4. *Full project proposal*: Often it is possible to use the agency's own forms. Be sure to carefully follow their instructions and note the date by which it must reach the donor.

While making contacts, we should prepare the following information which will be required for most proposal forms:

1. The name of the organization and any larger group to which it belongs, the director's name, and the programme address.

2. The names and brief qualifications of senior team members.

3. Details of the project area, including its location, terrain, and climate.

4. Details of the target population:
   - Number (approx.) of people and settlements to be served.
   - Social structure of the communities, including details of local employment, relative wealth, poor or neglected subgroups, etc.

5. Details of the people's health:
   - Current services available—government and private.
   - Serious illnesses and health problems.

6. Details of the programme:
   - Aims and objectives.
   - How these will be achieved.
   - Try to give an approximate framework. In a concept note this can be a short summary. For many larger agencies the project proposal will ask for a logical framework (or logframe); see the section 'Logical framework (logframe)' in Chapter 7.

7. Project Unique selling proposition (USP): how this project differs from earlier ones, or other programmes being carried out in the area.

8. Relationship with government:
   - Details of planned co-operation.
   - Whether written permission has been obtained.

9. Budget: give details of planned income and expenditure.

- Include detailed budget for one year, and an approximate budget for two further years.
- For income, estimate total from other sources.
- For expenditure, divide into capital (non-recurring one-off costs such as equipment) and annual (recurring).
- Under recurring costs include salaries, services, rent and buildings, and supplies, including medicines, travel and transport, training, and administration.
- Include in the budget items that are essential, but do not ask for expensive or unnecessary equipment.

There are more details on preparing budgets in the section on managing finance in Chapter 10. Figure 5.7 lists the questions used by one agency that supports a number of small-scale health programmes. Other information may be requested, such as the latest report and accounts of the parent organization, photographs of the area and people, results of a sample population survey, etc.

Finally, having received funds, we must maintain close, friendly links with the sponsoring organization:

1. Write a letter of acknowledgement and thanks.
2. Send in, on time, any regular reports, budgets, or other information requested.
3. Welcome any visitors from the funding agency.
4. Participate in any training seminars or capacity building which they arrange.

Setting up a base

Adequate accommodation

Many team members will live locally or nearby with their families. Those participating in urban programmes will often live in a neighbouring area but will need easy access to the programme's target community

Sometimes accommodation will need to be arranged for non-local health team members or for those visiting from outside for shorter periods to bring special skills. Ideally, accommodation should be adequately equipped, within or near the programme area, safe, and secure. It needs to be of a good standard to ensure the team members and any of their family feel comfortable.

To protect the programme and staff living in programme accommodation, an agreement should be drawn up that includes:

- length of tenure.
- list of items supplied with the accommodation.
- details of any rent and other charges, e.g. fuel, water, and electricity.

HEALTH PROJECT APPLICATION FORM

Project title ....

Contact person ....

Job title ....

Background to the project
1. How did this project begin and why is it needed?
2. Who have you discussed the project with?
3. Are any other organizations working on the same problems?
4. How does your project fit into government health plans etc?

Aims and objectives
1. Write your project aim in one sentence.
2. Write your project objectives, which should be SMART.
3. Include a logical framework if you have used one.

Does the project address priority health issues?
1. List what you think are the main health problems in your community.
2. What does the local community consider to be their main health problems?
   (Attach sample survey or statistics if you have them.)

Who will benefit from the project?
1. Who are the main beneficiaries?
2. Have they been involved in the planning? How?

How has the local church been involved in the project?
1. How will the project support the local church's ministry?
2. How has the church been involved in developing the project proposal? How
   has the church shown its commitment to this project?

Project plan/activities/risks
1. Anticipated start and completion dates of project.
2. For how long will you be seeking funds?
3. Which other funders have you approached?
4. What plans do you have to make the project self-sustaining?

Who will manage the project?
1. Who will be the main project leader?
2. Do you have a management team/committee?

Sustainability
1. Once funding has finished, what are your specific aims to enable the
   project to be self-supporting?
2. Has the project been discussed with local government? How does it fit in with
   their objectives and funding?

Monitoring
1. How do you plan to monitor the work of your project? What systems will you
   use?

Evaluation
1. How do you plan to evaluate the work of your project?
2. How frequently?
3. Will you use internal or external people to evaluate your work?

Budget and financial management
1. Detail all the items in your budget.
2. Do you have a financial manager?
3. Do you have someone to audit/certify your accounts?
4. Have you approached other funders, and do you have any funding secured
   already?

Additional Information

Figure 5.7 Simple health questions asked by one faith-based funding agency.

These should be agreed, written down, and signed by both parties. The agreement should include a clause that when the team member leaves the programme, they will no longer be entitled to stay in the accommodation. In practice, team members often live together on a campus or compound. This may be convenient but, where team members share work, leisure, worship and accommodation, relationships can easily become strained.

Office and stores

The programme base may be located in a primary health centre, health post, hospital, or town office. The simpler this is kept the better. Often three or four rooms will be enough to start with, one for the office, one for meeting and training, and one for storing equipment and medicines.

When allocating a room for storing medicines in particular, we should ensure that it is:

- secure against break-in.
- dry, even during the rainy season.
- large enough and well lit.
- accessible by vehicle for easy loading.
- rat-proof, bat-proof, and screened against mosquitoes.

The question of security is increasingly important now that attacks on 'soft targets' like health and development workers are becoming more common, and since many programmes will be working in insecure locations. It is worth asking a security expert to advise on the type and location of buildings used by the programme and what safety precautions should be taken, e.g. guard dogs or a night watchman. After setting up base, and at regular intervals afterwards, we need to make sure that arrangements continue to be safe and proportional to the level of threat or danger.

Ordering supplies

More details on receiving, storing, and issuing supplies are found in Chapter 13. This section focuses key items which may be needed at the start of a programme.

1. List what is required:
   a. Include all essential items.
   b. Decide on what type and number of items are needed.
   c. Discuss this list with the leaders of other programmes or anyone with suitable experience.

2. Identify where supplies can be obtained:
   a. Buy locally wherever possible (with the proviso in (g) below).
   b. For each type of equipment, compare prices and quality of different suppliers.
   c. Build a relationship with the main suppliers. Try to arrange discounts.
   d. Find an alternative supplier for important items in case the main supplier runs out of stock.
   e. Order supplies in plenty of time. There is often a long delay between ordering and receiving.
   f. Avoid poor-quality products, even if they seem helpfully.
   g. Set up careful systems to monitor the quality of medicines, especially in countries where fake or substandard medicines are known to be common.

Only obtain equipment from abroad if good-quality supplies are not available or manufactured within the country.

3. Carefully check all supplies on arrival
   a. Make sure they are complete and intact.
   b. Keep the receipts or confirmation of purchase, and guarantee of repair or replacement.
   c. Check where any servicing or maintenance can be carried out.

Two major items of equipment are usually needed:

1. Refrigerator

Solar powered fridges are increasingly used. They are most useful if solar power is also used for other community activities. Otherwise it is better to buy fridges that run on kerosene or electricity (via mains and/or generator). All fridges need regular maintenance, temperature monitoring, and defrosting.[5] If we are storing vaccines it is essential we have a regular electricity or other reliable power supply, and that any rise or serious fall in temperature can be seen on the fridge's thermometer, which needs to record maximum and minimum temperatures reached. In most countries electric fridges will need a back-up generator and a voltage stabilizer to protect the fridge from power surges.

2. Sterilizer

Unless we can arrange to use a nearby hospital's sterile supplies, a steam sterilizer, autoclave, or pressure cooker will be needed for sterilizing any non-disposable instruments used in the clinic or community. Needles and

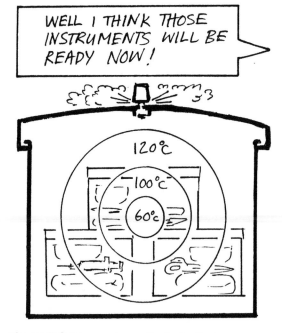

Figure 5.8 Take care that sterilization is effective.

Reproduced courtesy of David Gifford. This image is distributed under the terms of the Creative Commons Attribution Non-Commercial 4.0 International licence (CC-BY-NC), a copy of which is available at http://creativecommons.org/licenses/by-nc/4.0/.

* Steam under pressure (e.g. autoclave, pressure cooker) Required pressure: ⇒ 15 pounds per square inch (101 kilopascals)

Temperature	Time
115°C	30 minutes
121°C	15 minutes
126°C	10 minutes
134°C	3 minutes

* Dry heat (e.g. electric oven)	

Temperature	Time
160°C	120 minutes
170°C	60 minutes
180°C	30 minutes

Figure 5.9 WHO's recommended temperatures for sterilization.

Reproduced with permission from World Health Organization. Copyright © 2016 WHO. This image is distributed under the terms of the Creative Commons Attribution Non-Commercial 4.0 International licence (CC-BY-NC), a copy of which is available at http://creativecommons.org/licenses/by-nc/4.0/.

syringes should only ever be reused if it is impossible to obtain disposable items locally or from outside sources. Take great care that health workers who use sterilizers fully understand how they work and the length of time supplies need to be heated (Figures 5.8 and 5.9).

Ordering medicines

Decide which medicines are needed. Together with the programme medical adviser, draw up a list and then compare it with:

1. The list used by the nearest hospital (our list should be shorter), the list used by any well-regarded community health programme, or from a nearby health post.
2. The national Model List of Essential Medicines.
3. The latest WHO Model List of Essential Medicines.[6, 7]

When choosing the medicines, there are four areas that must be considered in the choice:

1. Appropriate for the health needs of the area.
2. Appropriate for the level of health worker who will be prescribing them.

3. Generic, meaning they should be ordered using the chemical, generic name, and not the trade name or brand name. There will be occasional exceptions.

By using only generic names, we can avoid confusion and save money. If medicine bottles with a branded name are placed in the pharmacy the generic name needs first to be written accurately and in bold on the containers. Otherwise the pharmacy can look increasingly confused and it is easier to make dispensing mistakes.

4. Good quality.

Many poor-quality or fake medicines are being made. Make sure that any medicines used are made by reliable companies licensed by the government. This can include multinationals. Only use foreign supplies if good quality essential medicines are not made within the country.

Then we must calculate how much medicine will be needed. This can be done in one of two ways:

1. Estimate the likely number of patients that may be seen per week or month (See Figure 5.10).

One way to do this is by discovering numbers attending clinics in any equivalent neighbouring projects. The proportion of a population attending a clinic is extremely variable. An approximate guide for communities with no other health facilities in the area might be an attendance of between a quarter and a half of the population within the first year for curative care (see also Chapter 11).

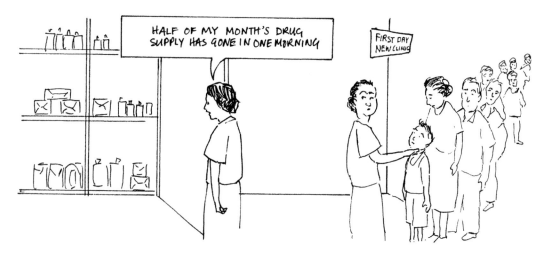

Figure 5.10 A common cause for lack of essential care.

2. Estimate the numbers of each medicine likely to be used per 100 patients seen.

Look through the records of patients seen in similar clinics or outpatient departments, and list the medicines used there that also appear on our medicines list. Total up the numbers of each medicine used, per 100 patients. Remember that most clinics overprescribe and that patients will only rarely require more than two or three medicines. If there are no similar clinics, we can work out from our knowledge of local illnesses the medicines likely to be needed.

It is also important to remember that medicines are ordered and received like equipment. Expiry dates must be checked. When we first set up a clinic it is helpful to have a reliable link either with a nearby hospital pharmacy, or a reliable supplier so we can have an initial stock of essential medicines.

Finally, keep a stock card, and keep a separate card for each item. Figure 5.11 shows an example stock card; it is

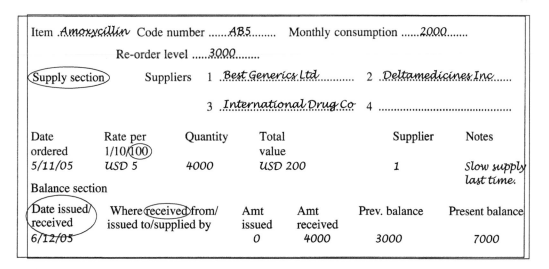

Figure 5.11 Example of a stock card.

divided into two sections: a supply section and a balance section. Cards (or sheets) can be filed alphabetically, and by subject, e.g. medicines in one card holder, medical supplies in another, laboratory supplies in a third.

Alternatively, computerized systems can be used. It is important to stock take at least once every month or quarter. This means checking that the balance of each item on the stock card is the same as the amount on the shelf. In the case of medicines, it is vital also to check expiry dates, making sure the oldest supplies are issued first.

Interested readers are referred to Chapter 11 for more information about ordering medicines.

Ordering a vehicle

Community-based programmes need to use the most economical and safe means for staff transport and for transporting equipment. This may eventually mean we need one or more programme vehicles but in many situations public transport, bicycle, motorbike, or other ways of travelling work adequately. A project vehicle may not be needed at the beginning, and may not be appropriate, as it suggests a project is wealthy or foreign. For as long as possible we should use local or public transport, a motorbike, bicycle, or walk.

Only order a vehicle if there is no alternative practical from of transport. If this is the case, then, when deciding whether to buy a vehicle, ask:

- Are funds available to buy it?
- Are funds available to maintain it?
- Are spare parts available to mend it?
- Is a skilled mechanic available to repair it?
- Is fuel available to run it at an affordable price?

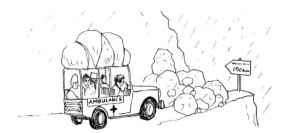

Figure 5.12 When choosing a project vehicle, consider the worst conditions it may have to encounter.

When choosing a vehicle, ask these questions:

1. Is it tough enough for the worst roads during the worst weather? (Figure 5.12)

2. Is it large enough to carry those likely to use it?

It will need to be large enough to carry programme members, CHWs, patients, visitors and equipment

3. Is it suitable for carrying seriously ill patients?

Does it sometimes have to be used as an ambulance; is it possible for a patient to lie flat?

4. Is it cheap to run?

In many countries, diesel is cheaper than petrol but is more polluting. Some vehicles do many more kilometres per litre than others, so fuel efficiency is an important question.

5. Is it reasonably dust-proof, and will it start well in cold weather?

6. Is it made in-country and can it be bought locally?

Where countries manufacture vehicles, those made within the country are usually more appropriate than foreign models because:

- They are cheaper to buy.
- They are cheaper and easier to look after and spare parts may be obtained more easily.
- They make the project look less foreign.
- They may be available at a discount for registered charities.
- There is no need for foreign exchange.

However, locally made vehicles may be less strong or durable than foreign models. Second-hand vehicles should be carefully checked by a skilled mechanic before being purchased.

7. Is it safe?

Ensure that seat belts have been fitted for both front and rear seats. This is essential even if it is not the local custom. Ensure the vehicle is regularly and expertly serviced. More development workers die in road accidents than from almost any other cause, often due to faulty vehicles, non-use of seat belts, and drunken driving.

Summary

When a programme first receives requests from a community or from government health services to start working, several activities must be carried out and co-ordinated before fieldwork is actually begun.

This includes developing a suitable team, upon which so much of the programme's future depends. Funding needs to be obtained wherever possible from local and national sources before foreign agencies are approached. The goal of becoming financially self-reliant should always be kept in mind. A programme base needs to be established for storing supplies and setting up an office. Accommodation for staff sometimes needs to be considered. The base should be within the target area or as near to it as possible so that the community can be involved in management at an early stage. Both accommodation and the programme base must be safe and secure, especially in insecure locations. In such areas we should ask for a careful risk assessment by a security expert and be guided about ongoing safe practices.

A list of essential equipment and medicines needs to be drawn up and supplies ordered in the correct amount, and from reliable sources. A refrigerator and sterilizer will be needed. Methods of travel and transport should be kept as inexpensive as possible. Sometimes a vehicle will become necessary, and if so, it should be bought locally or regionally where possible.

Further reading and resources

Battersby A. *How to Manage a Health Centre Store*. 2nd ed. London: AHRTAG; 1994. Available from: http://apps.who. int/medicinedocs/documents/s20951en/s20951en.pdf

The Directory of Social Change, 352 Holloway Road, London N7 6PA Tel: 08450 77 77 07 Email: cs@dsc.org.uk Website: www. dsc.org.uk. (The DSC produces a huge range of information on fundraising as well as comprehensive publications giving details of grant-making trusts, companies and other sources of financial support).

Funds for NGOs Website: www2.fundsforngos.org. Has guides on how to write funding proposals.

Kaur M, Hall S. *Medical supplies and equipment for primary health care*. Coulsdon: ECHO; 2001. Available from: http://apps. who.int/medicinedocs/documents/s20282en/s20282en.pdf

Skeet M, Fear M. *Care and safe use of hospital equipment*. London: VSO; 1995. Available from: http://www.frankshospital-workshop.com/organisation/biomed_documents/Care%20 and%20Safe%20Use%20of%20Hospital%20Equipment%20-%20VSO.pdf

Tearfund. *Fundraising, Roots book No. 6*. Teddington: Tearfund; 2009. Available from: http://tilz.tearfund.org/en/resources/publications/roots/fundraising/ (Practical strategies on all aspects of fundraising).

Tearfund. *Project cycle management, Roots book No. 5*. Teddington: Tearfund; 2009. Available from: http://tilz. tearfund.org/en/resources/publications/roots/project_cycle_management/

References

1. International Religious Health Assets Programme/World Health Organization. *Appreciating assets: The contribution of religion to universal access in Africa*. Cape Town: ARHAP; 2006. Available from: https://berkleycenter.georgetown. edu/publications/appreciating-assets-the-contribution-of-religion-to-universal-access-in-africa

2. The United Nations Water Decade Programme. *Implementing water, sanitation and hygiene (WaSH) information brief*. Zaragoza: United Nations; 2015. Available from: http://www. un.org/waterforlifedecade/waterandsustainabledevelopm ent2015/images/wash_eng.pdf

3. Cooperation Committee for Cambodia. *Practical guideline on human resource management*. Phnom Penh: CCC; 2013. Available from: http://www.ccc-cambodia.org/en/download?file_id=798&action=view&view_file_id=ea53c7cb ab9fcc3a79632dde195e53b53b76d868

4. Catholic Relief Services. *Institutional strengthening: Building strong management services, Chapter 8: Human resource management*. Baltimore, Maryland: Catholic Relief Services; 2011. Available from: www.crsprogramquality.org

5. Elford J. *How to look after a refrigerator*. London: AHRTAG; 1992. Available from: http://www.labquality.be/documents/LAB%20 MANAGEMENT/EQUIPMENT/MAINTENANCE/Elford_ 1992_How%20to%20look%20after%20a%20refrigerator.pdf

6. World Health Organization. *WHO model list of essential medicines*. 20th ed. Geneva: World Health Organization; 2017. Available from: http://apps.who.int/iris/bitstream/handle/10665/273826/EML-20-eng.pdf

7. World Health Organization. *WHO model list of essential medicines for children*. 6th ed. Geneva: World Health Organization; 2017. Available from: http://www.who.int/medicines/publications/essentialmedicines/en/

CHAPTER 6

Learning with the community

Ted Lankester

This chapter looks at the various ways we can get to know the community we are working with. How we do this will be different for each programme (Figure 6.1). It will depend on factors such as how much we already know about the area and the level of partnership already established with the community. It will also depend on how much information we need to gather. Sometimes the requirements of donors may affect the information we need to obtain.

This chapter discusses two broad ways of learning about the community. The first is the Participatory Appraisal (PA), which collects a wide range of qualitative (descriptive) information. The second is a community survey and diagnosis, which provides more detailed quantitative information. The term 'needs assessment' is commonly used, but the approach in this chapter is different. It aspires more to the description of Alex Fox of the charity Shared Lives:

A strengths-based approach to care, support and inclusion says 'let's look first at what people can do with their skills and their resources and what can the people around them do in their relationships and their communities'. People need to be seen as more than just their care needs—they need to be experts and in charge of their own lives.[1]

Participatory appraisal (PA)

What is participatory appraisal (PA)? A PA is a method of gaining information about a community in a limited period of time. PA is also sometimes known as rural or rapid appraisal (RA), participatory research and action, or participatory rural learning. PA has been described as 'a broad empowerment approach that seeks to build community knowledge and encourages grassroots action.

It uses a lot of visual methods, making it especially useful for participants who find other methods of participation intimidating or complicated'.[2]

From the outset we need to make sure this is a joint activity with the community, done with their full understanding. If we come as outsiders or as government health workers there may be suspicion of our motives.

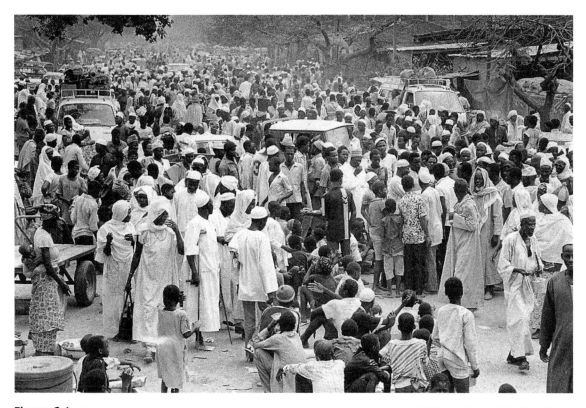

Figure 6.1 It is a challenge to learn about communities in an urban context where more than half the world population lives. The photograph shows Ouagadougou, Burkina Faso on a Friday.

This makes building trust and friendship even more important.

A PA is often used early in a programme to gain information to guide the way forward, write proposals, and make preliminary plans. A survey often follows later, especially when we need more detailed information about the type and extent of the problems which we need to work on with the community. PAs and surveys together provide the baseline information for everyone. The precise timing, sequence, and methods used are up to each individual programme. A PA works equally well in both rural and urban settings.

Some basic principles of the PA

When performing a PA, we must first explain to the community why we want to gather information. Members may be suspicious, or surprised that yet another group is coming to ask questions. We need to ensure that the community and its leaders understand why we have come (see Figure 6.2). Furthermore:

1. We must take care not to raise expectations.

In resource-poor communities, especially those who in the past have had donations and handouts, expectations can be raised at the mere mention of health centres, medicines or doctors. The community may jump to conclusions and then be bitterly disappointed. Before meeting anyone we need to explain that nothing has been decided on; that we are gathering information, so that we can make future plans together with the community.

2. We should only collect essential information.

For every piece of information we plan to gather we should ask: What is the reason I need this data? Will knowing this data make any difference? Sometimes donors will expect us to provide more detail information than we feel is necessary. This should not push us into asking for information that the community is unhappy to provide. Examples of useful but sensitive information amongst many include:

- details of deaths of infants and stillbirths;
- use of family planning methods; and
- enquiries about HIV and mental health.

Later, when trust is established, we may be able to find out more about these and other sensitive areas.

3. We need to carry out every stage of the process with the full participation of the community.

This includes planning, training, carrying out the appraisal, understanding the results, and drawing up plans. PA is a joint effort of team members, community leaders, community members, outside facilitators or experts, and, if possible, members of the district health team (DHT). In countries with strong central control, like the People's Republic of China, PA needs to be done in full partnership with government health workers and party cadres.

With the community involved at every stage, PA can generate interest and excitement as community members begin to see the real nature of their problems, and that the community is part of the answer.

PA can take anything from a few days to several weeks, depending on the depth and scope of the analysis. One to two weeks would be a typical period of time for new, small or medium-scale programmes. But shorter periods of time can produce valuable information if we already have strong community links.

For example, the author and two colleagues were allowed to spend only one day with a community where there was strong central government control. Within that day the team obtained sufficient information to help future planning of a village-based programme, using semi-structured interviews with a community leader, a younger and an older community member, a local healer, and a TB patient. In addition we made observations as we walked and talked in the village. We 'triangulated' our observations after the visit.

Deciding what information is useful

A PA needs to be planned carefully because unless it asks the right questions and strengthens links between the community and programme, it will have limited value. The information we are seeking may be about how the community functions, and its assets, needs, and wishes. Or, it may be looking more specifically at one particular aspect of health, such as child malnutrition, the prevalence of diabetes, or high blood pressure.

Table 6.1 shows various criteria relating to health and social determinants of health that it may be useful to ask about when doing a PA. It should be adapted to each programme's needs.

Planning for the PA

For a PA to be successful we need to think carefully about the best way to carry it out in our own particular context. For an in-depth PA we can follow the phases below. Using the term 'we' here refers to a joint community and programme method of working, and not to an approach landed on the community by a group of outsiders.

1. Defining the objective.

Why are we doing the PA? This will inform what information we collect and how we use it. A PA is an active tool designed for later community action, and (as mentioned) we must only gather information that is relevant and useful.

2. Choosing the most appropriate methods for the information we require.

Identifying sources of information and listing topics for questions or interviews will be part of how we choose the method(s) we use.

3. Forming and training the team.

Because the community will be fully involved with a PA, they should suggest suitable members to join the team. A combined programme/community team of three to six is a good number, ideally from different backgrounds and with differing areas of interest. The PA team will need training, preferably from someone with field experience of using and performing a PA. Training should include how the programme and community can best work together, effective and sensitive ways to ask questions,

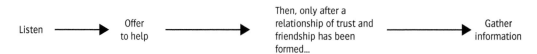

Figure 6.2 Follow this field sequence.

Table 6.1 **Information that may be useful to collect when doing a PA**

Family and community structure:
- Marriage customs, including age at marriage, polygamy, dowry customs
- Attitudes to the elderly, in-laws, and children
- Structure, hierarchy, and loyalties in the extended family or local tribes

Social patterns and power structures:
- Leadership—formal and informal
- Political, religious and economic groupings
- Caste, tribal groupings
- Inequality and its effect on health
- Ways of resolving disputes, making joint decisions
- Status and what determines it—wealth, land, education, or tradition

Spiritual beliefs and practices:
- How they affect lifestyles, attitudes to others, to the environment, and to health and nutrition
- How much spiritual leaders are involved or interested in health
- Local and national festivals: how and when they are celebrated

Daily routines of different family members:
- How work is divided among family members
- School attendance among children and attitudes towards it
- Employment and work patterns of men, women, adolescents and children

Yearly pattern of climate and farming:
- When the rainy season starts and finishes
- What times of year are made difficult because of flooding or extreme heat
- Months for ploughing, sowing and harvesting
- Crops grown
- Ways of coping with harvest failure
- Labour—migration in and out

Health-related beliefs and practices:
- Traditional beliefs about what causes and cures illness
- Attitudes to traditional healers and remedies; how and when traditional healers are used
- Use of modern medicines, health workers, hospitals, and private practitioners
- Whether health needs are a priority

Details of other programmes:
- Past and present government programmes in health, agriculture, and related development; how these are viewed
- Details of other CSOs currently or recently working in the community; achievements they have made and the community's perceptions
- Location and effectiveness of nearest health posts, primary health centres or hospital

Causes of poverty and inequality of wealth:
- Overall degree of poverty
- Difference in earning power, lifestyle, ownership of land, property, and animals between richest and poorest
- Outside constraints that lock the community into poverty
- Community problems that block solutions

(continued)

Table 6.1 **Continued**

Effects of disaster and crisis:
- how the community responds to social unrest, floods, drought, effects of climate change, acts of terror

In rural communities:
- Relation to the nearest city or large town
- Whether used for employment, leisure or crime
- Whether young people are leaving or wishing to leave their village or community

With urban programmes:
- Employment
- Environmental conditions including water, sanitation, garbage collection, and air pollution
- Specific hazards including to women and children

Levels of crime, violence, prostitution, drug abuse, people trafficking

Local power structures, slumlords and leaders

and how to use the various forms of PA (described later). Training in how to conduct interviews and focus groups is especially useful.

4. Collating information by category.

A PA generates large amounts of information. It is helpful if broad categories can be decided beforehand so that information can be written down under those categories. This helps systematic thinking and makes the analysis of information easier when the PA is completed.

Examples of categories might include causes of illness, reasons for low uptake of existing health services, or causes of economic hardship (external and internal). We can also use the broad headings shown in Table 6.1.

5. Practicalities.

This will include details such as timing, co-ordinating with community events, and deciding on convenient times of day and year. It also requires organizing liaison with the community about locations, facilities and people's availability.

Techniques used in PA

Whatever technique we use for a PA, participants should follow the '3Rs': *Remember* key information, *Record* details (use a notebook or a hand-held electronic device), and *Reflect* on findings from the day's work.

1. Simple, direct observation.

As we visit, drink tea, walk the paths and talk to community members, we are constantly observing,

raising questions and starting to ponder answers. We should record significant things we have heard and seen, as well as insights we have gathered. Later these will be compared with other observers.

For example, a transect walk is where we walk through a community from one side to another, carefully observing what we see. We may wish to make general observations, or to concentrate on specific aspects, such as the roles of women and men, the health of children, or how effectively a community seems to work together. We can form three pairs for the transect walk, where each pair looks at different aspects of the community and then compares findings. If we pair community and programme members, the community member can give their perspective on what is seen.

2. Semi-structured interviews.

These interviews are informal and based on a guiding checklist of questions, which can be altered as appropriate. By interviewing people of different backgrounds and age we can obtain information from different viewpoints. We may also select particular members of the community as *key informants*. For example, when carrying out a PA in a remote area of western China, we arranged for a Chinese government health official and programme member jointly to interview a village doctor, a traditional birth attendant, the village chief and the local teacher.

The interviewer must be fluent in the local language or have a skilled interpreter. Choose a quiet location, introduce yourself, and explain the purpose of the interview. It is helpful to have a checklist of questions to be answered, but allow the answers to emerge through free-flowing conversation; allow at least 45–60 minutes for the interview. At the end, thank the informant, and be sure to record answers during the interview or immediately afterwards. Key informant interviews tend to give an overall impression of the way things are—or of the way the informants wish they should be. Older informants may also give an idea of changes, good and bad, that have occurred over recent years. Information from key informant interviews needs to be checked and compared with information gathered from other forms of PA.

There are four groups of key community members that should usually be included:

Gatekeepers: those who decide what new people and new ideas are acceptable to the community.
Caretakers: those to whom people turn when they have problems.
Newscatchers: those who always know what is going on.
Brokers: those who know key people and can get things done.

Information from key informants can be checked by similar interviews with a cross-section of other community members.

There are also a few groups within a community that are important to interview because of the specific role they play within the community, or a special situation they have lived through. Most communities will have people who have chronic illness. A semi-structured interview with a person living with HIV/AIDS or TB can bring unique insights. In some communities, discussions with women may be hard to arrange. The viewpoints of women are essential to give a full and balanced view. It is often most appropriate to use woman-to-woman interviews.

Above all, we must be careful not to make those we interview feel threatened or intimidated. Sometimes one-to-one interviews are most appropriate, sometimes two-to-two, and the latter may allow for a livelier discussion.

3. Focus groups.

Focus groups are gatherings of six to twelve people from similar backgrounds who discuss a topic under the guidance of a trained facilitator. They are a valuable tool in CBHC at various stages in programme planning and evaluation and are especially useful in a PA. Three useful questions PA focus groups can ask are about the main problems affecting the community, the skills, assets, or abilities the community has to help solve these problems, and how those from outside the community can help in solving these problems.

PA participants should be people who are willing to discuss their ideas. They should be representative of specific sub-groups in the community, such as working men, women, those from a lower caste or income group, those with a disability, and elderly people. Sub-groups and participants are ideally chosen by the community, but be careful here to avoid bias.

The location should be quiet, comfortable, and convenient, and if possible, refreshments should be arranged. The facilitator should explain the topic, ensure it is adhered to, encourage all to participate, ask questions and record detailed notes. See Chapter 2 for more information about helpful ways to facilitate meetings.

Often the issues mentioned by the community are not specifically related to health. For example, they may have problems with drought, inaccessible roads, or fear of disasters. When this occurs, we need to remember that nearly all issues will affect health and well-being (see Chapter 1 on 'social determinants' of health). We may need to explain that we won't be able to tackle all issues directly, but that we may have contacts in government or civil society organizations who may be able to help.

4. Community mapping.

Mapping (see Figure 6.3) makes community health interesting and enjoyable for all. Many members can get involved, leading to a lively discussion and fresh insights into community life. Mapping provides a surprising amount of information and is an excellent tool for involving a wide range of community members.

Maps are best made on a flat piece of ground or, in the case of smaller groups, on a large piece of paper. Ideally, men, women, and children should join in together, although this is not always possible. At a recent mapping in Ethiopia, a crowd of up to 60 gathered spontaneously. Adults did the mapping and the map size grew to 10 x 15 metres. Meanwhile, children who had been chased away by adults started making their own map. The two maps when added together gave valuable insights: the adults tending to see the village from an economic viewpoint, and the children more from a human and educational viewpoint (Figure 6.3). A special form of mapping known as risk mapping can be very valuable in areas prone to disasters such as floods, hurricanes, earthquakes, or ethnic conflict (see Chapter 25). Buildings, water supplies, or vulnerable people and escape routes can be identified so that a community plan can be drawn up to help give special protection if a crisis occurs.

There are certain ways to make mapping easier, as well as an interactive experience for all those involved:

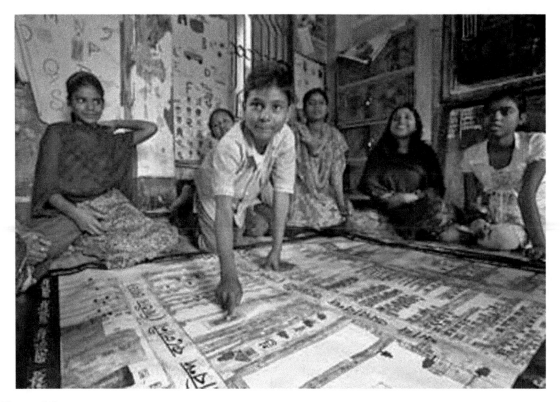

Figure 6.3 Children in Calcutta map their community.

Reproduced with permission from UNICEF. Children map their community using innovative technology in India. Available at https://www.unicef.org/statistics/india_58382.html Copyright © UNICEF India/2011/Crouch. This image is distributed under the terms of the Creative Commons Attribution Non-Commercial 4.0 International licence (CC-BY-NC), a copy of which is available at http://creativecommons.org/licenses/by-nc/4.0/.

- Choose an appropriate flat location, preferably out of the sun, wind, and rain.
- Gather materials (stones, coloured powders, leaves and twigs would be appropriate symbols in poor rural communities).
- While materials are being gathered, explain the purpose of making a map.
- Encourage the community to select two or three capable members who can draw the map and respond to instructions from the onlookers; this interaction allows for a feeling of collectivity.
- Agree on symbols for different village facilities, e.g. water sources, latrines, school.
- Make sure to allow at least one hour for the mapping, and up to two to three further hours if discussion follows.
- Have someone copy the map onto paper or into a notebook, and try, if the community agrees, to have it photographed, or even videoed, using a digital camera or mobile phone.

Issues raised during mapping can be further discussed in focus groups or community meetings and contribute to planning.

5. Seasonal health calendars.

Community members can construct these calendars, which are most useful when different variables, e.g. rainfall, food availability, levels of sickness, can be seen side by side. A calendar constructed in Sierra Leone (see Figure 6.4) showed that people often fell sick at three particular times: when there is most work to be done, least food to eat, and least money available for treatment. This information helps us to plan effective health programmes. Comparing calendars over a period of time can also show the effects of changing weather patterns and climate change and help people to readjust community planning to the best times of year.

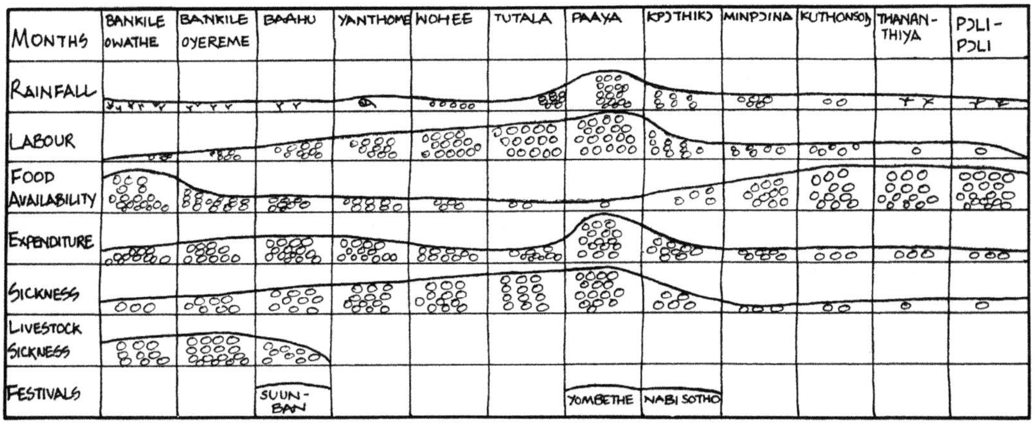

MONTHS	BANKILE OWATHE	BANKILE OYEREME	BAAHU	YANTHOME	WOHEE	TUTALA	PAAYA	KPJTHIKJ	MINPJINA	KUTHONSOJ	THANAN-THIYA	PJLI-PJLI
RAINFALL												
LABOUR												
FOOD AVAILABILITY												
EXPENDITURE												
SICKNESS												
LIVESTOCK SICKNESS												
FESTIVALS			SUUN-BAN				YOMBETHE	NABI SOTHO				

Figure 6.4 A seasonal health calendar made by young men in the village of Bubuya, Sierra Leone, through an Action Aid project.

6. Daily activity charts.

Women, men, adolescents, and older children can be asked to list their normal daily activities. This gives a powerful picture of village life and raises numerous ideas for discussion and action. Table 6.2 shows a report by the Swedish International Development Agency from an exercise carried out in sub-Saharan Africa.

7. Review of existing records and information.

All these methods involve using primary sources of information, i.e. gathered directly in the community. We can gain very useful details about disease patterns, etc., from secondary sources, i.e. reports and records made by other people. These may include hospital or clinic records and other information kept in the community (Table 6.3). Other programmes that have worked in our area may have information we can use. Sometimes outside researchers or anthropologists will have worked in the community and recorded valuable insights. We should seek these out.

We will need to decide whether or how much to use secondary sources before we do our own PA. It is often helpful to have some information to guide us before starting the PA, but by concentrating only on secondary sources may result in a skewed, outdated, or incomplete picture of current community issues. Also, a novel way of helping community members to share their abilities, needs, hopes, and wishes in an unthreatening way has been pioneered by the Salvation Army and Affirm Facilitation Associates. It follows what is known as a SALT methodology (see Chapter 2).

Analysing our results

It can be a challenge to analyse a mass of information collected by several people from a variety of sources. Here are some suggestions of ways to process information to ensure it is easier to understand, as well as useful for future planning:

● Daily recording

Each observer records information at the time of the activity or immediately afterwards. Where possible, they should use the categories discussed at the PA training.

● Triangulation

Ideally, important information collected from one source is validated or revised by checking data from at least two other sources.

● Using a problem tree

Using a problem tree for documenting and analysing can also be helpful in incorporating information into action plans (see Chapter 7).

● Ranking

Within twenty-four hours, observers rank or prioritize information under categories or using clear headings.

● Simple thematic analysis

Alongside ranking, picking out common themes or ideas that seem to be repeated or common across the various sources is helpful. Post-it notes are a useful tool

Table 6.2 **A woman's day or a man's day?**

Woman's day	Man's day
Rises first	Rises when breakfast is ready
Kindles the fire	
Breastfeeds baby	Eats
Fixes breakfast/eats	Walks 1 km to cotton field
Washes and dresses the children	Works in the field
Walks 1 km to fetch water	Eats when wife arrives with food
Walks 1 km home	Works in the field
Gives the livestock feed and water	Walks 1 km home
Washes cooking utensils, etc	Eats
	Rests
Walks 1 km to fetch water	Walks to village to visit other men
Walks 1 km home	
Washes clothing	Walks home
Breastfeeds baby	Goes to bed
Pounds rice	
Sweeps the house and compound	
Kindles the fire	
Prepares meal/eats	
Breastfeeds baby	
Walks 1 km to cotton field with food for husband	
Walks 1 km back home	
Walks 1 km to her field	
Weeds field	
Breastfeeds baby	
Gathers firewood on the way home	
Walks 1 km home	
Pounds maize	
Walks 1 km to fetch water	
Walks 1 km home	
Kindles the fire	
Prepares meal/eats	
Breastfeeds baby	
Puts house in order	
Goes to bed last	

for grouping and arranging pieces of information and for spotting patterns.

● Workshop for data collectors

This is the a forum where each individual presents findings as far as possible by category and rank. It is helpful if each person brings a legible summary of the main findings. During the workshop, information can be headlined and compared on flipcharts.

● Summary report

One or two members should document the information in report form using participants' written or electronic information and flipchart papers.

● Report finalization

Ideally, the draft should be shared with all main participants to make sure nothing important has been left out or that mistakes have been introduced before the final document is produced. This needs to be done with a quick turnaround; otherwise, information or interest may be lost.

How to use our findings

A PA can be a time-consuming exercise and the information we gain needs to be shared and used as widely as possible. The following groups can benefit from the data generated:

1. The community

Information needs to be shared and understood by the whole community. This will help them better understand the challenges and how they can use their assets and strengths to make tomorrow better than today. Sometimes new ideas, new information, and even worrying implications may arise, especially in urban settings. For this reason, it may be helpful to meet with community leaders first before meeting with the community as a whole.

As previously mentioned, it is important to manage any expectations during the PA (See Figure 6.5). One project in Nepal carried out a detailed PA in many villages, and the process lasted across several months. In the community feedback a village woman asked, 'Why have you brought an empty 'doko' [a traditional Nepali basket slung on the back] to our village?' The community's expectations were high that the PA would provide immediate change and progress within the

Table 6.3 A method for tabulating information about health facilities

Facility	Number	Where located	Distance from the community	Who owns/controls
Hospital				
Health centre				
Dispensary				
Mobile clinics				
Private clinics				
Village pharmacies				
Doctors				
Nurses				
Clinical officers				
Community health workers				
Traditional birth attendants				
Trained				
Untrained				
Herbalists				
Registered				
Unregistered				
Traditional healers				
Witchdoctors				

village; the drawn-out process of the PA resulted in feelings of resentment and disappointment.

2. Donor agencies

Donors often require the information we provide from PA. If this is well summarized it will win the project and the project team credibility. It may even help to secure initial or further funding.

Although ideally PA is done before programmes start, in modified form a PA can be repeated as part of a programme evaluation as required by donors (see Chapter 9).

3. Researchers

Furthermore, larger programmes may be able to use the information from the PA for research. For example, the team may benefit the project by linking with a college or university, or via a researcher visiting from a different country or region. However, this requires planning. In particular, ethics approval will need to be sought months in advance of the PA.

4. Government departments

The results of the PA can be shared, after gaining approval from the participants, with the District Medical Officer, District Management Team, or their equivalents. Other government departments covering areas such as agriculture, education, natural resources, and water and sanitation can also be informed. The data gathered from the PA will cross all developmental boundaries and help to stimulate a combined approach to problems of poverty.

At a high level PA helps us to understand the social determinants of health (see Chapter 1) in our project area. It also helps to bring about a key aim of CBHC, or 'intersectoral collaboration.' Finally, it helps us relate our work to the Sustainable Development Goals (see Chapter 1).

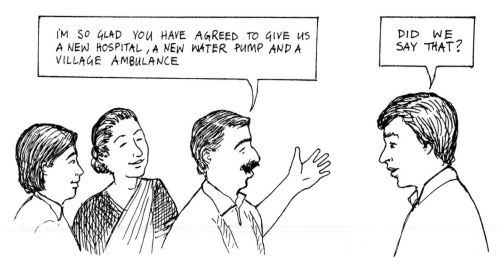

Figure 6.5 Ideas discussed in meetings are often taken as promises by the community.

Many excellent community-based programmes are not well documented or researched, often because everyone is so busy. PAs and community surveys can be valuable ways to inform and influence local and regional health policies. PA is also an opportunity to include the voices of the marginalized, e.g. those with disability.

The community survey

It is usually better to carry out some form of PA before we conduct a community survey, which is more detailed and usually more timeconsuming. Community health programmes will nearly always need a house-to-house survey to provide the more accurate, numerical information needed for planning. However, in remote communities or where resources are limited it can be helpful to combine PA and surveying. It is worth noting here that some communities have developed 'survey fatigue', especially if they are located in main cities or near main road or rail connections. As with a PA, a community survey is a community-owned initiative, ideally requested by them, and always done with their full understanding and involvement.

Why a survey is necessary

There are several reasons for doing surveys:

1. To discover the main health and development needs of the community before we start working.

Accurate baseline information on the community's health and population structure is best obtained before we work on solutions with the community. Then by resurveying after a period of time, say three or five years later, we can estimate how much progress has been made.

2. To discover which parts of the community have the greatest health needs.

They are usually:

*   children under five, especially those who are malnourished;
*   women who are pregnant and in the months following childbirth;
*   those with serious or chronic illnesses such as TB, HIV/AIDS, neglected tropical diseases, diabetes, hypertension, and other non-communicable diseases (see Chapter 22);
*   those with physical or mental disability;
*   those needing home or palliative care;

- a group, family, or individuals who are stigmatized, marginalized, or abusing alcohol or drugs; and
- families facing extreme stress or catastrophe for any reason.

We also use surveys to build relationships and to teach and create awareness. A survey done in a relaxed, friendly way will help to build friendships and create trust. It will prove a good 'starter project' for community participation (see Chapter 2). But, in addition to asking questions and completing the survey, we should make time to discuss health issues that families raise, and which create health awareness. For example, we can encourage families who have not received recommended vaccinations to do so. We can encourage people living with chronic illness to take regular medication, e.g. in epilepsy or with raised blood pressure.

Types of survey

These are the types of survey that can be carried out at this stage:

Comprehensive surveys

Every home is visited and questions are asked concerning all family members. The main advantages are that all individuals at risk can be discovered and comprehensive care can be recorded, thus minimizing delay in care and treatment. Information obtained is also more complete. The main disadvantage of using a comprehensive survey is the length of time it takes. However, in small- or medium-sized villages, or in city slums where households have already been grouped into appropriately sized clusters, e.g. 25–50 households under the guidance of a Community Health Worker (CHW), this is usually possible. A functioning village health committee (VHC), women's group, or Arukah Network cluster can also help this process.

Sample surveys

Some, but not all, households are visited. Every fifth or tenth house can be chosen or houses can be selected randomly using a random number chart. Sample surveys are used either if numbers in the programme are very large or if a quick, initial survey is needed at the outset of a programme or for completing a project proposal. This gives a useful, quantitative picture of the health of a community and can be seen as one component of a PA or as a useful addition.

Mixed surveys

Here we may visit each house to record certain important information such as the weight or mid-upper arm circumference of the children, but only some houses to record other information such as socioeconomic data

Pilot surveys

These are small-scale surveys carried out at the start of a programme, either to obtain an approximate census, or to pretest the technique to be used in a sample or comprehensive survey. All comprehensive surveys should be piloted first.

Who should do the survey?

Programme and community members should work together. For example, a community member can record answers, a programme member find out information.
Surveyors will need to be:

- open and friendly in manner;
- exact and neat in recording.

The community member could be one of the following:

- a CHW or VHC member;
- a responsible young person or high school student;
- any community member with a genuine interest and wanting to help for appropriate reasons.

In choosing team members we will need to follow good practice guidelines in the safeguarding of children and vulnerable adults, as there are opportunities for potential abuse in home-based surveying.[3] Usually the community should select their surveyors. They should each be asked to sign a simple confidentiality agreement.

When should the survey be done?

First and foremost, the survey should be conducted when the community is ready for it. We should make sure the community understands the reason for the survey and, more importantly, has welcomed us and is ready to participate. A suspicious or unwilling community may give inaccurate answers. Also, insisting on doing a survey or asking sensitive questions may result in damaged trust between the community and the health team.

If we have not done a PA, the survey can be done at an early stage and combined with some PA techniques.

If, however, a PA has been carried out and has led to agreeing some successful actions with the community, a more comprehensive survey can then follow. Community members are more likely to take part with greater enthusiasm as they will more clearly understand the reasons and value of doing the survey.

The survey should happen when the programme has enough resources. At the very least we will need:

- team member(s) who have been trained in surveying;
- survey materials, including forms or family folders;
- sufficient time to do the job properly;
- the ability to work with the community in response to the needs discovered; and
- sufficient funding to cover core costs.

In addition, many communities have scattered homes, which may require walking or cycling long distances. We need to ensure the team has sufficient time and energy, as well as that they are safe.

Finally, the survey should take place at a time of day and of year when most people are at home and not too busy with other activities, such as harvesting or seasonal employment. Ideally it should happen when the weather is not excessively hot, cold, or wet. In urban communities or insecure locations, it needs to be done at the safest time of day

What we need to do for a survey

Prepare materials

In order to prepare materials for a survey, we can follow a few guidelines. We need to decide what information needs to be gathered. This information should be:

- Useful.
  - Will it help in making plans?
  - Can it be used to bring about improvements?
  - Will asking questions raise unfair expectations for immediate solutions?
  - Avoid questions that are interesting but unnecessary for the programme's aims.
- Easily gathered.
  - Questions should be simple to ask and record.
  - Where possible, answers should be yes, no, a number or a single word. This makes it much easier to analyse the data (see Chapter 7).

Another way to prepare for a survey is to study and adapt existing survey forms. Find out if the government,

any voluntary health association, or nearby programmes have materials available. Appendix C provides a sample form, or other forms can be adapted and used. If we are planning to do research or a detailed evaluation later, it is worth designing the form with the help of someone who understands statistics and research design. Hand held electronic devices can be used (see Chapter 26) but we need to ensure that community members are happy to have their information recorded digitally.

Collect the materials needed

Each surveyor should have a list of questions. These will need to be carefully worded so that the answers obtained are valid. For example, if we are enquiring about TB prevalence, we could ask:

- Do you have a cough?
- Do you cough often?
- Have you been coughing for a long time?
- Have you been coughing for more than three or four weeks?

The last of these will give the most valid or useful answer in trying to discover whether people may have TB.

In order for all answers to be consistent, the same question must be asked to each community member with the same wording. If different team members use different questions (like those about coughing) answers cannot be compared and the results will not be accurate. Surveyors could also use the following:

- The Family Folder System see Appendix C.

These are made of stout paper and details about family members are filled in on the front. Other details such as questions on socioeconomic conditions can be recorded on the back or the inside. Each family has its own folder. This has proved to be useful in a number of programmes, but can be time-consuming when population numbers are high or when other documentation is needed for specific programmes.

The family folder system described was pioneered by programmes in India. A similar system has been adopted by Ethiopia's Health Extension Programme, where every household has a unique number and a family folder. Each family folder has a complete list of every household member and contains service cards for each person.

- Insert cards.

If we use the family folder system, these cards will be needed for comprehensive surveys. Whenever a family member is found whose health is at risk, details are recorded on an insert card, which is then placed in the family folder.[1]

- Tablet or smart phone surveying is increasingly done (see Chapter 26).

Before using this method instead of traditional ways of recording information, we must ensure there are definite advantages in terms of time, costs, accuracy, and consistency. Crucially, it must be acceptable to the community and not suggest that information is being recorded for ulterior reasons. Free and simple software, e.g. surveymonkey, Kobo, is available for surveying.

Finally, we need to obtain or make a community map of the community, if possible. Maps may be available locally or from the DMO.

Train the survey team

Allow adequate time for training, and surveyors should be trained in two basic skills: relating to the community, and obtaining the information needed.

Surveyors need to be friendly so that they are able to build relationships with community members, and tactful so that they can ask questions without causing offence. This is especially important when dealing with children and women, and they should be au fait with safeguarding guidelines. Additionally, surveyors should be comfortable in being persistent so that they obtain the answers they need. Lastly, they must be discreet, and able to observe confidentiality about health problems which requires both training and a signed confidentiality form.

Before asking questions, surveyors need to be trained to explain to each household who they are, where they are from, and why they are doing the survey. This will be easier when community members are part of the survey team and have been involved in planning and design. Survey skills can be effectively taught by role-play. In the author's experience this is essential to reduce mistakes made in obtaining accurate information (Figure 6.6). Surveyors will need to learn:

- Questioning: both what to ask and how to ask it, and they should carry a list of the questions.
- Recording: making sure that each answer is written down correctly
- Measuring: e.g. the mid-upper arm circumference (MUAC) of children aged 6 to 60 months, the child's weight, any other information needed. Skills should be practised until mistakes are eliminated.

This training will take place before the survey starts.

During the survey or in a pilot the supervisor should accompany surveyors until they are confident and accurate. After the survey the supervisor should check through the survey cards or computer records, and any

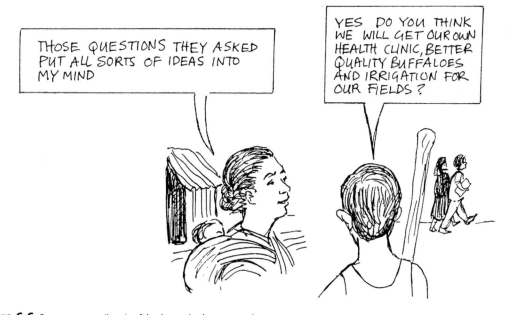

Figure 6.6 Surveys can easily raise false hopes in the community.

obvious mistakes or unanswered questions should be discussed with the surveyor. If accurate answers have not been obtained, the surveyor should be asked to resurvey the family in question. We should start by training several team and community members and then select those who show the greatest interest and ability to become future 'survey specialists'.

Carrying out the survey

There are three stages to the survey: arranging a date, forming the team, and deciding upon the parameters used to record information received. Firstly, arrange a date in advance, inform all those involved, and co-ordinate with community partners. Secondly, it is usually helpful to work in pairs: a team member and community volunteer together. Finally, decide on a numbering system for the houses before starting as numbering often causes problems. If this is forgotten, several houses can end up with the same code number. The difficulty here is that, frequently, houses have no numbers or numbers change as extra houses are built. If a permanent or formal numbering system exists, use that, but if there is no such system, devise one and make a careful record, e.g. mark numbers in chalk on the outside of houses (with the owner's permission).

When carrying out the survey, the model described here can be used as it is or altered to fit where needed. Each programme should adapt methods and forms to suit its own situation.

Data to be gathered

The following information is generally recorded when doing a survey. The letters in the sub-headings correspond to those in Figures 6.7, 6.8 and 6.9. These questions come from one example developed by a particular programme, and they will need to be adapted or constructed to form a set of questions entirely appropriate for each programme. Box 6.1 and Box 6.2 give examples of tally sheets used in gathering data.

a) *Name, address, etc.*
   1. Name, address, and occupation of the head of the family.
   2. Code number of the family.

A useful method is to construct a code with three sets of digits. The first set represents the health centre code, the second the community code and the third the house code, e.g. 03/10/46. A fourth set can be added for individuals, e.g. 03/10/46/01 would be the code number of the head of the family of the forty-sixth house in the tenth community of the target area of the third health centre.

b) *Felt problems.*
   1. What are the *main problems* affecting your family?

This is probably the best wording to use and is asked as the very first question of the survey before the answers have been influenced by other health-related questions. We could ask the question 'What are the main *health problems* affecting your family' but the broader we make this question, the more often we receive valuable information about factors that can influence health, e.g. shortage of food, distance from a water supply (See Figure 6.6).

c) *Family profile*
   1. Names of family members.

Enter these in a logical order by starting with the head of the family, partner, children, the next senior male,

(c) FAMILY PROFILE

No.	Name	Age/DoB	Sex	Relation to head	Relation to each other
01	MOHAMMED	65	M		
02	HASSAN	34	M	Son	
03	FATIMA	25	F	Daughter in law	Wife of 02
04	ALI	4 Nov'05	M	Grandson	Eldest son of 02 + 03

Figure 6.7 Family profile section of survey form.

No.	Name	Age/DoB	(d) DISEASES				(e) IMMUNISATION			Measles	Tet tox
			TB	Lep	Eye	<5nutr.	BCG	DPT	Polio		
01	MOHAMMED	65	1	0	0	0	0	0	0	0	0
02	HASSAN	34	0	0	1	0	0	0	0	0	0
03	FATIMA	25	0	0	0	0	0	0	0	0	1
04	ALI	4 Nov'05	0	0	0	1	1	0	0	0	0

Figure 6.8 Disease and immunization sections of survey form.

partner and children etc. Elderly relatives can be added either at the beginning or the end. In many communities this can be surprisingly difficult. There is large variety in communities about family structure. Children may be known by several different names, or only be given a permanent name after a certain age. Children under a very young age may not be mentioned by the family.

2. Ages

Children under five years should have the month and year of their birth recorded accurately to help in preparing growth charts. Those over five years can simply have their age recorded. If ages cannot be easily remembered, make a 'local events calendar' where seasons and annual events are marked to help parents remember the time of year their children were born. Check that the age the parents give broadly corresponds with the appearance of the child.

3. Gender

4. Relationships.

These can be written in two columns. The first records the relationship to the head of the family. The second need only be used for large extended families. It records how different members are related to each other, e.g. which wife is married to which husband, or which child belongs to which parents (Figure 6.7).

d) *Diseases and under-5 nutrition*
   1. Locally prevalent diseases.

We will need to decide on a small number of common (locally prevalent) illnesses to ask about, or we may wish to focus on certain illnesses about which we need

information. We should adapt our forms to have clear categories for the conditions we need to include. A comprehensive survey might ask questions about:

- Infectious and vector-spread illness such as malaria, dengue fever and TB;
- Non-communicable diseases such as diabetes, hypertension, cancer, stroke and chronic obstructive pulmonary disease (COPD);
- Neglected tropical diseases such as schistosomiasis (bilharzia) or river blindness;
- Mental health problems;
- Physical disability including blindness and hearing impairment.

We will need tact where a health condition has associated stigma. This is especially the case for people living with HIV/AIDS, or those with mental health issues or epilepsy.

2. Nutritional status of under-fives

This information can be found out only by careful measuring. There is limited value in asking questions or looking at the child. Children can either be weighed or children between six and sixty months can have their MUAC measured with a measuring strip (see Chapter 14).

e) *Immunization status*

This will usually include the original six diseases covered by the World Health Organization's (WHO) Expanded Programme on Immunization (EPI):

1. BCG (for TB), DPT (diphtheria, pertussis, tetanus), polio, measles—for children, and

2. Tetanus toxoid—for women of childbearing age.

Other immunizations currently recommended by WHO vary from country to country but usually include: hepatitis B, pneumococcus, haemophilus, and rotavirus (see Chapter 15).

In recording immunizations write positive answers only if certain that the complete course has been given. It is helpful to record the year in which each immunization was completed. BCG scars can be looked for. Many parents will be unable to give accurate answers. Where immunization has already been started by the programme, the immunization register, or other records, can be used to help fill in this part of the survey (see Chapter 15).

Usually the district medical team or immunization office will have their own immunization recording system, which may include records, computerized information, or self-retained record cards. Always avoid duplicating any system that is working well.

f) Family planning

This is usually a sensitive subject, in which case it can be done later when trust has been established and a Family Planning Worker trained (Figure 6.9; see also Chapter 18).

g) Addiction

Addiction covers smoking excess drinking of alcohol, or other drug abuse or concern in the community. Define the lower age limit appropriate for your community, e.g. from age twelve, and ask about every family member over that age. Be tactful when asking these questions; in some communities it will not be advisable during a first survey, especially in urban communities. We should be unsurprised if people are untruthful or evasive about these issues.

h) Education

When investigating and asking about adult literacy, it may be helpful to use UNESCO's common definition, which is people aged 15 or over who can read or write. Male and female will be separated later in the tally. Alternatively, we can ask for the highest level of educational attainment.

Primary school attendance commonly applies to children from the age of five to nineteen inclusive. Record either the grade attended at the time of the survey (or the highest grade attended if no longer at school). Alternatively, simply record if the child is currently enrolled at and attending school. The level of education, especially female literacy, has an important effect on health.

i) Deaths in the previous twelve months

Record the age, sex and cause of death. This information needs to be as accurate as possible. Deaths in the past year are often under-reported. The family may not want to talk about them; additionally, some may not consider deaths in the first few days of life worth mentioning or they may report only the deaths of sons. This means that, if we are using verbal reports of deaths within the last year to calculate mortality rates before the programme starts, we will need to ensure they are accurately reported. If under-recorded, the original state of health of the community will seem better than it really is, meaning that any improvements brought will be underestimated.

No.	Name	Age/DoB	Tub	Vas	O/C pill	Coil	If pregnant	Eligible FP	Alcohol ▼ Tobacco	Adult literacy	School	Remarks
01	MOHAMMED	65	O	o	o	o	o	o	o	/	/	o	Stroke 2 years ago. can walk in house
02	HASSAN	34	o	o	o	o	o	o	o	/	/	o	
03	FATIMA	25	o	o	o	o	/	/	o	o	o	o	
04	ALI	4 Nov '05	o	o	o	o	o	o	o	o	o	/	Twin Brother died at birth

(f) Family planning   (g) Addiction   (h) Education

Figure 6.9 Family planning, addiction, and education sections of survey form.

Box 6.1 **Community sheet used in SHARE project**

TALLY SHEET

Name of village	Date of survey	Name of surveyor
_____	_____	_____

Total population_____M_____F_____

			First Total	This column for later adjustments	Final Total
AGE OF POPOULATION	0 – 1	M			
		F			
	1 – 4	M			
		F			
	5 – 9	M			
		F			
	10 – 19	M			
		F			
	20 – 29	M			
		F			
	30 – 39	M			
		F			
	40 – 49	M			
		F			
	50 – 59	M			
		F			
	60 – 69	M			
		F			
	70 – 79	M			
		F			
	80 – 89	M			
		F			
DISEASES &UNDER 5 NUTRITION	TB				
	Leprosy				
	Eyes				
M	Don't know				
U	Green				
A	Yellow				
C	Red				
IMMUNISATION	BCG				
	DPT/Polio				
	Measles				
	Tet Tox				
FAMILY PLANNING	Tub				
	Vas				
	o/c Pill				
	Coil				
	Pregnant				
	Eligible FP				
ADDICTION	Alcohol	M			
		F			
	Tobacco	M			
		F			
EDUCATION	Adult	M			
	Literacy	F			
	School	M			
	Attendance	F			

Box 6.2 **Community diagnosis form used in SHARE project**

COMMUNITY DIAGNOSIS FORM

Name of village_____   Name of CHW_____

Name of supervisor_____   Name of Chief_____

Name of VHC members_____   _____

                    _____   _____

INFORMATION FORM FIRST HOUSE TO HOUSE SURVEY   DATE _____

(a)   Basic statistics

	Actual	Numbers Eligible	Percentage
Total population			
No. male			
No. female			
TotaJ numbsr of families			
SUBFFEKIEICI tuberculosis			
SUBFFEKIEICI leprosy			
Current eye problems			
Under 5 malnutrition (Red MUAC)			
(Yellow MUAC)			
No. BCG			
No. Completed DPT Polio			
No. measles			
No. completed Tat Tox			
No. Tubectomy			
No. vasectomy			
No o/c pill			
No. coil			
No. pregnant			
No. Eligible for family planning			
No. drinking (8 and over)			
No. smoking (S and over)			
Total number literate (15 and over			
No. male literate (15 and over)			
No. female literate (15 and over)			
Total number at school(5–15)			
No boys at school (5–19)			
No girls at school (5–19)			

Deaths in the last 12 month   Age   Cause

1_____
2_____
3_____
4_____
5_____

(b) Problems mentioned by villagers   Number who mention

1_____
2_____
3_____
4_____
5_____
6_____
7_____

(c) *Surveyor's observations*

_____
_____
_____
_____
_____
_____
_____
_____
_____

j) *Use of existing services*

Ask about who and where the family attends when there is illness or a need for medical help. This may be another programme elsewhere, a district medical office or hospital, a traditional healer or commonly one of a range of private practitioners.

k) *Water supply*

When recording information about water supply, make sure to include the type, distance from the community, and the number of months a year that a functioning main water supply (and any alternative) is available. Normal distance walked to collect water is a key piece of information. Note that distance may be given in terms of walking time if that is easier for respondents. Additionally, record how much water is collected daily per person or household. This may be best done by measuring the number of locally used containers, e.g. buckets.

l) *Sanitation*

Record the method of human waste disposal used by the family. Alternatively, this information can be gained by observation, or by asking key informants more general questions, e.g. 'how many houses have latrines/indoor toilets?'

m) *Diet*

For each main food source, record the number of months it is eaten by the family per year. Also record, if available, the number of months' supply grown by family, and number bought by family from outside the community.

n) *Estimated socioeconomic status*

When recording socio-economic status, using markers, e.g., 5 is the richest subgroup, 1 the poorest. Try to estimate this for each family, or ask questions like:

- Type of housing and number of rooms.
- Types and numbers of animals.
- Area and quality of land owned.

Note that urban communities and some rural communities will have other indicators of family wealth that can be used. This information helps us later to target resources to those most in need and shows which families might be eligible for reduced clinic rates or subsidies. It is important to understand that people may often under-report.

Symbols used in recording

There is no value in asking carefully worded questions unless the answers are also recorded accurately. Each surveyor must record with care and use the same symbols. For example:

- 0—a negative answer.
- 1—a positive answer.
- ?—answer is not known or a family member was absent (this can be altered when the answer is known).
- n/a—the question does not apply.

Numbers can be used, e.g. for school grade attained, and dates can be written, e.g. for year an immunization was completed. When writing dates, make sure that all members of the team use an agreed date format, as formats may vary between countries, e.g. in the US the date of 12 May 1981 would appear as 5/12/81, which, in the UK, would mean 5 December 1981.

Never leave blanks spaces in a form. Blank spaces on a survey form can mean several things, e.g. a family member was absent, someone didn't know an answer, didn't wish to answer, the surveyor forgot to fill in the answer. When blanks are left, statistics, such as those for child nutrition, quickly become inaccurate. Where an answer is descriptive (as under 'Felt problems' in 'Data to be gathered') the key words or ideas can be recorded.

Using the results for a community diagnosis

Having completed the survey, the results must now be used, not stored away and forgotten (See Figure 6.10). The results are analysed to make a community diagnosis and then discussed with the community to draw up a community plan (see Chapter 7).

Just as we question and examine a patient to help find a diagnosis, so we can do the same for a community. In this way we can discover the community's main health problems, their underlying causes, and explore possible solutions with the community.

Our main sources of information are the PA, which provides descriptive or qualitative information, and the community survey, which mainly gives numerical, quantitative, or 'hard data' about the health of the community. We may gain further information from secondary sources such as previous reports and District records (Figure 6.11).

Tally and tabulate the results

A tally is a simple method of adding up totals for each question that is marked on the tally. Using tally, or hash, marks is a simple way of keeping track of ongoing results. For example:

II means 2

IIII means 4

//// means 5

//// III means 8.

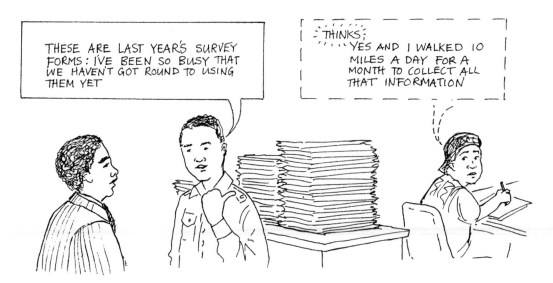

Figure 6.10 Being thoughtful about front-line workers.

Then the totals from the tally are tabulated on to a community diagnosis form. We need to choose a design appropriate for our own programme. For example, for each community we will need to know the total number of malnourished children under five. This will be the numerator (N) or actual number. We will also want to know the total number of children under five. This will be the denominator (D) or eligible number. Percentages (100 N/D) convey the most useful information. They give a picture of how serious a problem is at any one time. By comparing percentages over a period of time we are able to tell how much improvement has occurred. Often in practice the denominator is left out, which greatly reduces the value of any data and makes it harder to measure achievements.

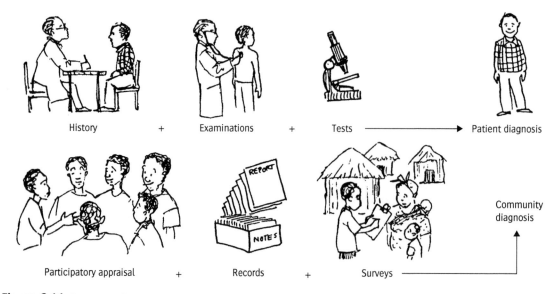

Figure 6.11 Community diagnosis.

List the problems

Draw up a list of serious problems in the community. The community diagnosis form contains space both for figures from the tally, and qualitative data from the PA and the survey. Both are considered when drawing up the problem list.

Analyse the results

We now have the basic information with which to start analysing results and drawing up plans with the community. For more information, see Chapter 7, which specifically discusses community plans.

If our programme is small scale and we have limited amounts of data, then we will probably be able to analyse this using skilled members of the health programme and community. In more detailed surveys we may collect large amounts of data. As programmes grow, the amount of data may become too large for us to analyse ourselves, in which case we may need to call in the help of outside experts, e.g. from a university department.

Using computers in data analysis

We need to be fully aware of the advantages and disadvantages of computerizing our data, but we will increasingly need good reasons not to go down this route. Table 6.4 shows the advantages and disadvantages of using computers in data analysis. Chapter 26 provides more information on the use of information technology, the Internet, SMS, and the use of apps.

Present the findings

We need to present information to the community. With permission, we will probably also pass on a summary of our findings to other stakeholders, e.g. donors, the government (usually to the DHT). We will need to present information in the most appropriate way for each of these groups, ideally using visuals, including graphs and charts. However, it is important to find creative ways to feed back the findings[5] to the community[6] so that illiterate members can also understand the results. For example, percentages can be described as cents in the dollar or pennies in the pound, etc. Pictograms are also helpful (see Figure 6.12).

Table 6.4 Advantages and disadvantages of using a computer in data analysis

Uses and advantages:

They can tally, tabulate, and process large amounts of information.

They can generate reports.

They can provide a range of support to the programme, e.g. 'due lists' for community and family care, e.g. immunizations, antenatal care.

They can produce graphs, bar charts, and other graphics.

They enable statistical analysis, tracking of infectious diseases, and research.

Disadvantages:

They can dominate the administration of a programme.

We may be working in areas where there is no capacity to input data.

Team members can become more interested in computers than people, with adverse effects on community partnership.

Data needs to be backed up reliably or it will be lost.

They may remove control from the community to the health team, thus limiting participation.

Computers depend on a reliable power supply.

They require training in how to use them and how to troubleshoot problems.

They require finance to buy hardware, update software, train programme members, and provide systems support from outside specialists.

They can crash, lose data, or develop viruses.

Information can easily be lost or corrupted, so a reliable back-up system has to be used or else data also has to be kept manually.

False information can easily be entered onto a computer.[*]

[*] Note that false information can also be entered into paper-based records. To overcome this problem when using a tablet or smartphone, a survey system produced by Kobo gives GPS readings of where the data is being entered, making it less likely that the information is being fabricated.

Summary

Before starting any health programme, we need to understand the communities and work in partnership with which we will be working. Having first established trust and friendship, we can carry out a PA using combined teams of observers. Training should be given to all involved and practical arrangements should be made that

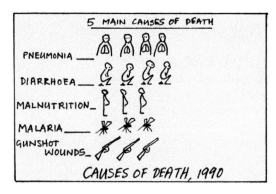

Figure 6.12 Pictogram to show causes of death.

are convenient for the community. The main methods of doing a PA include semi-structured interviews, focus group discussions, community mapping, and secondary information.

All information gathered must be carefully recorded and analysed. One of a PA's main values is to strengthen community partnership at an early stage in the development of a programme. The main purpose of the community survey is to gather numerical information for a community diagnosis. It is valuable for the ongoing prevention and management of illness, such as using the family folder system. It also provides a baseline for evaluating the programme at a later date.

The community diagnosis reveals the main problems affecting a community and is based largely on information from the survey and the observations of team and community members, including information from the PA.

Computers are increasingly used at both field level, both through hand held devices and in the programme office. Not all communities will be ready to fully computerize but a range of affordable devices, hardware and software makes this increasingly possible and affordable.

Having made a community diagnosis and enabled the whole community to understand its results and implications, we can move ahead and draw up more detailed action plans with the community.

Further reading

Chambers R. *From PRA to PLA and Pluralism: Practice and Theory. IDS Working Paper 286.* Brighton: Institute of Development Studies; 2007. Available from: http://www.oerafrica.org/FTPFolder/SharedFiles/ResourceFiles/36140/33527/33507/From%20PRA%20to%20PLA%20Chambers%202007.pdf

Chambers R, Kumar S. *Methods for Community Participation: A Complete Guide for Practitioners.* New Delhi: Vistaar Publications; 2003.

Narayanasamy N. *Participatory Rural Appraisal: Principles, Methods and Application.* London: SAGE; 2009.

Web resources

World Health Organization. Epi Info Computer Software. Available from: https://www.cdc.gov/epiinfo/ This is a public domain package with facilities for word processing, questionnaire design, data entry and analysis, and graphics. It is regularly updated and, though accompanied with excellent instructions, takes time and expertise for field programmes to use effectively.

United Nations Food and Agriculture Organization. Available from: http://www.fao.org/docrep/W3241E/w3241e09.htm A corporate document repository with a number of resources, such as a Chapter on Rapid Rural Appraisal

Work Group for Community Health and Development, University of Kansas. The Community Tool Box—an on-line resource. Available from: http://ctb.ku.edu/en/table-of-contents

The Institute for Participatory Practices, India. Available from: www.praxisindia.org The website has useful resources and publications.

References

1. Social Care Institute for Excellence. What is a strengths-based approach to care? Available from: http://www.scie.org.uk/care-act-2014/assessment-and-eligibility/strengths-based-approach/what-is-a-strengths-based-approach.asp

2. Participation Compass. Participatory Appraisal. 2012. Available from: http://participationcompass.org/article/show/137

3. Save the Children and Tearfund. Setting the Standards: A common approach to child protection for international NGOs. 2003. Available from: www.peopleinaid.org or from: https://resourcecentre.savethechildren.net/sites/default/files/documents/1603.pdf

4. MEASURE Evaluation. *Fact Sheet: Community Health Information System in Action in SNNPR.* 2012. Available from: https://www.measureevaluation.org/resources/publications/fs-12-72

5. Work Group for Community Health and Development, University of Kansas. Understanding and Describing the Community, Section 2, Chapter 3. In: *The Community Tool Box.* Available from: http://ctb.ku.edu/en/table-of-contents

6. McDavitt, B., Bogart LM, Mutchler MG, Wagner GJ, Green HD Jr, Lawrence SJ et al. Dissemination as dialogue: Building trust and sharing research findings through community engagement. *Preventing Chronic Disease.* 2016; 13:150473. Available at: https://www.cdc.gov/pcd/issues/2016/15_0473.htm

Drawing up plans

Ted Lankester

This chapter assumes we have formed strong links with the community, have gathered information, either through participatory appraisal, community survey or both, and that we are now ready to draw up a development plan for a one- to three-year period. One way of doing this is through using a logical framework analysis (LFA, or logframe), which is a useful way to help draw up an operational plan and is also used by most major donors.

What we need to know

Team consultation and discussion with the community

Discuss with the team

Before discussing the survey results with the whole community, the health team and all those involved in the survey will need to consult together. The purpose of the discussion is to understand and reflect on the findings. It is likely that we will have already gone through a similar exercise after the Participatory Appraisal (PA), but if not, the findings from the PA can be included now.

Usually any more detailed survey will have been done some time after the PA, meaning we need a further period of analysis and reflection as a programme team, to consider all the information we have collected with the community.

Prioritize the problems

Prioritizing or ranking the problems means rewriting the problem list using the information from the survey and other sources in order of priority, with the most important at the top.

One way of ranking problems is to ask four different questions about each problem:

- How serious is it?
- How widespread is it?
- How important is it to the community?
- How suitable is it for joint project/community action?

Each question has a score applied to it between 1 and 3, or 1 and 5 with a maximum possible total of 12 (20). Problems are then prioritized in order of their score (see Table 7.1). In the example shown, the resulting order

Table 7.1 **Prioritizing or ranking problems**

Problem	How serious	How widespread	How important to community	How suitable joint action	Total
Lack of clean water	3	3	2	3	11
Occasional malaria in wet season	2	1	1	2	6
Many deaths from neonatal tetanus	3	2	2	3	10
Heavy drinking of alcohol	2	3	1	2	8

of priority is: water: 11, HIV: 10, alcohol abuse: 8, and malaria: 6. It is worth emphasizing here that this prioritization is a way to prepare the team before they meet the community, and it is not a way for the team to impose a ranking on the community.

As mentioned in Chapter 6, the 'felt needs' that emerge from both the PA and the survey may not be health problems. However, nearly all problems will have an effect on health, i.e. they will be 'social determinants of health'. Some of these may be beyond the skill, capacity, or expertise of the programme, meaning that is important to link with experts in other CSOs or in government departments as soon as possible in order to address these problems.

Common top problems in urban slums are lack of employment, poor working conditions, overcrowding, violence, and poor sanitation. In rural areas, common top problems include distance from a water source, no adequate schooling, and lack of income.

Decide the process

It will certainly be our hope that planning can be a joint activity and that the community itself can help to lead or shape the process. In some communities there may be few people sufficiently well informed or educated to do this; the programme may therefore need to take the lead in the early stages. If this is the case, programme members should be trained to mentor and encourage members of the community in the leadership and other skills they will need. This will ensure that community members can play an effective part in planning and management as soon as possible.

How to meet with the community

It is helpful first to meet with the whole community in order to share results and ideas, and then with a village

health committee (VHC) or planning group to draw up specific action plans. If no such group exists this can be a good moment to help the community set one up, see the section on VHCs in Chapter 2.

Discussion and presentation of findings

We may already have had similar meetings, for example, when we were first invited to start a programme or to explain the results of the PA. Reporting

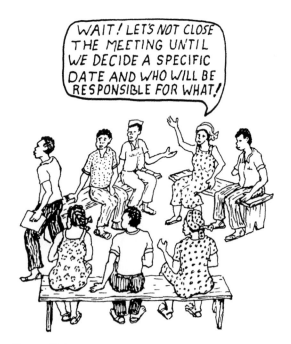

Figure 7.1 Before the meeting closes, make sure everyone knows what is to be done and who is to do it.

back the survey results can follow a similar pattern. If the PA and survey were close together, the meeting can combine both. It is important to report back findings from the PA or survey as soon as possible, as the matters involved will still be fresh in people's minds and their interest is aroused. Programme and community members involved in the PA or the survey can make a joint presentation.

Keep the presentation as simple as possible, and explain the main problems in a way that can be easily understood. The more responses and questions from the audience, the better. The purpose here is not merely to inform but to motivate community members to feel the seriousness of their problems and the urgent need to find solutions. For example, malnutrition in under-fives is common, but the community may not understand the seriousness of the situation as most children look much the same. Explain to those present that measurement is the only way to discover most cases of malnutrition, and how research has shown that malnourished children are more likely to die from common illnesses such as diarrhoea, measles and pneumonia.

Agree priority problems for joint action

During the meeting, talk about serious problems that are suitable for joint action. We will already have prepared our priority list but we must be flexible and ready to change if other priorities emerge. Make sure that any problems chosen are:

1. within the capacity of the programme (both in terms of money and expertise);
2. suitable for a joint community/programme approach; and
3. at least one or two are 'low hanging fruit', i.e. likely to bring quick results (see also Chapter 2).

Also agree with the community when tasks should be completed so that interest and commitment is channelled quickly and momentum is maintained (Figure 7.1).

Often the first action will be setting up and training a community action group (CAG).

Practical planning: village health committees (VHCs), community action groups (CAGs)

At this stage it is worth looking ahead in this chapter to the section 'Logical framework (logframe)' and in particular the template (see Table 7.7a). The headings on the logframe are a good place to start recording the main objectives and activities that emerge after agreeing priorities with the community. Some of the pros and cons of using a logframe as a planning tool are also mentioned.

For each problem selected in collaboration with the whole community, we can now start to draw up a detailed action plan. This is best done by the VHC or CAG, which will mainly comprise members of the community. Health team members will be involved as resource people or advisors. It will be helpful to also consider including a religious leader, a teacher, or senior member of any neighbouring health facility. Women must be fully represented, as should adolescents. One of our priorities is to encourage and train community members in management and leadership.

Chapter 2 describes how CAGs or VHCs can be set up and developed. Figure 7.2 shows ascending levels of community involvement, and we will obviously want to move up as fast as possible from 'Coercion' to 'Partnership' (coercion is the original title used in this diagram; it implies a sense of powerlessness). But moving up the ladder will require careful training and coaching of the CAG.

Table 7.2 gives some practical guidance on the roles and functions of CAGs and their leaders. In order for a CAG to carry out these functions, it will need training, mentoring and encouragement. During the earliest phases of a project the CAG will still be at a formative stage, so the health team will have a bigger role in facilitation.

Planning methods

There are five techniques that can be very helpful in drawing up a plan for any problem we have agreed to tackle.

Using a problem tree

Using a problem tree shows the causes and effects of problems we wish to address and to guide us towards solutions (Figure 7.3). For each problem identified we construct a problem tree, as follows:

Step 1. We identify *the causes* of the problem by asking 'But Why?' until we can go no further, and draw them as roots of the tree

Step 2. We identify *the effects* of the problem by asking 'So what?' until we can go no further (see Figure 7.3).

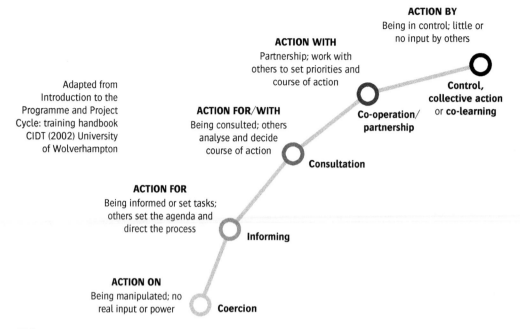

Figure 7.2 Levels of community involvement in planning.

Constructing a problem tree helps us to understand the root causes or social determinants of health problems. It is valuable to see these from the start, as the nearer we get to solving underlying causes of problems, the more effective our programme will be. This is often known as working 'upstream' or trying to identify and 'turn off the tap of ill health.'

SWOT Analysis

SWOT stands for *S*trengths, *W*eaknesses, *O*pportunities, and *T*hreats. A SWOT analysis helps us to examine available resources and potential obstacles. The *S* and *W* are the internal strengths and weaknesses of the community or action group; the *O* and *T* describe the external factors that may help or hinder a project.

We can list a number of entries for each category either by brainstorming onto a flip chart or having individuals write ideas down on post-it notes and then arranging them into the categories ranked by importance. Table 7.3 shows an example of a SWOT analysis from India which selected one Strength, Weakness, Opportunity, and Threat, and used them to develop a strategy and a plan.

SMART objectives

Clear objectives are essential for success. SMART is a set of criteria for ensuring that our objectives are clear. SMART stands for *S*pecific, *M*easurable, *A*chievable, *R*esults-orientated (or *R*elevant), and *T*ime-bound. Table 7.4 shows an example of constructing an objective using this technique.

The four 'Cs'

Part of good planning is gathering information about all aspects of an activity. One framework we can use is 'the 4 Cs':

- Community need and interest.
- Components or materials needed.
- Construction or carrying it out.
- Cost expected.

Table 7.2 Suggested tasks of the Community Action Group (CAG) in Project Planning

- Encouraging people to attend meetings
- Encouraging people to participate in community projects
- Agreeing venue and timing of community meetings
- Recording minutes and following up on action points
- Delegating tasks of gathering information, collecting resources, and organising work groups
- Meeting regularly to review progress and celebrate successes
- Involving the local church or other faith group and community leaders and reporting on progress
- Lobbying for local funds from businesses or regional grant-making authorities
- Monitoring morale of people involved in the project

Suggested roles of CAG Leaders

The Leader/Chairperson/Co-ordinator:

- acts as spokesperson for the programme within the community
- leads the group
- puts together an agenda and chairs meetings
- follows up on tasks to ensure they are done
- encourages people working on different tasks
- helps the group and community reflect on how the project is going and what could make it better
- helps the group solve challenges during the project
- helps the group think up ways of celebrating achievements.

The Secretary:

- writes letters, sends emails or WhatsApp messages on behalf of the CAG
- keeps copies manually and digitally of all records and correspondence

The Treasurer:

- oversees the money and other resources
- ensures that income and expenditure are recorded and controlled
- ensures that a petty cash system is running effectively
- helps with budgeting and is responsible for regular reporting of monthly or quarterly expenditure
- ensures that the petty cash book and the cash book are up to date and reconciled
- investigates and reports misuse of funds.

From Umoja Facilitators Guide Tearfund, see 'Further reading and resources'.

For example, in planning a programme to install smokeless cooking hearths and outside chimneys, one mountain programme in Asia (Figure 7.4) used this planning structure as follows:

1. Community:
   - Do the people *want* them?
   - Do the people *need* them?
   - How do they want them built?
   - Are they ready to do it themselves?
   - Will they need training?
   - Are they prepared to give their time and skills to this project?
   - Are they ready to pay some of or all the cost themselves?
   - What is the best time of year or season to carry this out?
2. Components:
   - What materials are needed?
   - Where can they be obtained?
   - How will they be transported?
   - Where will they be stored?
3. Construction:
   - What is the best way of making them?
   - What are the secrets of success that other projects have found?
   - What are the pitfalls to avoid?
4. Cost:
   - What will be the cost of components?
   - What will be the cost of labour?
   - What will be the cost of transport?
   - Will there be other hidden costs?

A similar framework of questions can be worked out for other community health activities (see Figure 7.4).

Using a what/who/how/when/where/ approach

Using this approach can be helpful as we try to work out the broad action plans needed for each task that needs doing. This approach helps us to think clearly about the problem and how it can be solved before we record it in more detail on the logframe.

Table 7.5 provides examples of this approach. Key steps in this technique are to decide: what should be

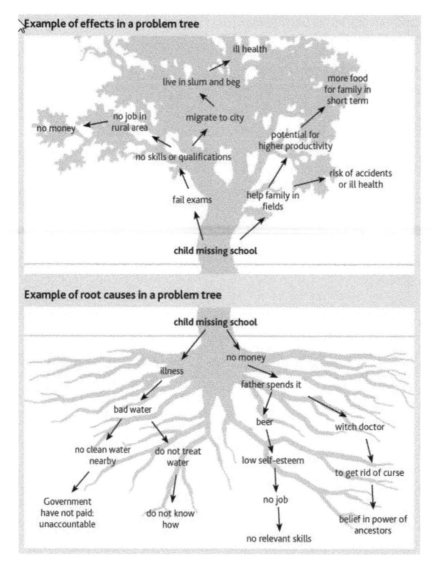

Figure 7.3 Example of a problem tree.

done, who does it, how it is done, when it is done and where it is done.

Before any meeting closes after using one of these techniques, make sure that any action decided on has been understood, agreed, and recorded and that it is circulated afterwards in summary. This summary is sometimes known as the action minutes. Key actions needed are recorded with the person responsible and deadline date. It is equally important that everyone involved knows what they are meant to do next, and the date of the next meeting or joint activity (see Figure 7.1).

Table 7.3 A SWOT analysis for a proposed community latrine complex

SWOT	Strategy	Plan
Strength: Community has several divorced or widowed women who are doing unskilled construction work.	• Train women in skills needed for latrine construction.	• Identify women • Arrange training. • Use them as resources when building latrines.
Weakness: Land is too marshy so pit latrines cannot be used.	• Persuade government to permit connection to municipal system. • Determine site that is close to municipal sewer lines.	• Visit government officials, agencies and politicians • Locate places where the sewer system runs closest to the community.
Opportunity: International funding agency is willing to provide training for making latrine slabs from locally available materials.	• Empower women's groups to be responsible for making low-cost slabs for sale to community.	• Motivate women's groups • Find production space.
Threat: Latrines will become dirty and then people will stop using them if government appoints and poorly supervises outside agency to maintain latrines.	• Community will hire cleaners, attendant and supervisor. • CAG will supervise. • Small user fee will be charged to cover expenses.	• Inform community; increase awareness of need for income to pay for cleaners, etc. • Hire latrine staff. • Train latrine staff. • Monitor that latrines are clean and working.

Table 7.4 Steps to construct a SMART objective

Step	Example
1. Restate the negative problem as a positive objective.	**Problem:** Some people living with AIDS (PLWA) are not getting good home care. **Objective:** To provide home care for PLWA.
2. Make sure the objective is **SPECIFIC**.	**Objective:** To provide home care for PLWA *in our community*.
3. Make sure there is a **MEASURABLE** indicator in the objective.	**Objective:** To provide home care for *thirty* PLWA.
4. Make sure the project is **ACHIEVABLE**.	Consider: Do we have *enough staff* to provide care to thirty patients? Are there at least thirty PLWA who will *require* and *request* care from us?
5. Make sure the objective is **RELEVANT**.	Is AIDS a *serious problem* in the community and is the community *concerned* about it?
6. Make the objective **TIME BOUND**.	**Objective:** To provide home care for thirty PLWA in our community *in the next year*.

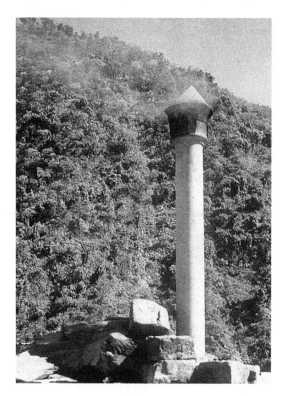

Figure 7.4 Successful management involving community, programme, and government: The first house to install a smokeless cooking hearth in a north Indian health programme.

Table 7.5 Problem: Twenty-five per cent of children suffer from moderate malnutrition

What causes	How solved	Who will solve	When to start
1 Lack of knowledge about correct feeding practices.	House-to-house health teaching; Teaching in clinic.	CHWs and health team members.	Immediately in community; In clinic when it opens in three months.
2 Irrigation channels broken and blocked leading to poor crop yields.	Repair of channels.	Community health committee with government development officer.	Liaise with government office now; Start repairs after harvest.

What we need to do

Recognizing common situations

1. Health problems are not a community priority: non-health problems are.

As mentioned, we must decide early on whether we can offer help in other development sectors such as micro-credit, literacy, forestry, water management, or agriculture. If we cannot help, it may be possible to link the community with others who can, thus stimulating 'intersectoral collaboration'.

In practice, the health programmes this book describes must integrate with the overall government health system at community, district, regional, and national levels. It must also work with other sectors and specialist agencies. See Chapter 21 for how environmental health shows the importance of a systems approach.

2. Gifts and skills of community members need to be recognized and used.

Traditionally we start with community needs and think of solutions. It is often better to start with 'assets', i.e. the gifts or abilities available in a community, and see how they can be harnessed to improve the community's health. This is known as an assets-based or strengths-based approach, and should increasingly be the starting point in working with communities (for more information on this subject, see Chapter 6).

Examples might include gifts in drama, singing, teaching, caring for the people living with disability, or organizing youth activities. If a community member is gifted or has a real 'passion' for a particular area it should be incorporated into the action plans. We should also be on the lookout for *champions*—those with a passion to get something done and to involve others.

3. Activities in different project areas need to be co-ordinated.

After a short time, we may be working with several different communities at the same time, each of which has its own list of needs and priorities. This calls for careful forward planning to make sure that plans and promises made are always followed up. Constructing a logframe for each community programme is an effective way of doing this.

Logical framework analysis (logframe)

Programme planning using a logical framework

At this stage, we will probably have identified problems in discussions with the community, and broadly agreed on plans for tackling them, perhaps using one or more of the techniques discussed earlier. It is important to record the goal, purpose (objectives), initial activities and outputs. As mentioned, the tool that does this well and which many agencies expect to be used is the LFA, or logframe, which is easier to use than people sometimes think. We can also use alternatives such as donor or community application forms that have questions constructed to produce much of the information that would be needed for a logframe.

Other alternatives to programme planning include Outcome Mapping[2] and the Benefits Realization Plan. The latter is not so widely used in CSOs but is a useful tool for use in larger programmes. For more information on both of these alternatives, see 'Further reading and resources'.

Why we use a logframe

The logframe is a system widely used by larger agencies and it is popular with donors. It helps us to do four main things: design a programme, describe a programme logically, structure a programme clearly and easily evaluate a programme.

Different terms are applied to various parts of the logframe by donors, but they largely mean the same thing. Helpful guides to writing a logframe can be found online (see 'Further reading and resources').

It is helpful to start filling in the logframe at an early stage in the planning process so we make sure we are thinking logically. This early start can help to capture all the ideas that are generated. We can think of it as a working template which becomes increasingly detailed as we progress with planning. Structuring and recording everything from the start can save a lot of time later when we come to monitor our programme (See Tables 7.8 and 7.9).

Advantages of a logframe

The advantages of using a logframe include that it is systematic, helps to focus team members in shared goals, provides a way of monitoring progress, and allows adaptations to be added as the programme evolves. It also helps us to identify any weakness in the design of the programme.

Disadvantages of a logframe

Before deciding to use a logframe it is helpful to consider some of the criticisms that have been made over the years. Firstly, a logframe can be complex, and using one effectively requires time, skill and training. It can also come across as rigid, and those using logframes must understand how to use it as a flexible management tool. Finally, logframes can lead to donor-driven approaches, where the ongoing needs, assets, and wishes of the community are not given priority (see Chapter 2).

If we do decide to use a logframe or if a donor expects us to use one, we need to be aware of these limitations and avoid the unwanted side effects they can cause if they are followed too slavishly. A number of different versions of logframes have been developed[3] and alternatives are emerging.[4]

What a logframe tells us

A logframe tells us the major things we need to know about a programme in order to plan successfully (Tables 7.5 and 7.6). These include:

- What the project aims to achieve;
- What activities will be carried out;
- What resources (inputs) are required;
- What the potential problems and risks are likely to be; and
- How progress can be measured.

Components of a logframe

The standard type of logframe is a grid with four columns and four rows. There are some differences in the way people name and use these columns and row, but the examples in Tables 7.7–7.9 show a commonly used format.

Filling in the logframe

Filling in the logframe can be done in different ways but we consider these three tips to be helpful.

1. Start using a logframe at an early stage in planning.

This helps us to get used to categorizing our plans according to the headings in the template.

2. Work down the summary column.

This helps us to define our goal (Table 7.6) and then list increasingly detailed ways in which we will actually try to achieve this.

3. Work across each row.

People good at thinking of concepts or the big picture may find it easier to start at the top; those who are good at thinking of practical details, i.e. field workers, may find it easier to begin at the bottom.

Table 7.6 **Problem: Five per cent of population with possible tuberculosis**

What causes	How solved	Who will solve	When to start
1 Lack of understanding.	Health education.	CHWs folk-drama group.	When CHWs have completed basic training.
2 No medicine available or affordable.	Ensure regular low-cost drugs.	Project director liaising with district medical officer.	At once.
3 Smoke from cigarettes and cooking hearths.	Health education; Install simple chimneys.	Representative from each house with instruction from health team member; Community leaders	Prepare now for community-wide project after rainy season.

Table 7.7a **Planning template to help complete a logical framework**

Goal	Objectives	Activities or Inputs	Outputs	Outcomes	Impact	Indicators	Means of Verification	Risks & Assumptions	Costs

From http://www.fundsforngos.org/free-resources-for-ngos/inside-the-logical-framework-of-a-grant-proposal

Table 7.7b **Explanations of the various terms used in a logframe**

Goal	The project goal is the general, high-level, long-term aim of the project. It is different from the project objective(s) because the latter are very specific and are only addressed by the project. However, the goal cannot solely be achieved by the project as there are other forces, e.g. government, other agencies, also working to achieve it. It is a major benchmark to compare work between different projects.
Objectives	Objectives are the specific objectives the project works to achieve within the stipulated time.
Activities or Inputs	Activities or inputs are actions undertaken by the project or the organization to achieve the set objectives.
Outputs	Outputs are immediate results that are achieved soon after the completion of the project or any specific project activity.
Outcomes	The outcomes are results that have been, or are to be, achieved after a period of time, but these are not immediate.
Impact	The impact is the longer-term result that happens because of the activities undertaken in the project.
Indicators	Indicators are a measure of the result. They give a sense of what has been, or what is to be, achieved.
Means of Verification	Data or information on which the indicators will be measured or monitored.
Risks and Assumptions	External factors affecting the progress of the project.
Costs	Budgetary explanations.

Checking the logframe

When checking the logframe, start at the bottom (activities) and ask: 'If we carry out this activity and assuming our assumptions are valid, will we achieve this output?'. In doing the same for each activity, we can make changes if the statements do not tally, if anything does not fit, or if anything has been omitted. We must also check that the wording and the various descriptions are clearly stated and not confusing. 'Further reading and resources' lists books, PDFs, and websites that explain this process in more detail. Finally, the logframe should be displayed as a working tool on a board in the programme office and recorded digitally so that it is accessible to all members of the team.

Summary

The success of our programme will depend partly on how effectively we draw up plans with the community and turn these into a workable format to guide our progress over a three-year period. Planning with the community uses material from either a community survey and diagnosis, a PA, or both. We must involve and inform the community in a way they can both understand and own. The main aim is to decide with them which problems to work on together. From an early stage it can be helpful to use the main headings in the logframe (see Table 7.7b) to record the emerging objectives and activities as they are agreed.

The programme should work through a CAG to draw up action plans for each problem identified. Various techniques can be used to help in this process, including problem trees and SMART objectives. Additionally, using the SWOT technique can help the project–community partnership analyse whether they have sufficient resources to undertake a planned activity. Using a what/who/how/when/where approach can help in planning tasks. The most detailed format for documenting the action plan is a logframe, which helps to clarify our goal and the ways we can attain it. For programmes unable to cope with a standard logframe, simpler versions can be adopted or forms constructed that draw out sufficient information to guide planning.

Table 7.8 **Example of a logical framework (logframe)**

	Summary	Indicators	Evidence	Assumptions
Goal	Decreased incidence and impact of diarrhoeal disease.	Mortality rate due to diarrhoeal disease reduced by five per cent by end of year 3; Incidence of diarrhoeal disease in diocese reduced by fifty per cent by end of year 3.	Government statistics; Local/health centre statistics.	
Purpose	Improved access to, and use of, safe water in diocese.	All households accessing at least 15 litres of water per person per day by end of year 3; Average distance of households to nearest safe water less than 500m by end of year 3.	Household survey report; Household survey report.	Health care does not decline; Diarrhoeal disease is due to unsafe water and hygiene practices.
Outputs	1 Participatory management systems set up for needs identification, planning, and monitoring. 2 Improved sources of safe water. 3 Raised community awareness of good hygiene practices.	Diocese and community joint plans and budgets in place by end of month 9. At least ninety per cent of WUCs raise local contributions by end of year 1. At least 90 improved or new sources of safe water established and in operation by end of year 2. Number of people washing hands after defecating increased to seventy-five per cent of target population by end of month 30.	Plans and budgets; WUC logbooks; WUC logbooks; Water quality test reports; Survey of knowledge, attitudes and practice.	Adequate quantity of water available; People are not excluded from accessing improved sources; Access not for potentially polluting uses; Hygiene practices are culturally acceptable.

WUC: Water use committees.

Table 7.8 **Continued**

	Summary	Indicators	Evidence	Assumptions
Activities	1.1 Established water user committees (WUCs).	30 WUCs established in 5 diocesan regions by end of month 3; Once established, WUC meetings held once a month.	Constitutions of WUCs; Minutes of meetings; Membership list.	Groundwater is free of arsenic; Communities have confidence that water sources can be improved; Committee membership will take responsibility to work for community.
	1.2 Provide training for WUC members in surveying, planning, monitoring, and proposal writing.	All WUC members trained by end of month 5.	Training records.	WUCs continue to function in everyone's interests.
	1.3 Communities carry out baseline and monitoring surveys of water use and needs and submit proposals.	All WUCs complete baseline surveys and submit proposals by month 7.	Survey reports and proposals.	Community prepared to work with WUCs.
	1.4 Hold joint Diocese, District Water Department and WUC regional planning meetings.	Agreement reached with Water Department and all WUCs by end of month 9.	Minutes of meetings; Letters of agreement.	
	2.1 WUCs select Community Water Workers (CWWs) and agree incentives.	2 CWWs selected by each community by end of month 9.	Minutes of meetings.	Incentive arrangements for CWWs are sufficient and sustained.
	2.2 Train CWWs to dig and cover wells and to maintain and repair handpumps.	All CWWs attend training by end of year 1.	Training reports including participants' evaluation.	Effective supply chain for spare parts.

WUC: Water use committees.

	Summary	Indicators	Evidence	Assumptions
Activities	2.3 Upgrade current wells and establish new wells.	60 current wells deepened, covered, and functioning at end of month 21; 30 new wells established and in operation by end of month 21.	Field survey; WUC logbooks.	District Water Department to be allocated enough resources to carry out water testing, and providing alternative testing if not.
	2.4 Arrange for District Water Department to test water quality.	All sources tested before use.	Field survey; WUC logbooks.	
	2.5 CWWs repair and maintain handpumps.	97% of handpumps in diocese function at end of year 2.	Field survey; WUC logbooks.	
	3.1 Train existing CHPs to increase their knowledge of diarrhoeal disease and the need for good hygiene practice.	Three CHPs per community attend training and score at least 90% in a post-training test by end of year 1.	Attendance records; Test results.	Community members apply the training they have received.
	3.2 CHPs train men, women, and children in good hygiene practice.	80% of community members trained by end of year 2.	Attendance records.	

CHP: Community Health Promoters, WUC: Water use committees.

Table 7.9 **Example of a simplified logical framework (logframe)**

	1 Project plan or structure	2 Indicators of progress	3 Risks and Assumptions	4 Outcome and Findings after Two Years
A Wider project aims	To eradicate measles from project area.	Incidence of measles falling.	Minimal civil strife; Rains not prolonged.	Incidence of measles falls by 50%.
B Immediate objectives	To immunize 30% of children under 12 months in year 1, 70% in year 2, in 10 villages.	Percentage of children under 12 months immunized per year, per village.	Villages will cooperate; No staff strikes.	Targets reached for 7 villages, (three still have coverage below 50%).
C Tasks or activities	Train team to immunize.	Health workers trained.	Training effective.	Team effectively trained to extend coverage.
	Train VHC.	VHC members actively participate.	VHC members have time and willingness.	VHC needing new challenge to avert boredom.
	Gain understanding of villagers.	Percentage of villages participating.	Villages overcome suspicion of measles vaccine.	7 villages well sensitized, 3 still resistant to change.
	Set target of four immunization days per village, per year.	Percentage attendance of those eligible per village, per day.	No unpredicted holidays and festivals on immunization days.	One out of four immunization days ruined by festival hangovers.
	Train CHWs to visit each child within one week of injection	Percentage of immunized children visited.	Partners of CHWs do not object to extra work.	Most families appreciated CHWs' concern.
D Resources or inputs	Salaries for staff	Salaries paid.	Funding continues.	New funds needed for extending to new area.
	Project vehicle	Vehicle in working order.	No serious lack of fuel.	Bicycles could be used for 5 villages.
	Visual aids	Visual aids bought and used.	Visual aids will be appropriate.	Visual aids used were wrong culture for village.
	Refrigerators and cold box	Fridge reliable, cold chain established.	Kerosene supply stable.	Solar fridge donated and maintained by another NGO.
	Needles, syringes, vaccine	Disposables purchased.	Price reasonable.	Disposable syringes available locally.
		Vaccine source secured.	EPI supplies available.	Time wasted as vaccine supply distant.

VHC: Village health committee, NGO: Non-governmental organization, CHW: Community health worker,

After a period of time we will need to evaluate with the community whether we have achieved the goals established at the start of the programme. The logframe provides a tool to track progress and make yearly adjustments to the project plan.

Further reading and resources

Benefits Realisation Plans https://www.finance-ni.gov.uk/articles/planning-programme-and-project-benefits-realisation

Blackman R. *Roots 5: Project Cycle Management.* Teddington: Tearfund; 2003. Available from: http://tilz.tearfund.org/~/media/Files/TILZ/Publications/ROOTS/English/PCM/ROOTS_5_E_Full.pdf

Chambers R. *Rural Development: Putting the Last First.* London: Taylor & Francis; 1983. A classic book which has helped to set the scene in participatory development over many decades.

Gosling L, Edwards M. *Toolkits: A Practical Guide to Assessment, Monitoring, Review and Evaluation.* London: Save the Children; 2003. Available from: http://www.savethechildren.org.uk/sites/default/files/docs/Toolkits_A_practical_guide_to_planning_monitoring_evaluation_and_impact_assessment2003.pdf

Njoroge F, Raistrick T, Crooks B, Mouradian J. *Tearfund Umoja Facilitators Guide.* Teddington: Tearfund; 2009. Available from: http://tilz.tearfund.org/~/media/Files/TILZ/Churches/Umoja/Umoja_Facilitators_Guide_-_Jan2012.pdf?la=en

Taylor L, Thin N, & Sartain J. *Logical Framework Analysis: Guidance Notes.* London: BOND; 2003. A step-by-step guide. Available from: https://www.gdrc.org/ngo/logical-fa.pdf

Web-based resources

Evaluation Toolbox. Available from: http://evaluationtoolbox.net.au/ This site provides information on problem trees, logframes, and other tools for community development and behaviour change.

Aid Delivery Methods. Volume 1:Project Cycle Management Guidelines. Brussels: European Commission; 2004 Available from: http://www.sswm.info/sites/default/files/reference_attachments/EUROPEAN%20COMMISSION%202004%20Project%20Cycle%20Management%20Handbook.pdf

Funds for NGOs. The website has a number of downloadable resources, including on logframes. Available from: http://www.fundsforngos.org/free-resources-for-ngos/

Outcome Mapping practitioners. Available from: http://www.outcomemapping.ca

Young J, Shaxson L, Jones H, Hearn S, Datta A, Cassidy C. *ROMA (Rapid Outcome Mapping): A guide to policy engagement and influence.* London: Overseas Development Institute: 2014. Available from: https://www.odi.org/sites/odi.org.uk/files/odi-assets/publications-opinion-files/9011.pdf

References

1. Arnstein SR. A ladder of citizen participation. *Journal of the American Planning Association.* 1969; 35 (4): 216–24.
2. Ramalingam B. *Tools for knowledge and learning: a guide for development and humanitarian organisations, Chapter 5—Outcome Mapping.* London: Overseas Development Institute; 2006. Available from: https://www.odi.org/sites/odi.org.uk/files/odi-assets/publications-opinion-files/188.pdf
3. Gasper D. *Logical framework: Problems and potentials.* Available from: http://www.petersigsgaard.dk/PDFfiler/gasper_logical_framework_problems.pdf
4. Fujita N. (editor). *Beyond logframe: Using systems concepts in evaluation.* Tokyo: Foundation for Advanced Studies in International Development; 2010. Available at: https://www.fasid.or.jp/_files/publication/oda_21/h21-3.pdf

The community health worker (CHW)

Ted Lankester

The community health worker (CHW) is increasingly centre stage in the theatre of community-based health care (CBHC). This chapter is, to some extent, the hub of this book. It is impossible to cover all aspects of CHWs; therefore, it looks at CHWs both from the perspective of government programmes and civil society organizations (CSOs), and considers the global health role that CHWs increasingly occupy, as well as the practicalities of how they work at the local level (Figure 8.1).

It is helpful to see this chapter in the context of the two preceding ones, as together they help to describe a valuable model which is proving effective in programmes run by governments and by CSOs, sometimes known "as the census-based impact orientated approach" (CBIOA).[1]

What we need to do

Defining a community health worker

A community based approach is increasingly seen as the best way to reach the remotest and neediest populations. The CHW is a local person trained to respond to those needs within his or her immediate community.

The use of CHWs is also in line with the global health priority of 'task shifting'. This is defined as the 'allocation of tasks in a health care system to the least costly health worker capable of doing that task reliably'.[2] With current estimates that the world is short of 17.4 million

trained health workers,[3] programmes need good reasons *not* to use CHWs.

CHWs have many names, including village health worker, lay health worker, accredited social health activists (ASHAs in India), and lady health worker (Pakistan); urban health worker is often used in cities. CHWs may be men or women. For ease of reference, this chapter refers to the CHW as female. With increasingly varied health needs in developing countries, CHWs must adapt to remain relevant and effective.

Their future role will continue to include common infectious and childhood illnesses, but also the care of

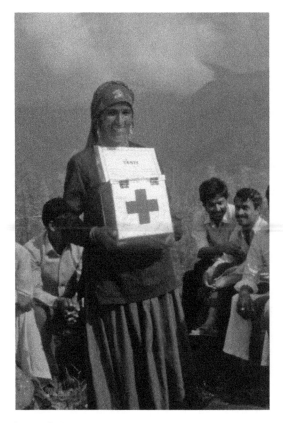

Figure 8.1 A CHW from the Himalayas.

Reproduced courtesy of Ted Lankester. This image is distributed under the terms of the Creative Commons Attribution Non-Commercial 4.0 International licence (CC-BY-NC), a copy of which is available at http://creativecommons.org/licenses/by-nc/4.0/.

those with non-communicable diseases (NCDs) such as hypertension and diabetes,[4] the people living with disability, and treatment of mental illness, including depression. In many places, the CHW is the main front-line health worker. Hospitals and primary health centres sometimes scarcely function, especially where HIV or other serious disease or civil unrest overwhelms the health system. But in other areas, as incomes improve, people will be increasingly drawn to hospitals or private practitioners as their first point of contact. In these situations, CHWs will need a higher educational background and more comprehensive training if they are going to meet people's increased expectations.

Some CHW programmes have not lived up to original expectations because of inadequacies in training, management, support, and supervision. Bearing this in mind, we must do everything possible to 'get it right' when we start a new programme, or scale up an existing one. It is helpful at this stage to give two examples of successful programmes—one NGO-led and one government-led.

The Bangladesh Rural Advancement Committee (BRAC) has been involved in grassroots programmes for over three decades and understands the needs of poor communities. This group alone has trained over 100,000 community health workers covering nearly one million people. As just one of their functions, these CHWs have trained millions of households in the use of oral rehydration therapy.[5]

As another example, the government health extension programme in Ethiopia has a dual cadre of CHWs: health extension workers with one year of formal training, and health development army volunteers (or community health promoters) who are trained to care for five to ten families, whom they visit in their homes. Most of the country has been reached.[6]

The majority of early CHW programmes were set up from the 1970s onwards by NGOs. Probably the most famous is the very successful Community Rural Health Project in Jamkhed, India, whose website is worth perusing in detail (http://www.crhp.jamkhed.org).

Later, especially during the 1990s and early 2000s, CHW programmes were questioned by health policy makers, donors, and governments. The emphasis switched to 'vertical programmes' (see Chapter 1). At the same time, some early CHW programmes failed to bring the hoped-for results, often because of poor leadership, supervision, and hospital support. However, more recently and especially since 2010, CHWs have become an increasingly central part of health policy in developing countries. The emphasis has moved from CHWs being mainly employed and led by CSOs to programmes led by governments, e.g. in India, Ethiopia, and Brazil.

CHWs will often play a growing role in helping to fulfil the objectives of universal health coverage and the third Sustainable Development Goal on health and beyond. Later in this chapter we look at some secrets of success in these 'new paradigm' CHW programmes. But committed government support and excellent management will be key.

Features of a traditional CHW: advantages and drawbacks

The CHW is selected by the community and ideally trained in the community. She lives in the community, serves the community, and may be paid by them. She 'belongs' and owes her allegiance to the community. Where governments take on CHWs, either as employees or as volunteers, there is a danger that these links to the community may be weakened.

The CHW has some *advantages* over other health workers, even those who are more highly qualified:

1. She is chosen and therefore accepted by the community.

2. She is available to the community because she lives there.

3. She understands the local language, culture, and everyday norms.

4. She is usually cost-effective, because she is inexpensive to train and can do many of the tasks traditionally done by doctors, nurses, and social workers.

5. She covers populations where other health workers are often unwilling or unable to work.[7]

6. She is cost effective. The return on investment in Sub Saharan Africa is estimated at $10 for every $1 dollar spent, compared to $44 for each child immunisation in LMICs.

It is also realistic to mention certain *drawbacks* of a CHW based programme so as to try and prevent them:

1. She may provide sub-standard care unless she is well trained, adequately supervised and regularly updated.

2. Any payment she receives for working as a CHW may be hard to sustain unless the community itself, or government, is involved in funding her.

3. She may have been incorrectly selected and may not have the right personality or sufficient motivation.

4. She may be insufficiently educated, though with appropriate training this can usually be overcome.

5. She may quite understandably be drawn by extra income, or status or future employment to gradually separate herself from the community. It can lead to high attrition rates of CHWs.[8]

This means, in practice, that a CHW programme that is well set up and well maintained can be highly successful, but a programme with poor planning and supervision may have little positive impact on the health of a community.

The roles and functions of the CHW

Roles

The CHW usually has a triple role in her community as health promoter, healthcare provider, and agent of change.

- *As health promoter* she will teach the whole community how to improve health and prevent illness (See Figure 8.2).

- *As health care provider* she will diagnose, and often treat, common illnesses early, before they become serious. She may also be expected to provide care and supervise medication for those with chronic illness.

- *As an agent of change* she will help the community change their knowledge, attitudes, and practice so that they lead healthier lives and tackle some of the social determinants of health.

Functions

The functions of the CHW will vary depending on many things, including the needs of the community, the availability of other sources of healthcare used by the community, government plans and policy, and specific local priorities—ideally those agreed upon between the community, the health programme, and the district health team. Above all, the functions of the CHW must follow national guidelines and any training curricula which the government has developed.

The following is a comprehensive list of a CHW's functions and *each programme will need to adapt and shorten this for its own use.* It shows the wide range of activities that can be carried out by a well-trained local community member. *A note of warning*: with governments increasingly drawing up curricula and guidance on the priority tasks expected of CHWs we must ensure our CHWs don't take additional responsibilities unless they genuinely have the time and inclination to do so. For example, the author was recently discussing with a West African health ministry the newly drawn-up curriculum for CHWs. He was disappointed not to see the inclusion of NCDs and mental health as part of their priority tasks. But with scarce resources and limited capacity it was clear that CHWs would not yet be able to take on these additional roles, important as they are Understanding "local politics" is a key skill (See Figure 8.4).

The functions of a CHW can be drawn from the following list.

1. Be first point of contact.

She must be willing to give appropriate care and advice to any community member as needed, within the limits of time, capacity, and distance agreed to by the community and her supervisor.

2. Educate about health.

She must be continually passing on knowledge in a practical and helpful way whenever the opportunity arises, both to individuals and to groups (Figure 8.2).

3. Care for children.
   a. Promote good nutrition.

The CHW can regularly weigh young children or measure the mid-upper arm circumference (MUAC) of children from 6 to 60 months of age (Figure 8.5). She will fill in a growth chart or other record card.

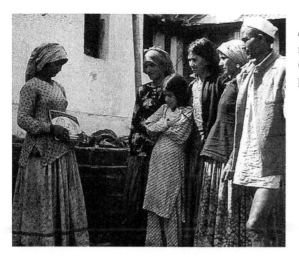

Figure 8.2 The CHW will teach at every opportunity

Reproduced courtesy of Ted Lankester. This image is distributed under the terms of the Creative Commons Attribution Non-Commercial 4.0 International licence (CC-BY-NC), a copy of which is available at http://creativecommons.org/licenses/by-nc/4.0/.

She will give practical feeding advice to parents, especially exclusive breastfeeding till the age of six months and complementary feeding from six months (see Chapter 14). She may help to arrange feeding programmes or help set up kitchen gardens.

b. Teach about oral rehydration solution (ORS) and other local forms of rehydration so that all community members know how and when to use this in the treatment of diarrhoea (Chapter 16).

c. Promote childhood immunizations according to the government's health programme

d. Distribute vitamin A, zinc, iron supplements, and worm medicine (anthelminthic) to young children (see Chapter 14 and Chapter 15).

e. Visit neonates and their mothers to advise on care or refer if serious problems arise (Chapter 17).

f. Ensure the supply of cotrimoxazole in children who are HIV-positive (Chapter 20).

A Cascading Health Promotion Model

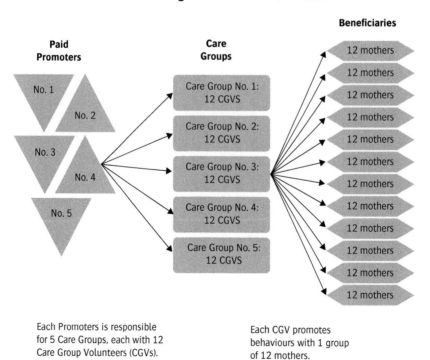

Figure 8.3 The Care Group Model as implemented by Food for the Hungry in Sofala Province, Mozambique.

Reproduced courtesy of Henry Perry, Care Groups: Experience and Evidence. Available at: https://www.slideshare.net/COREGroup1/care-group-presentation-29-may2014final. This image is distributed under the terms of the Creative Commons Attribution Non-Commercial 4.0 International licence (CC-BY-NC), a copy of which is available at http://creativecommons.org/licenses/by-nc/4.0/.

4. Care for mothers.

    a. Encourage antenatal care.

The CHW will motivate women to attend clinics or if sufficiently trained carry out checks herself.

She may distribute iron and folic acid to pregnant and lactating women, and, where relevant, antimalarials. She will promote tetanus immunization.

    b. Carry out deliveries.

The CHW if appropriately trained may do this herself or work alongside the traditional birth attendant (TBA) using clean and safe methods of delivery. She will refer women to skilled birth attendants where these are accessible and acceptable for facility-based deliveries or if problems arise in the pregnancy (Chapter 17).

    c. Give postnatal advice and care.

5. Promote child spacing and family planning and the prevention and treatment of sexually transmitted infections (Chapter 18).

6. Care for those with chronic infectious diseases, including HIV/AIDS and some neglected tropical diseases (see Chapter 16).

If this is programme policy she may identify cases of TB and supervise treatment schedules both for TB and for people living with HIV/AIDS. In doing so she will help to reduce the stigma of people living with HIV/AIDS.

7. Care in the community.

She will need to care for those with non-communicable diseases such as high blood pressure, cancer, diabetes, stroke and chronic obstructive pulmonary disease (COPD) (Chapter 22).

8. Care for the people living with disability.

This includes those with physical and mental disability, blindness, and hearing impairment (See Chapter 23). Also, The CHW should care for the elderly at home needing support and palliative care (Chapter 28).

9. Treat simple illnesses and give first aid.

Most CHWs will keep a stock of simple medicines, using them to treat common illnesses or severe symptoms, under the supervision of the health programme or District Health team. Where medicines are readily available, she may need to advise community members what medicines they need, including the dose and duration, and about avoiding unnecessary medicines and injections.

10. Know when to refer.

The CHW will learn how to recognize and refer serious illnesses and those she cannot treat herself.

11. Develop public health activities.

With the support of the village or urban health committee, the CHW may promote appropriate human and household waste disposal, safe water, smokeless cooking hearths, and other improvements.

12. Keep records that are needed by the health programme, or required by the government or donor agencies.

13. Work alongside her supervisor, other members of the health team or government health services.

This may include taking part in surveys, immunization programmes, care of school children, teaching and supervision, health centre activities, and community projects.

14. Help to develop community clubs.

Female CHWs may help to set up women's groups or teach female literacy, as well as help to set up adolescent or youth activities. CHWs may also play a role in microcredit schemes.

15. Encourage parents to send children to school.

16. Promote tobacco control and smoking cessation, and advise against alcohol and other substance abuse.

17. Promote the rights and safety of women, safeguarding of children and other vulnerable community members.

18. Carry out other activities as discussed between her, the community, the health team and the district health team.

19. Increasingly use smart phones (SMS technology) as a key means of communication (See Chapter 26).

20. Give alerts of emerging outbreaks of illness.

This is known as Global Health Security and the early tracking of Ebola in West Africa is a good example of the CHW's potential value in picking up early warning signs of serious epidemics.

Some programme examples

Uganda

Members of village health teams (VHTs) are selected by the community and are each responsible for between twenty-five and thirty households. They are volunteers who should be able to read and write in the local language.

They conduct health promotion activities and diagnose, treat and refer sick children to the nearest health centre. Initial training lasts for ten days and is carried out by health centre staff and NGOs following the national VHT training guidelines.[9]

Ghana

Where the eye disease trachoma is common, CHWs have been trained to distribute the antibiotic azithromycin to both adults and children and have encouraged face and hand washing.

Zanzibar

CHWs already trained in other community activities, e.g. polio eradication, can switch their skills to new priorities such as treating filariasis. Many thousands of CHWs have been trained to distribute ivermectin or albendazole to treat community members.

Iran

In the OR Iran's primary healthcare programme, CHWs known as Behvarz workers are effective in community treatment of NCDs including hypertension and diabetes, providing they are well trained and follow well-established guidelines.[10]

Pakistan

In rural Pakistan, CHWs with three days of intensive study and training had an impressive effect on recovery rates of mothers who had post-natal depression and this effect persisted for more than a year.[11]

Malawi

Orthopaedic clinical officers treat nine out of ten orthopaedic problems and injuries in some rural hospitals and health centres. They represent one group of what are known as non-physician clinicians (NPCs), a term used to include both CHWs and other more highly trained health care workers who are mainly based in health facilities but who have strong community links.[12]

The Care Model

More recently, an innovative and powerful new methodology based on peer educators is being put into practice in several countries (Figure 8.3). In Mozambique, about 50,000 households with pregnant women or children under two years of age are organized into blocks of twelve households. One volunteer peer educator (care group volunteer, or CGV) is selected for each block. Approximately twelve CGVs meet together as a group every two weeks with a paid project promoter to

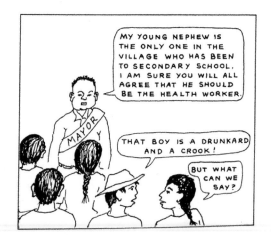

Figure 8.4 CHWs need to know how to handle community politics.

learn a new message or skill in child health or nutrition. Then the CGVs share the new message with mothers in their assigned blocks.[13]

One Million Health Workers Plan

This is a widely supported approach being used in Sub-Saharan Africa, which is being rolled out in several countries and is pioneering the use of Smartphones as a key part of enabling CHWs and CHW programmes to be as effective as possible.[14]

Evidence for an effective CHW

CHWs have been used for many years in a wide variety of both government-led and NGO-led programmes. It is only recently that solid evidence has emerged about just how effective CHWs can be. At the time of writing, one of the most detailed summaries of evidence for their effectiveness in maternal and child health and TB comes from a Cochrane review,[15] which found that CHWs are likely to bring about an increase in the number of women who breastfeed, an increase in the number of children who have an up-to-date immunization schedule, fewer deaths among children under five, fewer children who suffer from fever, diarrhoea, and pneumonia, and an increase in the number of TB patients cured. With the rapid increase in the use of CHWs, further evidence for their effectiveness is continually being published.[16]

What we need to do

Selecting a CHW

It is common to see programmes in some villages or slum areas where the community seems to make impressive health improvements while others stand still. This may be because one community has a more effective CHW than another. The correct selection of a CHW is of critical importance to the success of a community programme.

The CHW should be chosen by the community, unless there are strong government guidelines that insist on Ministry of Health involvement. Community choice can only be successful if the community and its leaders thoroughly understand what functions a CHW will carry out, and therefore, what personality and talents she needs to have. Two to three meetings or discussions may be necessary in order for the community to grasp these issues. Taking time over this stage can help the community to understand and own the CHW programme.

For example, in one Himalayan programme, community members assumed that the CHW would serve as a low-grade health aide. Because of this assumption, it was interpreted that her level of education and intelligence would be unimportant. As a result, inappropriate people were put forward for the role. This is a good example of how time taken in explanation is never wasted. The more community members understand the role and function of their CHW, the more they will support her and use her, and the greater the chances that the best person will be appointed to the role.

Each community has its own way of reaching decisions. Although the health team should not usually interfere in decision making, it must ensure that, in whatever way is appropriate, the CHW is acceptable to the majority of community members. Communities should be discouraged from suggesting a relative or friend of the local chief or mayor as this often causes problems for the programme (See Figure 8.4). Sometimes a community or village health committee (VHC) puts forward several candidates and allows the health team to make the final choice. If the health team or the government suggests a community member who appears very appropriate, the community still needs to confirm that choice.

Depending on the population density, and the CHWs functions, a part-time CHW can cover at most fifty families, but ideally not more than twenty-five. It is often a good plan for CHWs to work in pairs, especially where they function as unpaid volunteers or where communities are very scattered or less secure.

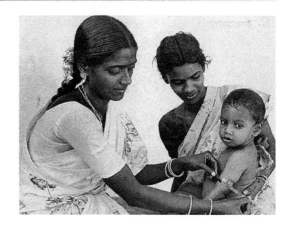

Figure 8.5 A CHW in south India measures a mid-upper arm circumference

Reproduced courtesy of John and Penny Hubley. This image is distributed under the terms of the Creative Commons Attribution Non-Commercial 4.0 International licence (CC-BY-NC), a copy of which is available at http://creativecommons.org/licenses/by-nc/4.0/.

For example, in a recent CHW training programme in Chin State, Myanmar, where health workers had to travel for up to five days to attend a month-long training programme, each village selected two health workers. This gave the trainees greater security and comradeship when walking long distances as well as during the training.

What type of person should be selected?

Male or female?

There is no absolute rule about whether a man or a woman takes the role of the CHW. Men are more appropriate in some communities, women in others. Some communities will expect men to care for men, and women for women. Box 8.1 shows some principles to consider when choosing a CHW, but there are many exceptions.

Well educated?

A CHW does not necessarily need to be literate or educated. However, in most communities, basic education is increasingly seen as important because of the range and complexity of tasks carried out by CHWs. Older CHWs, (See Figure 8.6) or those with little formal education, may struggle. The completion of ten years of schooling or at least primary education is a useful guideline but intelligence and eagerness to learn are just as important. Note that the remotest areas that

---

Box 8.1 **Aspects to consider when choosing a CHW**

Men:
- may be less busy than women.
- may be better educated.
- may find it easier to liaise with government officials and with other agencies.
- may be insisted upon in some societies.
- can more effectively prevent and treat sexually transmitted infections in men.
- may be more appropriate where security problems and personal safety cause concern.

Women:
- may be more appropriate in mother and child health.
- are often less eager to make money or set up as private practitioners.
- are more likely to be resident and available in the community.
- may be more compassionate and sensitive to people's needs.
- may be the only ones who can look after other women and children.
- as a CHW, may become a role model for female leadership.

A CHW should ideally be:
- a well-respected community member;
- friendly, approachable and kind;
- concerned for others' welfare;
- able to keep a confidence and not gossip;
- not primarily motivated by status or money;
- intelligent and eager to learn;
- hard-working;
- respected; and
- willing to visit any community member who is sick or in need of care, safety and security allowing.

---

are most in need of CHW programmes may have the weakest educational facilities as well. Many government programmes specify educational requirements.

Healthy and strong?

CHWs generally need to be healthy and strong. They will usually continue their other jobs at home or in the community in addition to serving as CHWs. However, the key question is based on occupational health principles: if appointed, would the CHW be in sufficiently good health to carry out the specific tasks she would be expected to do in the community, i.e. the tasks outlined in the job description?

For example, those suffering from infectious TB should not be chosen until the infection has cleared, although people who have been cured of TB and leprosy are often suitable. Those with mild forms of disability may be able to carry out most tasks needed. There are no valid reasons why people who are HIV-positive but otherwise well should not be chosen as CHWs, although they should be on regular antiretroviral therapy (ART) as an example to the community.

Mature in age and outlook

Younger people are usually quicker to learn. They are, however, more likely to marry and move away, or have young children, which may make them less available, unless they have a supportive family or can arrange childcare. Younger people may sometimes command less respect. Community members with previous experience as volunteers in another capacity often make suitable candidates.

Be supported by the family

It is important, especially for female CHWs, that they have family support for their work. Husbands, partners, mothers-in-law, and other family members need to understand their role, encourage them, and offer practical support when needed.

Already engaged in health work

TBAs make effective CHWs, providing they are flexible enough to change some patterns of ingrained behaviour (Figure 8.6). Their communities already know them and use their services, and they are usually respected. Other traditional practitioners can become effective CHWs, but there is some risk that after training they may use their new knowledge to prioritize their own earnings, or be so interested in curative care that they take little interest in preventative healthcare activities. In most situations, the ideal person to assume the role of the CHW is a kind-hearted woman, or man, aged between 25 and 45, in a stable marital relationship, and with atleast ten years of schooling.

Training a CHW

Many good books and guidelines have been written on the training of CHWs and some are listed in 'Further reading and resources'. Try to obtain a resource that is appropriate for your area or that is published nationally or regionally. Follow any national guidelines.

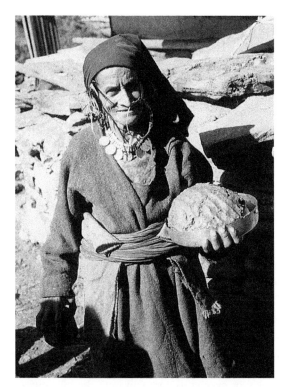

Figure 8.6 TBA in a remote mountain village. But will she be able to cope with learning the skills now needed by a CHW?

Reproduced courtesy of Ted Lankester. This image is distributed under the terms of the Creative Commons Attribution Non-Commercial 4.0 International licence (CC-BY-NC), a copy of which is available at http://creativecommons.org/licenses/by-nc/4.0/.

The personal development of the CHW

CHWs often come from poor or less-privileged backgrounds. When initially chosen they may lack self-confidence. This is especially common with women, who may have been less favoured as children and disadvantaged in education. But after a few brief months of training, they will be expected to treat illnesses, give health talks, and become agents of community change. A transformation will need to take place within the CHW to make this possible (See Figure 8.7).

The single most important part of CHW training is personal development so that the CHW becomes confident and caring (Figure 8.7). This will come about largely through the attitude of the health team and the respect with which she is treated. It can also be helped by specific leadership training or coaching.

There is no place in CHW teaching for the harsh and insensitive attitudes sometimes seen from overworked staff in higher level health facilities. Such behaviour may not only frighten and stifle CHWs but also teach them to treat their patients in the same manner. All

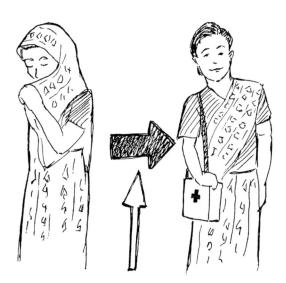

Figure 8.7 Effects of transformation.

Reproduced courtesy of David Gifford. This image is distributed under the terms of the Creative Commons Attribution Non-Commercial 4.0 International licence (CC-BY-NC), a copy of which is available at http://creativecommons.org/licenses/by-nc/4.0/.

health team members will need to be understanding and appreciative of the CHW—her gifts, her beliefs, and her fears. They should never despise or judge her for ideas that may be wrong or different, or for customs and habits that may seem strange. They should take an interest in her family, her community, and her traditions. This will involve learning from the CHW and adopting the good ideas present in her traditions and background.

This process of conferring dignity will happen both in training and day-to-day work. The health team must always show the CHW respect, and be careful not to ask her to do menial tasks that diminish her in the eyes of others.

Training locations

Different programmes will choose different places. A few will choose hospitals or central training sites, which may be convenient but are probably not the most suitable environments. Most will prefer local health centres or community rooms. Some remote areas depend on one location with trainees having to make their own way to the centre. Although it is less convenient for trainers, there are many advantages in training CHWs as near as possible to their own communities:

1. It is more convenient for the CHWs.

In poorer rural areas it may be hard for busy women to leave home for training. They may not be permitted by their husband or family to sleep away from their community.

2. CHWs can relate what they have learned to actual problems in their community.

They can take part in a community survey as part of their training.

3. Trainers can learn about the CHW's lifestyle and the day-to-day problems she is likely to face.
4. Practice in the field can be done more easily.
5. The community observes the training being given to the CHW, which increases their belief in her and her value.

There are also practical reasons why rural CHWs should not be taken for residential teaching to towns and cities, especially with male trainees. The more they participate in town-based training programmes, the more distant they feel from their villages. One health educator suggested that, in this scenario, 'all that is achieved in the end is just another set of unproductive workers in government service, or setting up in private practice' (Figure 8.8).

In practice, especially with government-led schemes, CHWs may not have much choice and frequently a hospital will be chosen as most convenient for the trainers.

The length of the training

The amount of time spent on training the CHW will depend on both the educational level of the CHW, and

the time she has available to undertake the training programme. CHWs who are illiterate or have only had very basic schooling may take a long time to learn basic knowledge and skills, as may older CHWs who have never studied or have not done so for a long time. Additionally, most female CHWs from rural areas are also mothers and farmers. Urban CHWs may have part-time paid employment in order to care for the needs of the family.

The length of training must fit in with their home commitments. Each programme should design its own timescale and pattern of training, but there are two commonly used training models. Regardless of which of these models is used, regular training and updates must continue for as long as the CHW is working. This culture of continuing professional development is essential. It helps the CHW to remain motivated, but it is important to ensure familiarity with new forms of treatment that become available, and as new programmes are implemented by the government.

Block training

Teaching initially occurs daily for a period of from one week to three months; three to six weeks is often an appropriate length. Regular lessons then continue once weekly or once every fortnight until the full course is completed. Alternatively, they can have further shorter block periods of training at regular, e.g. yearly, intervals. This method helps trainees develop fresh approaches and gain new knowledge that is regularly reinforced. Block training often takes place in a hospital or central training site, which, while convenient for teachers, is often inconvenient for rural CHWs who may have to

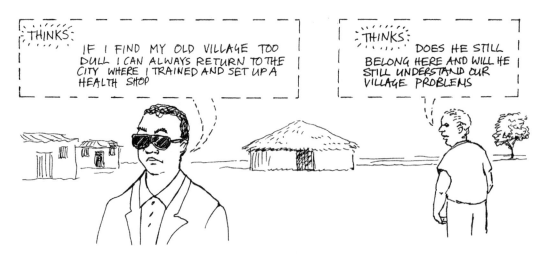

Figure 8.8 Disadvantages of training health workers away from their own communities.

travel long distances. One major advantage of block training is that CHWs may be able to start working in their communities within three months.

Weekly training

Weekly teaching occurs one or two days or half days a week until the course is complete. Although convenient for rural CHWs, the process of learning may be slower. With intermittent training, it may take six months to a year before the CHW has sufficient knowledge to be both safe and valued within the community.

Who should do the training?

When searching for a suitable candidate to train the CHW, often the answer in practice is 'whoever is available' However, those leading the training will need appropriate qualities, adequate qualifications, and have had excellent training themselves. Ideally, trainers should have an outgoing manner, and be friendly, lively, humorous, enthusiastic, and good at explaining and encouraging participation. They should also have an appropriate cultural background; the smaller the language and cultural gap between trainer and trainees, the easier the training.

Furthermore, ideally trainers should have practical experience in community health, as well as nursing, paramedical, or teachers' training. In practice, trainers will come from a great variety of backgrounds and will include doctors, nurses, lab technicians, teachers, medical assistants, multi-purpose health workers, and social workers. Trainers influence all those they train. This makes it essential that CHW trainers are themselves carefully trained to highlight affirming and positive attitudes towards those they teach, and use interactive, interesting, and varied teaching methods.

It may be helpful to inquire about Training of Trainers (TOT) courses. If not, it may be necessary to create a TOT course, ideally with other local CSOs or government programmes that may have the same training needs.

Aspects of successful teaching

Student-centred teaching

Traditionally, teachers stand at the front, look down on the class, and teach facts to their pupils. Pupils learn by rote, often failing to understand, and rarely participating because they are scared to ask questions. The training of CHWs should be the opposite of this (See Figure 8.9). Everyone should sit in a circle to reduce any hierarchy, and it is worth remembering that, in this type of programme, the teacher learns from the students and vice versa—everyone learns from each other. Teaching is not a one-way, nor a two-way but an all-way process. Each

class member is encouraged to take part, share ideas, and ask questions. Contributions from everyone are welcomed.

Problem-solving teaching

Lessons will often start with the student's problems and the community's concerns, rather than with the teacher establishing the agenda. For example, while many teachers traditionally start their health course with a lesson on human anatomy, the CHWs on the training session may instead be wondering about eye infections or recent deaths from malaria. A good teacher will choose a lesson relevant to the CHWs' current concerns, and not simply follow a syllabus from start to finish. In the context of community health, the purpose of knowledge is to help find effective answers to practical problems.

Using the trainees' knowledge

Before starting to teach a subject, we should first discover what the trainees know already, and how they might use that knowledge in practice. We need to discover if their knowledge of a health topic is correct, as well as understand the reasons behind any health beliefs held by them and their communities. For example, in many parts of the world, e.g. in parts of South Asia pregnant women believe they should eat less food so that their babies will be small and less likely to get stuck during delivery.

Good teachers will respect the reasoning behind beliefs and gently correct any wrong ideas which make an important difference to health. Many incorrect beliefs can be left uncorrected. For example, where custom prevents mothers from eating eggs during pregnancy, there is no immediate need to contradict this, providing the overall diet is adequate.

> Correct ideas are approved and built upon.
> Neutral ideas are left alone.
> Unhelpful ideas are pointed out and corrected.
> All ideas are listened to with respect.

Encouraging, friendly, enjoyable, and a multi-faceted approach

We should have an encouraging, not critical, approach, especially when CHWs may be unwilling to accept ideas that go against their own beliefs and traditions. The more CHWs enjoy the lesson, the more they will be open to new ideas. In turn, because they absorb attitudes as well as ideas, they are more likely to make their teaching to community members enjoyable and interesting.

A large tree is more quickly felled by three axes falling at different angles than by one axe always hitting at the same angle. So, for example, we can use different senses in order to encourage trainees to hear what is said, see what is shown, touch what is presented; finally, using role play or drama, they can act out any lessons that have been learned.

At the end of each lesson, ask the pupils to give a summary of what they have learned. Make sure they have really grasped one subject before going on to the next.

Structured lesson plans

Our plan for each lesson should include various components. This structure will not only keep us organized, but will create a sense of familiarity for those being trained. Each lesson should include:

1. Greetings, welcome, and introductions.

Sometimes it is helpful to start with an act of devotion that the group enjoys; members of the group may sometimes lead.

2. Discussion of problems that CHWs have recently come across in the community.

Minor points can be discussed at the time, while more major ones can form the basis of the day's lesson or be tackled later.

3. Review of the previous lesson.
4. Introduction of the day's subject.

Trainees should first share their own knowledge, attitude, and practice (KAP) on the topic for the day's lesson.

5. Consolidation of the day's topic.

This is the main part of the lesson. Use imaginative methods so the topic is really understood and learned. Use various methods here, including repeating back, role playing, storytelling, drama, songs, quizzes, interviews, etc. (see Chapter 4).

6. Practical use of the day's topic.

A skill may be learned in the classroom, e.g. bandaging or weighing. There may be a practical assignment to do in the community, such as teaching a lesson or checking for a symptom, e.g. night blindness or chronic cough.

7. Review and giving of reminder cards.

After reviewing the main points of the lesson, the CHWs are given special cards. These reminder cards summarize the main points—in words if the trainees can read, in pictures if they are unable to. The trainer can send a reminder by mobile phone after two or three days to remind CHWs of the main learning points.

Topics included in the curriculum

As CHW programmes become increasingly focused in global health, Ministries of Health will be drawing up a curriculum that is most suitable for the country, within

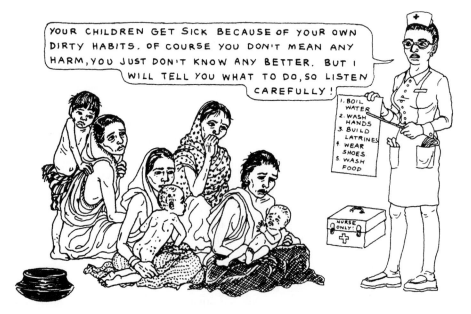

Figure 8.9 Teaching should be not like this.

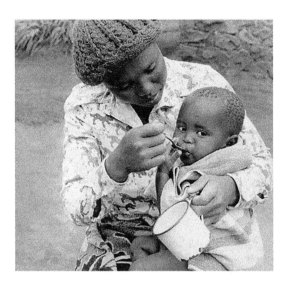

Figure 8.10 The CHW has taught the mother how to use oral rehydration solution, but does she also know how to make it?

Reproduced courtesy of John and Penny Hubley. This image is distributed under the terms of the Creative Commons Attribution Non-Commercial 4.0 International licence (CC-BY-NC), a copy of which is available at http://creativecommons.org/licenses/by-nc/4.0/.

the time and capacity of the CHW work force. This curriculum can be adapted or modified in agreement with the community and district medical team to be as relevant as possible within the local setting.

We need to move away from a situation where each different NGO uses their own curriculum (Figure 8.10). However, there are still widely used programmes that can sit alongside agreed curricula and add spark, interest, and new ideas. One example is Tearfund's Umoja programme, which has been used in Ethiopia with great effect.

If a government CHW training curriculum is not in place (or being developed), voluntary health associations, well-respected local hospitals with their own CHW programme, international sources such as the World Health Organization or respected CSOs may have valuable suggestions. The Arukah Network website and other resources at the end of this chapter provide further information. A suggested syllabus is shown in Table 8.1 but this should only be seen as a general guide.

Using new technology

A new, interesting but as yet unvalidated method for training CHWs in remote locations is through the use of information technology. For other uses of new technology in CHW programmes, see Chapter 26. For example, BBC Media Action has launched a breakthrough mobile health service to train 200,000 community health workers at a fraction of the cost of face-to-face training. It

aims to deliver hundreds of life-saving messages without reams of paper or expensive hardware. 'Mobile Kunji' and 'Mobile Academy' are accessible on any handset, on common short codes, and the lowest tariffs in India across six of the country's largest mobile operators. The services are initially being rolled out in Bihar, northern India, to educate 22 million rural families.

Notes on the curriculum

Subjects included

The list of subjects provided in Table 8.1 is a guide only—each project will customize its own curriculum. Also, it is not necessary to follow a strict order when teaching lessons. Start with subjects of interest to the trainees or that are relevant to the community. Mix teaching on diseases (often enjoyed most by the trainees) with other subjects like hygiene or practical first aid. Note that some subjects can be covered easily in one lesson; others may need two, or more.

Length and number of lessons

When deciding on length of the lessons, aim for about two to three hours per lesson, and ensure that there is plenty of variety of teaching techniques and that the trainees participate. Arrange breaks during the lesson for chat, refreshments, or games. When block teaching takes place trainees can become exhausted if they are expected to absorb too much information in one sitting. Regular breaks, interactive sessions, and energizers (see Chapter 2) can help. Providing opportunities for exercise, fun, prayer and other activities can make the whole teaching experience a rich and rewarding time. Importantly, don't ignore boredom. If trainees become bored, stop the lesson, change the approach, or arrange an activity: bored people don't learn.

Hospital experience for trainees

Whether or not a hospital or health centre is used as the teaching centre, CHWs will need to understand how a hospital works. A senior member of the health team should give trainee CHWs a tour of each department and introduce staff who are likely to see referrals from the community health programme. As well as benefiting CHWs, this will have several helpful results for patients who may be referred to hospital. CHWs will be able to give them advice and information before they are referred, and they may receive better care in the hospital because staff have met their CHW.

A transfer system can be set up between the CHW and hospital, which encourages continuity of care. In urban areas it can be much more difficult to make the personal contacts described here because of the size of

Table 8.1 Suggested syllabus for CHW training. Each programme needs to select and prioritize the most important topics

Care of under-fives:

1. How to recognize a sick child
2. How to care for a sick child
3. How to weigh children and use growth charts, how to measure the MUAC
4. Malnutrition: types, causes and prevention
5. Malnutrition: supplementary and therapeutic feeding
6. Hygiene
7. Immunizations
8. Diarrhoea and methods for rehydration including ORS
9. Acute respiratory infection (ARI) and its treatment
10. HIV/AIDS: its recognition and management, prevention of mother-to-child transmission

Care of pregnant mothers:

1. Human reproduction
2. Antenatal care: normal and abnormal signs, food supplements, preparation for delivery
3. Birth of the child: stages of labour, normal and abnormal deliveries, use of delivery kit
4. Postnatal care
5. Care of newborn: breastfeeding
6. Family planning and child spacing

Anatomy and physiology:

1. Parts of the body and how they work

Prevention and treatment of common illnesses:

1. Diarrhoea and worms
2. Abdominal pain
3. Chest infections
4. Tuberculosis
5. Malaria
6. Typhoid and cholera
7. Measles
8. Sexually transmitted infections (STIs)
9. HIV/AIDS: prevention, voluntary counselling and testing (VCT), home-based care, and use of ART
10. Health committees and women's groups
11. Anaemia
12. Eye diseases
13. Ear diseases
14. Mouth and tooth problems
15. Problems of menstruation
16. Urinary infections
17. Skin problems
18. Other locally important diseases, e.g. dengue fever, schistosomiasis, zika

19. Mental illness
20. NCDs: cardiovascular disease, COPD*, diabetes, stroke and cancer
21. Care of those living with disability, including the blind and hearing impaired
22. Care of the elderly: palliative care

First aid:

1. Cuts and bruises: bandaging
2. Burns
3. Bone injuries
4. Serious soft tissue injuries: shock
5. Animal bites and injuries
6. Snake and scorpion bites
7. Drowning
8. Poisoning
9. The unconscious patient
10. Cardiopulmonary resuscitation
11. Prevention of common accidents in home, community and the workplace, reducing the risk of road crashes
12. Treatment of drug reactions and collapse after injection

Environmental health:

1. Safe water
2. Sanitation and waste disposal
3. Healthy households and handwashing
4. Housing improvements: smokeless hearths
5. Tobacco, alcohol and drug abuse
6. Air pollution
7. Kitchen gardens
8. Appropriate development

General:

1. The role and function of the CHW
2. How a hospital works
3. How and when to refer patients
4. Record keeping and simple accounting
5. Healthy living
6. Keeping and using a medical kit
7. Methods of teaching and communicating
8. Leading discussion groups: raising awareness
9. Details of the health project to which they belong
10. Health committees and women's groups
11. National health problems, programmes, and priorities
12. Co-operating with others
13. SDGs, WHO, and UNICEF
14. Use of ICT including smart phones
15. Food and water security/disaster preparedness
16. Leadership and advocacy skills

most hospitals and their less personal atmosphere. In these situations, the most practical approach may involve the CHW accompanying the referred patient to the hospital.

Further training and examinations

After the basic curriculum has been covered, CHWs will need further development and instruction, including revision and updates on important subjects, classes or seminars on new health topics, and introduction to wider development issues. It is also worth considering providing Training of Trainers (TOT) so that CHWs themselves can become trainers, supervisors, or eventually trainers of trainers.

In addition to supplemental instruction and training, CHWs should have regular oral and practical tests to ensure their skills and knowledge are accurate and up to date. Before they receive health kits, arrange more thorough testing. For example, call in an outside 'examiner' who is familiar with the community who can test each candidate fairly and thoroughly.

The exam should be oral or written depending on the CHW's education, and needs to include questions on how to solve actual problems, including something practical (See Figure 8.10). Key topics should include how to recognize common illnesses and the correct uses of medicines. Where CHWs are supplied with health kits, the accurate use of medicines is crucial and will be a main factor in how safe and useful the CHW is for her community.

Supervising a CHW

There is no point training a CHW, encouraging her to work in the community, and then leaving her to her own devices. The quality of care a CHW can provide depends on how effectively she is encouraged, mentored, and supervised. Mentors should aim to visit at least weekly in the early stages unless communities are remote or scattered, the weather prevents it, or there is civil unrest. Once a CHW is established and confident, supervisors can visit less frequently as long as there is regular contact in other ways, e.g. in the health centre, training centre, or when submitting her monthly reports. The supervisor or mentor will often be the same person as the trainer. The use of Smartphones or other mobiles can revolutionize the connection, support, and encouragement a CHW receives from her mentor and from other CHWs (see Chapter 26).

The main tasks of a supervisor are to provide encouragement, support, and training, as well as both psychological and emotional support. The CHW will value her supervisor's advice about practical problems. She may also need help with personal troubles, especially if these arise from her CHW work. The supervisor must be willing to support and advise without fostering dependence. Significant issues are ideally handled face to face and not by phone.

Additionally, if the CHW needs correction or constructive criticism, the supervisor should do this gently, privately, and fairly. There should be ten words of praise for every one word of criticism. CHWs should never have their knowledge or approach corrected in front of community members. It is *essential* that their dignity is safeguarded in front of their peers.

Finally, when appropriate, the supervisor should make sure each CHW receives correct payment on time.

The CHW's health kit

Although some CHWs will be involved only in health promotion, curative care helps make a CHW more popular and more influential in health promotion. In some areas there will be no need for CHWs to carry health kits because there will be alternative suppliers, e.g. pharmacies, primary health centres. In other areas there is such a shortage of trained health workers and appropriate medicines that a CHW able to treat illness at village level is of great value and can save lives.

This use of health kits by a CHW also ties in with the global health priority of universal health coverage, of which CHWs are a crucial part. CHWs can visit patients in their community, preventing the need for sick patients to walk hours or even days to visit a health centre. There must be clear guidelines for CHWs who will be treating patients and will therefore need a health kit:

1. It must be legal in the country or district for the CHW to be able to dispense.
2. CHWs must be thoroughly trained and the community must have this assurance.
3. Medicines must be reliably supplied by the programme or government.
4. There should be no gaps in the supply chain so the community knows they can depend on their CHW, and that medicines will always be available.
5. CHWs need careful instructions about how to use each medicine reliably and safely. This is best done as a written protocol or group direction that, in effect, is a prescribing mechanism and enables the CHW to dispense. This must be in agreement with regulations and practices used nationally.

Medicines in the kit

The choice of medicines to include in the health kit is a top-level decision and a doctor familiar with work in the community should advise on it. As mentioned, we will need to be sure about national regulations on prescribing medicines, and whether CHWs are allowed to dispense, and if they are, that they are trained to do so. If an error occurs and a legal case is brought, it will be essential that the medicine prescribed has been recorded by name, dose, and date, and the reason for use is clearly stated, even if CHWs who have poor literacy have used simple symbols. Medicines chosen should be effective, simple, safe, as inexpensive as possible, and easily obtainable.

The exact choice of medicines to include will depend on local disease patterns, cost and availability of medicines, level of training of the CHW, availability of medicines from other sources, and prescribing regulations. Many government programmes list the medicines that CHWs are allowed or encouraged to prescribe (see also Chapter 11). Table 8.2 provides a suggested list of health kit medicines.

Equipment in the kit

Keep the equipment included in the health kit simple (see Box 8.2) and in accordance with the CHW's training (Figure 8.11). It could include bandages, tape and cotton wool; scissors and safety pins; gloves; alcohol wipes; MUAC measurer and/or portable weighing scale; simple health booklets and flashcards or teaching aids; delivery kits if used (see Chapter 17); record book and ball point pens; and a smart phone where appropriate.

Presenting the kit

This is an excellent chance for the district health team, the health programme, and the community to work together, and it needs to be planned with all parties involved.

The health kit should ideally be handed over to the CHW in a special presentation or 'passing out' ceremony. This has various benefits: the CHW is encouraged and affirmed in front of her people; the community has an opportunity to learn more about healthcare; and the project has a chance to raise community awareness. It is also a chance for a good celebration. The presentation itself should be festive, and can include cultural items such as health songs or a short drama. Community leaders can say a few words (preferably not political speeches). A guest of honour can present the boxes and certificates with each CHW being photographed in turn. A senior member of the district health team should attend.

The health committee chairperson or programme director can help the community understand more about the work of the CHW by explaining what she can and cannot do. The speaker can ask the community to

give her encouragement and forgive any mistakes she makes when she first starts work.

Keeping records

Records, whether digital or written, need to be kept as simple as possible with minimum duplication. Where CHWs have smartphones, these can be programmed beforehand with an info recording app for the essential information required by the programme and government. Using the app can be relatively simple but the CHW will need careful training. There may be someone from the VHC or woman's group who can help with this until the CHW is confident. Digitally recorded information must be kept secure.

There will often be a national system for CHW records, especially when programmes are government-led or government-funded. If we have made sure there is no appropriate digital system used by government (or CSOs), we can follow the system described here, which is appropriate if a CHW is literate or can work with a literate friend, relative, or colleague. Where this is not possible, a book with pictograms or symbols can be designed. There are vital pieces of information that should be recorded.

A list of patients seen and treatment given

A possible layout on a double page is shown in Table 8.3. Under 'Treatment' always record the name of any medicine used along with dose and total number of pills given.

An updated list of all 'at-risk' patients or families

This is the CHW's list of those needing special care or who need visiting on a regular basis. This list includes:

- under-five malnourished children;
- under-five children with any acute or chronic illness, and those who have not completed immunizations;
- pregnant and postnatal women;
- patients with TB, and people living with HIV/AIDS requiring home care;
- those with NCDs, e.g. diabetes, raised blood pressure;
- the people living with disability, very old, or anyone suffering social stigma because of an illness or condition;
- those with significant mental health problems, including depression; and
- those recently discharged from hospital.

These community members can be categorized or combined, but in both cases, include details as in

Table 8.2 Suggested list of medicines for CHW's health kit

Disease/symptom	Medicine**	Comments
1. Pain, fever	Paracetamol (500 mg/100 mg) Aspirin (300 mg)	Aspirin not suitable if stomach ulcers common, and not to be used in children under 16.
2. Pneumonia in children	Amoxicillin (or erythromycin)	With careful doses and protocols.
3. Stomach ache/ Indigestion	Aluminium hydroxide (500 mg)	Or omeprazole 20mg. If severe or persistent refer to hospital.
4. Intestinal worms	Mebendazole (100 mg/500 mg) Albendazole (400 mg)	Treatment of choice for pinworm, roundworm, hookworm, whipworm.
5. Diarrhoea, dehydration	Oral rehydration salts	Use cheapest available. Also, teach community how to make it up, or how to make sugar-salt solution, or use local liquid foods such as rice water.
6. Nausea, sickness	Prochlorperazine 5mg	Or other recommended locally
7. Malaria	Nationally recommended malaria treatment	Areas with high resistance need specialized advice. Ensure insecticide impregnated bed-nets are being bought and used.
8. Anaemia and for use in pregnant and lactating mothers	Ferrous salt (equiv. 60 mg Fe) alone or with Folic Acid (0.40 mg)	Warn that stools may turn black. Use iron with folic acid during pregnancy.
9. Serious bacterial infections*	Amoxicillin (500 mg) or erythromycin (500 mg)	Life-saving in Acute Respiratory Infections (ARIs). Valuable in many situations. Careful protocols needed for prescribing.
10. Allergy and itching, insect bites	Chlorphenamine (4 mg)	Warn about drowsiness
11. Vitamin A	Vitamin A tabs or syrup	Use as per info in chapter on nutrition. Ideally with zinc.
12. Eye infections	Tetracycline eye ointment 1% or gentamicin 0.3% drops	Cures most eye infections. Tetracycline or azithromycin cures trachoma if used early and correctly.
13. Scabies	Benzyl benzoate (25% lotion) or permethrin cream (5%) or lotion (1%)	May be alternative local remedy
14. Rub for muscles, bruises, headache, etc.	Local liniment or balm, e.g. Vicks, menthol	Usually popular
15. Antiseptic for cleansing skin	Chlorhexidine or local equivalent, soap	For cleaning skin infections/wounds
16. Hypertension	Bendroflumethiazide 2.5 mg	As part of an agreed programme, and often using other different or additional medicines.
17. Asthma	Salbutamol inhaler	With careful instructions
18. For umbilical stump	Chlorhexidine 1%	At birth

* These include chest infections such as acute respiratory infection, e.g. pneumonia and bronchitis, severe ear and skin infections, tooth abscess, severe sore throat or sinusitis, urinary infection, dysentery with fever, and some forms of sexually transmitted infection.
** Other commonly used drugs include: combined antibacterial and antifungal skin cream; ergometrine or misoprostol (blood loss after abortion or delivery, see Chapter 17); Senna (constipation); metronidazole (amoeba, giardia, trichomonas); multivitamins (food shortage conditions only); artesunate suppositories to treat malaria in children; phenobarbital (epilepsy). Some CHWs will also distribute oral contraceptives and condoms, see Chapter 18). Note: this is a fairly comprehensive list and many programmes may wish to shorten this depending on their situation, especially when CHWs first start using medicines.

Box 8.2 **Notes on medicines and equipment**

1. Medicines should be carefully packed into secure, damp-proof containers. Liquid medicines must be stored in leak-proof bottles.
2. Medicines must be clearly labelled. If CHWs are illiterate this can be done through symbols or pictures. For example, tablets to treat malaria can be labelled with the drawing of a mosquito. Normal doses can be recorded as a reminder.
3. Supplies must be regularly restocked. When seeing a sick villager, the CHW should never have to admit that her stocks have run out.
4. Re-ordering. A system should be set up with the supervisor
5. It is best to use the generic name of the medicine.

Both medicines and equipment can be kept in a box, which should be:
- large enough to contain all supplies;
- small enough to carry;
- strong enough for constant use;
- waterproof;
- divided into two or three sections, either arranged side by side, or one on top of the other;
- marked with a red cross or crescent, but remembering these exact emblems are copyrighted;
- fitted with a handle and shoulder strap;
- lockable and secured in a safe place when out of use.

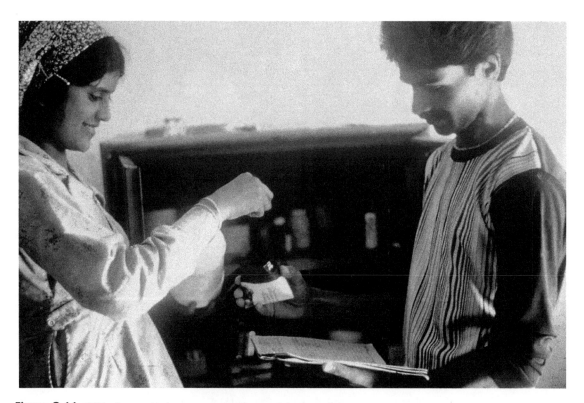

Figure 8.11 CHWs often need to become expert in the use of simple medicines.

Table 8.3 A chart showing the patients seen and treatment given by the CHW

Date	Patient's Name & No	Age	Problem	Treatment	Outcome	Money taken
January 4th 2017	Jose Lopez 01/04/19/05	46	Acute respiratory infection	Amoxicillin 250 mg 21 tablets	Much improved 48 hours later	30 cents

Table 8.4. An alternative system is to use a diary, recording patients' names and details on the date they are due to be seen. The two systems can be used together.

Vital events record

This records births, deaths, and migration in and out of the community (e.g. following marriage). The latter is often impossible to keep track of in urban centres, but is valuable information to collect in stable communities (Table 8.5).

Daily activity list

Some CHWs also keep a record of daily activities both for themselves and to show their supervisor. Books used should be strong with tough bindings, and should fit into the CHW's box. These three records can be kept in different sections of the same book. The supervisor can help to prepare this.

Monthly report form

Most CHWs will also fill in a monthly report form containing key data already mentioned. The purpose of this is largely for transferring data from community to programme office or computer, or to provide a report to the government, e.g. the district medical officer. There will often be national or official forms for these reports and we should enquire about these before designing our own. The form should be as simple as possible, easy to complete from other records, and appropriate for use alongside any computerized record system. Forms can be computer-generated and printed, making data entry simpler.

In some projects CHWs can enter data directly using hand-held electronic devices. Alternatively, forms known as due lists can be computerized and printed, on which the CHW records all information, and which act as a reminder of who she needs to visit, when, and why. This is an efficient system but, unless care is taken, it can shift the focus from the community to the office, and may disempower the CHW. If the CHW is also carrying out functions under any special programme, she should be trained to use record forms required for that programme. Examples include TB programmes using DOTs (see Chapter 19), the distribution of ivermectin in river blindness control, or praziquantel in schistosomiasis (bilharzia).

Supporting a CHW

Here, support means personal, not financial, support. In order for the CHW to become effective she needs confidence in herself and credibility in the eyes of her community. She will only succeed if she has an effective support system. Support will come from the various sources (See Table 8.6).

The health team

When first trained, the CHW will rely heavily on the health team and on her supervisor or mentor. The community may not have confidence in her, her family may misunderstand her, and she may scarcely believe in herself. The CHW will continue to receive regular lessons where she can ask questions, share concerns, and be encouraged. She can receive advice on how to manage tricky people or puzzling medical cases. The supervisor or other health team members should visit the CHW in her community, on a regular basis, initially weekly If possible.

Peer support from other CHWs

'A problem shared is a problem halved', and by meeting together regularly, CHWs can share their problems, and

Table 8.4 The CHW's list of all 'at-risk' patients or families

Date	Patient's Name & No	Age	Problem	Treatment	Date next visit
Nov 22nd 2017	Mary 12/03/84/06	28	Pregnant 32 weeks	Revisit or check in clinic	29th November 2017

Table 8.5 The CHW's vital events records: births, deaths, migrations

Births:

Date of birth	Name	Head of family	House No	Live, stillbirth	Name of midwife

Deaths:

Date of birth	Date of Death	Name	Head of family	House No	Age	Probable cause

For more stable communities include:

Migrations (permanent) in and out of the community					
Name	Head of family	House No	Age	In or out	Reason

may discover that their peers are facing similar situations. More experienced CHWs can give encouragement and practical advice.

The CHW's own family

The family may feel proud that she has been chosen by the community. However, they may also resent the time she spends away from the home and the extra work others have to do when she is absent. With this in mind, it is important to encourage and involve the family so that they can support the CHW. The support of the husband or partner is especially important. The supervisor should aim to build friendships with members of the CHW's family.

The CHW's community

From the CHW's viewpoint the community may seem more of a threat than a support system when she first begins her new work (See Figure 8.12). As she gains confidence and her treatment and advice are seen as accurate and successful, the community will come to respect and support her. In addition to this, community groups can have more formal support roles. For example, members of the VHC can accompany her to remote homes or at night, or they can help her to keep records. Women's clubs, young farmers' clubs, or youth clubs can give practical help and stand with her when others criticize or make complaints. Where women's groups have been set up (see Chapter 2), these will become the centre of a supportive team approach for many health issues (Figure 8.13).

We need to make sure that in supporting CHWs, issues of confidentiality stay within the boundaries expected by the community. In many rural settings this is usually not such a big issue, although there will be some health problems, e.g. those connected with sex or fertility, that must be kept private. In more divided communities and in some urban areas, confidentiality is a bigger concern.

The CHW herself

As she matures and becomes more experienced and knowledgeable, the CHW will learn self-confidence, and outside support systems will become less necessary. It is helpful to consider each CHW as needing ten support points in order to develop as an effective health worker. Table 8.6 shows two examples of how support points may add up.

How a CHW is financially rewarded

CBHC and the future of the CHW model depends partly on finding a range of practical answers about how to pay the CHW herself. Unsatisfactory planning and agreement over CHW salaries and excessive payment demands are one of the commonest causes of failure in CBHC programmes run by CSOs. However, they also occur in some government programmes where agreed salaries cannot be maintained or depended on.

Programmes led by the government

With an increasing number of CHWs involved in government-led programmes, a level of remuneration or payment for specific outcomes is often provided, A large-scale example of this is the Accredited Social

Table 8.6 **CHW's support points**

	Health team	Other CHWs	Family	Community	Self	Total
1st month	++++	+++	+	+	+	10
After 1 year	+	++	+	+++	+++	10

Health Activists (ASHAs, which are equivalent to CHWs) in India's National Health Mission.

Some government-led programmes, e.g. in Rwanda, use an incentive-based approach where CHW co-operatives receive performance-based rewards from the government, a portion of which are then reinvested in local income-generating activities.

Sometimes the government will 'contract out' CHW training and supervision to a CSO, with an agreed level of payment for the CHWs. This arrangement can work well, providing payments are made reliably. However, in all CHW programmes, a sense of voluntarism and community service continues to play a key part in motivating CHWs.

Programmes led by CSOs: sustainable support

A key dilemma for CSO-led programmes is that health programmes using CHWs need to be financially self-sufficient to maintain their existence, but CHWs understandably need a degree of financial support (Figure 8.13).

A good principle is that we should use government funds where available, request that these be paid as block grants with minimum conditions attached, and keep other funding options open. Where it is not possible for salary costs to be met by government, our ideal is to try and set up programmes in partnership with the community using sustainable options. See also Chapter 12 for more details.

Payment through the VHC

This is most likely to work if the community values its CHW so much that it is willing to pay her. If this is the case, the community must be able to work out a fair, honest, and efficient way of collecting money. Few poor communities are able to do this at the start, but may be able to later on, as faith in the CHW grows and community organization improves (Figure 8.14).

Payment through an insurance scheme

Community members each pay a fixed amount into a fund and receive certain health services in return. The CHW is paid out of this fund.[17] Schemes of this sort demand a good level of local organization in order to be effective, and, in particular, they will require a well-functioning and trustworthy health committee or equivalent.

Payment from individuals as they are treated

Payments from individuals is the system often used by TBAs, traditional health practitioners, and some remote

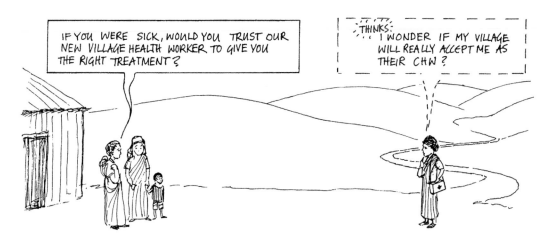

Figure 8.12 Newly qualified CHWs face big challenges.

144

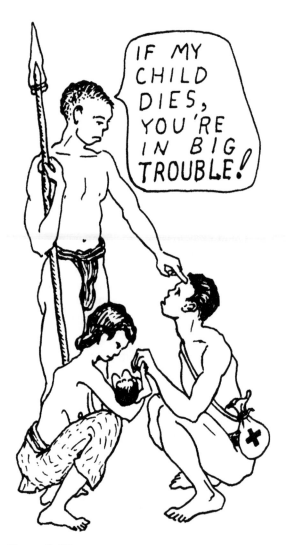

Figure 8.13 The CHW has less protection than most doctors and thus needs more support.

Reproduced from Hesperian Health Guides, www.hesperian.org. Copyright © 2017 Hesperian Health Guides. This image is distributed under the terms of the Creative Commons Attribution Non-Commercial 4.0 International licence (CC-BY-NC), a copy of which is available at http://creativecommons.org/licenses/by-nc/4.0/.

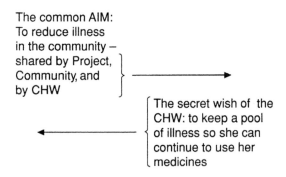

Figure 8.14 Conflict of aims when CHWs are paid by patients for each medicine dispensed.

Reproduced courtesy of Ted Lankester. This image is distributed under the terms of the Creative Commons Attribution Non-Commercial 4.0 International licence (CC-BY-NC), a copy of which is available at http://creativecommons.org/licenses/by-nc/4.0/.

Payment per medicine given is a bad model which leads to overprescribing and reinforcement of a 'pill for every ill' mentality in the community. The CHW must give medicines only as indicated, not just because the person coming to see them wants or even demands to have them (See Figure 8.14).

CHW volunteers

Although difficult, CHWs who volunteer their time may be successful in certain circumstances. Where CHWs work a maximum of, for example, eight to twelve hours spread across the week, each CHW will usually be able to care for up to twenty-five families. Programmes based on unpaid volunteers will therefore use a larger number of part-time CHWs rather than a smaller number of full-timers.

However, with the functions expected of CHWs continually increasing, there will be a tendency for remuneration to become more important and the numbers of people she can care for will fall.

Volunteer CHWs may possess strong motivation from a sense of social service or religious motivation. For example, recently in the Bodji area of Ethiopia, over 100 church deacons served as unpaid community health volunteers. Also, in the Adrokor Rural Clinic in Ghana, neither CHWs nor TBAs receive salaries. Being highly valued by the community, they are often brought gifts to supplement their income.

Finally, there may exist other means of support and affirmation for the CHW. A report from Malawi lists a variety of alternative rewards that reduce the need to pay CHWs. These include recognition and praise, exemption from user fees at the local health facility, free training and experience that may later help job prospects, and the

doctors in China, all of whom are paid in cash or kind for the services they provide. The local community is often familiar with this approach and can apply it to CHWs. However, we need to ensure fees are low so that community members can always access their CHW.

For example, the CHW can charge a fixed amount per consultation, as agreed with the programme or health committee. She can then keep part or all of this as payment, or return it to a pool from which fixed payments are made monthly to CHWs.

interest of community work as an alternative to work at home. In another example, an urban CHW from Delhi recently wrote, 'my family is much healthier now. None of us has become sick since I became a CHW. I also have more confidence in myself. I feel like a valued member of my community because people come to me for help and advice because they respect me.'[18] The rewards of community service can be emphasized to CHWs and their families when they are trained. It is worth noting, however, that it needs to be made clear that appointment as a CHW is not a path to fame and fortune either for the CHW nor her family.

Payments from funding agencies

This may seem the simplest or indeed the only solution at the start. The danger resembles that of a driverless car running downhill out of control. For example, outside donors may commit to funding a programme for a defined period, perhaps three to five years, with some funds specially set aside for CHW payments, and so the programme gives CHWs regular financial support. However, at the end of the three years, the donor has different priorities, and CHW support stops. This leads to ill-feeling and discouragement, making it difficult for any future programme to continue in this area because of feelings of mistrust on the side of the community. Before any programme starts, we need to think clearly and carefully about long-term sustainability (see Chapter 12).

This again raises a key strand in this book: the need for communities to increasingly lead their programmes, own their futures, and use their own talents and commitment in social enterprise so as to help provide the funds needed for programme activities.

Practical guidelines for paying a CHW

As mentioned, effective CHWs often serve because of their social or religious concerns, interest in the job, and personal commitment. On the other hand, CHWs often come from poor backgrounds and their families may depend on the work they do at home, in the field, or as wage earners. It may seem unreasonable for such CHWs to serve for eight hours or more a week and receive nothing tangible in return. Sometimes the CHW will be happy to give her services free, but her husband and family members may not agree, especially after initial enthusiasm wears off.

We must therefore find a balance between paying a CHW too much on the one hand and too little on the other, both of which may take away her sense of service.

If we pay the CHW too *high* a salary, her family may think of her simply as another wage-earner. Often, CHWs compare their salaries with those received by others, and if lower, may demand higher wages; a form of 'unionization' may even occur. Finally, money may replace service as the reason for working, and the quality of care given by the CHW may fall.

Conversely, if we pay too *low* a salary, the CHW and her family become discouraged or resentful. This resentment may lead to the CHW spending less time in the community and more time doing jobs in the home. Another potential problem may be that the CHW starts charging (or overcharging) for her services, which again may result in a drop in the quality of care provided.
In one central African project, volunteers were reported as saying: 'people are asking us "What sort of a job is this, that we do not get paid at the end of the month?"'

Government policy

There may be agreed levels in the country or district we should follow. Some countries recommend that CHWs should not be paid, while others expect that they should. As mentioned, if our programme is working with the government or is running a programme on the government's behalf, we will follow their payment policies.

Practical hints if payment is essential

- Avoid the term wages, salaries or income.

Use instead the name or idea of an incentive, contribution, stipend or compensation for time. Make sure that the payment method used does not break national labour laws.

- Payments must be punctual.

Make sure payments are in full and on time.

- CHWs should sign for payments received.

This saves argument later and will be needed by the programme auditor or health committee accountant.

- Training expenses and transport costs for training sessions can be reimbursed.
- Modest pay increases can gradually be given as agreed with the health committee.
- Equivalent grades of CHW are paid the same amount.

Where possible, use similar rates to those paid by neighbouring programmes.

- Encourage the health committee to take on the responsibility of managing these payments as soon as they are able—and dependable—to do this.

Some secrets for success in CHW programmes

Most of these have been mentioned in the course of the chapter, but because this is such an important subject they are summarized here, with examples.

High-level support from government

This is obviously important for government-led programmes, but all CHW programmes need to work in close connection with government and see themselves as part of the national health system. By demonstrating excellent models, CSOs can demonstrate the cost-effectiveness of good quality programmes.

Priority given to creating awareness in the community

If we go too fast, impose our ideas on the community, and then struggle to persuade them that CHWs are what the community needs, we are sure to fail. We must spend time in the community using a participatory appraisal, community surveys, and building relationships so people themselves come to suggest and own the CHW programme.

Care in selecting appropriate CHWs

We must explain to the community what a wide range of useful tasks a CHW can carry out. Often, people fail to grasp the significance of her role and the qualities needed in those they select. Again, this is a matter of taking time to create awareness and work together with the community in the early phases of our CBHC programme.

Encouraging family members to support the CHW in her role

Family members often don't fully understand the CHW's role and significance of what she does. Spouses or partners of both male and female CHWs may feel threatened or become suspicious. There may be resentment that the CHW spends less time as mother, cook, water-carrier, income earner, or farmer. Most of these problems can be prevented if we spend time with family members, such as mothers-in-law, at the start of the programme. We can help them to understand that the family will benefit through the CHW's knowledge, status, and any remuneration she may receive.

High-quality and ongoing training is essential

If we have given too little practical experience for CHWs to recognize and treat common illnesses, they may make mistakes in diagnosis, or use wrong medicines. This can quickly cause the community to lose confidence, and it may take a long time to regain it. We must continue to provide ongoing training and support to CHWs. It is also important that CHWs continue to learn new skills and to carry out different tasks. Otherwise they may become bored, or be unable to meet the changing health needs in their community.

Supervision and backup must be regular and supportive

Sometimes CHWs do not receive the support they need. Their supervisors fail to visit them, their health kits run out, and they become confused by the records they are expected to keep. Irregular or inadequate supervision is a common reason why many programmes start well but fail after two or three years. We must plan for long-term support and supervision of the CHW, and we may need to train the health committee progressively to take a role in her support and management (See Figure 8.13).

A performance system needs to be set up

Monitoring the performance of CHWs is vital. It requires accurate documentation and simple, agreed-upon indicators about how effective (and cost-efficient) their work is and how much they are respected and supported in the community.

Methods of support and remuneration must be agreed and understood

Disagreements about pay are one of the commonest reasons why CHW programmes fail. Usually CHWs (or their family) feel they are not paid enough. Issues about pay may not have been talked through at the start. A common situation is where CHWs assumed they would be paid, but the programme assumed the CHWs would be working as volunteers. Resentment will always be caused if payment is agreed but is then delayed or reduced. Funding may simply come to an end, leaving everyone bewildered and demotivated.

Make sure all issues to do with payment or remuneration are discussed in detail at the start of the programme and, if any problems develop, they must be solved before dissatisfaction spreads. Experience has shown that even when CHWs clearly understand they will not be receiving payment, they may later forget this or be persuaded by others they should expect to be paid. If CHWs are working as volunteers, they must receive thanks, public acknowledgement, and recognition.

Prioritize use of technology, ICT, and smartphones

Increasingly, ICT is centre-stage in the daily work of CHWs. Effective CHW health programmes need simple systems for trainers and supervisors and government to communicate, and for CHWs to maintain contact with each other. WhatsApp and similar communication groups are increasingly used (see Chapter 26). The use of Smartphones is already becoming the norm in many programmes.

CHWs need ongoing personal development

We need to understand this important expectation and make sure that CHWs continue to learn new skills and take on more responsibilities. Often this will lead to growing job satisfaction and a continuing sense of motivation and commitment. If we fail to provide opportunities for developing within the role, we may find that CHWs become restless and look for jobs elsewhere, meaning we have to recruit and train new CHWs. In turn, this turnover can cause delays and extra expense.

CHWs can continue to have a role in famine, war, or disaster

If this happens, it may still be possible for CHWs to use their transferable information and skills to new settings.[19] Sometimes the CHW can take on additional roles, such as helping at feeding centres or having a health care role in a refugee camp. Even though there may be turmoil at the national or regional level, grassroots programmes may still be able to continue, at least in part. Programme leaders and supervisors should show leadership to try to encourage maintaining the programme, and those that have to be temporarily stopped should be restarted as soon as possible. Even under the worst conditions, CHWs who have gained knowledge and confidence may often find a valuable role in the situations where they are. They can help to care for those around them, start health classes, and link with others to start informal programmes. In one programme in South Sudan, where there is long-term instability, many health facilities are more than ten hours away and unsafe to reach. CHWs carefully trained to use specific, field-tested materials improved the health of their communities, especially children under the age of five years.

Summary

In recent years, CHWs have played an increasing role as key members of primary healthcare programmes and in supporting universal health coverage. Increasingly, CHW programmes are being run by government, but CSOs can still play a valuable role providing they work with government, follow government guidelines, and adhere to an agreed national curriculum with agreed local variations. In turn, governments should be inclusive of new and existing programmes that are willing to work with them.

District health teams, the health programme, and the community need to work closely together in order for CHW programmes to function effectively. CHWs should be well respected members of a community, usually women, sometimes men between the ages of twenty-five and forty-five, and who are chosen by the community itself. They are trained appropriately using a comprehensive and practical syllabus in centres as near to their homes as possible. When basic training is completed, CHWs are given an exam and may then be presented with a health kit. They now start serving in the community where their tasks include giving health teaching, acting as agents of change, and, in many programmes, providing curative care. They also care for all community members whose health is at risk, liaising with the health team or nearest health facility to which they refer serious cases. They are encouraged to keep accurate records.

When CHWs begin working in the community they need encouragement and support from the programme, from the community, and ideally from their peers. CHWs ideally serve out of social concern, through religious motivation, or for other rewards apart from payment. If payment is necessary, the best sources are usually the community or government, and not donors or other outside agencies. There are several key aspects of successful programmes and common reasons why they fail or discontinue. By understanding these successes and failures, we can help to avoid them, and when problems do arise, we can take quick action to deal with them

The future of the CHW model will be assured as it develops ways of being sustainable and as CHWs are sufficiently well chosen, trained, and supervised so that community members have confidence in their services.

Further reading and resources

Abbatt F. *Teaching for Better Learning A guide for teachers of primary health care staff*. 2nd ed. London: Macmillan; 1992.

Abbatt F. *Scaling up health and education workers: Community health workers*. London: DFID Health Systems Resource Centre; 2005. Available from: http://www.hrhresourcecenter.org/node/616

El Arifeen S, Christou A, Reichenbach L, Osman FA, Azad K, Islam KS, et al. Community-based approaches and partnerships: Innovations in health-service delivery in Bangladesh. *The Lancet*. 2013; 382 (9909): 2012–26.

Haines A, Sanders D, Lehmann U, Rowe AK, Lawn JE, Jan S, et al. Achieving child survival goals: Potential contribution of community health workers. *The Lancet*. 2007; 368 (9579): 2121–2131. This is the most comprehensive assessment to date of the role of CHWs.

Jaskiewicz W, Tulenko K. Increasing community health worker productivity and effectiveness: a review of the influence of the work environment. *Human Resources for Health*. 2012; 10 (38). https://doi.org/10.1186/1478-4491-10-38

Kahssay H, Taylor M, Berman P. *Community Health Workers: The way forward*. Geneva: World Health Organization; 1998. Available from: http://apps.who.int/iris/bitstream/10665/42034/1/WHO_PHA_4.pdf A very useful review with areas to focus on for the future.

Laughlin M. *The care group difference: A guide to mobilizing community-based volunteer health educators*. Baltimore, MD: World Relief; 2004. Available from: https://coregroup.org/wp-content/uploads/media-backup/documents/Resources/Tools/Care_Group_Manual_Final__Oct_2010.pdf

Perry H, Crigler L, editors. *Developing and strengthening community health worker programs at scale: A reference guide and case studies for program managers and policy makers*. Washington, DC: USAID/MCHIP; 2013. Available from: http://www.mchip.net/sites/default/files/mchipfiles/CHW_ReferenceGuide_sm.pdf)

Perry H, Davies T. Effectiveness of the census-based impact-oriented approach in improving aid effectiveness in global health. In: Beracochea E, editor. *Improving aid effectiveness in global health*. New York: Springer; 2015. p 261–278. Can be purchased as an e-book chapter at: http://link.springer.com/chapter/10.1007%2F978-1-4939-2721-0_21

Perry H, Morrow M, Borger S, Weiss J, DeCoster M, Davis T, Ernst P. *Care Groups I: An innovative community-based strategy for improving maternal, neonatal, and child health in resource-constrained settings. Global Health: Science and Practice*. 2015; 3(3): 358–369. https://doi.org/10.9745/GHSP-D-15-00051

Scott et al. *What do we know etc*. https://human-resources-health.biomedcentral.com/articles/10.1186/s12960-018-0304-x.

The Technical and Operational Performance Support Program (TOPS). *Care Groups: A reference guide for practitioners*. Washington, DC: The Technical and Operational Performance Support Program; 2016. Available from: http://caregroups.info/wp-content/uploads/2015/08/Care-Groups-A-Reference-Guide-for-Practitioners-7-11-16.pdf

Werner D, Bower B. *Helping Health Workers Learn*. Berkeley, CA: Hesperian Foundation, 1995. This classic guide is unsurpassed and has been translated into numerous languages. Available from: TALC.

Internet resources

Arukah Network has details of a variety of CHW training programmes and curricula www.arukahnetwork.org.

Bangladesh Rural Advancement Committee (BRAC): http://www.brac.net.

CHW Central. A global resource for and about CHWs: http://www.chwcentral.org

https://www.wiltonpark.org.uk/wp-content/uploads/WP1447-Report.pdf This is a valuable set of evidence-based recommendations for CHW programmes written both from a governmental and community viewpoint.

References

1. Perry H, Davies T. Effectiveness of the census-based impact-oriented approach in improving aid effectiveness in global health. In: Beracochea E, editor. *Improving aid effectiveness in global health*. New York: Springer; 2015. p 261–278. Can be purchased as an e-book chapter at: http://link.springer.com/chapter/10.1007%2F978-1-4939-2721-0_21

2. Ferrinho P, Sidat M, Goma F, Dussault G. Task-shifting: experiences and opinions of health workers in Mozambique and Zambia. *Human Resources for Health*. 2012; 10 (34). DOI: 10.1186/1478-4491-10-34

3. World Health Organization. *Global strategy on human resources for health: Workforce 2030*. 2016. Available from: https://www.who.int/hrh/resources/pub_globstrathrh-2030/en/

4. Mishra SR, Neupane D, Preen D, Kallestrup P, Perry HB. Mitigation of non-communicable diseases in developing countries with community health workers. *Globalization and Health*. 2015; 11 (43). DOI: 10.1186/s12992-015-0129-5

5. Perry H, Zulliger R, Scott K, Javadi D, Gergen J, Shelley K, et al. Case studies of large-scale community health worker programs: Examples from Afghanistan, Bangladesh, Brazil, Ethiopia, India, Indonesia, Iran, Nepal, Niger, Pakistan, Rwanda, Zambia, and Zimbabwe. Washington, DC: USAID/MCSP; 2017. Available from: http://www.mcsprogram.org/wp-content/uploads/2017/01/CHW-CaseStudies-Globes.pdf

6. Perry H. *A comprehensive description of three national community health worker programs and their contributions to maternal and child health and primary health care: Case studies from Latin America (Brazil), Africa (Ethiopia), and Asia (Nepal)*. Boston: CHW Central; 2016. Available to download from: chwcentral.org

7. Kluge, H, Kelley, E, Swaminathan, S, Yamamoto, N, Fisseha, S, Theodorakis, P, et al. After Astana: building the economic case for increased investment in primary health care. *The Lancet*, 2018; 392 (10160): 2147–2152.

8. Nkonki L, Cliff J, Sanders D, Lay health worker attrition: Important but often ignored. *WHO Bulletin*. 2011; 89 (12): 919–23. Available from: http://www.who.int/bulletin/volumes/89/12/11-087825.pdf

9. Republic of Uganda Ministry of Health. *Village Health Teams: A handbook to improve health in communities*. Uxbridge: World Vision; 2009. Available from: https://www.k4health.org/toolkits/uganda-radio-distance-learning/village-health-team-vht-handbook

10. Farzadfar F, Murray CJL, Gakidou E, Bossert T, Namdaritabar H, Alikhani S, et al. Effectiveness of diabetes and hypertension management by rural primary health-care workers (Behvarz workers) in Iran. *The Lancet*. 2012; 379 (9810): 47–54.

11. Patel V, Kirkwood B. Perinatal depression treated by community health workers. *The Lancet*. 2008; 372 (9642).

12. Mkandawire N, Ngulube C, Lavy C. Orthopaedic clinical officer program in Malawi: A model for providing orthopaedic care. *Clinical Orthopaedics and Related Research*. 2008; 466(10): 2385–91.

13. Davis TP, Wetzel C, Hernandez Avilan E, de Mendoza Lopes C, Chase RP, Winch PJ, et al. Reducing child global undernutrition at scale in Sofala Province, Mozambique, using care group volunteers to communicate health messages to mothers. *Global Health Science and Practice*. 2013; 1(1): 35–51. DOI: 10.9745/GHSP-D-12-00045

14. One Million Community Health Workers Campaign. New York: Columbia University. http://1millionhealthworkers.org/about-us/

15. Lewin S, Munabi-Babigumira S, Glenton C, Daniels K, Bosch-Capblanch X, van Wyk BE, et al. A review of the effect of using lay health workers to improve mother and child health. *Cochrane Database of Systematic Reviews*. 2010; 3. DOI: 10.1002/14651858.CD004015.pub3

16. Vaughan K, Kok MC, Witter S, Dieleman M. Costs and cost-effectiveness of community health workers: Evidence from a literature review. *Human Resources for Health*. 2015; 13:71. DOI: 10.1186/s12960-015-0070-y

17. Mahal A, Krishnaswamy K, Ruchismita R, Babu BG. What is a health card worth? A randomised controlled trial of an outpatient health insurance product in rural India. *The Lancet*. 2013; 381(Supplement 2(0): S87.

18. ASHA. *Transforming lives in the slums of Delhi*. www.asha-india.org

19. Perry H, Dhillon RS, Liu A, Chitnis K, Panjabi R, Palazuelos D, et al. Health worker programmes after the 2013–2016 Ebola outbreak. *Bulletin of the World Health Organization* 2016; 94 (7): 551–3.

Community health management

CHAPTER 9

Monitoring and evaluating the health programme

Ted Lankester

What we need to know

The meaning of monitoring and evaluation (M&E)

Monitoring and evaluation (M&E) are the techniques we use to find out how well our health programme is achieving what it set out to do. We will originally have set objectives, i.e. the results we are aiming to achieve and may have recorded on the logframe (Chapter 7). M&E enables us to see how effectively we have reached those objectives. The techniques of M&E are one way to measure success, but other measures of success may be just as important.

Although M&E are bracketed together and are often confused, each has a specific meaning. *Monitoring* refers to ongoing assessment of our progress. It should be set up as part of our routine programme management and is ideally done by both programme and community members together. It uses the record systems we have built into the programme. *Evaluation* refers to a systematic review of the programme outcomes and impact often at the end of a funding cycle. It often involves an outside evaluation team.

One helpful way to distinguish between M and E is that monitoring asks the question 'Are we doing things right?', and evaluation asks 'Are we doing the right things?'. If monitoring is carried out well, evaluation will be easier.

Who benefits from M&E?

The programme itself

We often start with good ideas and ambitious objectives. As time goes on, these may get lost in day-to-day activities or problems (See Figure 9.1). M&E can highlight whether the programme is still on the right road, how far it has travelled, and how far it still has to go. In this way M&E forms part of the planning cycle (Figure 9.2). Regular monitoring will also identify problems early so they can be corrected, and improvements can be suggested.

The community

M&E helps the community to see how the programme is working, and shows the benefits it is bringing. Community members will work with us in this process. We will also regularly feed M&E reports back to the

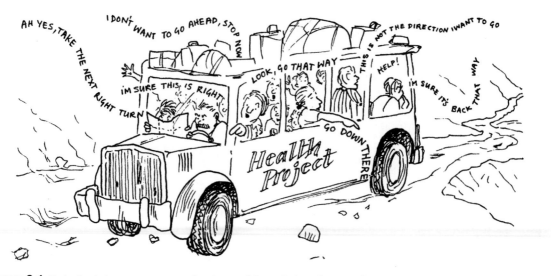

Figure 9.1 Evaluation helps everyone to see what they are doing and where they are going.

community as a means of promoting understanding of the whole process. Findings and results will need to be presented in such a way that the community sees the benefits (and problems) and is motivated to participate in improvements (see Chapter 2).

Donors, sponsors and a wider audience

In practice, evaluations are often carried out because donors want confirmation that their money is being well spent. But all stakeholders—programme, community,

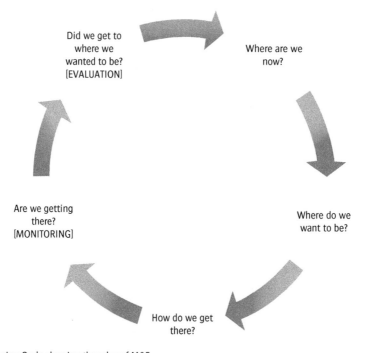

Figure 9.2 The Planning Cycle showing the roles of M&E.

donors, and government—should benefit from evaluation if it is well planned and carried out.

An evaluation showing good results can help our programme to become better known and a model for other programmes. We can use Twitter, Facebook and other forms of social media to make findings known to wider audiences. If it uses a rigorous methodology it can be published to share the learning and raise the profile of the programme.

Government

Governments may want to know what results the programme is achieving and whether it is reaching district and national targets. If we are involved in specific programmes, e.g. End TB, Roll Back Malaria, their coordinators will need our results. Civil society organizations involved in community-based health care (CBHC) are often able to achieve more effective results at community level than government. Evaluation (and the return of regular monitoring figures) should enable us to demonstrate this and increase our credibility (Figure 9.3). In turn, this will enable CBHC as part of civil society to

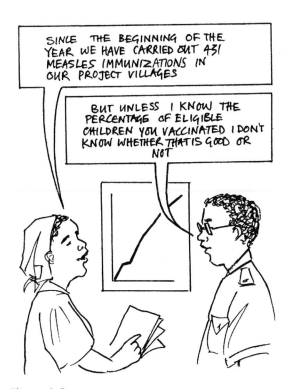

Figure 9.3 Know the percentages.

be entrusted with more health tasks in national health programmes, which will be to everyone's benefit.

Some useful definitions

The definitions in Box 9.1 each have examples from a well-building programme.

Who should perform M&E?

The section on participatory appraisal (PA) in Chapter 6 should be read alongside this section. As the project moves into M&E, PA can give rise to participatory M&E (PM&E).[1]

The title of the book *Nothing about us without us*[2] provides a slogan to remind us that the community needs to be involved closely at every stage, rather than being marked by outsiders as though they were taking an examination. This is especially important when vulnerable community members are monitored, as with the people living with disability and those with mental health issues. It is essential that these community members are involved in, and feel empowered by, the processes of M&E.

Monitoring can be done by the health team and the community together, but it will need to be planned carefully using appropriately simple participatory techniques.[3] For example, A well-digging programme in Myanmar asked the community to make a chalk-mark each time they used the well to record what times of day it was being used.[4] Evaluations can sometimes be done by community members alone. To be effective, these 'insider evaluations' need to be small scale and analyse a limited number of programme activities. The team would need to have, or be taught, necessary skills and good monitoring systems would need to be in place to feed into the evaluation. The term *community-based participatory evaluation* is sometimes used.[5]

In practice, final impact evaluations usually involve outside experts who come to work alongside the health team and community. The success of using outsiders depends on several conditions.

Firstly, the evaluation must be planned in advance. It may last one or two weeks, and will need to be done at a time of year when neither the health team nor community is overworked, nor the weather too extreme. Essential programme activities should continue, not least because evaluators will want to observe the programme at work.

Secondly, the evaluators must have clear terms of reference, i.e. know exactly what they are meant to be doing, and also what they are *not* meant to be doing. They should be sensitive to the local culture, and have an affirming attitude. Terms of reference should be

> **Box 9.1 Useful definitions for M&E using examples from a well-building programme**
>
> **Activities: What is actually done**
> - Building wells.
> - Hygiene education.
>
> **Evaluation: An assessment, at a specific time, of a programme's outcomes and impact**
> - How water use in the village has changed.
> - How the wells have influenced household hygiene and sanitation.
>
> **Monitoring: Continuous process to record, reflect and use information regarding progress**
> - Use of resources, activities completed, progress towards programme objectives.
>
> **Indicators: Evidence or signs that change has taken place**
>
> **Quantitative indicators are those that can be measured or counted**
> - Number of people using the wells.
>
> **Qualitative indicators are those gained by observation**
> - Local people's views about the wells.
>
> **Goals: Long-term aims for impact**
>
> - To improve health in target population.
>
> **Objectives: Results the programme is expected to achieve**
> - To increase the amount of clean water used in village households.
>
> **Inputs: Physical and human resources used within the programme**
> - Tools, bricks, labour.
>
> **Outputs: What is produced as a result of completed activities**
> - Functional village wells.
>
> **Impact: Long-term and sustainable change resulting from an activity**
> - Long-term improvements in the health of local people, social relationships in the village, and the position of women.
>
> **Outcomes: The effect on the original situation due to the programme**
> - Increase in health through fewer households experiencing water- and hygiene-related illnesses.
>
> Source: data from CSSDD Myanmar/Myanmar Baptist Convention. This box is distributed under the terms of the Creative Commons Attribution Non-Commercial 4.0 International licence (CC-BY-NC), a copy of which is available at http://creativecommons.org/licenses/by-nc/4.0/

agreed between evaluator, programme and any donor agency or government department involved, written down and signed by all involved. Evaluators should be carefully briefed both by donor and programme before starting work.

There are several advantages of using outsiders these include involving experts with special skills who will be able to advise on effective methods of carrying out the evaluation. Because of their lack of bias, results from outsiders may be more accurate as the evaluators have no personal interest in the achievements of the programme. Finally, outsiders may receive more accurate feedback from the community, and community members may be readier to tell outsiders how they really feel.

Disadvantages of using outsiders include higher costs in terms of time and money, although a donor agency often funds the evaluation. Also, the visiting experts

may not know the local customs, language, or situation. It is therefore helpful if evaluators are familiar with the country, region, and type of programme they are evaluating. Finally, published material from evaluations or visits may be politically insensitive or unhelpful to the community. If the evaluation includes any research that may be written up, this must be clearly discussed beforehand.

Some pitfalls to avoid

Monitoring too little

Many programmes go from year to year without M&E. Annual reports are still written, with patient numbers, immunizations and procedures carried out. Such figures may accurately record the activity being carried out, but have little to say whether the programme is effective or meeting its objectives.

In practice it is quite easy for a programme to get 'out of control'. It is easy to become overwhelmed by challenges and needs; record systems and reports can turn into a nightmare. Obviously, any lack of quality in reporting or recording information is serious and we need to act, including being honest with any agency that is helping to fund the programme. The list of questions in Box 9.2 was designed by one funding agency to help programmes in this situation to focus on key reporting criteria and develop their forward planning.

Monitoring too much

Some programmes go to the opposite extreme, which can happen especially if they are very bureaucratic or run by managers interested in statistics. Collecting figures and producing good reports becomes more important than working for long-term improvements in the community.

Sometimes programmes are required to provide huge numbers of reports. This happens particularly if they are involved in special programmes such as EPI (immunization), End TB, or Roll Back Malaria. We must therefore ask donors to request only vital information, and we should only agree to evaluations that are genuinely useful for the programme. Programmes should clearly negotiate with donors, and consider refusing funding if it is tied to a very heavy monitoring schedule or to many new indicators.

Note that the quality and value of M&E decreases with every additional indicator, while the cost in terms of money, time and distraction increases. Thus, the role of a programme manager is to resist adding indicators. One suggestion is that indicators should be reviewed every year for usefulness and any ineffectual or burdensome ones discarded.

Ignoring the needs and opinions of the poor

When we gather qualitative information, the articulate and well-off usually do most of the talking, while the poor may have less chance to express their views. The process of identifying those who do and don't benefit is known as 'equity-based disaggregation', a term often used by donors. Sometimes the overall health of a

---

Box 9.2 Informal evaluation questions

Project impact on local community

What effect does the presence of the project have on the local community? (If the project did not exist, what would happen?) A story may help to show the project impact.

Disease prevalence and project impact

What do project staff consider the three most common diseases in the project area? What effect has the project had on the prevalence of these diseases during the last three years? (Is there any statistical evidence?)

Community involvement in project

Is the local community involved in this project? If yes, how is their involvement facilitated e.g. through village health committee, community volunteers, etc. How often do project staff meet with community members? If there is no community involvement, why? Are there any plans to increase this? If not, why?

Community volunteers

Do volunteers from the community work in the project e.g. as voluntary health workers (VHWs) or HIV/AIDS home-based care workers (HBCWs)? Approximately what number are there currently active and newly trained in the last year?

Current project problems and challenges

What are the three most serious problems which have a negative effect on the running of the project? How have these problems been addressed? How successful have these efforts been? What do project staff consider would be needed to solve them?

Do you expect any future changes in project area?

E.g. economic or political changes, climatic changes, staff 'brain drain' e.g. to rich countries, or changes in disease prevalence e.g. HIV/AIDS, etc.

Future plans and priority objectives for the next year

What are project staff's 3 priority objectives for the project? What may stop them implementing these objectives? How do they plan to overcome these problems?

Thank you for completing this form.

community improves but the health of the most vulnerable stays the same, or worsens. We can monitor this by keeping separate figures for different socio-economic groups. Similarly, we can keep separate figures for men and women, or for different language groups, or for those living with disability. We will need to think carefully about the most appropriate categories to use for our situation. Most importantly, we must ensure that any evaluation considers the impact of the programme on those in the community who are the most marginalized.

We should also be aware of the term 'cross-cutting themes' or 'cross-cutting issues' in evaluation. Many large donors identify certain cross-cutting themes that should be integrated into project design and evaluation.[6] Typical themes are gender, equity, inclusion, disability, environmental sustainability, etc. Even if cross-cutting issues are not part of our programme's funding requirements, it is often useful to assess what cross-cutting

issues are most important in terms of the community's health, then apply these to the programme's objectives, and measure them effectively.

Results of the evaluation are used wrongly or not at all

If an evaluation produces negative findings, these should be shared fully with the team. Only then can everyone acknowledge the issues raised, learn from them, and make improvements. At the same time, blame and criticism must be avoided. Any positive findings should be shared more widely, especially with those who are mainly responsible. In some circumstances, it is prudent for the programme leaders to shoulder any blame, and for the community, government, or political leadership to receive any praise. In terms of negative findings it is worth asking whether these are simply the result of unrealistic goals, and consider creating new, more attainable goals.

What we need to do

How to choose what to monitor or evaluate

There is a long list of programme activities we could monitor or evaluate. Usually, however, we need to choose some key activities that reflect our programme objectives. Most chapters in this book set out aims for various programme activities and give ideas of what to evaluate. Table 9.1 is a sample M&E chart that includes some of these and lists more. Whatever the scale of our programme, we must be careful to set up simple but precise recording systems at the very beginning. These systems will lay the foundation for evaluation in the future.

We will probably have constructed a logframe (see Chapter 7) or a similar, less-detailed framework, and this can be used as a guide to help set up monitoring. We can then adjust the logframe based on the results of monitoring. We must remember the logframe not only sets out our goals and objectives but is also meant to be descriptive, so it must be updated with changes and developments on a regular basis. The logframe will need to be revised or even rewritten after evaluations.

For evaluation, we should compare our current position with our baseline situation or conditions, which we will have established at the time the programme started. Alternatively, we can compare how things are in the programme area with how they are in a 'control' area that we also surveyed originally but in which we have not been

working. In practice this can be difficult as it is usually inappropriate to make measurements without making improvements. One way of doing this is to plan a roll-out to the 'control area' as the second phase of the programme.

In summary, for M&E we need to select a few important areas that are important to monitor, easy to record, and helpful for planning and evaluation. This is best done at the planning stage of the programme.

Select the most appropriate indicators

Having chosen criteria for the M&E, we must now decide how to measure it. Indicators are best defined as a measure or evidence of progress towards an agreed target. Table 9.1 provides examples of indicators.

Ideally, we should find out from either the district health officer or a local civil society organization programme those indicators that are most widely used where we are working. This avoids duplication of effort and helps make comparisons across programmes. We can use other sources, e.g. if we are engaged in a national HIV/AIDS programme, we should be aware of the indicators drawn up by UNAIDS in 2016.[7]

If our programme is large and well established we will need to be aware of the indicators used for the Sustainable Development Goals (usually Goal 3) that relate to our activities. Often however these are 'big

Table 9.1 **A sample M&E chart**

Subject	Examples of indicators	Possible sources of information, written or digitized
CHW work (Chapter 8)	Percentage of all patient attendances seen by CHW. Percentage of community homes visited on average once per week. Level of CHWs' knowledge about prevention and cure of common illnesses. Percentage of families or individuals able to prevent and self-treat selected illnesses e.g. diarrhoea, scabies. Level of satisfaction of community with their CHW.	CHW records Clinic attendance register Spot survey Questionnaire Questionnaire Questionnaire PA methods
Use of essential medicines (Chapter 11)	Percentage of CHWs or health centres with at least x number of doses of all medicines present and in-date at time of inventory. Percentage of CHWs or health centres with regular supply of essential drugs, e.g. antibiotics, antimalarials. Percentage of population with reliable access to affordable essential drugs. Percentage of population reporting that they went without a medicine in the previous six months because unavailable or unaffordable.	Inventories Spot surveys Special surveys CHW and clinic records
Child nutrition (Chapter 14)	Percentage of under-fives who are underweight. Percentage of children between six and sixty months with MUAC under 125mm.	Child's growth card CHW notebook MUAC charts Family folder insert card
Immunizations (Chapter 15)	For selected immunizations, e.g. measles, DPT, rotavirus, etc., percentage of under-fives who have completed course (in past one, three, or five years). For BCG, percentage of under-fives with BCG scars. For tetanus toxoid, percentage of women at delivery who have had three or more injections. Incidence rates of some diseases for which there are immunizations available.	Immunization register IMCI returns Family folder and insert card Mother's home-based record card Immunization register CHW/TBA records Returns from Partnership for Safe Motherhood Disease register Clinic and CHW records Special survey
Control of diarrhoea, malaria (Chapter 16)	For diarrhoea, percentage of families using ORS as first-line treatment. For malaria, number or percentage of children five or under who slept under a bed net the previous night. Number or percentage of five or under dying from malaria.	Special survey Roll Back Malaria records Clinic records
Maternal heath (Chapter 17)	Percentage of mothers attending for four or more antenatal checks in clinic or with trained midwife. Percentage of newborns weighing 2500g or less or with MUAC of 8.7cm or less. Percentage of babies delivered by midwife, trained TBA, or skilled attendant, using sterile delivery pack.	Mother's home-based record card TBA/CHW records Returns from Partnership for Safe Motherhood Mother's home-based record card

(continued)

Table 9.1 **Continued**

Subject	Examples of indicators	Possible sources of information, written or digitized
Family planning (Chapter 18)	The contraceptive prevalence rate. $$\frac{\text{Number of women aged 15–49 (or partners) using contraception}}{\text{Total number of women aged 15–49}} \times 100$$ Average space between children	FP Register Family folder and insert cards Family folder
Control of TB (Chapter 19)	Follow the National TB Programme Aims and Targets, recording TB cases and recording outcomes,	
Use of clean water, waste disposal (Chapter 21)	Percentage of families using clean water source within fifteen minutes' walk from house. Percentage of families with all family members using latrine.*	Family folder Other surveys
Abuse of tobacco, alcohol, drugs (Chapter 22)	Percentage of population aged e.g. 10 or 15 and over who admit to use.*	Family folder Special surveys

Note: the section following is more complex and many of these topics will only be possible to carry out in larger programmes with good outside support and technical help. Further indicators for large-scale programmes can found in the indicator list of Sustainable Development Goal 3.

Infant mortality rate	This is: $$\frac{\text{Number of deaths under 12 months}}{\text{Number of live births}} \frac{\text{per year}}{} \times 1000$$	Vital events register Family folder CHW records
Under-five mortality rate	This is: $$\frac{\text{Number of deaths of children under 5}}{\text{Total number of under 5 children at mid-year}} \frac{\text{per year}}{} \times 1000$$	Vital events register Family folder CHW records
Maternal mortality ratio	This is: $$\frac{\text{Number of maternal deaths with pregnancy-related cause (during pregnancy, delivery and up to 42 days after delivery)}}{\text{Number of live births}} \frac{\text{per year}}{} \times 1000$$	Vital events register Duplicate mother's home-based record Family folder and insert cards Clinic and hospital records Partnership for Safe Motherhood
Adult or Female Literacy Rate	This is: $$\frac{\text{Number of adults (or women) aged 15 or over who can read and write}}{\text{Total number of adults (or women) aged 15 or over}} \times 100$$	Family folder Special survey
Cost effectiveness	This is, broadly: $$\frac{\text{Total cost of project}}{\text{Number people covered by CBHC}}$$ But needs calculating with the aid of a health economist.	

Notes:
1. * = Accurate definitions needed according to culture of programme
2. Family folder refers to the survey or resurvey done using the family folder. Full information on each family appears on the outside of the folder (see Chapter 5; Appendix C). Much of the most useful information for evaluation is best collected during house-to-house surveys using the folders.
3. There are several different record systems used by different programmes. Clinic records refers to any records or registers kept in clinics not otherwise specified. Most will now be computerized.
4. For some subjects more than one indicator is usually listed, although in practice only one would normally be chosen for any single evaluation.
5. Most information, from whatever source, would be tabulated annually and stored in the master register or computer.
6. For national programmes, official data collecting forms should be used.

picture indicators' and more useful for population-wide measurements. If we are involved in any national programmes we will need to follow the indicators set up by these programmes.

The way we collect data for our indicators is also important. It may be paper-based, but can increasingly be done digitally (see Chapter 26).

It is helpful at this stage to distinguish between two different types of indicator. The first is quantitative, numerical, or 'hard' data (numbers, rates, and percentages) and the second is qualitative, descriptive, or 'soft' data (knowledge, attitudes, practice, satisfaction levels, stories). Both types are important in CBHC. We must absolutely not disregard soft indicators as being inferior; on the contrary, they are increasingly seen as essential.

An example of quantitative indicators

Let us say that we want to monitor our DPT immunization programme over the past year. The indicator chosen must give the most accurate measurement of what we really want to know. Some possible indicators we could use include a) the total number of DPT injections given during the past year; b) the total number of *children under five* who received DPT injections during the past year; c) the total number of children under five who *completed* courses of DPT during the past year; and d) the percentage of children under five *in the community* who completed courses of DPT during the past year (See Figure 9.3).

As we move from the first to the fourth indicator, it becomes increasingly specific, and therefore, increasingly useful. While the first indicator (a) is commonly used in annual reports it has only limited value. What we really want to know is how completely we have immunized our target population, which means that (d) is therefore the most appropriate. These four indicators are all examples of *input indicators*—i.e. they measure activity carried out. But we could use a very different indicator.

We could also measure *output* or *impact indicators*, which measure the effectiveness or impact of the programme. Thus, we could measure e) the number of children who suffered from the diseases diphtheria, pertussis, and tetanus during the past year, or f) the percentage of children in the community who suffered the same diseases in the past year. Because our ultimate aim is to eradicate these three diseases from the population, f) is therefore the best indicator of all.

Impact indicators often take time to show any improvement, so they may not be useful in indicating achievements over the shorter term. However, in CBHC, we aim, with the community and government, for long-term sustainable and impactful programmes, so ultimately our indicators should reflect this.

It is worth bearing in mind that quantitative indicators are more useful if it is possible to segment the data to make comparisons, e.g. whether more boys are immunized than girls.

Examples of qualitative indicators

The use of qualitative indicators is especially valuable in CBHC. Measuring the community's perception of the improvements and interventions, i.e. community response, is important and not difficult to do.

For example, we want to measure the extent to which people value their community health worker (CHW). We can ask a question like 'What do you think of your CHW?' or, more specifically, 'What do you think of the way the CHW provides services for mothers and children?' Instead of a free-form response, we ask for a ranking from 1 to 5, where 5 is 'Very helpful', 3 is 'OK', and 1 is 'Unhelpful'. Answers can be tabulated as set out in Table 9.2.

In another example, perhaps we want to evaluate ways in which women's status has changed as a result of the programme's work. We would provide statements to the community members about how women's status has changed, and these statements might include:

- Women are better able now to participate in family decision making than when the programmes started.
- Women have a better opportunity to take on leadership roles in the community.
- Women are better able to participate in village affairs.

Community members are asked to select one of the following options to indicate their response to each of the statements: strongly agree, agree, not sure, disagree, strongly disagree. Furthermore, questions like 'What do you think about the following statement?' are useful. Make sure to accurately record any response. Alternatively, a question could simply invite a yes or no answer.

It is worth noting that there are some differences in how programme evaluators use the words qualitative and quantitative. The above examples that rank responses or are yes/no questions could be seen as semi-quantitative because they can generate numerical data, such as satisfaction levels. Note that the term *quality indicator* is also sometimes used and it refers to measuring the quality of a programme, regardless of what method is used.

Table 9.2 Differences in community member assessments of their CHW over a three-year period; numbers indicate the total number of people choosing that category (i.e. 2=two people)

Attitudes to CHW	very helpful	helpful	OK	not very helpful	unhelpful
One year after appt	2	5	6	8	4
Three years after appt	11	9	7	4	1

Collect the data

The way we collect data will depend on our indicators, but for qualitative indicators there is a variety of methods we can use other than asking questions, such as transcripts, interviews, indicator surveys, focus groups and stories.

We may want to collect more wide-ranging views from the community about the value of the programme. We may use focus groups or interviews to ask people about their feelings regarding the community health programme, and then transcribe their responses and analyse the words or phrases that recur. This way of analysing descriptive evidence is often known as coding, and is especially useful in drawing comparisons or showing improvement over a period of time. Adding quotes and comments is very valuable in finding a full picture of the community's assessment.

When we are able to gather information in different ways and from varied sources it is known as triangulation, which helps to paint the most accurate picture. However, we must not make the process complicated as it can become very time-consuming.

Photos or videos of improvements, especially 'before and after' pictures, along with stories and anecdotes, can sometimes speak louder than words or statistics. A novel, participatory, and fun approach to evaluation is to use photovoice or videovoice. This is a structured method whereby community members are asked to take photos that represent what we are interested in (e.g. change in mental health, or attitudes to mental health) and this can stimulate some interesting discussions and even help to bring about behavioural change.

For further ways of gathering and processing information, see Chapters 6 and 7.

Analyse the data

Having completed our data collection, we must now analyse the data as quickly as possible so that it can be fed back to the various stakeholders, especially the community. A simple step-by-step approach would be as follows in Box 9.3.[8] Other chapters such as Chapter 6 describe these processes in more detail.

Act on the result

Unless action is taken on the findings of M&E, the whole process is a waste of time and money. A good evaluation raises hopes that issues will be better understood by all partners, but lack of change in the situation will create disillusionment. The participatory evaluation[9] process described earlier and under 'Further reading and resources' can help M&E become an effective learning process for the whole community, leading to change and improvement.

Use results widely

The results of regular M&E should be used as widely as possible and made known to any who will benefit from seeing them. It is common practice to provide different report versions for different purposes. A donor may not need the specifics and names. At the programme level specifics might be needed, e.g. the names of those who have not completed immunizations. But the community might need a summary that is depersonalized, or is written in simpler language than an official report.

Respond to recommendations

Regular monitoring gives evidence that helps to fine-tune the programme. We should respond to any unexpected findings and change course if necessary. Reports from evaluations need handling with care as the health programme and community will be eager to hear results, may be anxious about new ideas and suggestions, and must be involved in the process through a range of discussions.

Before releasing any final report, a further meeting should be held with the programme team to go through the main findings and recommendations. This allows them to agree and validate the findings and discuss the issues in a safe environment. This also

---

Box 9.3 A simple step-by-step guide to analysing data from the evaluation.

1. Reflecting

Think back to your evaluation questions, why you are doing the evaluation, who it is for, and what they want to know about your project.

2. Collating

This involves bringing together the information into a workable format. Quantitative data may need to be organized through statistical analysis or using basic calculations (e.g. total numbers, averages, percentages of the total). Qualitative information needs to be organized thematically; the term 'thematic analysis' is used to describe the process of identifying key themes or patterns.

3. Describing

You should provide a description of the facts which have emerged from the information gathered e.g. what was delivered, how much, to whom, when, and where. Remember to describe both positive and negative findings.

4. Interpreting

Interpreting goes beyond describing the facts. Rather, it is about trying to understand the significance of your data and why things happened as they did. Look at internal and external factors that contributed to the project's achievements; also consider any challenges or difficulties encountered.

5. Conclusions and recommendations

Draw out conclusions based on the strengths and weaknesses of the project. You can then begin to make recommendations for building on these strengths as well as addressing areas for improvement.

---

helps them to start thinking through changes that need to be made. Bearing this in mind, any outside evaluation should comment on successes and failures, recommend courses of action, suggest how changes can be carried out, and propose specific follow-up to ensure any recommendations are acted upon in some form.

The health team, with the community and guided by the evaluation, will replan the programme or any parts of it that need changing. Usually this will mean rewriting part of the logframe for a new programme phase. This will need to include revised objectives, inputs, budgets, and plans.

We may find it hard to respond positively if some of the findings are discouraging. We should aim to be organized enough to do something about it, brave enough to face up to failure and acknowledge any areas that need changing, and flexible enough to modify our programme.

Further reading and resources

Bates G, Jones L. *Monitoring and evaluation: A guide for community projects*. Liverpool: John Moores University Centre for Public Health; 2012. Available from: http://www.cph.org.uk/wp-content/uploads/2013/02/Monitoring-and-evaluation-a-guide-for-community-projects.pdf

Carter I, editor. Increasing our Impact. *Footsteps*. 2001; 50. Tearfund. Available from: http://tilz.tearfund.org/~/media/files/tilz/publications/footsteps/footsteps%2041-50/50/fs50.pdf

Community Sustainability Engagement Evaluation Toolbox. Available from: http://evaluationtoolbox.net.au/

Gosling L, Edwards M. *Toolkits: A practical guide to assessment, monitoring, review and evaluation*. London: Save the Children Fund; 1995. Available from: http://www.savethechildren.org.uk/resources/online-library/toolkits-practical-guide-planning-monitoring-evaluation-and-impact

International Federation of Red Cross and Red Crescent Societies. *Project/programme monitoring and evaluation (M&E) guide*. 2011. Available from: http://www.ifrc.org/Global/Publications/monitoring/IFRC-ME-Guide-8-2011.pdf

WK Kellogg Foundation. *W.K. Kellogg Foundation Evaluation Handbook*. Battle Creek, MI: WK Kellogg Foundation; 2004. Available at: http://cyc.brandeis.edu/pdfs/reports/EvaluationHandbook.pdf

Participatory impact monitoring: Selected reading examples. Eschborn: GATE; 1996. Available from: http://www.sswm.info/sites/default/files/reference_attachments/GTZ%20ny%20Participatory%20Impact%20Monitoring%20Selected%20Reading%20Examples.pdf

Rubin F. *A basic guide to evaluation for development workers*. Oxford: Oxfam; 1995. Available from: http://policy-practice.oxfam.org.uk/publications/a-basic-guide-to-evaluation-for-development-workers-121038

United Nations Development Group. *Monitoring and evaluation: UNDAF companion guidance*. New York: UNDG; 2005. Available online from: https://undg.org/wp-content/uploads/

2017/06/UNDG-UNDAF-Companion-Pieces-6-Monitoring-And-Evaluation.pdf

U.S. Department of Health and Human Services Centers for Disease Control and Prevention. Office of the Director, Office of Strategy and Innovation. *Introduction to program evaluation for public health programs: A self-study guide*. Atlanta, GA: Centers for Disease Control and Prevention, 2011. Available at: https://www.cdc.gov/eval/guide/cdcevalmanual.pdf

Valadez J, Weiss W, Leburg C, Davis R. *Assessing community health programmes: A trainer's guide*. Lusaka: TALC; 2007. A participant's manual and workbook are also available.

World Bank. *Sleeping on our own mats: An introductory guide to community-based monitoring and evaluation*. Washington, DC: World Bank; 2002.

References

1. Sustainable Sanitation and Water Management. *Participatory Monitoring and Evaluation*. Available from: http://www.sswm.info/content/participatory-monitoring-and-evaluation

2. Charlton J. *Nothing about us without us: Disability oppression and empowerment*. Berkeley: University of California Press; 2000.

3. Rietbergen-McCracken J, Narayan D. *Participation and social assessment, tools and techniques, Module IV, Section 2*. Washington, DC: World Bank; 1998. Available from: http:// www.sswm.info/sites/default/files/reference_attachments/ WORLD%20BANK%201998%20Participation%20and%20 Social%20Assessment.pdf

4. Tearfund. Increasing our Impact. *Footsteps*. 2001; 50. Available from: http://tilz.tearfund.org/~/media/files/tilz/publications/ footsteps/footsteps%2041-50/50/fs50.pdf

5. Braithwaite RL, McKenzie RD, Pruitt V, Holden KB, Aaron K, Hollimon C. Community-based participatory evaluation: The healthy start approach. *Health Promotion Practice*. 2013; 14 (2), 213–19.

6. Funds for NGOs. *Crosscutting Themes—Common Questions in Proposal Writing*. New York; 2012. Available from: https:// www.fundsforngos.org/free-resources-for-ngos/crosscutting-themes-common-questions-proposal-writing/

7. UNAIDS, Joint United Nations Programme on HIV/AIDS. *Global AIDS Monitoring 2018: Indicators for monitoring the 2017 United Nations Political Declaration on HIV and AIDS*. 2017. Available from: http://www.unaids.org/sites/default/files/ media_asset/2017-Global-AIDS-Monitoring_en.pdf

8. Community Evaluation Northern Ireland. *Prove & improve: A self-evaluation resource for voluntary and community organisations*. Belfast: CENI; 2008. Available from: http://www.ceni.org/sites/default/files/ProveandImprove.pdf

9. Work Group for Community Health and Development, University of Kansas. *The community tool box, Section 6, Chapter 36: Participatory Evaluation*. Available from: http://ctb.ku.edu/ en/table-of-contents/evaluate/evaluation/participatory-evaluation/main

Managing personnel and finance

Ted Lankester

This chapter considers how to manage personnel and finance, especially from the viewpoint of small and emerging organizations. Most chapters of the book include ideas on management for the topics being discussed. In addition, Chapter 4 also gives further thoughts on recruitment and seeking funding.

Many health programmes that start well eventually fail through poor management. Management skills are important not only for programme directors but also for all health team and community members who share responsibility. It is important that we see the topics in this chapter (and the others) as key skills needed by the community and the health team. Eventually outsiders will depart and the health programme will be led by the community, usually in association with government services. Leadership overlaps with management and is also crucial for success. This chapter tries to cover both, and considers the various aspects of governance which need to be put in place in the early stages of any programme.

In community-based healthcare (CBHC), management skills are as important as clinical skills. Good management is key to making programmes efficient, effective and sustainable.

What we need to know

A contented, motivated team is the basis for a successful health and development programme. This will depend in large part on those in charge using appropriate leadership styles and being effective managers.

The meaning of leadership and management

Leadership and management are different skills but have many areas where they overlap. Leadership is the role and set of skills that helps to propel a programme forwards. It depends on personality, vision and determination to see what can be achieved and how obstacles can be overcome. At its best it inspires the team. One definition of a leader is someone that people want to follow.

Management refers more to the systematic, efficient organization of processes, so that plans are enabled to happen and brought to fruition.[1]

In CBHC, leadership and management are both essential for success. In new or small-scale programmes the leader will often be responsible for most of the programme management. Later the leader may be known as the chief executive (or president for larger organizations in the US) or programme director. This person works with senior managers responsible for different aspects of the programme or organisation, or in smaller programmes with an operations (Ops) manager. Together, the leader and managers form a leadership team, a better and more inspirational term than a (senior) management team.

Abilities in leading and management partly stem from personality and natural talents. But both can be hugely helped by training, coaching, and mentoring. We are aiming for leaders and managers who are excellent at their jobs, have good relational skills, and a commitment to fairness and justice.

Models of leadership

Some people follow the autocratic or authoritarian command and control approach. They make the decisions, keep control, give the orders, and block discussion. The result is a feeling of disempowerment of team members. Others follow a facilitative or consultative approach where everyone contributes, authority is delegated, jobs are flexible, and self-discipline is encouraged (Figure 10.2). The leader is first among equals, and the result is a motivated team and community that share ownership of the programme's successes and challenges (See Figure 10.2).

Many natural leaders tend to be authoritarian in style, and others become so when put in positions of power. For this reason, leaders in CBHC will need actively to learn and maintain a more facilitative style, and

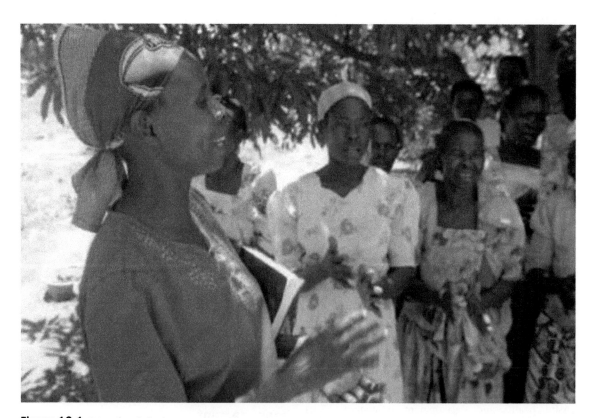

Figure 10.1 Future female leaders.

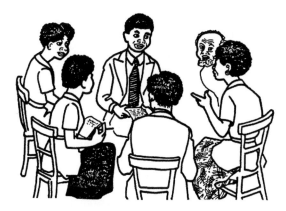

Figure 10.2 The facilitative approach to leadership.

develop a non-hierarchical, evolutionary culture where leadership is more distributed.[2] However, finding this type of leadership is far from simple.

Even though a facilitative style is usually the preferred one in CBHC, we need to be aware of a few issues that may arise. Excessive team involvement can lead to perpetual discussion and delayed decisions, but conversely, some team members have little interest in discussion and decision-making and simply want to get on with their job. Additionally, quite often there is a danger that too much consultation will slow the project down.

Importantly, leadership must be free to lead in order for programmes to be effective. In difficult, dangerous, or uncertain situations, clear, decisive leadership from the front is sometimes needed.

Guidelines for leading

Leaders at all levels in the programme and the community should follow a certain list of guidelines in order to be effective. Because they head a team, they must be *consultative* in the day-to-day running of the programme (Figure 10.2), but decisive when the situation requires. They must also be *facilitators* and empower other team members to learn new skills and grow in self-confidence. On the back of facilitating, they will also need to be *talent spotters*, and learn how to recognise, use, and develop team members' innate talents and skills.

A successful leader will be *credible*—leaders must be competent and fair so they win people's trust, and they must also be unbiased and avoid favouritism. Everyone in the team, from the lowest to the highest in the pecking order must be treated with equal fairness and respect, as favouritism can cause jealousy and sow the seeds of infighting, which may seriously damage the programme (Figure 10.3).

Finally, a good leader must be *patient* ready to listen and support even when this can be time-consuming. Being available and supportive, spending time with the team and with individuals, helping with work tasks, and providing support for personal problems will create a feeling of inclusiveness. By being accessible, even at inconvenient times, the leader will show that he or she is truly part of the team.

Ways of encouraging the health team

Team and community members will perform best if they know what they are aiming for, so it is always important

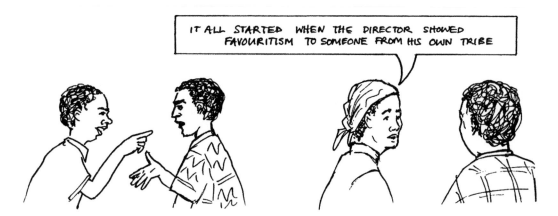

Figure 10.3 Leaders need to treat all team members with equal respect and dignity.

for the team to share the same objectives and, when objectives are reached, to reward people for their achievements. Other ways of encouraging the health team include:

- Delegating responsibility for specific tasks, with training, and with the authority to act;
- Ensuring salaries are paid on time and that increases and promotion are given when due;
- Arranging in-service training and regular opportunities for personal and professional development;
- Handling problems directly and fairly, seeking the root cause of the trouble and trying to solve it; and
- Affirming and supporting team members, especially those for whom we have line management responsibility.

This includes such simple things as remembering birthdays and being thoughtful during times of crisis. For example, the father of a Congolese team member working in Kenya died. The manager, knowing that this man was the oldest son and would have many family duties to perform, gave him ten days' compassionate leave, even though he had no contractual right to it. The man was able to arrange the funeral and support his family, and then returned able to work effectively and satisfied he had fulfilled his family duties.

Things that discourage the health team

Poor administration, and leaders who are forgetful, who delay or overwork staff, or who plan inefficiently will frustrate their teams. Other things that discourage the health team include:

- Lack of respect for others;
- A domineering attitude;
- Giving work that is too easy, too hard, too much, or too little;
- Cancelling leave unless there is an urgent reason,
- Reluctance to delegate or giving responsibility without clearly communicated authority, and
- Lack of training and development opportunities.

It is important to follow good leadership patterns from the beginning. It is easier to keep a team happy than to make a team happy.

Understand personal and financial pressures on team members

In areas where health needs are greatest, we must understand two background factors that will often affect management of the programme. The first is the shortage of health workers, often because of migration to better paid jobs elsewhere. The second is the personal and financial pressure many team members will be under. In many instances they will have multiple home duties, including caring for the family. They will often be under serious financial pressure as relatives expect their salary to pay for the needs of the wider family members. We need to understand this when we face poor attendance, stress, and petty corruption among our staff. We will still need to follow management and disciplinary procedures, but act from a position of understanding.

What we need to do

Write job descriptions

Job descriptions (JDs) list the details and tasks of a job—either for a paid staff member or volunteer. When a programme first starts it may be unhelpful to define jobs too tightly as there is often a phase when team members are discovering how best they can match their skills with the tasks needing to be done. Later, as different team members take on specific tasks, it will be useful to define them, often formalizing what team members have already been doing.

Established programmes should include JDs in the recruitment process, and they must all have a flexibility clause—health workers should be ready to do any reasonable task. A well-written JD helps people know what is expected of them and give a sense of security. It may help to prevent or solve disputes.

A job description should include the following:

1. Job title.
2. Who the job-holder reports to, i.e. their line manager.
3. Those team workers which the job-holder works with and that they supervise or manage.
4. The main purpose of the job.
5. The tasks and duties of the job.

In addition, a contract of employment or a less formal agreement can be drawn up. This should include:

- grade and salary;
- length of contract;
- details of appraisal; and
- terms and conditions of service.

Sometimes it is helpful to list the components of a particular task in more detail, either in the JD or separately. For example, a CHW supervisor's job might include:

1. Visiting CHWs regularly in order to:
   - give encouragement;
   - check that she is carrying out her duties;
   - teach skills and knowledge;
   - plan future tasks;
   - refill her health kit;
   - complete her records;
   - pay her expenses.
2. Assessing how well the CHW is functioning and to decide on appropriate guidance for her.
3. Keeping the team leader informed of a CHWs' progress (See Figure 10.4).

Induct new team members

When a new team member joins, they will need to go through an induction process. This helps the team member to learn as much about the programme as possible. Induction not only raises the confidence of new team members but also enables them to be effective from an early stage. Induction needs to be planned carefully, and will depend on the time available and the experience and seniority of new team member(s).

Induction should include an overview of the history, present situation, and future plans of the programme, including its values, beliefs and principles. It should also provide a clear explanation of all relevant aspects of the programme, an opportunity to meet other team members, and an opportunity to observe various programme activities, e.g. to understand the working of the finance team. Finally, it should provide the opportunity to ask questions.

Inductions need to be planned in advance so that time is set aside for members of the team involved. Never assume it will just happen in the course of a busy day.

Carry out appraisals

An appraisal is a yearly meeting between a team member and their manager. It does not replace the need for regular meetings nor for meetings to address significant problems as they arise.

The purpose of an appraisal is to review the past year, looking at what the person has accomplished and comparing this with the objectives set in the previous appraisal. It also provides a forum in which the team member and manager agree on personal objectives or a personal development plan for the coming year. It gives the appraisee an opportunity to raise any issues and concerns related to their job. It gives the manager the opportunity to identify areas needing improvement, to identify training needs, and to recognize and affirm good performance.

Appraisals need to be regular, confidential, affirming, and relational, not disciplinary in character. They must be planned in advance so that both the appraiser and appraisee can prepare beforehand. The advantages of regular appraisals include strengthening of mutual trust and understanding between the team member and the manager, identifying and addressing problems and weaknesses before they cause problems, and affirming the appraisee.

It is helpful for a form to be filled in by the appraisee before the appraisal, with guidance notes. The manager can make notes, comments, and suggestions, and both then agree on the final appraisal document and sign it off. The appraisee can hold a copy along with the person responsible for HR. In busy programmes appraisals are often forgotten, delayed, or ignored. Carried out regularly, and fairly, they can be motivational for both team members and managers.

Resolve conflicts

Preventing disputes is easier and quicker than solving them. From the beginning, we must write clear job descriptions and give clear task instructions. We can prevent disputes by being fair and meeting regularly to plan together, contribute ideas, express feelings, and discuss problems. If we recruit team members with friendly and tolerant attitudes, these positive aspects will influence the whole team. In teams where members of different ethnic or language groups work together, we must do everything possible to encourage mutual trust and respect (see Figure 10.4). Those in positions of leadership need to set an example and avoid favouritism. Assure the team that no one has 'special access' to the person in charge. Do not listen to gossip, and avoid too many members of one family belonging to the programme (See Figure 10.5).

It is also important to provide spiritual input. There can be a regular time for prayer or meditation, with which team members need to feel comfortable—otherwise it should be optional. We can encourage apology and forgiveness if disputes have occurred or there has been

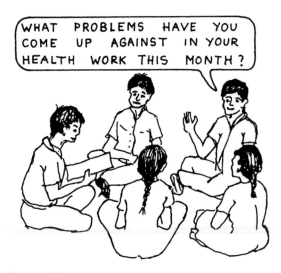

Figure 10.4 Part of the job description for a CHW supervisor.

Reproduced from Hesperian Health Guides, www.hesperian.org. Copyright © 2017 Hesperian Health Guides. This image is distributed under the terms of the Creative Commons Attribution Non-Commercial 4.0 International licence (CC-BY-NC), a copy of which is available at http://creativecommons.org/licenses/by-nc/4.0/.

perceived unfairness. Even in the most contented teams, conflicts will arise. If they are handled quickly and sensibly, they can usually be solved. If they are ignored or mishandled, their effects can continue for years.

Guidelines for solving disputes

As mentioned, it is far easier to prevent disputes in the first place. We should also act early, drawing on friendship, fairness, and common sense so that problems are less likely to become serious. For serious disputes between team members we must respond quickly. See each party separately, and listen carefully, making every effort to understand each person. We can then ask each party if they are ready for mediation. If they seem willing, they are encouraged to do this on their own. If they fail or are unwilling, we can offer to be a mediator or invite them to name someone else acceptable to both parties.

If a problem is complex or there is a sense of injustice, encourage each complainant to have someone accompany them for support and to interpret their needs. It is important to remain unbiased and slow in giving judgment. We must also be ready to act as scapegoat. One of the causes of the dispute may be our poor management!

Finally, keep careful documentation and record the outcome and what was agreed, and if appropriate, ask both parties to sign. Correct any problem that might cause the dispute to recur.

Managing more major disputes between team members and managers are beyond the scope of this book.

Manage change

It has been said that it is normal for organizations continually to go through processes of change.[3] It is helpful for all new members of staff to know and understand this. In a rapidly changing world, programmes need to respond to new and unpredicted challenges, and they may not be able to continue in the same way indefinitely.

Any change in a programme leads to increased stress. Many people will be frightened by the unknown or worried by loss of control. They may be concerned they will lose their job or be asked to take on new responsibilities against their wishes. If there is a shortage of money or personnel they may be worried about workload. It is worth noting here that some people find change more difficult to cope with than others, especially if they are facing problems in other aspects of their life or have an ongoing illness. Box 10.1 shows different examples of job stresses and questions that can occur in programme change.

Because of underlying anxiety, there may be more arguments and complaints than usual, more absences due to illness, or a general decline in morale. We can support the team through change by understanding the stresses they are feeling. We must inform the team promptly and fully about any developments, and think carefully about timing. Any planning and discussion to show the reasons for change must happen with the team, and the change(s) should be carefully planned and communicated (we can use mobile phones, WhatsApp, etc., in addition to in-person chats). Make sure all team members know what is happening and how their working conditions will be affected. Having an 'open door' policy enabling people to talk about any concerns will help, as will having a culture of welcoming the suggestions and ideas of all team members, both in operational areas and in strategic planning.

Delegate to others

Delegation is the art of enabling others to use the talents they possess, and do as much as they can. Learning to delegate is essential for health workers, managers, leaders, or anyone who has responsibility for others' work. The two main advantages of delegation are that it gives the person delegating more time to spend on important, strategic tasks, and gives others an opportunity to learn new skills and to develop confidence.

Box 10.1 Situations and questions associated with programme change

Stressful situations associated with programme change include:

- The appointment of a new director, team leader or line manager.
- Converting a programme from a curative, clinical approach to a participatory, community approach.
- Starting in a new area or beginning a different type of work.
- Uncertainty about funding, or about the programme's future.
- A change in management style.
- Changes and development in information technology, especially if training and IT support is not available.
- Changes in location of the office or programme.

During programme change, team members may ask themselves questions like:

- How will this affect me?
- Will I have more or less money?
- Will I have more or less status?
- Will I enjoy the job as much?
- Will I be able to do the new job?
- How will I get on with my new colleagues and with my new boss?
- If the project closes, where will I find employment?

Delegation is the basis of task-shifting (Chapter 1) and an important principle in community health: 'A job should be done by the person *least* qualified who can do it well.' However, before delegating we need to ensure that the task is appropriate and the person to whom we are giving the task is willing and able to do it. We will often need to arrange training. While we need to delegate, we must also teach others how to delegate. We need to resist the notion that it is quicker to do something ourselves than teach others to do it. In delegating a task, we need to pass on information and skills needed to do the task, the responsibility for the task – with the assurance that final responsibility remains with us, especially if anything goes wrong – and the authority to carry out the task. If any of these three principles are left out, conflict is likely to develop in the team. Although delegation is an important part of management, leaders can become isolated from their team members unless they regularly join in with team activities, as well as day-to-day or menial tasks.

Manage staff in the day-to-day programme

Apart from planning major programme activities, we also need to set up a system for managing day-to-day activities. This will involve matching the staff available with tasks that need to be done in the field. At an early stage in the programme, health committee members can share in day-to-day planning. A chart can be made that lists out the days of the month, with each day divided into columns either by programme area or by activity. The chart can have a plastic surface, and coloured, erasable, felt-tip pens can be used to mark different activities and personnel involved. Planned activities are filled in, with names of the key people involved.

Final details are completed at least a week ahead with instructions about time and place and other important information, e.g. equipment needed. This board is displayed in the programme headquarters. Any last-minute changes due to illness, severe weather, security concerns or civil conflict etc. is communicated, e.g. by mobile phone, to all those involved as soon as possible (see Figure 10.6).

Give variety and keep a sense of balance

Balance and variety help to keep people contented. When team members do identical tasks day after day, especially under pressure, it is easy for them to become bored, stressed or demotivated. Where possible, we need to give variety so that tasks are shared and more than one person is trained to do any specific task. For example, two or more people can be trained to dispense medicines, while the main dispenser can be trained to do other tasks, such as registering patients. It helps if our team culture supports the idea that team members are multipurpose, e.g. programme drivers can be involved in a range of activities between driving assignments. For individuals and teams, balance might include being involved in prevention and cure, community and hospital, field and office, serving the better-off and the poor, health and development, or working with men, women, and children. Most important of all is work–life balance. We must ensure that work is not excessive and that safeguards are built into the programme's planning and budget.

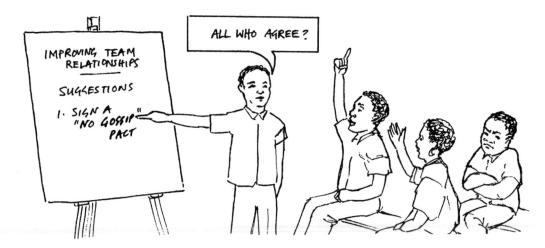

Figure 10.5 Trust between team members is one key to successful programmes.

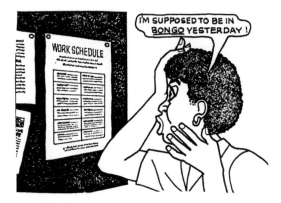

Figure 10.6 Ensure that everyone is fully informed when plans change.

Set up good governance systems

Many programmes fail through poor governance, and at an early stage of the project we will need to start setting up a simple and effective governance system.[4] Many small- and medium-sized projects have found Box 10.2 a helpful guide. We can use this at the start of our programme so we are aware of all the areas that need to be covered. Then, at regular intervals we can check through the list and use it to rank how well we are doing in the different areas.

A well-governed programme will need to have all these systems in place. However, when first starting out we must concentrate on those areas which are simplest and most important. For programmes starting from scratch, this will include the setting up of a board of management or trustees.

Box 10.2 **Board of Trustees or Directors**

There is an independent group governed by a documented constitution, with at least six voluntary (unpaid) members, each with limited terms of office. This is called the Board.

The Board has good representation from relevant stakeholders with relevant skills and expertise.

The Board meets at least twice a year to provide strategic direction to the organization.

The organization is properly registered and compliant with local reporting, tax, and labour requirements.

The organization has a strategic plan and it monitors progress against planned goals.

The strategic plan has been developed in consultation with the board, staff, and other relevant stakeholders.

The organizational structure is effective for delegating responsibility and sharing information between staff.

Box 10.2 *continued*

Does the organization have sufficient controls around anti-bribery? For example, what are the procedures if staff are asked for/offered a bribe? Does the organization have zero-tolerance towards bribery?

Financial management and accountability

The organization has standard financial policies and procedures which are understood by all staff members.

The organization has sufficient good quality financial/accounts staff to handle further funding.

The organization reports expenditure of projects separately to more than one different donor and for several different budgets.

Accounts and supporting documents are filed securely and are retained for the period specified by the relevant donor.

The organization has a bank account with a stable and reputable bank.

At least two signatories are required for all payments.

The organization financial records are audited annually by an independent audit firm.

What percentage of total costs are core costs (e.g. salaries, fixed overheads)? Is this reasonable?

An annual budget for the whole organization is prepared and monitored on a regular basis.

The organization has a medium- to long-term fundraising strategy.

All fixed assets are adequately safeguarded, e.g. insured, usage monitored.

Human resources and administration

The organization has standard documented procedures for managing human resources (e.g. HR manual).

Recruitment processes are clearly defined, transparent, and fair.

All staff have clear job descriptions that are documented and reviewed on a regular basis.

All staff have contracts setting out the terms and conditions of their employment.

The contracts are in line with relevant labour laws and are transparent and fair.

All staff have adequate skills and experience to carry out their role effectively.

Staff are given opportunities for training and career development where possible.

Administrative procedures are documented in up-to-date manuals and are understood and followed by all staff.

All volunteers are given an induction and clear training for their role within the organization.

Volunteers receive sufficient support and their roles and responsibilities are clearly documented, e.g. volunteer agreements.

Programme management and reporting

Workplans, activities, and expenditure are reviewed and compared against proposals and budgets at least every three months.

Programme reports are always completed and sent to donors and other stakeholders on time.

The organization has a clear system for managing restricted grant monies against budgets.

The organization maintains adequate documentation to support all programme activities, e.g. minutes of meetings, receipts, attendance registers.

Organizations working with children and vulnerable people have a suitable policy in place to protect these individuals.

Credibility and advocacy

Staff are familiar with the national framework for TB and any national co-ordinating mechanisms.

The organization actively participates in relevant local and national networks/forums.

Key stakeholders including CSOs and government sectors respect the organization and believe it has significant expertise in its area of work.

There are productive contacts with at least one relevant decision maker in national government.

If advocacy work is undertaken, the organization has conducted national level advocacy projects to change the policy or practices of targeted influential individuals or institutions.

If advocacy work is undertaken it is evidence-based and systematic research is used to compile the evidence.

Research, learning, and dissemination

There is an adequately skilled individual or team with specific responsibility for M&E.

All project proposals include evaluation and dissemination of lessons learned.

The organization has undertaken an evaluation of its overall impact in the last three years.

Managing finance

Who should handle finance?

Anyone involved in handling money will need to be sufficiently well-trained. They must also be thorough, efficient, and trustworthy. It is important that we think of our health programme as including both health team members and community members. The community will need to be involved at an early stage in how to handle finance as community members will become increasingly involved in areas of financial administration as they develop their skills through training and mentoring.

A warning: many otherwise excellent programmes falter, fail, close, or cause a scandal because of poor financial management.

Two grades of people are needed in order to ensure the financial success of the programme: a bookkeeper and an accountant. A bookkeeper will enter cash received and money spent on a daily basis. This can be a relatively junior person, provided they are taught exactly how to do it. They should enter transactions at the time they are made and never delay entry until the following day (or week).

An accountant will oversee finances and prepare management accounts at the end of each month, quarter, half year, and year. They will also need to estimate cash flow for the following month, quarter, and half year. An accountant must also prepare a budget in discussion with the programme leaders, and prepare end-of-year accounts for the auditor.

Sometimes the programme director will do the accounting, especially when the programme first starts. As the programme expands, an accountant can join the team, possibly working part time at first. At each stage of the programme, someone should take responsibility for financial management, whether it is the programme director, an accountant, or a finance manager. Members of the community can be involved in specific financial tasks, initially with a title such as financial assistant. Excellent accounting software is available, including specialized non-profit packages, as and when a programme has the time, capacity, and training to use them reliably.

We will need to have the following in place before computerizing accounts:

- Good-quality manual systems that have been well set up and are working efficiently.
- One, preferably two, trained staff members able to manage the system, and do basic troubleshooting.
- Access to expert backup, advice and repair.
- A reliable electricity supply, including voltage stabilizer, backup generator, etc.
- No other more important priorities on which to spend staff time and resources.
- A user-friendly software package that can run alongside manual systems for a number of months.
- Protection against computer viruses, adequate data backup, and security against fraud and theft.
- A well-planned process for buying, induction and training. This must be built into project planning so as not to cause undue stress to staff or add to workload.
- Backup arrangements so that key tasks, e.g. paying bills and salaries, can still be carried out if no computer systems are working.

With increasing skills in computing and financial enterprise in the Millennial Generation, young and gifted community members can often take a role using computers in financial management. Box 10.3 provides a glossary of terms used in financial management.

Source: Footsteps 11, Tearfund, p. 11.

Box 10.3 **Glossary of financial terms**

Asset Any item that keeps its value is known as an asset. For NGOs, these are normally stocks of goods, office equipment, vehicles and property.

Bank statement A report produced by a bank listing all the receipts and payments made into or out of a bank account.

Book-keeping The process of recording the basic details of each transaction.

Budget The best possible estimate of the future cost of activities over a given period of time, and of how those activities will be paid for.

Cash advance A sum of money entrusted to someone to use when precise costs are not known in advance.

Cash book A book or spreadsheet that lists all the transactions made into and out of a single account.

Reconciliation The process of comparing and checking information held in two sets of records that describe the same transactions.

Supporting documents The original documents that describe each transaction. They include receipts, invoices and authorizing documents.

Transaction Any exchange of goods, services or money in return for other goods, services or money.

Doing the accounting

The following are the basic start-up tasks for a small-scale programme (See Box 10.3). Many of these can be computerized or make use of an accounting software package:

1. Buy and prepare cash books and files.

These will vary depending on the size and style of accounting. Typical books would include:

- A cash book or register to enter all money received and paid out, with a column to record current balance;
- A ledger to list expenditure by category of goods and services bought, and income by source;
- A petty cash book or register where minor day-to-day spending is recorded, with details of each entry also recorded on a petty cash voucher with receipt attached;
- A salary register, where details of salaries for each programme member are recorded and where payments can be signed for;
- Files to keep receipts for items bought, with attached invoices, and details of money received with documentation. All should be kept in strict, usually chronological order or by category.

2. Open a bank account.

Unless banks are distant or unreliable, we should open accounts and place funds not immediately needed into an account that earns interest. Remember that cheques,

especially from foreign sources, may take weeks to clear. Also, in many countries, suppliers want to be paid in cash or by money order, rather than by cheque or credit card.

3. Prepare management accounts.

These will need to be prepared monthly, quarterly and half-yearly. They include summaries of income received, expenditure by category, amount of money owed by the programme (creditors), and owed to the programme (debtors). Income and expenditure are compared to the budget for the period under consideration. The purpose of management accounts is for understanding and control. They are essential to monitor the programme finances and plan for the future.

4. Prepare cash flow forecasts.

An example is given in Table 10.1. Programmes frequently have a 'cash flow crisis' at some point during the year. The best way to know if funding is sufficient for the coming months is to prepare monthly cash flow forecasts. This involves calculating the amount of money we are likely to spend and to receive each month over the next six months. This helps us to know when income may be especially low or expenditure may be higher than usual, so we can make appropriate plans. Each month we can put in the actual figures for the previous month to replace the forecasted amount for that month. This 'rolling forecast' is an accurate and timesaving way of doing cash flows.

Management accounts look backwards to the previous few months; cash flow forecasts look forward to

Table 10.1 **Example of cash flow forecast**

Women's income generating project
Cash flow forecast for the period 1 January to 30 June 2015

	Jan #	Feb #	Mar #	Apr #	May #	Jun #
Estimated money coming in:						
Sale of honey	7,500	7,500	7,500	7,500	7,500	7,500
Grant for major equipment					30,000	
Other	600	600	600	600	600	600
Total money coming in [A]	8,100	8,100	8,100	8,100	38,100	8,100
Estimated money to be paid:						
Purchase of equipment					30,000	
Materials		5,350		3,970		
Wages	2,625	2,625	2,625	2,625	2,625	2,625
Rent of premises				13,200		
Vehicle expenses	230	230	230	230	2,190	230
Office expenses	575	575	575	575	575	575
Telephone, electricity	1,517		1,033	1,517		1,033
Total money paid [B]	4,947	8,780	4,463	22,117	35,390	4,463
Opening cash/bank balance	2,340	5,493	4,813	8,450	(5,567)*	(2,857)*
+ Total money coming in [A]	8,100	8,100	8,100	8,100	38,100	8,100
− Total money paid [B]	4,947	8,780	4,463	22,117	35,390	4,463
Closing cash/bank balance	5,493	4,813	8,450	(5,567)*	(2,857)*	780

* Figures in brackets are negative cash amounts
# = their currency symbol
Adapted with permission from Tearfund. Managing Cash flow. *Footsteps*. (57). Copyright © Tearfund. Available at http://learn.tearfund.org/en/resources/publications/footsteps/footsteps_51-60/footsteps_57/managing_cash_flow/. This table is distributed under the terms of the Creative Commons Attribution Non Commercial 4.0 International licence (CC-BY-NC), a copy of which is available at http://creativecommons.org/licenses/by-nc/4.0/

the next few months. Together they help us to keep accurate financial control.

5. Consider setting up an imprest system.

Any team member who regularly spends project funds is advanced a fixed sum of money (the imprest) from which purchases are made. When this becomes low, the programme member presents his or her receipts for money spent to the director or accountant, who replenishes the imprest up to the original amount.

6. Prepare annual accounts for the auditor.

These will include as a minimum:

- Details (with documentation) of income, debtors, creditors, and details of any loans.
- Clear separation of income allowed for any purpose (general funds) or limited funds given for a specific purpose.
- Donations from overseas, separately listed and accounted for.
- A profit and loss sheet, and a balance sheet.

Table 10.2 is a useful checklist of basic standards for finance management.

Table 10.2 **Checking your financial management: monitoring good practice**

Supporting documents. Every financial transaction should be backed up by a 'supporting document', such as a bill, invoice or receipt.	Always	Mostly	Sometimes	Never
1. A supporting document is available for every payment.	5	4	1	0
2. A supporting document is available for every item of income.	5	4	1	0
3. Supporting documents are neatly filed, so that it is easy to find any document when it is needed.	5	4	1	0
4. Bank statements are neatly filed.	5	4	1	0
5. Supporting documents and bank statements are kept for the previous seven years.	5	4	1	0
Cash books: Every transaction should be written down in a cash book. A cash book is simply a list of the money that an organization has spent and received. It can be kept on paper or on a computer.				
6. The date, description, and amount of every transaction are recorded in a cash book.	5	4	1	0
7. All cash books are updated at least once per month.	5	4	1	0
8. A separate cash book is kept for each bank account.	5	4	1	0
Cash records				
9. All cash is kept in a locked cash box or safe.	5	4	1	0
10. Petty cash records are checked every month by a different person from the person who writes them up.	5	4	1	0
11. The balance in the cash book is checked against the balance on the bank statement every month.	5	4	1	0
12. The balance in the cash book is checked against the actual amount of cash in the office every month.	5	4	1	0
Budgeting				
13. Budgets are prepared every year.	5	4	1	0
14. Budgets include enough income to pay for all planned expenditure.	5	4	1	0
15. Each month, a cash flow forecast is prepared for the next six-month period.	5	4	1	0
Add up the numbers you circled, to give your score:				

Preparing budgets

All programmes will need to prepare budgets, i.e. listing out the amounts we expect to spend (expenditure) and to receive (income) by different categories. We should do this as accurately as possible for one accounting year, and in outline for two further years. If we are receiving money from donors, we should prepare budgets the way they advise and according to any conditions they set down. They will often suggest the expenditure headings to use. Sometimes we will need to devise our own headings, especially if our categories of expenditure are different from the donor's or if we have other funding sources that use different headings. As our budgets become more detailed we will probably want to computerize our accounts and add codes to different categories of income and expenditure through accounts software.

Meanwhile we can simply list items under specific categories.

1. Capital items

This refers to larger sums of money that are received and spent on items lasting a number of years, e.g. buildings, vehicles, computers, high-cost items of equipment.

2. Recurrent items

This refers to income and expenditure for items or services, and includes staff salaries. Typical simplified headings might include:

- Expenditure
  - Staff salaries
  - Services
  - Rent and buildings
  - Health care supplies including medicines
  - Travel and transport
  - Training
  - Administration
  - Maintenance of equipment
  - Depreciation (an annual amount to cover the reduced value of capital items bought in the past)
  - Contingency (to cover the unexpected).
- Income
  - By source and amount.
  - How allocated against expenditure.

We need to make sure that the budget, along with plans for the coming year, is submitted well before the deadline set by any funding agency.

Setting up a reserves policy

If our organization is a registered business or charity we should develop a reserves policy sooner rather than later. If we are passionate about making a difference to our community's well-being and allow our enthusiasm to run ahead of our resources, we may face serious danger. We may quickly and unexpectedly run out of money, and be informed by our auditor or accountant that we are no longer a going concern. All the enthusiasm can be wasted because we have not saved surplus as a buffer for when we need extra unexpected money.

From time to time, all organizations will find they need more money than they have budgeted for. This may because of a new opportunity, an unexpected debt or expense, maternity cover, failure of a donation to arrive,

or insecurity in our location. A sensible estimate for the reserves we may need is equivalent for the normal day-to-day expenses of the programme for at least 4 months and ideally longer. It is an important challenge to make this a priority.

Smaller-scale and more recent programmes often find it difficult to build up reserves as there is usually little extra income to set aside. Also, donors are not willing to give money to build up reserves. This means that whenever we receive undesignated income it is good practice to put a small proportion of this into a reserve or coded account so that a fund gradually accumulates.

It is helpful to look at what is involved in setting up reserves in a bit more detail:

- *Reviewing existing funds*: how they were built up and what they are used for.
- *Analysing current and potential income streams*: how much is definite and how much is merely hoped for.
- *Analysing expenditure patterns and cash flow needs*: making sure we have made accurate estimates based on reality and not on unfounded optimism.
- *Assessing the need for reserves*: working out realistically the likely highest unexpected sum we may be faced with in our particular circumstances.
- *Calculating the reserves level*: Using the best evidence we have of the above points, and aiming for and maintaining reserves at that agreed level.
- *Presentation of the reserves policy*: to our stakeholders and above all to our board of directors or trustees, both for their information and their agreement.

There is more helpful information on this on the Humentum website.[5]

Who needs details of the programme accounts?

- The programme itself, for its records, and to sort out any questions or problems later on.
- Any donor agency supporting the programme.
- The government, who may inspect them, especially if foreign donations have been received.

Further reading and resources

Aga Khan Health Service. *Managing a health facility: A handbook for committee members and facility staff.* Oxford: Macmillan; 2007. Available from: TALC

Cammack J. *Basic accounting for small groups*. 2nd ed. Oxford: Oxfam; 2003. A very useful step-by-step guide to accounting and bookkeeping. Available from: http://policy-practice. oxfam.org.uk/publications/basic-accounting-for-small-groups-121164

Davies A. *Managing for change: How to run community development projects*. Bradford: IT Publications/VSO; 1997. A valuable book covering aspects of importance to both small and larger projects.

Gaw H. Leadership. *Footsteps*. 2011; 84. Available from: http://tilz.tearfund.org/en/resources/publications/footsteps/footsteps_81-90/footsteps_84/

McMahon R, Barton E, Piot M. *On being in charge: A guide to management in primary health*. 2nd ed. Geneva: World Health Organization; 1992. A definitive guide on project management covering all aspects. Still very useful. Available from: http://apps.who.int/iris/handle/10665/37015

People in Aid. *Code of best practice in the management and support of aid personnel*. London: People in Aid; 2003, Available from: http://www.dochas.ie/sites/default/files/People_In_Aid_Code.pdf Highly recommended.

Websites

BOND is a network of development agencies, which runs training courses. http://www.bond.org.uk

People in Aid. http://www.peopleinaid.org.

References

1. Covey S. *The 7 Habits of Highly Effective People*. New York: Free Press; 1989. A good exposition of the difference between leadership and management.
2. Laloux F. *Reinventing organizations*. Fleet: Nelson Parker; 2014.
3. Tsoukas H, Chia R. On organizational becoming: Rethinking organizational change. *Organization* Science. 2002; 13 (5): 567–82.
4. Blackman R. Organisational Governance. *Roots Guides 10*. Teddington: Tearfund; 2006. Available from: http://tilz.tearfund.org/~/media/Files/TILZ/Publications/ROOTS/English/Governance/ROOTS_10_E.pdf
5. Humentum. Available from: https://www.humentum.org/free-resources/guide/free-downloads

CHAPTER 11
Using medicines correctly

Ted Lankester

What we need to know

The discovery of effective medicines and vaccines has been one of the most significant developments in recent world history, and has saved more lives than any other single advance. It means that many infectious diseases can be cured or prevented and many non-infectious diseases can be controlled.

Traditional medicines are still used widely (see Chapter 3). This makes it all the more important that we help communities gain access to essential supplies, and that we learn to use medicines in the most effective way, and above all, that good practice becomes embedded in our programme and our communities. In this chapter, the use of the word medicine is preferred to the word drug. The correct storage of medicines and vaccines is explained in Chapter 5.

The dangers of misusing medicines

This section looks at why we need to exercise care in prescribing. Later, the chapter looks at positive ways of using medicines effectively.

Overuse of antibiotics

Medicines are dangerously misused in many countries, with antibiotics topping the list. The overuse of antibiotics is becoming a public health emergency, as microbial resistance to antibiotics grows. Our health programmes must ensure that antibiotics are used only when needed and according to strict guidelines. For example, a recent study in the United States showed that one in three antibiotics are prescribed unnecessarily.[1]

World Health Organization (WHO) surveillance figures show that in developing and transitional countries, about half of all acute viral upper respiratory tract infection and viral diarrhoea cases receive inappropriate antibiotics.[2]

Too many injections

Each year more than sixteen billion injections are given worldwide. In some countries more than ten injections per person per year are being used.[3] One project in south India calculated that, on average, 150–200 injections were given each morning by a single nurse in each of the primary health centres studied. Figures from Ghana have shown that eight out of ten prescriptions include an injection.[4] About ninety-five per cent are used for curative care, so only five per cent are immunizations.[5] Many of these injections are entirely unnecessary.

Unsafe injections

Many injections are carried out in an unsafe manner, using non-sterile equipment. One study indicated that each year unsafe injections cause an estimated 1.3 million early deaths, a loss of twenty-six million years of life, and an annual burden of 535 million USD in direct medical costs. This includes twenty-one million cases of hepatitis B, two million cases of hepatitis C, and 250,000 cases of HIV/AIDS.[6]

Polypharmacy

Just as serious as the overuse of injections is the use of far too many medicines that are wrongly prescribed, ineffective, or dangerous. Patients are prescribed (on average) nearly three medicines per prescription, and up to five per patient in some countries; over forty per cent of primary care patients in low- or middle-income countries receive antibiotics.[7] This leads to huge sums of money being wasted each year. Moreover, patients come to believe the dangerous myth that only multiple pills, an injection, or an intravenous drip has any effect.

For example, the author once witnessed a patient collecting twenty-one separate medicines and injections from an urban pharmacy in South Asia. They had been prescribed by a local doctor, and included three different antibiotics. They were all for one patient, who was sufficiently strong to load these into a large carton and carry them out of the door.

Here is another story from Asia. When we arrived at his house the patient was really struggling; he was exhausted, tired, depressed, and short of breath when walking. After an extensive history and reading of the ECGs and results, we concluded that he had not a heart attack as he had been told, but was suffering from polypharmacy. He was on ten medications, including six for blood pressure. After a staged cut back of medicines from ten to two, he said 'I feel like a new man.' His monthly medicine bill fell by ninety per cent.[8] This shows that overuse of medicines is not only wasteful, but harmful.

Substandard, mislabelled, and counterfeit medicines

A growing and deadly problem is the use of substandard and counterfeit medicines. Substandard medicines are of such poor quality that they may be ineffective or dangerous. Counterfeit medicines are fraudulently manufactured and labelled, but do not contain the active ingredient they claim to possess. They may contain starch or chalk. Sometimes they are made in unhygienic conditions. One estimate of the scale of the problem was that one in ten medical products used in resource-poor countries are substandard or falsified.[9] Exact figures are difficult to confirm, but it is an escalating world-wide problem. Antibiotics and antimalarials as life-saving medicines are especially targeted.[10]

When checking medicines for counterfeits, examine the packaging for condition, spelling mistakes, or grammatical errors, along with the manufacturing and expiry dates; ensure that any details on the outer packaging match the dates shown on the inner packaging. Make sure that the medicine looks correct, and is not discoloured, degraded, or does not have an unusual smell. Finally, listen to patients as they are often the first to detect counterfeit medicines.[11]

The use of and ordering of online medicines is also dangerous. There are multibillion-pound scams increasing at a fast rate. The WHO estimates that fifty per cent of medicines ordered from illegal online sites are fake.[11] We should advise against all use of online medicines.

Self-medication

It is also thought that, in many poorer countries, patients buy or obtain half their medicines without seeing a health worker. This is especially harmful in the case of antibiotics or drugs used for treating TB or HIV. However, this practice is understandable, as seeing a doctor or health worker can add hugely to the expense of medical treatment. This again points to the importance of our health programmes ensuring that essential medicines are easily affordable, and that trained health workers are able to prescribe and provide them quickly at low or no cost.

Side effects and drug resistance

Misuse of medicines causes not only dependency, but also serious or fatal side effects. When antibiotics are misused there is an even greater danger: drug resistance. As mentioned, increasing numbers of dangerous germs are rapidly developing resistance to antibiotics. Some diseases are becoming very difficult and expensive to cure. Multidrug-resistant TB (MDR-TB) and extensively drug-resistant tuberculosis (XDR-TB) is just one example (see Chapter 19). Another is the development of Meticillin-resistant Staphylococcus Aureus (MRSA), a dangerous infection spread mainly in hospitals with poor hygiene control. *Clostridium difficile*, often referred to as *C. diff*, is another dangerous pathogen that is difficult to treat and is largely caused by the overuse of antibiotics. Each year, new antibiotic-resistant germs are emerging.

Wastage leads to poverty

The combined effect of all these bad practices leads to enormous wastage. Medicines absorb up to forty per cent of national health budgets. At the grassroots level, overprescribing increases poverty. The poor and

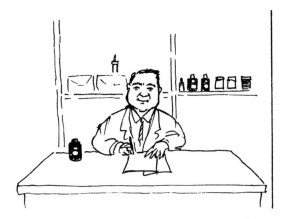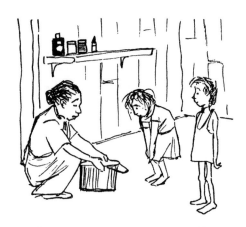

Figure 11.1 PPNN: A Pill for every problem, a needle for every need: An effective way of robbing the poor to pay the rich.

uneducated are charged for injections and medicines they often don't need (see Figure 11.1). Manufacturers and suppliers of these medicines profit at their expense. The poorest may have no money left when they really need essential medicines.

It is tragic when families sell their only cow or buffalo, on which they depend, to buy medicines they may not really need, or sell their daughters to pay for ineffective treatment.

The idea of a rational drugs policy

These multiple effects from incorrect prescribing have led experts to develop the idea of a rational drugs policy, in part driven by WHO estimates that fifty per cent of medicines globally are used 'irrationally'.

Rational use of medicines requires that patients receive medications appropriate to their clinical needs, in doses that meet their own individual requirements, for an adequate period of time, and at the lowest cost to them and their community.[12] The WHO has produced guidelines on the appropriate use of essential medicines as well as their manufacture and quality control. The use of ineffective and dangerous medicines is actively discouraged.

The WHO drew up the first *Model List of Essential Medicines* in 1977, which is now regularly updated and comprises a formulary giving details on each medicine listed. Different countries use this list to draw up their own national medicines policies and essential medicines lists. One government that has been successful in doing this, thanks to strong medical leadership, is Bangladesh.

However, the pressures against developing these policies and carrying them out are extremely strong.

Each year some irresponsible medicine manufacturers develop new, clever ways of persuading people that a whole range of medicines and injections is necessary when they are not. With freer global trade and weaker regulation, the situation becomes ever more difficult. Although many medicines are of good quality, an increasing number, especially those made locally without careful checks, are poor quality, altogether fake, or dangerous and contaminated.

Two examples illustrate the pressures against rational drug use. One drug company offered Peruvian pharmacists a bottle of wine if they ordered three boxes of its cough and cold remedy. Another company told doctors to suspect *Giardia* or amoeba in all cases of diarrhoea and treat it immediately with metronidazole. In fact, this drug is only needed in a very small proportion of diarrhoeal cases.

For those in community-based health care (CBHC) these trends have two main implications. First, we must follow rational drug policies and only use medicines on an essential medicines list. Second, we must help protect members of our community against unethical promotions of medicines or breastmilk substitutes. We must educate them in ways of preventing illness and in accepting treatment with one or two medicines, rather than injections and multiple prescriptions.

One important footnote: although some pharmaceutical companies are guilty of unethical advertising, many are not. We should try to build positive relationships with medicine manufacturers and suppliers as this can reduce our costs and make it easier to maintain regular supplies of essential medicines.

Problems with access to life-saving medicines

Nearly two billion people lack access to essential medicines, including life-saving drugs.[13] A recent International Labour Organization report shows that fifty-six per cent of people living in rural areas worldwide lack access to essential health care services, more than double the figure in urban areas, where twenty-two per cent are not covered.[14]

There are many reasons for this gap, which include insufficient domestic manufacture of medicines, particularly to treat neglected diseases (where profit margins are low), high prices, lack of competition between generic suppliers, trade tariffs and other restrictions, corruption, and the collapse of health systems, but above all, poor local access owing to distance, understaffed health centres, and inadequate infrastructure.

The third Sustainable Development Goal has as one of its targets 'To achieve universal health coverage, including access to safe, effective, quality and affordable essential medicines and vaccines for all'. In our health programmes, we must ensure that all community members have access to life-saving medicines and that we identify and tackle anything that prevents it.

The most important life-saving medicines for many areas of the world include antibiotics, treatment for tuberculosis, artemisinin-combined therapy (ACT) to cure malaria, and antiretroviral therapy (ART) to treat HIV/AIDS. Wider availability of medicines is also needed for non-communicable diseases and mental health problems (see Chapters 22 and 24).

One of our roles in CBHC is to make sure these medicines are reliably available at community level. This may involve us in advocacy at local, district, or even national level. An effective strategy is to join existing campaigns to make life-saving medicines available and affordable, both nationally and locally. At the time of writing the 20th *Model List of Essential Medicines* dates from April 2017 and is revised every few years.[15] For relief and emergency situations the WHO has put together a detailed list and guidance document.[16] A new Model List for maternal care has recently been introduced.[17]

The difference between medical care and health care

Most health workers enjoy using medicines and many will expect to relieve symptoms and cure diseases simply through prescribing medicines and giving injections. This is medical care as opposed to health care. It is summed up in the slogan PPNN: A Pill for every Problem, a Needle for every Need.

Good practice follows a different model. It aims to promote good health and to prevent ill health in a variety of ways at individual and at community level. Medicines are still used but only when necessary. This is health care as opposed to medical care. Those who are more interested in profit will wish to offer a medical model of care, but CBHC actively opposes this.

One of our main tasks as community health workers is to educate people about the correct and incorrect use of medicine. If we succeed, communities will become healthy and self-reliant. If we fail, communities will become poorer, more exploited, and more dependent, and we will have become part of the problem.

Keeping medicine use safe

We need to grasp the importance of prescribing medicines safely: in the right dose (according to the patient's age and weight) and for the correct period of time, according to evidence-based guidelines. Each medicine has its own therapeutic range, i.e. the dose and duration which is most effective and minimizes unwanted side effects. Among private practitioners in particular these principles are often not followed.

There are two other main faults in prescribing: over-prescribing and under-prescribing.

Over-prescribing: using too much of what is not needed

There are some common *reasons* for overprescribing. First and foremost, health workers may have been wrongly trained to follow a medical model, not a health model. Additionally, while some health workers gain a feeling of satisfaction from prescribing, others may get a handout from the drug company. Finally, many CHWs and some village doctors, for example in China, receive payment according to medicines prescribed: the more they prescribe the more they earn. We need to find a different way of remunerating CHWs.

It is often easier to prescribe for each symptom than discover the cause and treat the illness. Subsequently, those lacking knowledge or confidence often use several medicines in the hope that something will work, i.e. the 'scattergun approach'.

However, the commonest reason why doctors overprescribe is that patients expect many medicines and an injection. If they don't receive these, often they seek out another doctor willing to provide them (Figure 11.2).

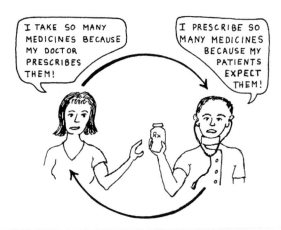

Figure 11.2 The vicious circle that leads to the overuse of medicine.

There are some common *results* of over-prescribing as well. For example, patients can become psychologically dependent on medicines and doctors. This in turn means that they spend more and more money on medicines, and they develop a demanding attitude.

For example, one programme decided not to pay money to its CHWs but instead to provide free medicines both for the CHWs and their families. The heads of these families soon came to realise they could obtain a profit by reselling such medicines. Encouraged by their families, the CHWs demanded ever-increasing amounts of medicines, refusing to co-operate when medicines were refused. The project was forced to close down.

Sometimes patients may go into debt to pay for medicines but take little interest in disease prevention. Yet when essential medicines are needed, supplies may have run out. Finally, patients may pass on this kind of consumerist thinking to their children.

Under-prescribing: using too little of what is really needed

There are some common *reasons* for under-prescribing. To begin with, medicines may not be available, e.g. they may be hard to obtain, or deliveries may not be ordered in time (Figure 11.3). Stocks may have been used up because of previous overprescribing. There may be a lack of supplies at country and international level. Patients may be unable to afford the full course of medicine. Finally, health workers may not follow the correct treatment schedules.

Thus, it follows that there are some common *results* of under-prescribing. For example, people die from curable diseases such as malaria, pneumonia and TB. People lose faith in the hospital, health centre or programme when they fail to get better. Lastly, money is wasted and people endanger their health by buying useless substitutes.

The importance of expiry dates

Medicines can only be kept a certain length of time before spoiling. This is known as the shelf life. Usually

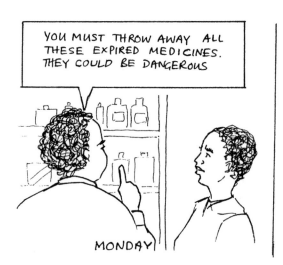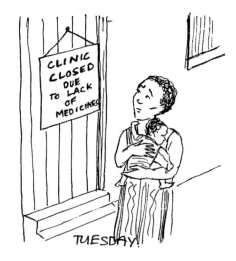

Figure 11.3 A common dilemma when both medicines and good management are in short supply.

a printed expiry date shows when the shelf life ends. But after the expiry date, a medicine may become less effective: this is the case with many antibiotics. Sometimes, e.g. with tetracyclines, it may become more toxic, or it may become more likely to cause an allergy, e.g. with penicillin. However, medicines will often continue for a time to be both safe and effective after their expiry date. Drug companies may record early expiry dates to protect themselves from legal action if adverse effects occur.

Normal practice is to see if the expiry date has passed. However, under bad storage conditions, some medicines may spoil before their expiry date. Always check all medicines to make sure they are not damp or sticky, discoloured, or broken. In addition, check certain drugs and supplies for specific problems, e.g. tetracycline often turns brown when ineffective; aspirin may smell unpleasant; condoms may dry out; vaccines must be kept cold (see Chapter 15); ergometrine requires refrigeration and protection from light; and epinephrine (adrenaline) has a very short shelf life.

We can help medicines last longer by keeping them in a dry place, at an even temperature, and out of direct sunlight. This means that any store room will need to be shielded from direct sunlight and have adequate ventilation. All containers must be airtight and lids firmly closed. We should use sugar-coated or foil-wrapped tablets where cost allows. Packing medicine carefully reduces breakages in transit, and we must store supplies in peripheral health centres for as short a time as possible, unless storage and safety concerns are carefully managed. The 'cold chain' for all vaccines must be maintained, and we must buy only high-quality medicines that have been recently manufactured.

There are a number of reasons against using expired medicines. They may be less effective or unsafe. If it is discovered that we are using out-of-date medicines, it may anger the local people; we may be accused of dumping dangerous medicines on the local community. However, there are reasons in favour of using expired medicines, too. There may be no other supplies available, or it may mean throwing away supplies that are desperately needed. Large sums of money may be wasted if supplies are discarded. Furthermore, many expired medicines still work and are still safe (See Figure 11.3).

Some suggested guidelines for using out-of-date medicines include only using medicines past their expiry dates when absolutely essential, i.e. when no alternatives are available, but *never* use medicines that show signs of having spoilt. Always order the correct amount of medicines in plenty of time so as to have sufficient in-date supplies, and check expiry dates on arrival, then store in date order and use those with earlier dates first (see Chapter 5). Finally, be sensitive to the community's opinion about expired drugs. Some will be greatly concerned, while others will not mind at all.

What we need to do

Model List of medicines: what it is and why we need it

The WHO list is comprehensive and we must narrow it down to what is essential for our own programme and area. We should use the WHO list to draw up our own Model List of medicines, which will be different for each country, each region, and most importantly for each programme.

CHWs may need approximately twelve essential medicines, although this is variable and will depend on the level of training of the CHW or other health provider, and to the degree of access to life-saving medicines (see Chapter 8). Clinics, hospitals, and facilities for safe delivery will need considerably more.

When involved in vertical programmes such as End TB or Roll Back Malaria we should always use the nationally recommended essential medicines. Essential medicines for children are especially important and are often not available in correct doses and formulations. We need to ensure we obtain the best possible supplies for this most important group of community members.[18] The *ideal medicine* has all the features shown below in Figure 11.4, and is clearly labelled with its generic name, strength, and expiry date, in the locally used language or script.

Who or what should be consulted about the Model List?

The project doctor or medical advisor may have valuable suggestions, but these may include more medicines than are needed if the doctor comes from a hospital background (Figure 11.5). Other programmes working in the area may also provide suggestions, although we must make sure we consider the specific needs of our community. In addition we must follow any national

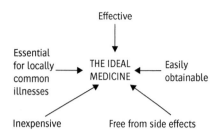

Figure 11.4 The ideal medicine.

Reproduced courtesy of Ted Lankester. This image is distributed under the terms of the Creative Commons Attribution Non-Commercial 4.0 International licence (CC-BY-NC), a copy of which is available at http://creativecommons.org/licenses/by-nc/4.0/.

guidelines for the treatment of any prevalent health condition in our locality, including TB, HIV, or neglected tropical diseases if our clinic is involved in treating these conditions. The District Medical Officer may have a national Model List or a list specifically recommended for primary health centres. Ultimately, we should check the latest WHO Model List of Essential Medicines, from which all our medicines must be selected.

> EXCUSE ME, DOCTOR, BUT ONLY 3 OUT OF THE 8 MEDICINES YOU PRESCRIBED FOR THE LAST PATIENT ARE ON OUR ESSENTIAL DRUGS LIST

Figure 11.5 Doctors must be accountable in prescribing.

Reproduced courtesy of David Gifford. This image is distributed under the terms of the Creative Commons Attribution Non-Commercial 4.0 International licence (CC-BY-NC), a copy of which is available at http://creativecommons.org/licenses/by-nc/4.0/.

The final list should be worked out between the programme director (who will know how much medicines cost) and the medical advisor (who will know which medicines are necessary) and of course a responsible member of the community or the village health committee.

Training the health team about prescribing

All those who will be prescribing need careful instructions on the following subjects:

The dangers of over-prescribing

We will need to correct any wrong ideas or practice, pointing out the extent of current overprescribing and the dangers.

For example, we can arrange a simple survey, visiting homes to find out what medicines have recently been used and where they were obtained. Alternatively, patients who come to the clinic are asked which medicines they have been prescribed in the last few months. Often wads of old prescriptions or bills will be produced. Unless the whole health team understands and practises rational medicine use at all times, community members will never change their expectations.

Correct prescribing and dispensing

There is a difference between prescribing and dispensing. Prescribing is when a doctor, or person legally entitled to prescribe, writes down a recommended medicine or treatment for a patient. Dispensing is the handing over to the patient of the prescribed medicine after due checks that the details are correct. Prescribing should usually be done by a doctor, but some medicines can also be prescribed by other authorized health workers such as pharmacists and nurses. In many countries other health care workers can also prescribe if they follow treatment protocols, standing orders, patient group directions or similar guidelines. Dispensers don't always need specific accreditation, but they will need careful training.

In smaller scale programmes the prescriber will often also be the person who dispenses the medicine. *Prescribers* will need to:

- Understand and use the programme's own Model List;
- Know the correct amount of the correct medicine for each condition, according to best practice and evidence-based guidelines. This is important for all conditions but especially vital in TB and HIV and the use of antibiotics and antimalarials;

- Write the prescription correctly and clearly;
- Use generic medicine names;
- Be aware of possible side effects and medicine inter-actions, always having available an online informa-tion source or up-to-date formulary;
- Know the approximate cost of each medicine so pre-scribing can be affordable for the programme and the patient; and
- Use existing protocols such as the Integrated Management of Childhood Illness (IMCI).

A study from Nigeria has shown that treatment costs are five times higher using traditional ways of prescribing compared to guidelines laid down by IMCI.[19]

Dispensers will need to:

- Understand and recognize the names of medicines being prescribed;
- Check the number and dosage of each medicine being dispensed;
- Check the name of the patient and any ID number or date of birth (if known), especially in societies where many people share the same name;
- Check the expiry date; and
- Know how to answer simple questions from the pa-tient about how the medicine should be used or taken.

Those learning to dispense medicines need careful training and supervision until they do it correctly. Equally, those prescribing medicines need to have regular updates and continuing professional de-velopment from sources other than drug company representatives.

Using medicine correctly: creating community awareness

Correct use of medicines is one of the most important subjects the community needs to understand. Among health workers and practitioners, there will often be a hidden struggle between those who want to prescribe as many medicines as they wish and those who want to prescribe only essential medicines. Both sides will be trying to win the hearts of the community. In creating awareness (Figure 11.6), we can use a variety of methods (see Chapter 4). Drama is one of the most effective.

In order to use the correct medicines in the correct way, here are some Dos and Don'ts.

Do:

1. Use as few medicines as possible.

Fight the belief that, if one pill is good, lots must be better. Some patients will need no medicine at all; few will need more than two.

2. Spend time explaining rather than prescribing.

Explain why medicines are not always necessary (Figure 11.7). Simple advice may not only cure the problem but also prevent it from recurring. For example, a doctor working in North Africa decided that, instead of pre-scribing for every symptom, he would spend time giving advice instead. The new method seemed to work well until a tribal chief appeared with headache. When re-fused tablets, the chief angrily left the clinic, warning all the waiting patients that the doctor was useless. A few days later the chief reappeared, smiling. He explained how the headache had gone when he followed the doctor's simple advice. He would now encourage others to do what the doctor suggested.

3. Treat causes rather than symptoms.

If the illness is cured, the symptoms will go. If only symptoms are treated, the disease may continue.

4. Use generic preparations

Usually use single generics, rather than combinations of medicines. There are a few important exceptions to this, e.g. iron and folic acid in pregnancy, fixed dose com-binations in TB, antiretrovirals to control HIV/AIDS, and artemesinin combined therapy (ACT) in malaria and sometimes combined preparations to reduce blood pressure.

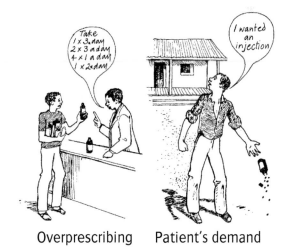

Overprescribing   Patient's demand

Figure 11.6 Spend time correcting expectations.

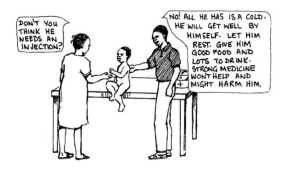

Figure 11.7 When medicines are not needed take the time to explain why.

5. Buy good-quality medicines at the cheapest possible prices.

- First choice: reliable, quality-tested local manufacturer.
- Second choice: multinational company making good quality, inexpensive drugs in-country or in-region.
- Third choice: obtain from abroad, through reliable suppliers.

6. Try to obtain medicines from government sources for any national programme in which the project is involved, e.g. End TB. These will usually be quality-assured.

7. Make sure that all prescribers use the programme's Model List.

8. Avoid wastage through carefully assessing the stock needed, bulk buying, checking supplies on arrival for breakage and discoloration, using older stock first, and ensuring safe storage and transport.

9. Discourage self-prescribing.

Don't:

1. Give injections when medicines taken by mouth work just as well.

We will need to explain gently each time why a medicine by mouth is more appropriate.

2. Give injections for common colds.

They don't help and they can be dangerous. There is no cure for the common cold.

3. Give antibiotics unless they are really needed.

4. Give intravenous glucose for dehydration unless the person is unable to drink.

5. Use tonics or enzyme mixtures. Only use vitamins if the patient is seriously ill or malnourished, there is lack of food security, or it is official government policy. Give nutrition education instead.

6. Give medicines just because people want them, expect them, or threaten to go elsewhere.

7. Be discouraged if this advice seems hard to follow: health workers throughout the world are all facing similar problems.

Further reading and resources

BMJ Publishing Group/Royal Pharmaceutical Society. *British National Formulary* (BNF). London: Pharmaceutical Press; updated annually. Provides clear and precise details of which medicines to use for which conditions. Also useful for doctors involved in hospital medicine. Available from: https://www.pharmpress.com/product/9780857113382/bnf76

Christian Medical College Vellore. *Hospital Formulary 8th Edition*. Dept Pharmacy CMC Vellore, 2018.

Fountain D. *Primary diagnosis and treatment: A manual for clinical and health centre staff in developing countries*. revised ed. London: Macmillan; 2008. A valuable book. Available from: TALC.

Goldacre B. *Bad Pharma: How Medicine is Broken, and How We Can Fix it*. Fourth Estate; 2013.

Kaur M, Hall S. Medical supplies and equipment for primary health care: A practical resource for procurement and management. Coulsdon: ECHO International Health Services Ltd; 2001. Essential for all health programmes. Available at: http://www.who.int/management/resources/procurement/MedicalSuppliesforPHC-Introduction.pdf

Pinel J, Weiss F, Henkens M, Grouzard V. *Essential Drugs Practical Guidelines*. 3rd ed. Geneva: Médecins sans Frontières; 2006. Available from: http://psfci.acted.org/images/PSF_dossiers_pdf/pdf_eng/essential%20drugs%20partical%20guidelines%20msf%202006.pdf

Shann F. *Drug doses*. 17th ed. Victoria, Australia: JR Medical Books, 2017. Available from: http://www.drugdoses.net

Werner D, Thuman C, Maxwell J. *Where There is no Doctor*. 9th ed. Berkeley, CA: Hesperian; 2011. Translated into a variety of languages. Available from: http://www.burmalibrary.org/docs12/Where_there_is_no_doctor-2011(en)-red.pdf

World Health Organization. Essential medicines and health products information portal: A World Health Organization resource. Available from: http://apps.who.int/medicinedocs/en

World Health Organization. *Immunization in Practice: A Practical Guide for Health Staff—2015 Update*. Geneva: World Health Organization; 2015. Includes a module on the cold chain. Available from: http://apps.who.int/iris/bitstream/handle/10665/193412/9789241549097_eng.pdf;jsessionid=C6E2AAE0F7BF6DD2589EC6C16AE929BC?sequence=1

World Health Organization. *Safe Injection Global Network advocacy booklet*. Geneva: World Health Organization; 2011

Available from: http://www.who.int/injection_safety/sign/sign_advocacy_booklet.pdf?ua=1

World Health Organization. *WHO Model list of essential medicines*. 20th ed. Geneva: World Health Organization; 2017. Available from: http://apps.who.int/iris/bitstream/handle/10665/273826/EML-20-eng.pdf

World Health Organization. *WHO Model list of essential medicines for children*. 6th ed. Geneva: World Health Organization; 2017. Available from: http://apps.who.int/iris/bitstream/handle/10665/273825/EMLc-6-eng.pdf

References

1. Centers for Disease Control and Prevention. *1 in 3 antibiotic prescriptions unnecessary*. 2016. Available from: https://www.cdc.gov/media/releases/2016/p0503-unnecessary-prescriptions.html

2. World Health Organization. *The World Medicines Situation 2011: Rational Use of Medicines*. Geneva: World Health Organization; 2011.

3. Hutin YJF, Hauri AM, Armstrong GL. Use of injections in healthcare settings worldwide, 2000: Literature review and regional estimates. *British Medical Journal*. 2003; 327 (7423): 1075.

4. Bosu W, Ofori-Adjei D. An audit of prescribing practices in health care facilities of the Wassa West district of Ghana. *West African Journal of Medicine*. 2000; 19 (4): 298–303.

5. World Health Organization. *Safety of Injections: Questions and Answers*. Geneva: World Health Organization; 2006. Available from: http://who.int/injection_safety/about/resources/en/QuestionAndAnswersInjectionSafety.pdf

6. Miller M, Pisani E. The cost of unsafe injections. *Bulletin of the World Health Organization*. 1999, 77 (10): 808–11.

7. World Health Organization. Medicines use in primary care in developing and transitional countries, The World Medicines Situation 2011. Rational Use of Medicines. Available from: http://apps.who.int/medicinedocs/documents/s18064en/s18064en.pdf

8. Morris J, Stevens P. *Counterfeit medicines in less developed countries: problems and solutions*. London: International Policy Network; 2006

9. World Health Organization. *Substandard and falsified medical products: Fact Sheet*. Updated January 2018. Available from: https://www.who.int/news-room/fact-sheets/detail/substandard-and-falsified-medical-products

10. Royal Pharmaceutical Society of Great Britain. *Counterfeit Medicines Advice for Healthcare Professionals, DAD, MHRA*. 2009. Available from: https://www.fip.org/files/fip/counterfeit/national/UKCounterfeitadvice209.pdf

11. World Health Organization. Growing threat from counterfeit medicines. *Bulletin of the World Health Organization*, 2010, 88 (4): 247–8.

12. Grover A, Citro B. India: Access to affordable drugs and the right to health. *The Lancet*. 2011; 377 (9770): 976–7.

13. Scheil-Adlung X, editor. *Global evidence on inequities in rural health protection: New data on rural deficits in health coverage for 174 countries*. ESS Document No. 47. Geneva: International Labour Organization; 2015.

14. World Health Organization. *WHO Model list of essential medicines*. 20th ed. Geneva: World Health Organization; 2017. Available from: http://apps.who.int/iris/bitstream/handle/10665/273826/EML-20-eng.pdf

15. World Health Organization. *The inter-agency emergency health kit for use in relief and emergency situations*. Geneva: World Health Organization; 2011. Available from: http://www.who.int/medicines/publications/emergencyhealthkit2011/en/

16. World Health Organization. *Priority medicines for mothers and children*. Geneva: World Health Organization; 2011. Available from: http://www.who.int/medicines/publications/A4prioritymedicines.pdf

17. Robertson J, Forte G, Trapsida J-M, Hill S. What essential medicines for children are on the shelf? *Bulletin of the World Health Organization*. 2009, 87(3): 231–7.

18. Wammanda R, Ejembi C, Lorlian T. Drug treatment costs: Projected impact of using the integrated management of childhood illnesses. *Tropical Doctor*. 2003; 33 (2): 86–8.

CHAPTER 12
Making a programme sustainable

Ted Lankester

What we need to know

Central to all we discuss in this chapter is our priority of focusing on the poorest and most vulnerable in the community. As we pursue the important aim of sustainability, we must never turn away those who are in greatest need. For example, Table 12.1 gives us a reality check and highlights catastrophes that frequently affect urban slum dwellers.

Sustainability is a joint venture between the health team and the community. Only with major input from the community, with ideas described in this chapter, can any programme remain vibrant and confident about its future.

What we mean by sustainability

Sustainability has been a 'buzz word' in health and development circles for many years. Many programmes are short lived. Outsiders enter with promises, raise expectations and work hard to bring about lasting change. Then, often from lack of funds, the programme falters and fails, leaving the community little better (and sometimes worse) off than before, and disillusioned.

To minimize the risk of this happening, we must, think carefully and creatively from the start about how the health programme can be sustained far into the future. It is helpful to try to define what sustainability actually is. One definition describes sustainable programmes as those whose internal and external methods of raising finance and other resources are likely to ensure their long-term survival. In addition, they need to have appropriate staff, effective infrastructure, and good governance.

A sustainable programme does not have to be entirely self-sufficient, using no external resources. Rather, they are self-reliant and able to assume responsibility for their own futures. This will usually be through a combination of cost recovery from users, income generation, and selected support from outside.

Understanding the difference between self-sufficiency and self-reliance is important. Few, if any, programmes will manage to be entirely self-sufficient (free from any dependence on outside funding) especially in the poorest areas where community-based health care (CBHC) is of such special value. All programmes must work towards self-reliance, always making sure that the poorest have priority. However, we should not think of sustainability purely in financial terms. From a holistic viewpoint, there are other ways in which a programme must be sustainable

The first way relates to the local community feeling connected to the programme, and demonstrating long-term commitment. This will largely come about when the community is involved as widely as possible in the programme, including shaping it from the beginning. This will help people to feel the programme belongs to them. Community 'ownership' may be the single most important factor for long-term sustainability.

Table 12.1 A reality check for those living in slums

Serious or fatal accidents, on the road, in the house, or at work	Domestic violence
Fire	Sudden illness or death of breadwinner
Flood	Family members turn to crime
Electrocution or electrical burns	Demolition of homes
Medicine costs, e.g. TB and HIV	Civil disorder
Demands from creditors	Corruption in government
Loss of job	Severe weather
Loss of land forced migration	Drug addiction
Imprisonment	

Adapted with permission from Booth, B., et al. Urban Health and Development. Copyright © Macmillan, TALC and Tearfund. This table is distributed under the terms of the Creative Commons Attribution Non-Commercial 4.0 International licence (CC-BY-NC), a copy of which is available at http://creativecommons.org/licenses/by-nc/4.0/.

The second way relates to protecting the environment. A programme must not exploit, undermine, or degrade the local environment and ecology. It must take care to preserve the local flora and fauna. This is especially important in areas such as tropical forests, coasts, and mountain areas where environments are fragile and any ecological damage is hard to reverse. For example, every year in hill areas in Bangladesh, soil erosion caused by deforestation or overgrazing leads to floods and widespread devastation, but it is possible to counteract these kinds of damage. For example, on the Kenyan coast the Muhindi project aims to provide cooking fuel from cheap sustainable resources so as to reduce using indigenous trees for charcoal burning. At the same time, trees are being replanted by community members to reverse the destruction of past years.

The third relates to the culture and customs of the population. A correct approach to CBHC must ensure that we tackle the root causes of poverty. We can do this by pursuing equality in women and children's access to services, promoting girls' education, and working towards behavioural change, such as reducing alcohol and tobacco use. But we must be careful not to disrupt the culture, customs, and distinctiveness of the community. For example, only if a health behaviour or custom

is harmful to health do we suggest alternative ways of thinking and behaving.

The fourth way relates to the personal welfare of staff and community members working with them. We should set up and maintain employment practices that protect people from overwork, exploitation, dangerous practices, or prolonged separation from family members. It is vital to set up and maintain an ethical personnel policy.

Some important historical background

It is useful to understand some historical background to funding health and development. After the 1978 Alma-Ata Declaration (see Chapter 1), the number of health programmes set up by NGOs increased dramatically. In the 1970s, there was a general belief that poverty could be tackled successfully and that donors would be able to help achieve this. But by the mid-1980s economic hardship had already started to affect many countries. Governments in low income countries started to cut back on health and social welfare spending.

At about the same time, the western world began to elect more right-wing governments with less sympathy for the plight of the poor. In the 1980s, the World Bank and International Monetary Fund introduced Structural Adjustment Programmes, with the idea that if countries could strengthen their economies, then the poor would automatically benefit. Unfortunately, an effect of these policies was that countries spent less on basic services and the gap between rich and poor widened.

In 1987, the Bamako Initiative was launched, which tried to combine the idea of cost recovery with the genuine needs of the poor, and introduced the idea of revolving drug funds (RDFs) to finance essential community drug costs. It was hoped that, as users paid for their medicines, sufficient funds would become available not only for drugs but also to improve health services in general.

During the 1990s, the concepts of sustainability and cost recovery, i.e. patients paying towards the cost of their health services, became key slogans. Evidence since then has shown that many cost recovery schemes, and in particular user fees, seriously reduce the number of poor people using health services.[1] Other priorities, such as animal husbandry, often reduces to very low levels the money available for user fees.

It is difficult to raise a large proportion of costs through user fees; even the original guideline figure of fifteen per cent is an ambitious target. If fees are introduced for a previously free service, users must see an improvement in the service; otherwise they will stop using the service. This might be overcome by dialogue with communities, e.g. if the community realizes that user fees can result in more reliable medicine supply, people may use the health services more, but the poorest may be unable to afford to use them.

All these factors make it difficult to combine sustainability with a just and open-handed approach to the poor. Currently there is a global move away from charging user fees, but the debate is likely to continue. However, the fact remains that if programmes prove sustainable, they will survive. If they can't, they will close, perhaps leaving people without basic services.

Some of our programmes will be receiving funds from government or international donors. This is fine for the present but it is no guarantee for the long term. Civil society organizations (CSOs) will need to have several options to ensure they are able to continue their work. Also, in order to attract start-up funding, we will need to persuade donors that we have practical ideas for ensuring long-term sustainability.

Financial sustainability consists of two essential parts: reducing costs and raising resources.

What we need to do

Ways to reduce programme costs (See Figure 12.1)

Programmes are more likely to survive if they are run as efficiently as possible. Cost-cutting can save the equivalent of large annual donations. There are a few ways we can do this.

Firstly, we can cut costs where possible in all programme areas. We need to carry out an audit of all programme activities to understand our costs, which includes fuel and transport costs and buying supplies. We can then look at ways to reduce spending and any wasteful activity.

Next, we can increase efficiency of the programme by ensuring good time management and the best use of staff time and skills. Because salaries are usually the largest single programme cost, anything that increases productivity will improve sustainability. But we must ensure that efficiency is never at the expense of staff health and welfare, nor of the environment. By recruiting staff with high motivation, appropriate training, and the willingness to take on tasks outside their main job description, we can increase the number of tasks done by each individual.

We can also reduce costs through task shifting, i.e. not just more flexible working practices, but where legal and possible *using the person least qualified to do the job well* (Chapter 1). Staff should be working within the top of their skill range, rather than within its lower end. This can save considerable staff costs if introduced across the programme. Additionally, if we consider limited-term contracts for team members coupled with career development plans and ongoing training, we can encourage staff to see their time with the programme as *part* of their career, not a job for *life*. Finally, whenever dealing with staff, we must make sure that they are affirmed and motivated, that any disputes are minimized, and, if they occur, they are handled swiftly and appropriately (Chapter 10).

Huge amounts of money are also wasted by overprescribing. We can reduce this by using a Model List of Essential Medicines (see Chapter 11), and prescribing only medicines on our own adapted list. We must also refuse gifts of unwanted or expired medicines which waste time and can cause staff confusion. Staff must be trained to prescribe the minimum amount of medicine necessary for effective treatment, and to use patient group directions, disease protocols, or standing orders to treat common ailments, and banning alternatives or additions.

Furthermore, we should obtain any free supplies to which we may be entitled. Depending on country and district these might include:

- TB medicines;
- antiretroviral therapy for people living with HIV;
- immunizations;
- Vitamin A and zinc supplements;
- iron and folic acid supplements; and
- any medicines donated free for mass distribution for locally prevalent diseases, including neglected tropical diseases, e.g. praziquantel for schistosomiasis.

Sometimes, however, these sources suddenly cease to be available. We should not become overly dependent on them.

We must prevent wastage of medicines through poor storage and theft. Buy medicines with as long an expiry

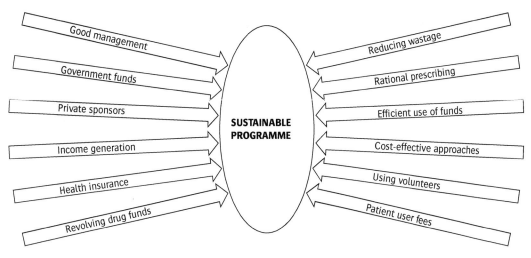

Figure 12.1 Twelve ways to help a project become sustainable.

date as possible and use previously ordered stocks first. If we concentrate on low-cost approaches, and think of curative care and the use of medicines as only one part of CBHC, a great deal can be done to raise health awareness and work towards behavioural change at low cost. This might include training community health workers (CHWs), raising health awareness in the community through meetings, focus groups, drama, and puppet shows, starting female literacy classes (ideally in the context of women's groups or using microloans for small business enterprises; see Chapter 2).

Planned Preventive Maintenance (PPM) refers to proactively maintaining equipment so it keeps functioning rather than breaking down. It involves auditing equipment, obtaining the funds and expertise needed for repair and maintenance, and setting time aside for repairs and maintenance. Vehicles, water pumps, and office and clinical equipment will be priorities. PPM avoids crisis breakdowns, which can be expensive and discouraging. For example, the NGO Transaid works in some African countries to build the capacity of programmes to maintain vehicles and motorbikes in good working order. It also supports other ideas for sustainable transport.[2]

Finally, we can use volunteers—many communities have members who are willing to volunteer. The creative use of volunteers can reduce salary costs. However, it is important not to exploit volunteers, and to be sensitive to their needs. Volunteers, unless welcomed, affirmed, and valued by other team members, can become demotivated, especially if their families do not approve of their volunteering.

Volunteers need to be well managed like other team members, and it is helpful to draw up an agreement with them. The programme should offer to pay transport costs, other out-of-pocket expenses, and, where appropriate, a small stipend. CHWs are an example of the use of volunteers (see Chapter 8), but the concept can be extended to other programme workers.

In some countries the use of interns and apprentices is increasingly popular. They are usually young people with enthusiasm and a desire to learn. Interns usually have some qualifications or specific skills. Apprentices often come straight from school with no experience. Both need either a basic salary or living expenses and can be taken on for a six- to twelve-month period (or longer for apprentices).

It is important that the experience they gain is helpful and affirming and nurtures them in their future career, whether they eventually join as team members or not. Ways of recruiting and paying interns and apprentices must follow national labour laws and at least minimum standards for payment amounts and working conditions.

Ways to increase programme resources

Cost recovery is where users of the health facility, i.e. patients, pay for at least some of the costs of the service, in particular, medicine costs. This may be through paying user fees at the time they visit the health centre, or through regular payment to an insurance scheme.

In making any decision we must consider the crucial goal of universal health coverage (Chapter 1), whereby patients receive the treatment they need at a fee they are able to afford.

Of course, it is not only the cost of medicines that need to be covered. However, community members are usually more willing to pay for curative care (Figure 12.2) than other aspects of CBHC where benefits are longer term and less obvious. Cost recovery for medicines may generate a small surplus. This can be used to cross-subsidize other parts of the programme, e.g. the training and payment of CHWs. However, this process will hopefully be overseen by a well-functioning village health committee (VHC) so that the community understands it.

There is a strong move in many circles to abolish user fees altogether. But unless we have a clear alternative, abolishing user fees may jeopardize the future of the programme. If we are unable to afford reliable supplies or salaries, the number of patients declines and community members either receive no care at all, return to traditional healers, or attend private practitioners. Curative care may cease altogether.

Over recent years much experience has been gained worldwide on how best to encourage communities to contribute to their health care. There is a general move away from user fees towards insurance premiums, i.e. from paying at the time of illness, to paying annually at a time of year when a patient's income is highest.

The guidelines suggested here are taken from a variety of successful programmes, and most of these can apply to both user fees and health insurance premiums.

Involve the community at all stages

This is the key to success. The community will not make contributions, especially to insurance schemes, unless they understand how the cost recovery scheme works and why it is needed to keep their health programme running.

- Make use of payment schemes already familiar to the community.

For example: ,in parts of Tanzania, traditional healers have sliding scales of the amount they charge, based on ability to pay. Other communities have traditions of contributing to community activities such as funerals or festivals. These systems can be used as models to explain and guide fair user fees or insurance premiums.

- Make sure the community has confidence in the health facility.

Health workers must be friendly and competent. Essential medicines must be always available. Nothing undermines a health service like a frustrated health worker turning away the mother of a seriously ill child because antimalarials have run out. Community members will only pay premiums if they have a high level of trust in the health services provided (See Figure 12.2).

- Investigate other schemes being used nearby.

We should find out about cost recovery systems used in other parts of the country or health district. We can join them, use them, or adapt them to our situation.

- Consider the use of cross subsidy to help pay other programme costs.

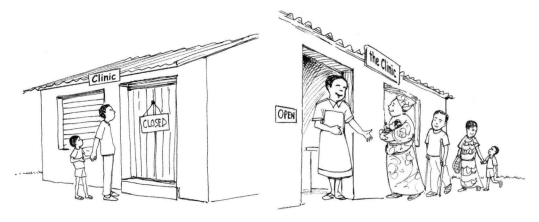

Figure 12.2 Clinics must be affordable, friendly, accessible, and have reliable supplies.

For example, in Ghana, one slightly controversial project made a profit from sales of vitamin B complex, which people really wanted (despite little clinical need and ensuring that the health programme did not actively promote it). This helped to subsidize (expensive) snake anti-venom.

- Manage the scheme at the most local level possible.

Schemes work best when user fees and insurance schemes are managed at community level, ideally by a VHC, if they have sufficient skills to manage it. This demonstrates to the community that the fees paid are being used locally. Note that this committee will need careful training, outside support, and encouragement.

- Make sure that finances are honestly managed.

Large sums of money may be generated, which can be daunting to handle and a temptation. There will need to be systems and audits to guard against mistakes and theft.

Collecting user fees

We will need to devise careful, practical methods of fee collection. It is helpful to work through three steps.

1. Decide on how much money needs to be recovered.

To help us fix fees and premiums we will need to calculate two things.

- How much will patients be able to afford?

This will be a range, depending on people's circumstances. One place to start is discussion with the community, including the poorest groups. Another is sliding scales used by similar programmes locally.

- How much does the programme need in order for the clinic to be viable?

We have to decide whether we aim to recover the cost of medicines in full or in part, or in full plus extra to contribute towards staff salaries and other costs. Obviously we cannot charge a fee or premium that is more than people can afford, but we still need to know the amount we are aiming to recover. Then we can calculate the balance to be raised from other sources.

2. Set up a policy on fee levels and exemptions.

This needs to be done by the VHC or other group representing both community and programme. If policy is clear there is less cause for argument or disagreement when it comes to payment.

A policy will need to have clear statements on categories, exemptions (and how they apply), what happens if fees or premiums are not paid, and what level of health centre staff have authority to make decisions.

For example, a programme in Bangladesh uses a system of four categories where each is charged a different rate. We can use this as a model and adapt it for our situation.

Group 1. Families with no male earner or with a people living with disability male earner. Lowest user or membership fee.

Group 2. Families that cannot afford two meals per day throughout the year.

Group 3. Families that can afford two meals per day all year but do not have a surplus.

Group 4. Families that have an agricultural or financial surplus.

A family survey can be used to set sliding scales and exemptions (see Chapter 6).

3. Put our policy into practice.

We will need to decide questions such as:

- Who collects the fees or premiums?
- How will money be handled, stored, or banked?
- How will the fee or premium category and exemption be identified?
- What forms will be needed?
- Who will arbitrate if a dispute arises?

User fees continue to cause a lot of discussion and disagreement. They have become a standard, simple way of recovering at least some of the cost of providing health care. However, experience has shown that user fees dissuade certain people from attending. These include women needing antenatal care, people with certain infectious illnesses (in particular, sexually transmitted diseases), couples needing family planning, and the very poor. In many communities the number of women attending falls.

An example of a successful health centre that charged user fees is Mabuku in the Democratic Republic of Congo. Factors leading to success included:

- A competent and respected head nurse who was able to balance immediate needs with long-term development;
- A community with high confidence in its health workers, both clinic and community based;
- An active health committee, meeting regularly and representing a wide range of the local population; and

- People who can't pay in cash can contribute in produce or livestock, which is either sold or contributes to staff salaries.

The Mabuku Health Centre is an example of cofinancing where the community had a strong input in setting up the scheme, both in decision-making and management.

Two contrasting examples of abolishing user fees comes from Sierra Leone and Burkina Faso. The Free Health Care Initiative (FHCI) was set up in Sierra Leone in 2010 after eighty-eight per cent of citizens said that user fees were their greatest barrier to accessing curative care. The FHCI ensures that children under five, pregnant women, and breastfeeding mothers receive free healthcare. In its first few years it has been successful and is a valuable model to study.[4] In Burkina Faso, two health districts eliminated user fees for pregnant women and children under five. They were able to show that eliminating these fees contributed to reducing child mortality.[5]

If after careful consideration we decide to charge user fees there are two common ways of collecting them.

1. Fees can be collected per clinic attendance as a charge taken on registration (see also Chapter 5).

One main *advantage* of this method is simplicity: a single charge is taken at each visit. A further advantage is that people know in advance what they have to pay, which also reduces disputes. Exemptions can be made, e.g. the very poor, children under five, antenatal visits, or immunizations. The main *disadvantage* is that patients want their 'money's worth' of medicines for the fee they have paid. They may expect unnecessary injections or medicines, and feel cheated if they don't receive them. This can be overcome by partial reimbursement if no medicines are necessary and training staff to explain why medicines are not needed (see Chapter 11).

2. Fees can also be charged per medicine or procedure.

The *advantage* of this is that patients are charged according to the actual medicine or procedure they receive. A *disadvantage* is that collecting the fees and accounting can be more complex and time consuming.

Revolving drug funds (RDFs)

RDFs are a long-term method of funding medicine costs. Medicines are sold to patients, via clinic or CHW, and the money received is used to buy more medicines. A grant or loan at the start of the programme buys sufficient essential medicines to last, e.g. six months. Schemes, if carefully managed, can reinvest the original money to buy replacement medicines so that little or no outside funding is needed.

There are several *advantages* of RDFs. It is an attractive option for donors, and a good way to learn self-sufficiency for the community. The *disadvantages* are that administration can be difficult, especially at local level, as large sums of money may be involved. RDFs have a high failure rate unless they are carefully planned.[6]

The secrets of success are the same as for cost recovery generally. RDFs work best when there is simplicity in paperwork, and careful training for administrators of the scheme. If there are too many exemptions the fund runs out of money. Unless there are good procedures, monies received and banked can get lost, confused, or stolen, which causes loss of confidence in the scheme, and the programme. Setting up RDFs involves considerable time and expense. Ongoing monitoring and training are essential for success (Figure 12.3).

Community health insurance schemes

Health insurance is also known as a prepayment scheme. Community members pay a regular amount into a fund, and only those who have paid this premium or membership fee are eligible for benefits. In practice, insurance schemes work better the more members they have, as the risk is spread over a wider group of people. In some countries or districts there are national, not-for-profit insurance schemes, such as the mutual health insurance schemes in Rwanda,[7] or community-based health insurance schemes in India and elsewhere. Guidelines for success are largely those already mentioned, and there are numerous case studies available on the Internet.[8] These will help the scheme to get off to a good start, but a major problem with pre-payment schemes is that people are reluctant to pay in advance for something that may not happen (Figure 12.4).

There are various ways of increasing uptake of community health insurance schemes. For example, people who have not yet paid can be charged a penalty when they attend the clinic, or more appropriately, they can pay their annual premium, plus the price of the immediate medical care together, thus becoming members at the same time as receiving treatment. Difficult-to-persuade community members can be encouraged to join the scheme as a way of guaranteeing their children's healthcare (Box 12.1). Premiums can be set by household.

For example, Micro Insurance Academy in India have had some success with a process they call CHAT: Choosing Healthcare All Together, whereby the

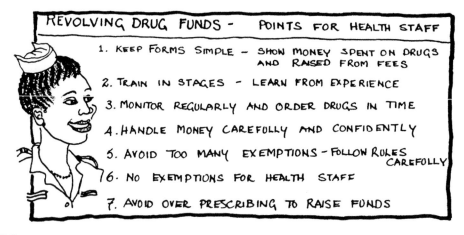

Figure 12.3 Revolving drug funds.

community meets with expert facilitators and decides together on a community health insurance scheme at the level of benefits and premium that suits them.[9] For example, a low premium would pay for care (including medicines) from the CHW. A small extra premium would cover additional care from the nearest health post or clinic by referral from the CHW. For a larger premium, the primary health centre or referral hospital could be included, again by referral. However, this will work only where there is good integration between different levels of the health service.

A bypass fee can be levied if people go straight to the primary health centre or hospital without visiting the CHW or health post. This can help to deter people from seeking care for health problems which can be adequately seen at a lower level, rather than going directly to the local district or referral hospital.

The main *advantages* of health insurance schemes are that people pay into the fund when they are well and at a time of year when their resources are greatest, e.g. harvest or payday. When illness occurs, they have no worry about paying.

However, there are also several *disadvantages*:

- It may be difficult to persuade fit people to pay when they have no felt need;
- If people pay a premium they may be tempted to overuse the health facility and expect medicines for trivial illnesses. *Solution*: charge a small co-payment at the time of attending the clinic;
- Members may only pay their premium when they first start feeling ill. *Solution*: people may not use insurance-paid healthcare within two weeks to a month of buying their insurance;
- Sometimes CHWs overprescribe, knowing that the insurance scheme will pay for the medicines;
- As with RDFs, there can be quite high failure rates. Schemes that have been carefully thought through, have community ownership, and are efficiently and honestly managed can be very successful.

Figure 12.4 Health insurance is becoming a key part of community health.

Dear Friends,

The main reason for the death of people in our villages is lack of money to pay for healthcare. In 1995 health unions (Mutuelles de Santé) were begun in Nikki, bringing together farmers and health staff. The health unions help people to face together the problem of illness by improving the health of members and helping people to plan for possible illness in the future. They raise funds from entrance fees and annual subscriptions collected from the member families. The health unions are small groups—there may be several groups or just one in each village. There are also district unions and a regional association, which co-ordinate all the health unions. In the last year over 10,000 members registered in health unions. Members receive a membership card which gives their family the right to one year's free healthcare for childbirth, treatment of small wounds, snake bites, malaria, diarrhoea, vomiting, and surgery. Minor illnesses and the cost of doctors' consultations are not included in the free treatment

Yours sincerely

Finally, we must guard against the development of a two-tier system: those who are insured and those who are not. There must be strong encouragement to enlist as many community members as possible. At the same time, those genuinely unable to afford premiums must be protected.

Other ways to raise funds

1. Income generation.

An increasing number of programmes are now raising income to make themselves sustainable. The skills of social entrepreneurs can be very useful in creating new income streams. Many communities have younger members with such skills and ambitions—people who no longer feel satisfied with a dependency mindset, but believe they can own their future through start-ups, income generation schemes and cooperatives.

There are various methods of income generation that are currently used in health and development programmes. For many of these schemes, capital grants are necessary to set up the income-generating activities but set-up costs can sometimes be raised through crowdfunding on social media or other platforms. Examples of social enterprises that can raise valuable funds over a period of time include:

- Making and selling handicrafts.
- Setting up market gardens and nurseries and selling fruit and vegetables.
- Using funds from private patients in a neighbouring or attached hospital to subsidize the community health programme

- Running bakeries.
- Hiring out vehicles (with priority to the needs of the programme).
- Running a petrol/diesel station (which also gives opportunities for HIV education for long-distance truck and bus drivers).
- Obtaining capital funds to set up a tourist lodge and then using the profit.

The website of Arukah Network (www.arukahnetwork.org) and others provide examples in addition to those given here.

In addition to year-round income generation, some programmes arrange special fund-raising events. For example, one company in Delhi with personal links to a slum development programme arranged an evening banquet for top industrialists in the city. Large numbers attended, paid a high price for tickets, and during an enjoyable evening learned about the programme through meeting the programme director and slum community volunteers. Considerable funds were raised and much goodwill and understanding generated and the press was invited in order to further increase the impact.

2. Microfinance.

In many countries, schemes are being set up to provide loans for community groups to help them develop their own businesses and income generating activities. These microfinance schemes are usually managed by programmes with special expertise in this area or by banks and other institutions with trained field workers that provide the loans and help communities use them

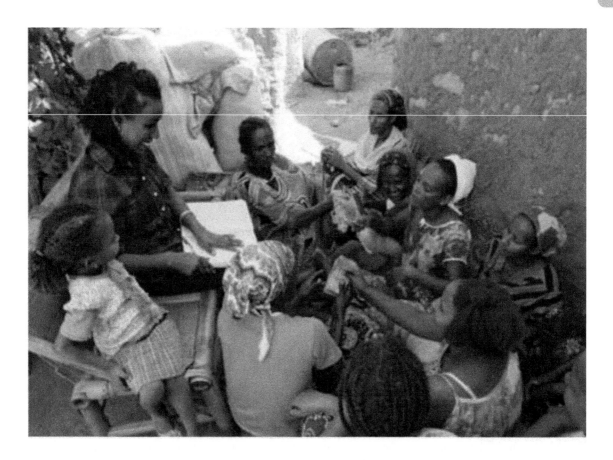

Figure 12.5 Self-help group pass their savings to the group leader during a weekly meeting

successfully. The Grameen bank in Bangladesh is a well-known example.[10] In another type of microfinance, 'self-help groups' are run as savings clubs initially; as savings grow they make small loans to members (Figure 12.5). Sometimes we can work alongside such groups so that income raised can be used to help fund essential healthcare for the family. Any such programme needs to be carefully set up with built-in safeguards and clear agreement between the stakeholders.

There have been some programmes, notably in Ghana and the Philippines, where microfinance officers have received basic health training so they can include health education in their programmes. For example, one urban programme has set up a Financial Inclusion Programme which has received special funding. Members of the slum community who combine a severe financial need with determination to overcome it are able to apply. Many have been able to turn their lives around. Poonam, a thirty-four-year-old woman who took a loan to buy a sewing machine, learned how to sew and made sufficient profit to support her children's studies and other family needs.

3. Working with donors and funding agencies.

We are likely to be entering a more prolonged era when funds from some established sources, e.g. from wealthy countries, are less willing than previously to support overseas aid. Donor fatigue (Chapter 5) is likely to become an increasing restraint. However, most programmes will take several years at least to become self-financing, so they still need to establish partnerships with donor or other support agencies. Such agencies often help with start-up costs, grants for new initiatives and capital expenditure. We need to find out various funding agencies' priorities and success criteria in order to target them more successfully.

Increasingly, funds are available in-country rather than from offices in the global north. One example of this is the Country Coordinating Mechanism used by the Global Fund. It is worth our time visiting the offices of bilateral and multilateral funding agencies of the country where we work before making an application so that any proposals are fine-tuned and realistic.

Receiving too much money can be destructive to community health programmes as it leads to dependence. Equally harmful is when short-term funding 'falls off the cliff' leading to disappointment and frustration. Ideal partnerships with funding agencies should go beyond finance. They should be a two-way learning process, with visits, training, and technical help from, or sent by, the funding agency.

4. Strategic alliances with the private sector.

Local industry, pharmaceutical companies, and philanthropists may be interested in supporting programme activities. For example, several drug companies distribute free medicines for special illnesses (e.g. albendazole for intestinal worms). We will need to scrutinize any commercial links for ethical standards and any ulterior marketing agenda. However, valuable links with the private sector sometimes come about through personal networking of programme leaders, board members, or trustees. There also may be a major employer nearby who has an interest in the improved health of its workforce and may be able to subsidize our services.

5. Accessing government funding for specific programmes

As discusses in Chapter 3, we should link up with national programmes and develop relationships with government at district level. Funds may be available for specific programmes, such as TB control, impregnated bed nets, and vaccines, sometimes through multilateral aid.

6. Contracting out

Governments are increasingly contracting out services to CSOs. For example, in the Uttarakhand cluster of Arukah Network, India, some health programmes have been contracted out to the cluster itself or to cluster member organisations, e.g. working with the people living with disability and providing disaster relief after severe flooding in mountain communities. When programmes work together towards common objectives it becomes easier to attract both donor and government funding.

7. National health insurance schemes

Some developing countries are now setting up national schemes, as opposed to community schemes. For example,

Thailand has successfully pioneered this on a nationwide scale. Some national schemes cover only secondary care. Most plans for national health insurance are 'work in progress'. We should find out what schemes might be under discussion for our country or region. We should also be aware of any services that could be contracted out to programmes like ours so members of national schemes could use the services we provide, and the programme receive reimbursement under the scheme. For most programmes in most countries this is a potential way forward.

8. National cash transfer schemes.

For low- and middle-income countries this is a relatively new system in global health. In national cash transfer schemes, the government makes regular or one-off cash transfers to poor or vulnerable families. Although this might seem a patronizing approach, there is evidence that, in many instances, this proves valuable. It helps to smooth out the difference between times of the year or times in a family's life which are relatively well-off and those which are lean. It enables enterprising families to set up their own microbusinesses. It helps cover important health expenditure, especially for children. There is also evidence that it has a 'next-generational' benefit, i.e. greater financial stability leads to a positive impact on the health, well-being, and accomplishments of children. Around almost one billion people worldwide are involved in such schemes.[11] We should find out if any such system exists in our country, region, and district and if so, work with community leaders in making these benefits available.

Further reading

Banerjee AJ, Duflo E. *Poor economics: A radical rethinking of the way to fight global poverty*. New York: Public Affairs; 2011.

Jamison D, Summer LH, Alleyne G, Arrow KJ, Berkley S, Binagwaho A, et al. Global Health 2035: A world converging within a generation. 2013; *The Lancet*. 382 (9908): 1898–1955.

Lafond A. *Sustaining primary health care*. London: Save the Children; 1995. This is more a useful policy document than a practical manual.

The World Bank. Universal Health Coverage Study Series (UNICO). Washington, DC: World Bank; 2018. Available from: https://www.worldbank.org/en/topic/health/publication/universal-health-coverage-study-series

World Health Organization. *Research for universal health coverage: World health report*. Geneva: World Health Organization; 2013. Available from: http://www.who.int/whr/2013/report/en/

References

1. Lagarde M, Palmer N. The impact of user fees on access to health services in low- and middle-income countries

(Review). *The Cochrane Database of Systematic Reviews* [online]. 2011; 4. DOI: 10.1002/14651858.CD009094

2. Transaid, London, UK. Available from: http://www.transaid.org/

3. Johnson A, Goss A, Beckerman J, Castro A. Hidden costs: The direct and indirect impact of user fees on access to malaria treatment and primary care in Mali. *Social Science & Medicine*. 2012; 75 (10): 1786–92. Available from: http://www.sciencedirect.com/science/article/pii/S0277953612005564

4. UNICEF. *Case study on narrowing the gaps for equity, Sierra Leone. Removing health care user fees to improve prospects for mothers and children*. 2011. Available at: http://www.unicef.org/equity/files/ICON_Equity_Case_Study_Sierra_Leone_FINAL15Nov2011.pdf

5. Johri M, Ridde V, Heinmüller R, Haddad S. Estimation of maternal and child mortality one year after user-fee elimination: An impact evaluation and modelling study in Burkina Faso. *Bulletin of the World Health Organization*. 2014; 92 (10): 706–15.

6. World Health Organization. *Managing Access to Medicines and Health Technologies. Chapter 13: Revolving drug funds and user fees*. Available from: http://apps.who.int/medicinedocs/documents/s19589en/s19589en.pdf

7. Saksena P, Fernandes Antunes A, Xu K, Musango L, Carrin G. Mutual health insurance in Rwanda: Evidence on access to care and financial risk protection. *Health Policy*. 2011; 99 (3): 203–9.

8. Duncan E. *Community-based health insurance in India: what are the critical success factors?* MBA [dissertation]. Newcastle, UK: Newcastle University; 2016. Available from: http://www.openthesis.org/documents/Community-based-health-insurance-in-603082.html

9. Dror D, Panda P, May C, Majumdar A, Koren R. 'One for all and all for one': Consensus-building within communities in rural India on their health microinsurance package. *Risk Management and Healthcare Policy*. 2014; 7: 139–53.

10. Yunus M. *Building social business: The new kind of capitalism that serves humanity's most pressing needs*. New York: Perseus Books Group; 2010.

11. DIFD Policy Division. *DFIC cash transfers evidence paper*. 2011. Available from: http://www.who.int/alliance-hpsr/alliancehpsr_dfidevidencepaper.pdf

SECTION 3
Community health topics

CHAPTER 13

Setting up and improving a community health clinic

Ted Lankester

What we need to know

A report from the International Labour Organization[1] shows that 56 per cent of people living in rural areas worldwide do not have access to essential health care services.

This chapter describes the setting up of a clinic with the emphasis on starting a community-based clinic, e.g. health post or equivalent where nothing effective exists. Although it does not include how to set up inpatient facilities in a hospital or primary health centre, some sections in this chapter will still be useful in those situations.

The chapter also provides ideas on how to improve or scale up existing clinics, ranging from district hospital outpatients, through primary health centres down to peripheral health posts. Our emphasis must always be involving the community so that their needs and ideas shape how the clinic develops. The community should increasingly share in and where ever appropriate take over its management.

What health services already exist?

We must remember that the government of the country has the prime responsibility for setting up health services. In the poorest areas with the most vulnerable populations, this may hardly happen because of weak health systems. Any programme we set up needs to help and strengthen existing health systems. Only in exceptional circumstances should we be duplicating any existing services, clinics, or health centres.

Of course, there are many gaps, and if we have a collaborative attitude the government will often welcome civil society organizations (CSOs) to work with them or manage services on their behalf.

This means that before starting any new clinic, as part of our needs assessment, we must find out what services already exist in our programme area and meet the district health team.

Also, because we are interested in community health, not simply curative care through clinics, we must ask about 'turning off the tap of ill health', e.g. training Community Health Workers (CHWs) in prevention and tackling root causes. Unless we keep this focus, we end up with patients returning to the same clinic, to get the same medicine, to return to the same environment, to get the same illness.

We need to enquire how government health centres are arranged in our country, region and area. Countries are usually divided into different health 'districts', or equivalent, and then into smaller subdistricts; often, they are divided into smaller zones below that. We must discover the terminology used. Where sufficient resources exist, districts will have a district hospital, usually run by the government, but sometimes handed over to a voluntary, private or religious agency to run. Subdistricts and their equivalents usually aim to have primary health centres with basic inpatient and maternity facilities. They serve an approximate population number or a defined geographical area. At more peripheral levels there will be dispensaries or health posts, usually with few or no overnight beds. There may also be mobile clinics (see also Chapter 3).

We must also ask how effectively government health facilities are functioning. This will vary greatly not only between countries but between districts. Many factors make it difficult for governments to keep up standards of health care, e.g. high demand of growing populations, conflict and displaced people, ageing populations with chronic diseases, low government resources, shortage of personnel, weak infrastructure. For these and other reasons, resources are stretched, staff unpaid and demoralized, drugs in short supply and buildings and equipment not maintained. In some areas there may almost be a complete shut-down of health care services.

In addition, we need to ask what other health-related programmes are functioning in the project area. There may be programmes run by CSOs, e.g. charities or faith-based organizations (FBOs)—in practice these are often church or mission hospitals. In many areas, private practitioners, or the private sector in general, are becoming the main providers of curative care. Traditional medicine remains strong in many areas. There may be vertical or disease-specific programmes organised by the government or a multilateral agency, which concentrate on specific tasks such as childhood immunization or the Integrated Management of Childhood Illness (IMCI). Examples are End TB, Roll Back Malaria, and the control of locally important illnesses, e.g. schistosomiasis. There may be overlap, duplication, and confusion between these programmes, making an integrated community-based approach even more important.

Other agencies may be concentrating on development, e.g. sanitation or water, or on other sectors involved in literacy, control of soil erosion, micro-credit, and housing, all of which have a direct effect on health.

As mentioned, governments have the prime responsibility for health care of their populations but often have insufficient resources. CSOs may offer innovative ways of providing good quality health care. It is important that government and CSOs recognize each other, acknowledge any government responsibilities, build partnership, and discuss in detail how they can work together.

CSOs will need to make sure they co-operate with government and integrate their services wherever they can. It is valuable if CSOs can become partners in the scaling up of existing or successful services. At the same time, they need to make sure their own values, approaches, and priorities are recognized in any collabotration with the government.

Here are some ways we can develop collaboration and integration:

- Think carefully about how any new clinic fits in with existing facilities in the area. What gaps need filling? What areas are under-served?
- Consult the community thoroughly about the services they wish to have, the appropriate location and their willingness to share in managing the clinic (Figure 13.1).
- Build relationships with government at district and local levels, and with any other organizations working in the same area. In particular, have discussions with the district medical officer (DMO).
- Clusters such as those set up by The Arukah Network (previously Community Health Global Network) can help to bring collaboration and much greater efficiency (Chapter 2).
- Decide whether it is possible to strengthen an existing clinic, e.g. by working with existing staff, or even offering to run it on their behalf.
- Consider starting a new centre in areas where there are no services.
- Secure written permission, a contract, or agreement from the government and/or the DMO for any new clinic you plan to set up.
- Arrange to collect and send statistics to the DMO in line with national guidelines.

Choosing the type of clinic to set up

This should be decided in partnership with the community, and in discussion with the DMO or equivalent. We

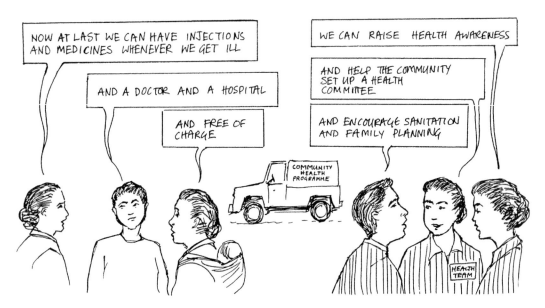

Figure 13.1 A case of differing expectations.

will need to understand the specific needs of the community, e.g. through a Participatory Appraisal (PA) and survey (Chapter 6) and this should shape our plans. Occasionally, donors may specify their wishes but we need to avoid being 'donor-driven' in our approaches (see Chapter 2). In practice, some programmes will develop general clinics, also known as multipurpose or polyclinics. Here, any person can attend with any problem. Others will run specialist clinics such as Maternal and Mother/Child Health (MCH) clinics on one day of the week, TB clinics on another (if they are part of the national TB programme).

General clinics are usually more convenient for patients. These can be used where access is easy, or patient numbers large and also in established refugee camps.

Moreover, each individual can use the same visit to have all problems seen on one occasion. For example, a mother may come to the clinic with sore eyes, a chronic cough, needing a final antenatal check, and requesting advice about family planning. Sometimes the type and frequency of the clinic will depend on what health personnel are available.

Who will use the clinic?

Unless the clinic is part of a genuinely community-based programme the least needy may use it most, and the neediest will use it least (Figure 13.2). Often this is due

to various barriers to accessing health care, which can sometimes be surprising and varied. Focus groups with women or other community groups can give insights into what the barriers are. For example, in South Sudan, a health centre was set up with a clean, white-washed delivery room, but women were not willing to deliver in a place where blood might show on the walls. The clinic had to paint the lower half of the walls dark brown to resemble a local hut.

The least needy who use it most may include those with minor health problems wanting injections and pills; those ill a long time who have already seen many doctors, and arrive clutching sheaves of reports; or those living nearby who can easily attend, who are well enough to reach the clinic, or who have relatives able and willing to bring them. Finally, men in poor communities

> ### Box 13.1 **Health team members**
>
> Health team members should never develop clinics at the expense of being involved at community level. It is usually far more useful to spend half the week teaching CHWs or improving a community water supply than spending five days within the walls of the clinic.

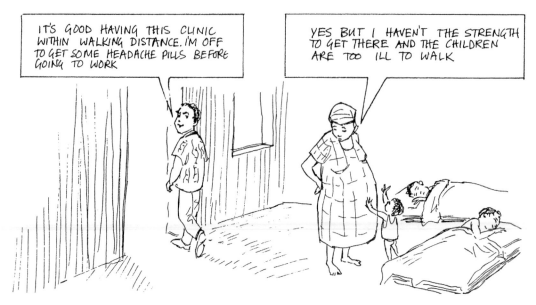

Figure 13.2 The least needy may use the clinic most, and the neediest may use it least.

often have more time to attend than women, and are less willing to tolerate pain.

The neediest who use it least may include the very poor, the most vulnerable, people living a long distance away, and those too timid to attend; women unable to leave home because of household duties, the needs of their children, or harsh words from their partner; children too sick to walk, or with no one to carry them; the very ill, the very old, people living with disability; and those with mental illness.

Our clinics must work hard to reverse this pattern. Clinics must be user-friendly, sensibly priced, appropriately sited, and run in partnership with the community. In addition, our clinics must genuinely contribute to the global health priority of Universal Health Coverage (UHC). It will be important to monitor use of the clinic and find out reasons why those most in need may not be using it, i.e. discovering any barriers to its use. Of course, there may be positive reasons for low attendance such as effective CHWs who deal with most of the community's problems. But often there are other reasons which are not obvious.

For example, a Ugandan study asked community members why they did not take sick children to the health unit. The responses included lack of money (90 per cent), transport problems (26 per cent), and other children at home to care for (15 per cent). Also

mentioned were that the health services were substandard, the father was sick at home, the husband was absent so unable to give his opinion, an ill child improved after the first treatment, or that there was no alternative but to remain at home.

How many people should the clinic serve?

There are several factors to consider. For example, a clinic may serve one large village, one cluster of smaller villages, a plantation, a factory, or a refugee camp. It may serve a certain section of a city slum. Usually the clinic will tie in with our survey area, existing government facilities, our CHW training programme, and other community activities (See Box 13.1).

In addition to any barriers described above many factors contribute to the numbers attending the clinic. One example is the effectiveness of the CHW. If our clinic is serving a definite target area and CHWs are working effectively, it will affect numbers attending. As mentioned before numbers may decline if CHWs are diagnosing and treating more people. But they may also increase if CHWs are ensuring that more people attend the clinic for immunizations, antenatal care, children with severe malnutrition, and with other illnesses requiring referral. Numbers may also increase when clinics become well known, e.g. for excellent care or because the local media has been promoting them. Over a period of time older populations and those with non-communicable diseases may increase the numbers and type of patients.

Over the short term, large changes in those attending a clinic may be caused by local epidemics or closures of neighbouring services. In rural areas especially, times for sowing and harvesting the main crops can greatly affect attendance rates, as can festivals. Another factor is how much the centre is perceived as being able to care for the seriously ill and to handle emergencies.

Assessing how many people may attend a clinic is therefore very difficult as it has to consider all the complex factors in a particular area. In practice, assessing likely attendance through a sample questionnaire or community meeting can be helpful. There must also be flexibility to respond to variation in numbers. The author remembers two successive Mondays where for no obvious reason forty people attended one week, and one hundred thirty-four the next.

When clinics find they routinely have more patients than they can manage, curative care tends to take over. There is no time to look at a fuller range of health needs or underlying causes a patient or family may have.

Where should the clinic be located?

Clinics should be set up within the community or as near to it as possible. Ideally no one should need to travel more than about one hour on foot, although this is difficult to achieve where households are scattered. It should also be located in a place convenient, safe, acceptable to the majority and near a transport route.

If one clinic serves different villages, tribal groups, religions, or castes, it must be in a location that everyone is happy to attend. A roadside or pathside building is often appropriate.

The clinic and its waiting area must be safe for children and other vulnerable people. In city slums, clinics should ideally be situated in areas known to be safe, e.g. those that are well-used and well-lit.

When the clinic should start

This can be a difficult decision and should be discussed with community leaders. It may have to be started before training CHWs or carrying out any other community activity. Remote or poor communities may have so much illness or so little understanding of community involvement that they are not prepared to work in partnership with the health team until basic health services are provided.

If possible, we should delay starting a clinic until after CHWs have been selected by the community (see Chapter 8). In this way the community understands that CHWs are the first point of call when illness strikes. If people become used to visiting a clinic for day-to-day health problems they may later bypass their newly trained CHW (Figure 13.3).

If we do delay starting a clinic, there must be some alternative the community is able to use for curative care.

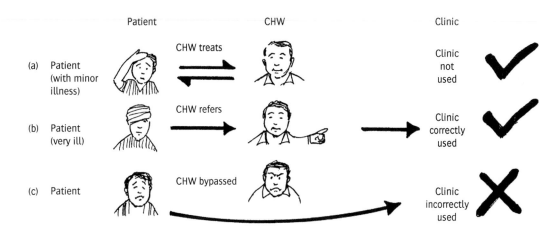

Figure 13.3 The correct (a) and (b) and incorrect (c) relationship of the CHW and clinic.

In practice this may be the facilities and practitioners they have been using before we started the programme. But we will need to help strengthen any nearby effective

referral service until our clinic is ready for use, which in turn could be used as our main referral centre later.

What we need to do

Designing the centre

This will depend on many factors, e.g. urban or rural settings and the expectations of the community. For example, the Accord project in Tamil Nadu, India, planned and implemented an entire health system with full community involvement. In the health centre patients slept on mats, not on beds, nurses spoke only the tribal language, and most staff were trained vocationally from the community. After ten years, antenatal coverage reached 90 per cent, and childhood immunization increased from 2 per cent to 75 per cent.

In rural areas, we should rent or construct the simplest building that is able to fully support the services we are planning to give. In doing this we must remember the main functions of a clinic building, which are to protect patients, health workers (HWs) and equipment from excessive heat, rain or cold and to provide a safe and clean environment where patients can gather. A well-known community health doctor has commented that 'There is nothing that discourages health professionals from getting out into the community more than an expensive health centre building'!

In designing a centre, we need to consider the number of people being served, the services being offered, its proximity to a referral centre and any local preferences. At the upper end of the scale, a community clinic is a permanent, purpose-designed building, with some inpatient or overnight beds and a delivery room. It serves the function of a typical primary health centre. At the most basic level, a room or a veranda in a CHWs

home can act, with certain safeguards, as a place where patients can be seen. A layout which works for many communities is shown in Figure 13.4.

Some communities will be better served by a mobile clinic. Regardless of the size or design of the clinic, there will usually need to be a confidential space where more intimate examinations can be carried out.

Clinics ideally should be made of local materials in the local building style. They can be purpose-built with community members contributing. For example, the community can help to clear the land, provide labour and materials, and set up rainwater catchment systems on the roof. This involvement helps the community 'own' their clinic from the start. Alternatively, an appropriate local building can be adapted and used. Where possible, solar power should be used.

Make sure that the different parts of the health centre are clearly signposted in the local language(s). Outside, display opening times and where relevant which clinics are held on which day (NB: we must still be willing to see seriously ill patients or those who have walked long distances, outside clinic hours). Inside, have clear, friendly notices explaining where people should sit, the functions of the various rooms, and a simple arrow system. Make sure any health posters are easily understood and relevant for the majority of clinic users. Discuss with local people how notices can be designed with symbols for those unable to read, or consider other options to help non-readers, such as having community volunteer guides.

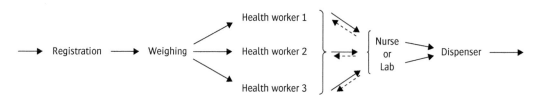

Figure 13.4 Flow pattern for a typically sized clinic.

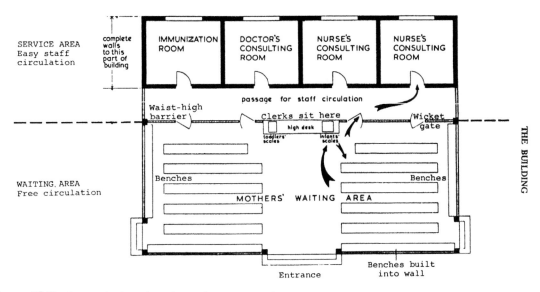

Figure 13.5 A basic under-fives clinic plan used in many countries.

Figure 13.4 shows a suggested flow pattern for a typically sized clinic. Waiting space out of the sun and the rain needs to be available, either centrally or adjoining each clinic station. Figure 13.5 shows a design that can be adapted for a general clinic, e.g. one of the nurse's rooms can be the dispensary. An oral rehydration solution (ORS) demonstration corner can be added in the immunization room.

Set up the clinic stations

The registrar or receptionist has two main jobs: to welcome and to register. It is important that registrars have a friendly and welcoming attitude towards everyone who comes to the clinic, including the poor, the people living with disability, and those who are late or come on the 'wrong day' (Figure 13.6).

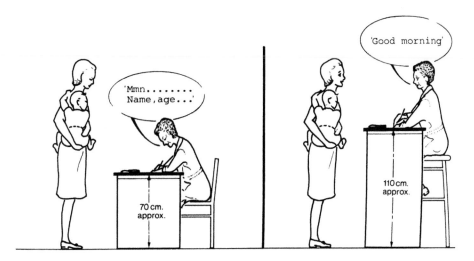

Figure 13.6 Registration is the first and perhaps the most important contact with the health service.

At the time of writing, a UK report showed that 40 per cent of potential clinic users were discouraged or put off from using the clinic because of the receptionist.

To do their job well, registrars need to understand how patients may be feeling. Imagine the situation of a mother who has never visited the centre before: she gets up early and walks a long way carrying a sick child. She is worried. She does not know how the clinic works. She is not sure if she can afford the charges. When she arrives, there are many people sitting looking anxious. There is a notice giving information but she can't read it. A friendly smile or a welcoming word from the registrar can be extremely reassuring.

Before recording details, the registrar does basic 'triage' making sure that sick children or the people living with disability, frail, or seriously ill are seen as soon as possible. Each programme will need to work out an appropriate system for registering patient details. Assuming that patients do not come by appointment, the registrar should arrive in plenty of time, and get organized before patients arrive.

When the patients arrive to register, various methods can now be followed. For example, existing patients place their self-retained record or registration card on the desk, and then sit and wait until their name is called; new patients report to the registrar. Another option is that all patients queue (preferably sitting out of the sun or rain) and are registered and seen in turn. If there are large numbers of patients, all take a number on arrival, sit, and wait until their number is called.

For each patient, the registrar records details. In a clinic register or computer screen registration may include:

Patient Name	Family Name	Patient No.	Age	Sex	Village or urban area	Money paid

For existing patients, the registrar will date and stamp the card. New patients (or those who do not have their card with them) will be issued a new card with their name, age, village/area of city, etc., in addition to the date and stamp. The card is put into a protective envelope along with the number given to the patient by the registrar. If patients prepay a fixed amount, the registrar will take the money. If a family folder is being used the registrar includes this (see Chapter 6 and Appendix C).

Self-retained record cards (plus the family folder, if used) are placed in a pile in the order in which the patients arrive. If different Health Workers (HWs) are seeing different patients (Figure 13.7), separate piles are made for each HW. The registrar ensures that, where possible, patients who have recently visited the clinic see the same HW as before. A clinic assistant, e.g. a CHW or health committee member, collects the pile of cards from the registrar's desk, places them on the HW's desk, and calls out names in turn. Meanwhile, patients sit waiting their turn (except for certain categories; see Figure 13.7). Finally, after the last patient, the registrar totals the entries and any money taken, hands this over to the person in charge of the clinic, who checks and countersigns the

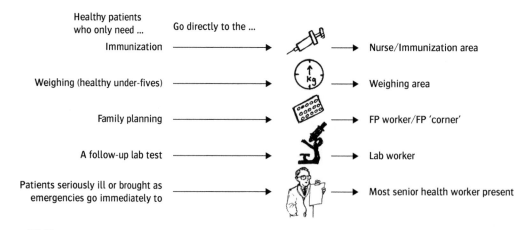

Figure 13.7 Saving everyone's time in a busy clinic.

register. Lastly, a check is made that there are sufficient cards, stationery, etc., for the next clinic.

Registrars can be drawn from health team members, responsible members of the community, or from the village health committee or women's group. The more this role is community-owned, the better, but confidentiality needs to be carefully considered. Efficient registrars who ensure patients know where to go and who to see save everyone a great deal of time.

Setting up weighing stations

All children under five, pregnant women, TB patients, people living with HIV/AIDS (unless weighing provokes stigma), any malnourished patients on a feeding programme, and any seriously overweight patients on a weight-reducing plan should be weighed. Alternatively, time allowing, everyone can be weighed—which provides a chance for the HW to share snippets of useful health information with her captive audience. A suitable place for weighing can be a separate room, a convenient place near the registrar, or a veranda. Suitable equipment, especially for children, includes round-faced spring balances or tubular scales. Stirrups or a pair of small 'weighing trousers' slipped over the clothes worn by the children are needed for children under three years, baskets for newborn babies. Adults can use simple 'stand on' scales.

As in all community health activities, the least qualified person who can do the job well should be given the task. With careful training, family members such as parents or older siblings can do the weighing (Figure 13.8). All CHWs should be able to weigh accurately. Nurses, in their role of teacher, should allow others to learn the weighing process, rather than regularly doing the weighing themselves.

Common mistakes in weighing include times when there are many children waiting but only one pair of weighing trousers is available. In a rush to speed up the weighing process, children's excess clothes are not removed, which skews the reading. Other times, frightened children are left to hang on the scale while adults and onlookers unsuccessfully try to cheer them up. Weights can be misread through carelessness, e.g. the child is bouncing, the scales are not at eye level, or because the mother fails to let go. Weights that don't seem correct should be rechecked. Often, growth charts are wrongly filled in (see Chapter 14). Finally and importantly, the community culture may not be understood. For example, in some traditional areas, people consider weighing children as wrong, dangerous, or bringing bad

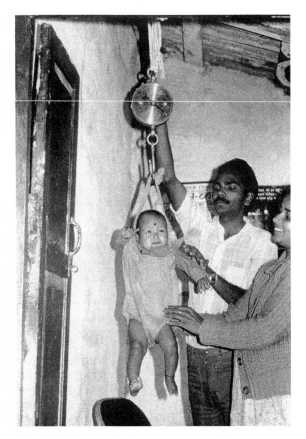

Figure 13.8 Family members weigh their own children, with guidance.

Reproduced courtesy of Ted Lankester. This image is distributed under the terms of the Creative Commons Attribution Non-Commercial 4.0 International licence (CC-BY-NC), a copy of which is available at http://creativecommons.org/licenses/by-nc/4.0/.

luck. Such beliefs need to be understood and gently corrected. Clinic weighing should not necessarily replace weighing in the home by the family or CHW.

If time is limited it may be more useful to give nutritional advice than spend time weighing and plotting this on a weight chart. A general rule is that feeding advice should always be given and that weighing should be done whenever time allows, ideally using a weight chart. Any feeding advice must be entirely appropriate for the culture of the community and should only recommend foods that are available and affordable locally.

The consultation

One model of a health consultation, originally described by Stott and Davis[2], lists four key elements in any consultation between a HW and a patient:

1. Dealing with the acute problem, i.e. the felt reason the patient attends.

2. Dealing with any underlying or chronic problems—often the most important reason for attending.

3. Helping the patient to change their health behaviour so in the future they are less likely to attend.

4. Promoting one aspect of good health related to the reason they attend.

HWs who see patients must be trained carefully and be supervised by doctors or senior experienced HWs until they have reached a safe and competent standard. They should follow guidelines prepared by doctors, such as standing orders, treatment schedules, group protocols, or patient group directions. The IMCI gives details on how to assess and manage sick children. We should use this where possible along with any national adaptations.

In many countries, HWs will need to demonstrate they have completed training and registration before they are able to treat patients or prescribe medicines, especially when no doctor is present. In government programmes, these procedures are usually in place, but CSOs are not always aware of official regulations.

Box 13.2 shows a system that can be followed by any well-trained HW who sees patients (see also Figure 13.9).[3] Simplify this for your situation. The process will speed up with practice. The questions can be adapted by each programme according to local disease patterns and the time available. In specific situations we can ask for more information, e.g. malnutrition (Chapter 14) and antenatal visits (Chapter 17). Obtain full details; for women of childbearing age ask whether they are pregnant (in order to offer antenatal care and also know what medicines are safe to prescribe).

Box 13.2 **The steps a health worker should follow when seeing a patient**

1) Health worker warmly greets the patient.
2) She consults the patient's record, notes the patient's status, and any relevant family or ethnic information. The health worker looks for details of any previous illness or treatment. If a family folder is being used, she takes note of the size, structure and socioeconomic status of the family.
3) The health worker asks the patient what the problem is—listening carefully without interrupting.
4) Based on the patient's answer, based on any important symptom described, the health worker now asks questions:
   a) *For diarrhoea*:
      • How many stools per day?
      • How many days have you had it?
      • Is there fever? blood? mucus? vomiting? excess flatus? significant pain?
   b) *For pain*:
      • Where is the pain?
      • How long have you had it?
      • Have you ever had it before?
      • What makes it better or worse?
   c) *For cough*:
      • How long have you had it? More than 3 weeks?
      • Is there sputum, blood, fever, or chest pain?
      • Have you ever had TB treatment or been diagnosed with TB??

   • Does anyone else in your family have a cough; has anyone been treated for TB?
   d) *For fever*:
      • How long have you had it?
      • Is it continuous or does it come and go?
      • Is there sweating, shivering, vomiting, or headache?
   e) *For cuts, bites, accidents*:
      • When did it happen?
      • How did it happen?
      • If an animal bite, what was the animal, is the animal alive, and if so, where is it?
   f) *For any other symptoms*:
      • How long have you had it?
      • Have you had it before?
5) Other questions we can ask if the diagnosis is still unclear:
   • Have you lost weight?
   • Do you drink alcohol, smoke, or use other drugs?
   • Ears: any pain or discharge? Is the patient deaf?
   • Eyes: any pain, soreness or difficulty seeing?
   • Throat: any soreness or loss of voice?
   • Chest: any other symptoms?
   • Bowels: any other symptoms?
   • Urination: pain, frequency or trouble passing urine? Any urethral discharge?
   • Periods: pain, heavy loss, discharge, bleeding between periods?
   • Skin: any sores, itching, rash, or swellings?

Box 13.2 *continued*

- Genitals: any sores, ulcers, or other problems? (NB: in many cultures this is best asked by a health worker of the same gender as the patient, and in private.)
- Bones, joints, muscles: any swelling, pain, or stiffness?
- Mind: any sadness, agitation, confusion, or fits?
- Any other symptoms not mentioned?

6) The health worker examines the patient by *looking*:
- General appearance: anything unusual?
- Well or ill?
- Depressed, anxious, confused?
- Thin or dehydrated?
- Normal colour? pale? yellow? flushed with fever?
- Breathing normally? wheezing? child with fast breathing (If yes, suspect pneumonia; see Chapter 16.)
- Eyes: infection? pale mucous membranes? yellow? vitamin A deficiency? trachoma?
- Tongue: pale? dry? sore or smooth?
- Part of body where symptom located: anything to see?

7) The health worker examines the patient by *touching* and *feeling*:
- Pulse: rate? regular? strong?
- Part of body where symptom located: any swelling, warmth, pain, or tenderness?
- Listening to the chest: any unusual or added sounds over lung? heart murmur?
- Measuring temperature and blood pressure, if necessary.
- Checking the urine (this can also be done at the nursing station).
- Checking respiration (a pulse oximeter and peak-flow meter is useful in older populations and where asthma, COPD, and air pollution is a problem).

8) Health worker diagnoses the problem.
9) Health worker treats the patient.

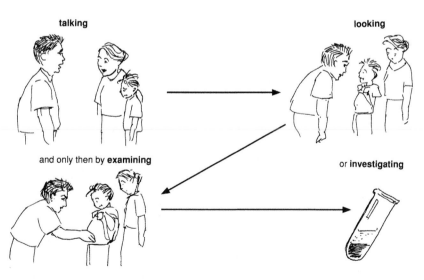

Figure 13.9 Learn to diagnose patients mainly by …

Where TB is common we ask whether there has been cough for more than three weeks (increasingly two weeks is used). Where HIV/AIDS is common we sensitively enquire whether the person is interested in voluntary counselling and testing (VCT) and if so explain where and when it is available. If they are HIV-positive, we follow any local procedure (Chapter 20).

With the result of any tests (if the clinic has a field laboratory) and helped by the standing orders or IMCI algorithms, the HW makes the diagnosis. If the HW is uncertain what the problem is or how serious it is, advice should be sought from a doctor, nurse, supervisor or colleague.

Having dealt with the patient's felt needs, the HW now searches for any 'real' need(s) of the patient. While patients nearly always come because of 'felt' needs—a pain or problem for which they want a cure, we must also try to find the equally important 'real' or underlying need (Figure 13.10). This can be thought of as a problem, disease, or lack of health that affects the long-term health of the patient, family, or the community. Underlying needs might be:

- Malnutrition found by weighing or observation.
- Incomplete immunization.
- Presence of serious illness such as possible TB, AIDS, schistosomiasis, etc.

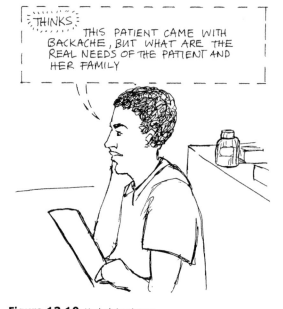

Figure 13.10 Underlying issues.

Reproduced courtesy of David Gifford. This image is distributed under the terms of the Creative Commons Attribution Non-Commercial 4.0 International licence (CC-BY-NC), a copy of which is available at http://creativecommons.org/licenses/by-nc/4.0/.

- Environmental exposures to unclean water, untreated waste, indoor smoke, or unhealthy hygiene practices.
- Pregnancy needing antenatal care.
- Family planning.
- Recent discharge from hospital.
- Chronic illness, e.g. diabetes, hypertension.
- Mental illness.
- Physical and mental disability, which may be open for stigma reduction or treatment.

The HW may discover these needs by asking appropriate questions, checking the blood pressure and urine, checking the patient's record card (in particular the family folder and insert cards). If patient records are computerized, the HWs should check any follow-up notes that may have been entered. If time allows, the HW should also check for any real need of any other family member. For example, if a child is accompanying the patient, the HW makes sure that the child has been recently weighed and completed immunizations. If a mother is accompanying a patient, could she be pregnant and need antenatal care? If a coughing father is accompanying another family member, has he been tested for TB?

The family folder and insert cards should be checked to make sure immunizations are complete and that any important follow-up to previous problems has been carried out. Any family members needing to be seen can be brought to the next clinic. Additionally, there may be a seriously ill family member at home or one who is housebound who needs home-based care and a visit from the CHW.

- When clinics first start or cover too large a population there may be so many patients attending that there will be little time to search for real needs or wider family needs.
- Remember, however, that health projects should be set up in such a way that CHWs can deal with routine problems in the community.
- This frees clinics for treating serious illness and caring for the real, underlying needs of patients.

Unless this is prioritized, clinics will spend all their time treating minor, felt needs and the real needs of the individual and community remain unmet. The overall health of the community fails to improve.

In treating the patient, the HW prescribes any medicine necessary, writing down the generic name, the dose, how often the medicine should be taken and for how long, to guide the dispenser. The HW should also mention any precautions, special instructions, or side effects.

It is important to keep the number of medicines prescribed to the minimum needed, and always follow the correct treatment protocol. In particular, antibiotics must only be used if there is a definite need, not just simply to please the patient, so as to avoid overuse (Chapter 11). Two other areas need care: firstly, the use of abbreviations for medicines, which may not be understood by all team members (especially new recruits), and secondly, dosages for children, which are often incorrectly calculated.

The HW also needs to advise the patient about how to help prevent the condition from recurring. For example, a method that has proved successful in some projects is the use of health drills. These are carefully worded summaries of health advice that are listed alphabetically for each common health problem. The HW seeing the patients, the nurse, and the dispenser all have copies. The HW should explain the relevant health drill to the patient, and then 'prescribe' it in the notes. When the patient later sees the nurse or dispenser, this health drill, i.e. identical instructions, will be explained again.

Once the diagnosis and the advice has been given to the patient, the HW arranges any procedure such as bandaging, tooth extraction, or immunization. She will refer the patient to a more senior HW if not sure of the diagnosis or treatment. She makes sure the patient understands the condition, prescription, and/or treatment, and asks the patient to repeat back any important instructions. For example, a project in Tansen, Nepal uses body diagrams as part of the medical consultation so that patients can better understand their health problems (Table 13.1). The diagrams doubled the number of patients who gained understanding, and took only a little extra time. Finally, the HW recognizes if the patient does not seem satisfied and tries to discover the reason. At the end of the consultation, the HW provides a follow-up appointment date for the patient to return to the clinic.

It is vital that the HW records any important information on the patient's record card, the family folder insert card, and any relevant register. There is an increasing expectation that HWs record and provide weekly/monthly reports in a regional or central HIMS (Health Information Management System). Donors and major funders or health system strengthening programmes (and vertical programmes) often shape these for their own agendas. These can be quite burdensome for local HWs, but we can help in our supervision times to make this as speedy and accurate as possible. If the programme is computerized, the HW should enter any data from the hard copy or use a hand-held device in the clinic.

Expanding the consultation's benefit

Patients learn as they wait

In mother and child clinics, patients can wait in the consultation room, or just outside it, so that they 'learn by overhearing'. CHWs can gather groups of waiting mothers and give appropriate health messaging (see Chapter 4). This approach must be guided by how confidentiality is understood in the culture.

Each one teach one

Use the consultation as a time to teach other HWs, especially CHWs. Encourage other health team members to pass on their knowledge and skills whenever they have a chance.

Respect patients' beliefs

Patients may have ideas that may seem strange or incorrect. They may be more interested in *who* caused the disease than *what* caused it. We should instruct them gently without causing offence.

Continuity

Ideally, the same patient should see the same HW for all visits. If a patient comes to know and trust a HW they are more likely to follow their advice and return for follow-up.

Respect the need for privacy

Make sure there is strict privacy when necessary, e.g. when discussing HIV/AIDS, STIs, infertility, TB, leprosy, or other stigmatized conditions. In most cultures, family planning is also a private matter.

Table 13.1 **A model of a health consultation**

In	Investigate using the protocol
Every	Explain the disease using the body diagram
Case	Counsel about non-drug treatment
Follow	Follow up/refer according to protocol
The	Treat according to protocol
Protocol	Preventative health issues: discuss one

The field laboratory

A small field laboratory is quite easy to set up and greatly adds to the value of a community clinic. Advantages of setting up a field laboratory include: helping to confirm the diagnosis, i.e. clinics can concentrate on curing illness rather than simply treating symptoms, increased accuracy (especially when HWs without formal qualifications are seeing patients), providing 'customer satisfaction', and cost-effectiveness. By reducing the number of visits to hospital, the field lab saves time and money.

Types of test available

There are many tests that can often be handled by a well-managed field laboratory with simple equipment, and staffed by a carefully trained worker. Blood tests, including haemoglobin, white cell count and differential, erythrocyte sedimentation rate (ESR), malaria smear plus Rapid Diagnostic Test for malaria antigens, and HIV testing in the context of VCT (with careful training and control) can all be done in the field lab. In many situations, haemoglobin levels and malaria slides are the most valuable tests. Without testing, malaria is commonly underdiagnosed or overdiagnosed, either of which can be dangerous for patients. Sputum tests can be done for acid-fast bacilli (AFB) in TB (Chapter 19), but treatment should not normally be started unless a patient is sputum positive. The quality control of sputum testing for TB needs to be in line with national guidelines, but on-site testing is very valuable. Any diagnosis and treatment of TB must only be done if the programme is officially integrated into the national TB programme.

Other tests include stool tests for worms (e.g. hook, round, whip, tape), protozoa (e.g. amoeba, *Giardia*) and Schistosoma ova. These tests still miss a number of affected stools. Urine tests can include microscopy for pus cells, bacteria, and Schistosoma ova where relevant, or dipstick (or other method) for sugar, protein, bile, and blood. Skin tests (scrape for fungus), vaginal swabs (gonococcus, Trichomonas, or Candida), and voluntary counselling and testing (VCT) for HIV/AIDS can all be done, and the latter is a valuable service, providing it follows good practice guidelines and is offered in such a way that clients feel comfortable using it.

The laboratory worker

Tests can be done either by a qualified laboratory technician with basic training, or by a health team member who is carefully trained and regularly supervised by a qualified technician. Laboratory workers must be accurate, reliable, thorough, and aware of their own limitations.

Unless carefully trained and supervised, workers may be tempted to 'fudge' results, especially if they are rushed for time or lacking confidence, or want to record a result that they believe the doctor or HW is expecting.

Equipment needed in a field laboratory

Disposable needles and syringes are used unless they are completely unavailable. Sterilizing, e.g. by using a steam sterilizer for any reusable items, must be done with care (Chapter 5) and supervisors should make regular spot checks on how accurately steam sterilizers and fridges are both functioning and being used. A suggested list of general equipment appears in Appendix B. For further details on setting up a field lab and the equipment needed, see 'Further reading and resources'.

Laboratory procedure for patients

Patients needing laboratory tests will usually be referred by the HW they have just seen. They will go to the laboratory, bringing either their self-retained card or a separate laboratory request slip, on which the lab worker will record the result. Patients should wait their turn, both for the test and its result, preferably sitting in an area near the lab. They can then report back to the HW.

The clinic nurse

Larger clinics may have fully qualified nurses. Smaller clinics will often use a variety of HWs with different levels of training. Wherever possible, a qualified nurse should be present. Nurses who have been trained in hospitals and then join community health programmes often need a complete reorientation in approach and outlook. In practice, HWs well-trained on the job are sometimes more suitable than nurses who may wish they were back in the hospital.

The nurse's varied functions

Nurses typically have a role in quality control and good practice, such as in maintaining hygiene, infection control, and storage and stock management of equipment and medication. Many clinics will be led by nurses, who may also function as the senior HW seeing patients. Nurses also tend to give immunizations and other injections if really needed (Chapter 10). Furthermore, their tasks tend to include dressing and bandaging, cleaning skin infections and wounds, lancing abscesses, giving family planning advice and supplies, running an ORS corner, assisting the doctor or the HW, taking temperatures, weights, blood pressures, urine checking, measuring oxygen saturation with a pulse oximeter if available and teaching.

The dispenser or pharmacist

Any HW with a particular gift or interest can be trained as a dispenser. Dispensing is different from prescribing, which needs to be done by a specially trained HW who may need formal qualifications or training. The person prescribing will usually be responsible for setting up procedures for dispensers, training them, and monitoring accuracy. The dispenser is usually the last HW whom the patient will see. A smile, or a sharp word, may linger in the patient's mind, affecting future compliance.

It is good practice in smaller health centres for two or three people to be trained in dispensing so that in busy clinics no one person has to count pills and give instructions for hours at a time, leading to boredom and inaccuracy. It also makes the clinic more flexible when staff are absent or ill. The dispenser's job can include both dispensing and stock-keeping. However, combining this role opens an easy route for corruption. There is value in a different team member checking and ordering stock, if the team is large enough.

Dispensing

This includes:

1 Reading the doctor or HW's handwriting.

This may be difficult! If in doubt the dispenser should ask, not guess (Figure 13.11). If a medicine has run out or is not available, the HW or doctor should be asked if an alternative can be used.

2. Counting. The exact number of pills must be given.

Use of a pill counting triangle can help with speed and accuracy. Any broken, dirty or discoloured medicines should be thrown away. Medicines past their expiry date should not normally be used unless there is a genuine shortage of supplies (see Chapter 11).

3. Explaining. For each medicine the patient will need to know:
   - How many?
   - How often?
   - How long for?
   - How? With water, before or after food, etc?
   - What side effects?
   - What food, drink or activity needs to be avoided if any?

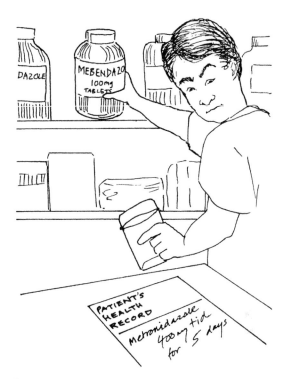

Figure 13.11 Mistakes are easy to make when a doctor's writing is unclear or a dispenser is overworked.

In the case of eye drops, ear drops, ORS packets, asthma inhalers or capsules that have to be opened and mixed on a spoon for children, the dispenser should be ready to demonstrate, as well as giving verbal instructions.

Before leaving, patients should repeat back the instructions, to make sure they have understood. Many patients who leave clinics clutching pills and medicines will not take them as instructed. They may fail to understand the instructions given, forget what they have been told, or think their own ideas are better (Figure 13.12). For example, a doctor greeted a leprosy patient by the roadside who one month previously had been diagnosed at a clinic and given thirty white dapsone tablets. The dispenser had instructed him to take one per day. Asked now how he was feeling, the patient replied: 'I took all thirty tablets together—and now I feel well.' Other patients may not be so fortunate. Exit surveys of patients can be useful to check if patients can understand the dispenser's instructions.

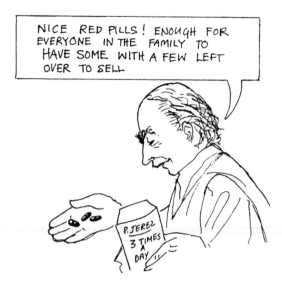

Figure 13.12 Remember what happens after patients leave the clinic.

Reproduced courtesy of David Gifford. This image is distributed under the terms of the Creative Commons Attribution Non-Commercial 4.0 International licence (CC-BY-NC), a copy of which is available at http://creativecommons.org/licenses/by-nc/4.0/.

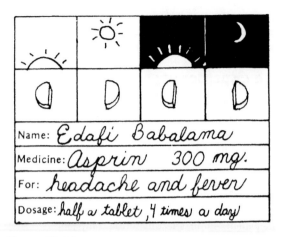

Figure 13.13 If patients cannot read, use pictures to explain amounts and timings of pills and medicines.

Reproduced from Hesperian Health Guides, http://hesperian.org/wp-content/uploads/pdf/en_hhwl_2012/en_hhwl_2012_18.pdf. Copyright © 2017 Hesperian Health Guides. This image is distributed under the terms of the Creative Commons Attribution Non-Commercial 4.0 International licence (CC-BY-NC), a copy of which is available at http://creativecommons.org/licenses/by-nc/4.0/.

4. Labelling the packet or bottle.

Any container or envelope must be well labelled. If the patient is illiterate, we should use symbols. For example, one aspirin to be taken four times a day can be represented as shown in Figure 13.13. Even these symbols must be explained.

5. Repeating the health drill.

6. In areas with high malaria incidence, dispensers can provide impregnated mosquito nets for children.

Stock-keeping

Stock-keeping is an important task that dispensers must perform on a regular basis. They will need to check all medicines for quantity remaining, at least once monthly, for expiry dates at least once quarterly, and they should use an alphabetical stock list (Figure 13.14). The purpose of this system is to re-order in plenty of time so that stocks never run out unless there is a national shortage. Clinics must always keep an adequate supply of essential medicines in stock.

If the clinic is being run in partnership with the Ministry of Health or part of a national system, medications may be supplied in generic batches as an essential drug kit. This might need to be supplemented or redistributed from quieter to busier clinics to prevent stocks

running out in busy clinics. Some programmes find the system explained here useful (see also Figure 13.14):

1. The dispenser uses a re-order sheet.
2. Two copies are made:
3. Copy 1 is sent with the order.
4. Central stores returns Copy 1 with the new supply, filling in (b).
5. The dispenser then writes down the amount actually received in (c).
6. Copy 2 is put directly into the dispenser's file and is attached to Copy 1 when this is returned.

Labelling, storing, and packing supplies

Each medicine may have several different brand names but only one generic name. In order to avoid any confusion, the generic name should always be used, even though it may be longer, difficult to remember, and can have minor variations in spelling. Always avoid using abbreviations.

The storekeeper in central stores should always send out supplies with labels attached. The label can include the details indicated in Figure 13.15. Where supplies are sent out in bottles labelled by drug companies, a bold ring or circle can be made around the generic name instead of sticking a new label on to each bottle. When semi-literate CHWs help in counting out tablets, colour

Stock list

Drug name	Code No	Unit of issue	Full stock level	Stock level when re-order necessary
Asprin	P 40	Bottle 100	2000	500

Re-order sheet

Name of health centre		Date ordered		Date received	
Item	Code No	No ordered (a)	No sent (b)	No received (c)	Remarks

Figure 13.14 Example of a stock list and reorder sheet.

codes can be used, e.g. green labels for antibiotics, orange for antimalarials, etc.

Supplies should be arranged neatly, in alphabetical generic order, with the newest supplies (or those with the longest expiry date) at the back of the shelf. The front of the shelf itself can be labelled either with the medicine name or with a letter of the alphabet. In practice it is easy for new supplies to be put at the front and for old supplies to get pushed to the back and expire. Huge amounts of medicines are wasted in this way.

The following system can prevent this:

1. For each medicine, storage space is divided into two sections side by side labelled A and B (see Table 13.2).
2. At the beginning, A is existing stock and B is empty.
3. When the amount remaining in A reaches the reorder level, new supplies are requested and these are put in B.
4. The new supplies are not used until all of A has been used up.
5. When B gets low, new stock is put in A but not used until supplies in B are finished.

Supplies also need to be stored at the correct temperature, which in practice means avoiding buildings or rooms in full sun and having a good means of ventilation even when the building is closed.

In busy clinics where medicines come in bottles and need to be counted out much time can be saved if standard courses of commonly used medicines are then prepacked and prelabelled. Use bottles or rain-proof envelopes during the rainy season, or in very resource-poor areas paper envelopes, e.g. folded from magazine paper, but only in dry climates and if no other containers are available. In many pharmacies, both in hospitals and smaller health facilities, labelling is often unclear and untidy, which adds to the risk of making mistakes in dispensing. One measure of the quality of our programme is how reliably we record, stock and display medicines in a clear and simple way.

Keep and transfer clinic records

Many programmes will develop their own system of records but we should use any national or government recording systems so data can easily be collected and compared. However, we have to guard against any system that is too complex or time-consuming, and we should avoid duplication. Most centres can use patient retained record cards, the family folder and insert cards, clinic registers, or computerized record forms.

Health programmes should have one central location where key project data is stored either manually or on computer. Usually this will be in a programme base, rather than in a community health clinic. In insecure

Generic name of drug	Code No.	Number of tablets when container full

Figure 13.15 Example of a drugs label.

Table 13.2 **A system to help prevent medicine waste**

A B	A B	A B	A B
Drug 1	Drug 2	Drug 3	Drug 4

locations it is wise to have backup data stored in two separate places. Different programmes may use different systems. The following points may help programmes in developing a system:

- Add a column for a chief diagnosis to the clinic register.
- Complete a clinic report form listing numbers of patients seen by gender, community, diagnosis etc. An alternative is to take photos of the pages used by the registrar and return them to base after each clinic. Many programmes will design their own forms or use the reporting forms needed by nationwide programmes, e.g. IMCI, End TB.
- Call in all registers from clinic to base either monthly, quarterly, or half-yearly for key data to be transferred from clinic registers to an HQ Master Register, or Health Management Information System.
- Design or use a computer-based system that can print off clinic stationery, e.g. register pages, family folders, insert cards etc. This stationery would be used for each clinic, taken back to base at the end of the clinic, and entered into the computer. This system leads to less duplication of records and is a step towards full computerization. Some programmes will use hand-held electronic devices to enter data and which will automatically update the central computer records.

If we use any computerized records and systems in our programme we must make sure this will increase efficiency. Above all, it must not detract HWs from following a patient-centred approach. It is all too common to see heath workers staring and struggling with screens and computerized records rather than giving full attention to the patient.

Patient retained record cards

Record cards will have separate designs for adults, and for children under five (which ideally have a growth chart on the back). Those with chronic diseases, e.g. TB, can have a special additional card, but the national TB programme will have their own record system, which we

should use. Those using antiretroviral therapy will have specially designed cards.

Patients keep their cards in plastic (or better, a biodegradeable alternative) envelopes and bring them whenever they come to clinic, see the CHW or go to hospital. Members of the team can make entries on these cards as follows:

- The registrar writes down the date and any fee paid.
- The person weighing children fills in the growth chart.
- The HW seeing patients will make brief, accurate, legible notes.

The family folder and insert card

This section applies only if a family folder system is being used (see Chapter 6). The family folder system is recommended as an ideal way to see most at-risk patients regularly, with the CHW playing a major role.

The family folder itself

With the exception given, nothing is written on the family folder itself unless a mistake is discovered. The folder is a record of the state of health of the family on the day of the survey (see Chapter 6). If the folder has a section 'Vital Events Since Survey' this can be completed for births, deaths, or if anyone permanently joins or leaves the household.

The insert cards

These should only be used for patients considered at risk. This includes all children under five, pregnant women, and those with serious or chronic illness such as TB, diabetes, and other non-communicable diseases. For people living with HIV/AIDS, even if taking ART, cards should only be kept if confidentiality is secure and/or stigma is not a major issue. Make brief strategic notes for the purpose of follow-up. Insert cards are placed in the family folder and can be prepared either when the person in question attends the clinic or a member of their family comes. Some programmes fill out cards at the time of the community survey. Self-limiting or trivial problems should not be recorded on the insert card, as this wastes valuable time.

Family folders and insert cards should be kept at the health centre and not given to the patient. They are too bulky and will get lost or damaged. Instead, the patient should keep their own small self-retained record card. Clinic registers and report forms should be kept as simple as possible. The HW seeing patients fills in any special register or report form. The nurse can fill in the immunization or family planning register or report form. A record of patients referred is kept.

Decide on a system of payment

How much should we charge our patients? Under the global health priority of UHC, user fees are actively discouraged.[4] In many instances, user fees have dissuaded the poorest people, whose need is the greatest, from seeking treatment. See Chapter 12 for a fuller discussion. However, most patients can make at least some contribution for the services and medicines they receive. This is in the interest of the patient (who often values the treatment more), is helpful for covering the programme's medicine supply costs, and makes the programme more sustainable. However, we must ensure that any user fees are not too high (Figure 13.16) and do not discourage the most needy from attending.

Payment levels need to be fair, acceptable to most of the community and affordable for the poor. Despite setting up an appropriate system, we may still have patients who claim they can't pay. When this happens, we have several options. First, we can check the socio-economic status on the family folder, and give a concession to the genuinely poor. We can also ask for advice from the CHW or health committee member who will probably know the patient's true situation. Finally, we can encourage patients to pay as much as they are able, or to pay in kind, e.g. by bringing grains, fruits, vegetables, or poultry, which can be used or sold by the programme (see also Chapter 12). No one should be turned away because they are genuinely unable to afford the modest fees charged.

Fixed prepayment to the registrar

In the fixed prepayment system, a set amount is paid to the registrar at the time of registration. Patients must understand this is to pay for services, whether or not any medicine is prescribed. Children pay less than adults, or ideally nothing. Other categories of patients can receive free care, e.g. women having antenatal checks, family planning, TB patients, and people living with HIV/AIDS.

One variation on this is sometimes useful. Patients coming to a clinic from villages who have their own CHW pay a lower, 'A' rate, if they bring a referral slip. If they have no referral slip, they pay a 'B' rate. Patients from villages who haven't sent people for CHW training also pay a 'B' rate. This encourages 'B' villages to send someone for training or, if the village is too distant, to request CHW training for their area.

When using a pre-payment system, there should be four columns in the registration book: rate, amount paid, any amount refunded, and total.

Payment by item of service

This system is commonly used in hospital outpatients and can be adopted for larger clinics. When paying by item of service, the registrar gives each patient a registration or payment slip. As the patient goes from one clinic station to the next, each service, medicine, or test is written on this slip, along with the cost. Before leaving

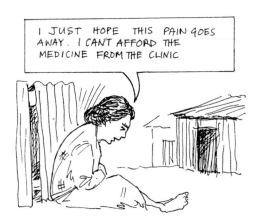
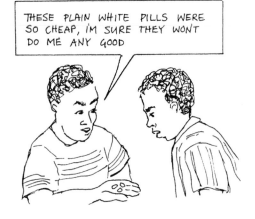

Figure 13.16 A problem of charging too much or too little.

the clinic, the patient hands the slip in to the cashier, dispenser, or registrar, who totals the charges, takes the money from the patient, enters the amount received in the clinic register or computer, and gives a receipt to the patient. In practice, charges per station often tend to work out higher, making it more difficult for the poor. It also takes more time, but may be needed for insurance schemes (Chapter 12).

Set up a referral system

Without a good referral system, CBHC is incomplete and unsafe. In addition, patients can waste a huge amount of money, and HWs a great deal of time. Primary health care is a system of simple but effective services near to people's homes, with referral to the next tier in the health system if the problem cannot be resolved (Figure 13.17).

Unless a good referral system is set up, patients wander from one practitioner to another, accumulating medicine, advice, and reports. They receive partial treatment from many doctors, but often no effective treatment from anyone. In a recent study, caregivers (mainly parents) of severely ill infants in South Africa were interviewed after their children had died. Despite free public health services, urban caregivers attended up to eight different health practitioners, and rural caregivers up to four. Referral systems were chaotic or absent.[5]

Who should we refer?

1. Any seriously ill patient who needs specialist advice or tests to find the cause of the illness.
2. Any patient needing treatment or surgery that cannot be done in the clinic.
3. Anyone demanding a 'second opinion'.
4. Emergencies that cannot be handled at the primary level.
5. Anyone with suspected serious infectious disease. This varies from place to place but TB patients need to be seen by comprehensive services following specific protocols. Those feared to have dangerous illnesses need careful referral, e.g. cases of viral haemorrhagic fever such as Lassa, Marburg, or Ebola. Those with special concerns, e.g. pregnant women in areas with Zika virus, may want referral.

How should patients be referred?

1. Give patients a referral letter.

One copy should be given to the patient, the other kept in a clinic file or the family folder. Alternatively,

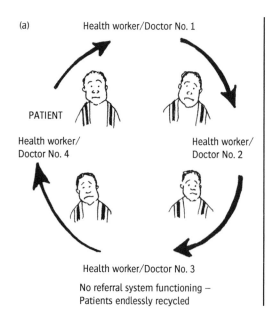
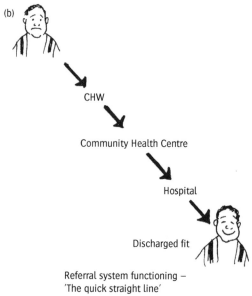

Figure 13.17 Recycling illness or a correct referral system.

a note can be written on the self-retained card. For example, one health programme uses this system if patients can't afford hospital referral and if subsidy may be available, e.g. through an insurance scheme (Chapter 12). They discover how much the patient can afford, agree this with the patient, record it at the foot of the referral letter, ask the patient to sign and a HW to countersign, and undertake to arrange payment of the rest.

2. Give patients a careful explanation.

All HWs must be trained to recognize the patients they cannot treat or diagnose themselves. Unless they refer these patients reliably, the community will lose

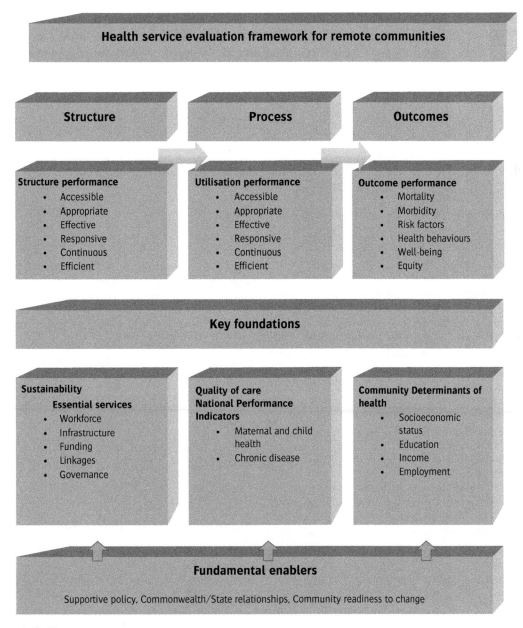

Figure 13.18 Health service evaluation framework for remote communities.

confidence in the clinic and the programme. The HW must take time to address the patient's fears and to answer any questions.

3. When necessary, accompany patients to hospital.

In addition to relatives, many patients need someone to go with them who knows the system, particularly when travelling to larger hospitals or hospitals in cities. This might be a health team member, an experienced CHW, or a member of a health committee who will support them through the frightening world of white coats, queues, and demands for illicit extra payments.

Programmes with their own referral hospitals still need to ensure that the poor are treated with dignity and respect. Seriously ill patients should be transported in a programme vehicle or accompanied on public transport (or light aircraft). For the poor, sick, or timid, going to a crowded hospital is a terrifying experience. They may wonder: Can I afford it? What will they do to me? Will I need an operation? What if I die?

Who should patients be referred to?

Many programmes will have their own linked or preferred hospital to which patients are referred. If this is not the case, the health programme and community together need to decide on the nearest, best quality, and most acceptable centre. Building links with this centre can make a big difference to the quality of care that patients receive. Often it will be the district general hospital or an equivalent, e.g. a mission hospital. In practice, the success of a referral system often depends on making a network of contacts and friendships beyond the programme.

Concentrate on teaching and health promotion

Clinics give great opportunities for health promotion. Sick or worried people are often open to new ideas. Before deciding to teach about health, it will help to read the section in Chapter 4 on behavioural change. Teaching will only be effective if it helps to change behaviour, and in clinic settings, when patients have specific health needs, we have a good entry point for this. In turn, patients can be encouraged to share the new information and changes in behaviour with their families and friends.

When clinics are busy, health teaching is the first activity to get squeezed out, unless everyone makes teaching a priority. When time allows, there are some proven teaching methods that are appropriate to use in clinics (see also Chapter 4).

1. Person-to-person.

This occurs at each station and 'health drills' can increase its effectiveness.

2. Health talks, dialogues, and demonstrations.
3. Learning through overhearing.
4. Patient support groups.

TB patients, people living with HIV/AIDS, or those wanting to stop drinking or abusing drugs can form support groups, with a HW acting as facilitator. Groups of overweight patients with confirmed or 'likely to develop' Type 2 diabetes (see Chapter 22) can also benefit from support groups.

5. HW demonstrations using patients.

A HW can request a patient to give emphasis to a health message.

6. Patients can teach other patients.

Cured TB patients can teach those who have been newly diagnosed. Mothers of once-malnourished children who are now at the recommended weight on the growth chart can share how they successfully fed their children. Those who have been HIV-positive for some time or are recovering through ART can help lead self-help groups.

7. CHWs can teach health songs.

They can also do this in schools or churches or other social groups or community settings (for other examples, see Chapter 4).

8. Use of YouTube, videos, and DVDs.

For example, one project in a mission hospital in Uganda made a video using local people and in the local language, which was shown while patients were waiting. This approach can cause intense interest and convey health messages very effectively.

Preparation for serious illness

There are three obvious reasons why clinics must be prepared for serious illness. The first is the need for a contact point for each community when serious illness or accidents occur. The second is that clinics that deal successfully with emergencies gain credibility and are utilized more by the community. The third is because communities often expect a clinic to provide emergency care.

For example, a survey among two communities in Sri Lanka showed that people expected to receive emergency care from the primary health system, including treatment for their seriously ill children, but used traditional home remedies for more minor ailments.[6] Examples of actions that can save lives before we refer seriously ill patients include first aid in accidents or acute conditions, e.g. Airway, Breathing, Circulation (ABC). Our clinic HWs should be able to:

- Use naso-gastric tubes for severely dehydrated children who are unable to drink.
- Inject benzyl penicillin in children with suspected meningitis.
- Use rectal diazepam in children with convulsions.
- Use rectal artesunate in children with suspected malaria.
- Start antibiotics in children with severe acute respiratory infection, providing they are able to swallow.
- Use misoprostol in women with post-partum haemorrhage.

To deal effectively with emergencies and serious illness, three things are needed at community level:

1. Recognize emergencies in the home.

Examples are early signs of serious illness in children and signs of life-threatening complications before or after delivery. For example, in a Mexican project the training of mothers and CHWs in recognizing postnatal haemorrhage and breathing difficulties in children under one year of age almost halved death rates.

2. Ensure emergency transport is available.

For example, in one remote Himalayan valley community members with access to a vehicle arranged to make it available to anyone in the valley requiring emergency transport to hospital. The journey would take a whole day by bus, but only two hours by jeep.

3. Emergency medical care must be available at the first contact health centre.

With simple equipment and basic training many conditions can be treated or first aid can be provided until referral is arranged. Simple systems should be in place for immediate response when seriously ill patients are brought to the health centre. One way to reduce death rates in children is to use the IMCI approach to severe childhood illness (Chapter 16). Finally, we need to have a plan outlined in case there is an outbreak of a serious infectious disease locally that puts health care staff at risk.

Understand the role of mobile clinics

Mobile clinics have been used for many years and are an important part of health care in remote or poor communities. Eye camps, family planning camps, and surgical camps where mobile teams spend longer periods in one location are variations on this idea. We should actively consider whether this approach might be useful in our area.

Some smaller clinics are almost mobile clinics. Often there is a simple building or room that a visiting team uses weekly or monthly. The team brings most of its supplies, although some equipment can be stored there. Mobile clinics are usually fully equipped vehicles (or occasionally a small aircraft or boat) with an appropriately trained team. They visit a circuit of remote villages on a regular basis at pre-arranged times and locations. *The advantages of mobile clinics* are that remote patients can be examined, treated, and, if seriously ill, brought back to a hospital. They enable communities to receive basic health care, that would otherwise have nothing. There are usually no costs for buildings. *The disadvantage of mobile clinics* is that they tend to deliver health care services rather than involve communities. They concentrate on curative care and may make little impact on underlying health problems. But there are ways of using the advantages, and avoiding the disadvantages.

Only visit communities with a mobile clinic if this is part of a CBHC programme. Get to know the community, carry out a Participatory Appraisal (Chapter 6), encourage them to identify needs and solutions, consider setting up a CHW training programme. We can use the mobile clinic for health promotion, training, involving community members and routine vaccinations, not just curative care. For example, all communities within one hour of the mobile clinic locations come for vaccines, and communities beyond that are visited regularly by vaccinators on bicycles with vaccine cool boxes. Deworming and other mass programmes can also be carried out.

Before visits are made by the mobile team the community can be informed, e.g. by text messages, to make sure the visit is as effective as possible. With this in mind, the mobile clinic visit could also be combined with village meetings, CHW training, or a community survey. This depth of visit would usually mean staying two or three days. In order to make the visit as successful as possible, health committees can be taught how to organize the site, remind people when the mobile clinic is coming, and do registration and crowd control. Also, traditional birth attendants and other traditional health practitioners can attend and learn. Finally, empower the community to build its own simple health post where CBHC activities can be carried out on a regular basis under community leadership. The mobile clinic would continue to visit but the emphasis would be on support and training in a locally run health post. Any patients too sick for CHWs to manage would be seen when the mobile team visited.

Mobile clinics can also be used in urban areas. For example, the ASHA project working in the slums of Delhi recently bought a vehicle and enabled the programme to provide mobile services in several slum colonies. The vehicle does not just bring curative care. Visits are a chance to mobilize the community, build relationships, give health teaching, move towards setting up CHW training and form community action groups (www.asha-india.org).

Monitoring and evaluating the clinic

We need to have some way of measuring the effectiveness, success and acceptability of our clinic. Larger programmes can use some of these ideas and create their own ways of measuring them. Figure 13.18 can be used as a guide for larger or more established programmes.

For smaller programmes, here are some suggested indicators:

- Numbers of patients attending the clinic each working day, week, month, year
- Number/type of illnesses being treated
- Number of patients seen daily, or weekly in the community by the CHW
- Proportion of the community who are able to access care in the clinic. This can be done by a questionnaire which can also ask about barriers to access e.g. finance, distance.
- Community opinions of the quality of care, friendliness of staff, and overall satisfaction. Can be measured by 1 to 5, 5 being the highest.
- Number of clinic days a year when essential medicines weren't available including name of medicine and reason.

There are many other topics which can be measured and each programme needs to decide which are the most important in terms of its objectives and the expectations of the community.

Further reading and resources

AMREF. Africa's leading health development organization, saving and transforming lives in the poorest and most marginalized communities. Their website has a variety of research papers and a video gallery related to Africa. Available from: http://www.amref.org.

Austin M, Crawford R, Klaassen B, editors. *First Aid Manual.* Revised 10th ed. 2016, London: Dorling Kindersley; 2016.

Burns A, Neimann S. *Where women have no doctor: A health guide for women.* Berkeley, CA: Hesperian; 1997.

Cheesbrough M. *District laboratory practice in tropical countries: Part 1.* 2nd ed. Fakenham: Tropical Health Technology; 2009. Available from: http://www.tht.ndirect.co.uk

Cheesbrough M. *District laboratory practice in tropical countries: Part 2.* 2nd ed. Fakenham: Tropical Health Technology; 2010. Available from: http://www.tht.ndirect.co.uk

Cheesbrough M. *Tropical medicine microscopy.* Fakenham: Tropical Health Technology; 2014. Available from: Tropical Health Technology, http://www.tht.ndirect.co.uk

Fountain DE, Vergera Art R. *Primary diagnosis and treatment: A manual for clinical and health centre staff in developing countries.* 2nd ed. London: Macmillan; 2008.

Grouzard V, Rigal J, Sutton M, editors. *Clinical guidelines: Diagnosis and treatment manual.* Geneva: Médecins sans frontiers; 2016. Available from: http://www.refbooks.msf.org/msf_docs/en/clinical_guide/cg_en.pdf

Kaur M, Hall S, with Attawell K, editor. *Medical Supplies and Equipment for Primary Health Care.* Coulsdon: ECHO; 2001.

Schull C. *Common medical problems in the tropics.* 3rd ed. Oxford: Macmillan; 2010.

Werner D, Thuman C, Maxwell J. *Where there is no doctor.* Revised edition. Berkeley, CA: Hesperian; 2011. Available from: https://warriorpublications.files.wordpress.com/2015/03/where-there-is-no-doctor-2011.pdf

References

1. Scheil-Adlung X, editor. *Global evidence on inequities in rural health protection: New data on rural deficits in health coverage for 174 countries.* ESS Document No. 47. International Labour Office, Social Protection Department. Geneva: ILO; 2015. Available from: http://www.social-protection.org/gimi/gess/RessourcePDF.action;jsessionid=wJJfYtqhFSsh6y2nwLdqQpgm5gy7hjK9QGZ4vBZ3z7hHKNWd6Tnx!-1211598784?ressource.ressourceId=51297

2. Stott N, Davis R. The exceptional potential in each primary care consultation. *Journal of the Royal College of General Practitioners.* 1979; 29 (201): 201–5.

3. SkillsCascade.com. *Models of the consultation: A summary, 2000–2003.* Available from: http://www.skillscascade.com/models.htm

4. Lagarde M, Palmer N. The impact of user fees on access to health services in low- and middle-income countries (Review). *Cochrane Database of Systematic Reviews.* 2011; 4. DOI: 10.1002/14651858.CD009094

5. Sharkey A, Chopra M, Jackson D, Winch PJ, Minkovitz CS. Pathways of care-seeking during fatal infant illnesses in under-resourced South African settings. *Transactions of the Royal Society of Tropical Medicine and Hygiene.* 2012; 106 (2): 110–16.

6. Wolffers I. Illness behaviour in Sri Lanka: Results of a survey in two Sinhalese communities. *Social Science and Medicine.* 1998; 27 (5): 545–52.

CHAPTER 14

Preventing and treating childhood malnutrition

Ted Lankester

What we need to know

Why adequate nutrition is important

In 2016, UNICEF issued a statement that 'nearly half of all deaths in children under 5 are attributable to undernutrition. This translates into the unnecessary loss of about 3 million young lives a year'.[1] Malnutrition weakens children's immunity, making it much more likely they will die from diseases in childhood. The three infections that cause most deaths are pneumonia, diarrhoea, and malaria (Chapter 16). Measles is still common in many parts of the world and is much more dangerous in malnourished children. Malnourished children are more likely to catch infections, more likely to become severely ill, and take longer to recover Figure 14.1).

A well-fed child will get ill sometimes—but usually recovers on its own.

A malnourished child will get ill frequently—but recover more slowly and is more likely to die

Childhood malnutrition diminishes adult quality of life

Poor nutrition in the womb and during early childhood, especially the first 1000 days of a child's life, leads to stunting. This has serious long-term consequences. Children who are stunted grow up to be shorter and weaker than those who are well fed in childhood. The World Bank estimates that nearly a quarter (159 million) of the world's children under five are stunted,[2] over a third of whom are in India.[3] WHO's Global Nutrition Report gives more details.[4]

Stunted children tend to do less well in school. They are likely to become less productive farmers and earn lower wages.

Malnourished children often have impaired mental development. This means they do not reach their full intellectual potential as adults, are less likely to get good jobs and so are less able to provide for their children.[5]

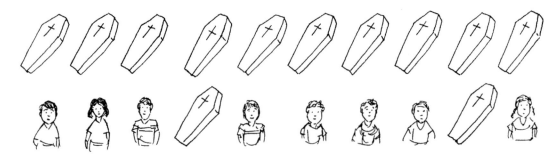

Figure 14.1 In low-income countries, five out of ten children can have their lives saved by good nutrition, and a further three by actions at community level.

Thus, reducing malnutrition in this generation of children will contribute directly to greater health and wellbeing in the next. Of course malnutrition can affect people of all ages. Chapter 28 has some details on this.

Different forms of malnutrition

Severe acute malnutrition (SAM)

This form of malnutrition is commonly associated with severe food insecurity during famine, civil conflict, failure of rain or crops, or other natural or man-made catastrophes. However, it can also occur in more stable circumstances, especially in cases of HIV[6] and disability.[7] Children with mild or moderate malnutrition may also become severely malnourished for various reasons,

including infections, intestinal parasites, and poor absorption of food from other causes.

SAM is defined as infants and children who are 6–59 months of age and have a mid-upper arm circumference (MUAC) less than 115 mm, and/or a weight-for-height/length less than -3 Z-scores of the WHO Child Growth Standards median, and/or have bilateral pitting oedema.

For an explanation of Z scores see the section 'Measure malnutrition'. SAM is a life-threatening condition. Without effective treatment, case-fatality rates in hospitalized children range from 30% to 50%.[8]

Severe wasting or marasmus means extreme thinness, which is most visible over the shoulders, ribs, upper arms, buttocks, and thighs. The skin on the buttocks may look like 'baggy pants' (Figure 14.2).

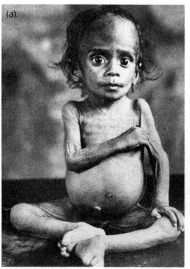 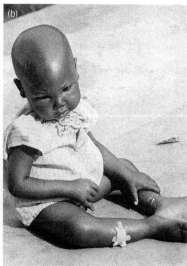 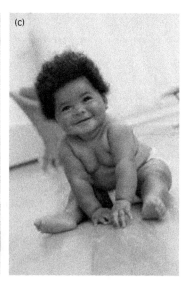

Figure 14.2 (a) Marasmus and (b) kwashiorkor (oedematous malnutrition) and (c) child obesity are three forms of dangerous malnutrition

Malnutrition with oedema, or Kwashiorkor, usually occurs first in the lower legs and feet. To test for oedema, grasp each foot with thumb on top and press gently for ten seconds. The child has oedema if a dent remains after removing the thumb.

(a) Marasmus and (b) kwashiorkor (oedematous malnutrition) are two forms of SAM and can overlap and be present in the same child.

It is not fully understood why some children tend to develop one form of malnutrition rather than the other.

SAM in practice nearly always results from a combined lack of energy foods, protein, and micronutrients, especially Vitamin A and zinc.

Moderate malnutrition

Moderate malnutrition is far more widespread and less easy to recognize than severe malnutrition. It is defined as an MUAC ≥ 115mm to < 125mm and/or weight-for-age between -3 and -2 Z-scores below the median of the WHO child growth standards.

It can take the form of wasting (low weight for height—indicating acute malnutrition) or stunting (low height for age—indicating chronic or recurring malnutrition), or a combination of both.

Faltering growth is an early sign of malnutrition, and unless urgent action is taken, the child may become severely malnourished very quickly. This underlines the importance of regular weighing (or MUAC in children over 6 months) so malnutrition can be picked up early. Most cases of mild or moderate malnutrition are not obvious to the mother or even to the health worker. This 'hidden' group of malnourished children has higher than average health risks.

Childhood obesity

The World Health Organization (WHO) declared that:

Childhood obesity is one of the most serious public health challenges of the 21st century. The problem is global and is steadily affecting many low- and middle-income countries, particularly in urban settings. The prevalence has increased at an alarming rate. Globally, in 2015 the number of overweight children under the age of five, is estimated to be over 42 million. Almost half of all overweight children under 5 lived in Asia and one quarter lived in Africa.[9]

Obesity usually continues into adulthood and greatly increases the risk of Type 2 diabetes, hypertension, heart attacks, and stroke (Chapter 22) and also (See Figure 14.2).

Anaemia or iron deficiency

This is nearly always present in undernourished children, and often also in apparently well-nourished children. Anaemia is defined as less than 11 g/dl, unless severe anaemia as below 8 g/dl.

There are few obvious signs of anaemia. Pallor is not an accurate way to identify it. However, anaemic children will often be tired, catch infections easily, and perform poorly at school. Anaemia is usually caused by insufficient iron in the diet, but especially in Africa, malaria, schistosomiasis (bilharzia), hookworm (also In South Asia), and whipworm can make it worse. Infections can reduce iron absorption. Iron-rich foods include meat, eggs, lentils, and green leafy vegetables.

Vitamin A deficiency or blinding malnutrition

An estimated 250 million preschool children worldwide are vitamin A deficient. Pregnant women are also affected, especially in the last trimester of pregnancy. It is the commonest cause of blindness in children. An estimated 250,000 to 500,000 vitamin A-deficient children become blind every year, half of them dying within twelve months of losing their sight.[10]

Vitamin A deficiency, even if not low enough to cause eye problems, lowers immunity, and increases the danger from diarrhoea, respiratory infections, measles, and probably malaria, meaning that Vitamin A supplementation reduces mortality rates. Many infections such as measles further reduce Vitamin A levels. Eating green vegetables and yellow fruit helps but oils are also needed in the diet to help absorption.

Zinc deficiency

Zinc deficiency is often associated with Vitamin A deficiency and lowers resistance to diarrhoeal diseases and acute respiratory infections. In addition to its effect on the immune system zinc deficiency harms the intestinal tract leading to greater volumes of stool and to malabsorption. This is why zinc is now included in ORS (Figure 14.3).

Iodine deficiency

Iodine deficiency is still the commonest cause of mental impairment worldwide, and continues to affect people in 54 countries.[11] People in mountainous areas are especially likely to develop symptoms. Low-lying flood-prone areas, such as Bangladesh, are also affected, as iodine is washed out of the soil. The use of iodized salt is gradually reducing the number of people affected, though some areas still have a significant problem.

For example, in Nepal, where salt is still transported by yak to very remote areas, about one quarter of Nepali school children have actual or borderline iodine deficiency despite the widespread use of iodized salt.[12] One reason is that salt is not properly iodized by the companies despite legislation. There are simple testing kits that can be used at community level, and indeed some child health programmes have tested salt in the markets for their iodine level.

Goitre (a swollen thyroid gland) is the most obvious sign of iodine deficiency and is most commonly seen in women. The most dangerous effect, sometimes known as cretinism, is found in children born to iodine-deficient

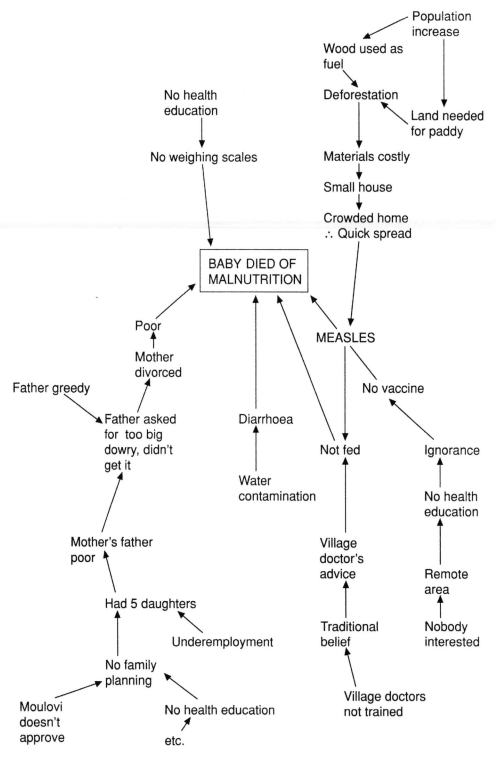

Figure 14.3 Some causes of malnutrition from a community workshop in Bangladesh.

mothers. These children will typically be deaf, dumb, slow, have a 'puffy' appearance, and a tendency to constipation. Importantly, iodine-deficient babies may show very few signs, yet grow up suffering cognitive impairment.

Other deficiency diseases

These include:

- Lack of vitamin B leading to pellagra and beriberi.
- Lack of vitamin C leading to scurvy, commonly found in refugee camps and among displaced people.
- Lack of vitamin D or calcium leading to rickets—found mainly in women and girls where custom forbids exposing their skin to sunlight. This can lead to a malformed pelvis and extra dangers in giving birth.

Mild degrees of insufficient vitamin D levels are very widespread, even in resource-rich countries and may increase the likelihood of fractures and hip pain, especially in the elderly.

The root causes of malnutrition

It is helpful to understand the wider causes, or 'social determinants' of malnutrition because sometimes we can address these 'upstream' causes. Look at the causes below to see if they are locally important and if there are solutions within reach (See Figure 14.3).

1. Famine, war, and disasters lead to food insecurity where food supply is unreliable or unaffordable.
2. Poverty and illness—where people are unable to grow or buy sufficient food; lack adequate water supplies and sanitation; live in overcrowded conditions; and are unable to afford health care.
3. Lack of relevant knowledge—where food is available but diet and feeding practices are inadequate.

The starting point in understanding the levels and causes of malnutrition will usually be information found in our Participatory Appraisal or community survey. If our programme focuses on malnutrition because of current food insecurity, we will need to do this by gathering information in greater detail from the community or from other information sources for our region.

We will now look at some causes of malnutrition in different groupings.

Causes of malnutrition in the child

- Low birth weight.
- Exposure to parasitic infections, e.g. hookworm, roundworm, whipworm, *Giardia*.
- Measles and failure to vaccinate against it.

- Bottle feeding with infant formula, which is less nutritious, may be over-diluted and often causes diarrhoea.
- Inadequate complementary feeding after six months.
- Feeding practices such as giving watery gruels, giving too few meals, no encouragement or assistance at meal times.
- Frequent drinking of dirty water with damage to the intestine, leading to poor absorption (enteropathy) and stunting, even without diarrhoea.
- Exposure to frequent infections such as diarrhoea, coughs and malaria leading to poor appetite, loss of weight and decreased resistance to further infection (see Figure 14.4).
- AIDS contracted from the mother, or other infections, including TB, heart disease, kidney disease.
- Disability, which is a growing issue as neonatal care improves and survival increases and as more children survive diseases such as meningitis and cerebral malaria.
- Being a 'fussy eater' can add to the above problems.

Causes of malnutrition in the mother

- Mother herself tired, ill, depressed, or malnourished.
- Mother unable to establish adequate breastfeeding routine.
- Overwork in home, the daily need to collect fuel and water, and demands of other children.
- Work outside the home to supplement family income.
- Mother illiterate and uneducated, so follows incorrect practices, such as withholding food from an ill child and fluids in diarrhoea.
- Mother divorced, separated, widowed, or otherwise unsupported.
- Mother married as minor rather than adult.
- Adolescent pregnancy contributing to low birth-weight children and subsequent malnutrition.

Causes of malnutrition in the family

- Shortage of food due to poverty.
- Husband or partner chronically unwell, uncaring, absent, drunk, addicted, unemployed, overworked, violent.
- Too many children to feed and care for, no access to or use of family planning, no child spacing, multiple pregnancies
- Disagreement between family members on how to feed the child.

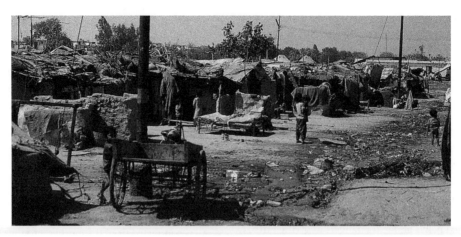

Figure 14.4 The circle of infection and malnutrition in an urban slum.

- Tensions with mother-in-law and other family members.
- Cash crops replacing food crops, meaning less food for children. Extra money spent on cigarettes, tonics and soft drinks rather than better food.
- Daughters not wanted.
- One or both parents living with untreated HIV/AIDS.

Causes of malnutrition in the community

- Insufficient land or employment.
- Poor farming practices, soil erosion and deforestation, no irrigation, unproductive land, no land at all.
- Remote area with poor transport and little access to markets.
- Poor water supply and sanitation leading to diarrhoeal illnesses.
- Inappropriate advice from some traditional practitioners recommending 'holy food' or 'holy water', which may be contaminated
- Debt, bonded labour; threats from landlords and moneylenders.
- Money overspent on weddings, religious ceremonies, and dowries.
- Tribal, class, and religious conflicts.

Causes of malnutrition in the country

- War, civil unrest, famine, seasonal floods or hurricanes, drought.

- Effects of climate change giving unpredictable weather.
- Depressed economy, national debt, lack of foreign exchange.
- Education and health not government priorities.
- Previous food aid leading now to attitude of dependence. Depressed prices for locally grown food and commodities and so no incentive to grow. Seed grain used up.
- Corrupt, inefficient, or extreme political system causing the poor to suffer the most.
- Unjust trading laws that favour wealthy countries.
- Structural adjustment programmes.
- High levels of HIV/AIDS or lack of access to antiretroviral therapy (ART), leading to premature death and illness, in turn affecting the local and national economy.

The common ages for malnutrition

The key period for malnutrition is the first 1,000 days of a child's life, from conception to two years. This includes in-utero malnutrition, classically seen in war zones and sieges, but also with any significant reduction in maternal intake.[13] More specific at-risk periods partly depend on local customs, the season of the year, and the types of food available in the community. The greatest risks usually occur at specific times.

1. In the first month of life in poorer communities, the child will often have a low birth weight.

More than two-fifths of all deaths in children under five occur in the first month.[14] Low birth weight often contributes to this. It has been shown that intermittent preventative treatment of malaria in pregnancy where malaria is common can improve the birth weight of neonates.[15]

2. Between the ages of six and 24 months.

In many communities, complementary feeding occurs either too early, too late, or is insufficient, which can have a major impact on nutrition. Ideally, children should be fed on breast milk alone for the first six months, except in special situations such as when the mother is HIV positive (see Chapter 20). Breastfeeding should then be continued until at least two years of age. Furthermore, breastfeeding is often stopped early, which may happen either gradually, or suddenly if the mother becomes pregnant, develops an illness, or has to start working or travelling to work—a common situation in urban areas.

- Inadequate amounts of food may be given, and contribute to the problem, and foods may be contaminated with germs, leading to diarrhoea.

- Infants may get infections by placing objects in their mouths and through dirty feeding bottles, or from infant formula that may itself be made with untreated water.

- Toxins in food can also contribute to malnutrition.

For example, in parts of West Africa aflatoxins from stored peanuts infected with a fungus can affect health and nutrition. However, this is probably overstated and peanuts remain an excellent source of food, providing they are well prepared and well stored, as is necessary with all foods.

3. Whenever a new child is born.

After the birth of a new baby, the mother will then give her time, attention, and breast milk to the newborn. The result is that the next-to-youngest child receives less of each. This effect is most important when the birth interval is less than three years.

4. Any time of family crisis.

What we need to do

Measuring malnutrition

There are a variety of useful ways to measure malnutrition, and the most important ones are listed here.

1. In community health programmes, the weight for age chart (growth chart) is most commonly used. The WHO has recently revised its growth charts, which set an overall universal standard of how infants and children should grow, using a choice of percentiles or Z-scores. Z-scores (also known as standard deviation scores) are a measure of the distance between the child's value and the expected value of the reference population. Many national health ministries have used WHO data to develop their own country-specific growth charts.

2. In situations where SAM frequently occurs, it is also important to measure Mid Upper Arm Circumference (MUAC)—this can be done by community health workers (CHWs) and even by mothers and carers themselves.

3. Finally, in adults and older children, the weight to height ratio (weight divided by square of the height) is used to calculate the Body Mass Index (BMI) which is currently defined as between 18.5 and 24.9. This is the commonly used measure in adolescents and adults and increasingly in younger age groups also.

A warning: Measuring malnutrition does not improve matters by itself. Some programmes spend a lot of time measuring without doing health teaching or involving parents and carers. But if time is limited and problems are severe, we should concentrate on educating and training mothers about nutrition, rather than on measuring the problem. There are two methods of measuring malnutrition: weighing scales and MUAC (Figure 14.5).

Weighing scales

The advantages of scales, if used carefully, is that weighing shows us accurately the degree of individual and community-wide malnutrition. Disadvantages include that scales are expensive, may be difficult to obtain, and many brands are heavy to carry and break easily if dropped. Unless everyone is trained how to use them, mistakes can easily be made, especially in completing the growth chart.

How often should weighing be done?

Usually once per month in healthy children under three years of age. It should usually be done weekly in community-based management of acute malnutrition (CMAM) programmes.

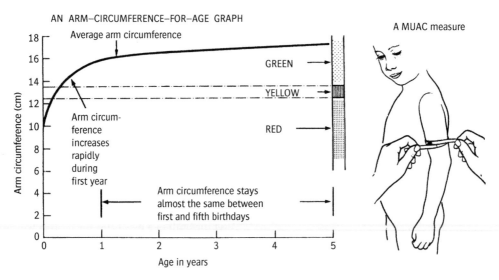

Figure 14.5 Measuring mid-upper-arm circumference (MUAC).

Since this classic image was first drawn newer evidence suggests that MUAC measurements can be started from 6 months (see note in text).

Where should it be done?

Weighing should be done in health centres, clinics, or feeding centres. It can also be done by mothers in small community-based groups (see Figure 14.6), or in homes, but if time is limited, home visits should concentrate on education rather than weighing.

Who should do the weighing?

At first, probably a nurse, other health worker, or CHW will teach the procedure. Then, weighing can be done by the mother, father, or older sibling. Also, members of women's clubs or health committees can weigh children either from house to house or as a community

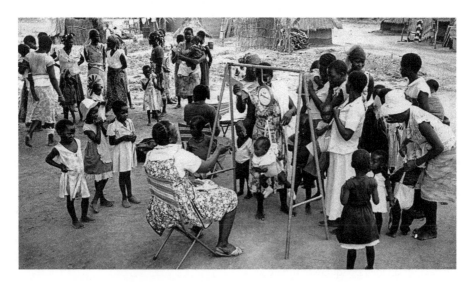

Figure 14.6 Community weighing session in Zimbabwe.

activity, giving feeding advice at the same time. All those involved in weighing will need careful teaching and supervision until they can do it quickly and accurately, leaving time for identifying problems and explaining better ways of feeding.

Safeguarding is an important concern in any community activity which involves children or vulnerable adults.

How to weigh very young children

1. The child sits on the parent's or guardian's lap and a pair of specially designed strapped trousers (pants) which fit reasonably well are fitted onto the child.
2. The parent lifts the child by the body, not by the straps, and hangs the child on the weighing scales.
3. The child hangs just long enough for an accurate weight to be measured, and is then lifted down.
4. The weight is plotted on the growth chart.
5. The card is explained to the parent. Feeding advice is given where necessary.

Arm measurers

Measuring the mid-upper arm circumference (MUAC) is increasingly taking over from the use of weighing scales. This is for two main reasons. It is accurate and reliable. It is also quicker, easier to use, and cheaper than weighing scales. See Figure 14.5 with the comment below it.

In children, the MUAC hardly changes between the ages of 6 months and 60 months (previously thought to be between 12 months and 60 months) WHO standards for MUAC show that in a well-nourished population there are very few children aged 6–60 months with an MUAC less than 115 mm. Children with an MUAC less than 115 mm have a highly elevated risk of death compared to those who are above that level. Thus, it is recommended to increase the cut-off point from the previous 110, to 115 mm to diagnose SAM using the MUAC.[16]

Revised measurements are therefore as follows:

- Well-nourished child: MUAC from 125mm
- Acutely malnourished child:
    moderate: MUAC 115-125mm
    severe: MUAC 115 mm or less.

UNICEF has now incorporated these into colour-coded tapes: severe, red: moderate, yellow, well-nourished, green.

Locally appropriate colours can be used instead.

Tapes can either be bought, e.g. from UNICEF, or made, e.g. from strips of X-ray film.

Using the MUAC

When using the MUAC, the child should be sitting or standing with the arm hanging unsupported from the shoulder. Wrap the tape firmly but not too tightly around the left mid-upper arm, i.e. half way between the tip of the shoulder and the tip of the elbow. The CHW, mother, or older siblings can make this measurement, but will need supervised practice, and training to interpret measurements and act.

Advantages and disadvantages of MUAC measuring

The MUAC strip is cheap and easy to carry, and it is quicker and easier than scales, allowing more time for health education. It is ideal to use in homes, scattered communities, and refugee camps. It can be used by those who are unable to read, write, or understand numbers.

Disadvantages include that it does not measure stunting, and mistakes can be made if the person measuring is in a hurry or if the child is fretful (NB: this is also true for weighing).

Further use of the MUAC

MUAC measurements can also be used at birth to give an indication of whether the newborn has a low birth weight.

An MUAC of 8.7 cm at the time of birth is approximately equivalent to a birth weight of 2500 grams, although this level has not yet been finally agreed. If a tape is marked at 8.7 cm, any measurement below this gives a probable indication of low birth weight (Figure 14.7).

Measuring the MUAC enables illiterate CHWs (or traditional birth attendants) to discover low weight children at the time of birth and target care towards them. There is even discussion about using a variant of this in schoolage children instead of BMI but no conclusions yet.

Recording malnutrition on growth charts

Having weighed a child or measured MUAC, we need to record it on the child's record, retained by the family. For recording weight, we should ideally use the Growth Chart used in the country or region where we are working, and we should teach all team members and CHWs (where literate) how to use them. Many growth charts are completed incorrectly. Health workers should not start training others until they no longer make mistakes themselves.

When using a growth chart (see Figure 14.8):

- Fill in the month and year of birth.
- Fill in the month and year or highlight this each time the child is weighed.

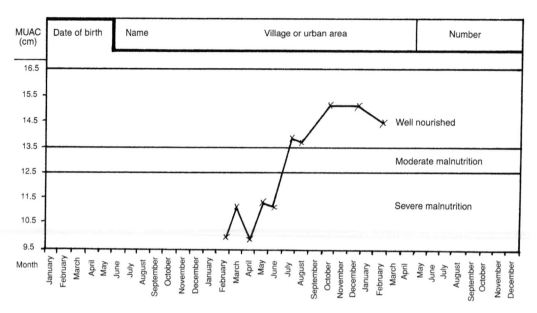

Figure 14.7 Mid-upper arm circumference (MUAC) measuring card.

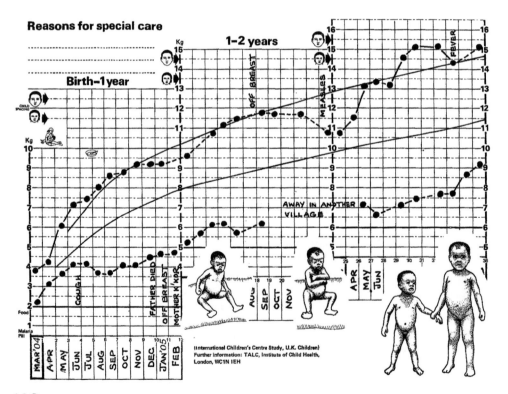

Figure 14.8 Growth chart for two children born in the same month in the same village. From an example of one of the original growth charts developed in Nigeria by the late Professor David Morley.

- Put a dot (and a ring), or a (x) for the measurement, checking and rechecking that it is in the right place, and linking it up with previous measurements using a pencil.

Learn to interpret the findings, and explain these to the parents, family members and other carers.

The direction of the growth curve is the most crucial.

- If it is rising—good. Reinforce teaching.
- If it is flat—this is a warning. Find the cause, act, and give suitable teaching to the parents. If the line is flat for two months or more, this is known as growth faltering. Recognizing this and acting is one main reason why we monitor weights.
- If it is falling—there is a serious problem. We must discover and treat the problem as soon as possible.

The actual weight itself is also important. However, if a child is stunted, in other words periods of malnutrition in the past have reduced child's growth in height, then this will be shown by persistently lower actual weights on the chart. The most common causes of poor weight gain are that child is not getting enough food or that the child has an infection.

Remember the purpose of the chart: it is an early warning system. The growth chart tells us if things are going wrong before we (or the mother) would otherwise notice them. This means we can find and treat the cause at an early stage, which reduces the danger of related health problems in the future. It also helps us to evaluate whether parents have understood and successfully followed the nutrition guidance we have given.

Ensure the mother keeps the card. She should bring it whenever she visits the CHW, the clinic or the hospital. Other points to note:

1. The card can help us to correct any common mistakes: for example, mother forgets the date of birth—often has forgotten the month, sometimes the year, of the birth, or she may never have known it.

We can help by purchasing or making a local events calendar. This has festivals, seasons, etc., marked on it, which serve as a reminder. Using this, we can take time to work out the date with the mother. Always consider if the child appears and behaves the age the mother says.

2. The health worker may also get confused, and need plenty of supervised practice. A ruler or straight edge helps in plotting the correct weight.
3. The mother may not understand the chart.

It can seem complicated and she may think that it belongs to the health worker. Include the mother and, where possible, other family members or carers at every stage in weighing and recording, taking time to explain how the card works and how it shows the progress of the baby. She will soon start taking a pride not only in the card, but also in the weight gain of the child.

Most mothers, even those who are illiterate, will be able to understand a growth chart. At the very least, they will see whether the line is rising, flat, or falling. Many mothers or other family members will be able to weigh children themselves. However, if a mother is slow to understand the chart, spend time in health education instead.

4. The mother may forget the card or spoil it. Try to provide a protective envelope for any self-retained card.
5. The health worker must never show anger or be irritable when weighing as a mother may get discouraged and stop coming to the clinic. Teach the team to be patient and to make sure that weighing is enjoyable, and always praise the mother for something done well.

Understand parents' response to advice

A mother, father or older family member will only improve feeding practices if they follow this 'chain of action'.

- Understanding that the child is malnourished. How? *By our patient explanation*, ideally with a growth chart, and, where possible, also to other family members.
- Being able to do something about it. How? *Foods we recommend must be locally available and affordable*. The family must give time to feeding and be prepared to alter some of their practices. Older siblings may be able to help.
- Having knowledge and skills to prepare and store food correctly, feed it appropriately and give it in sufficient amount. How? *Our teaching must be based on insight into community lifestyle, foods available and how families function*. Home visits fine-tune our advice and are a chance to answer questions.

We must always ensure we listen to the mother or family caregiver and respond to any concerns. We need to discuss action plans with her and make sure she understands, agrees and is able to carry them out.

Prevent and cure malnutrition

There is a well-known health programme in north India where many children attend local clinics and parents

Table 14.1 **Children from ages 1 to 5 with MUAC of 12.cm or less**

Village name	April 1985		January 1988	
Parogi	4/16	25%	0/17	0%
Bell	7/21	33%	0/17	0%
U. Sarab	1/17	6%	0/17	0%
L. Sarab	13/30	43%	0/30	0%
U. Kandi	10/19	53%	2/19	11%
L. Kandi	6/24	5%	0/24	0%
Total	41/127	32%	2/128	2%

hear health talks. Yet studies here have shown that children who attend these clinics continue to have levels of malnutrition little different from those who do not attend. The health teaching does not lead to behavioural change (see Chapter 4). In contrast, in a small Himalayan health programme (SHARE) 32 per cent of children aged one to five were found to be severely or moderately malnourished when the programme started (Table 14.1). After CHWs were trained to give nutritional advice by visiting house to house, using foods grown by each family, only two severely malnourished children remained two years later. From these examples we learn that giving health talks in clinics is unlikely to be effective in itself. Where food supplies are adequate, one key method of curing and preventing malnutrition is to train CHWs to make regular visits to each home. In that environment they are able give practical advice according to the exact needs of the family, and ensure that any advice is put into practice. This is explained in some detail in Figures 14.9 and 14.10.

The six rules of good nutrition

1. Ensure pregnant mothers have adequate nutrition.
2. Promote exclusive breastfeeding for six months and regular breastfeeding till at least the age of two.
3. Introduce mixed feeding at six months.
4. Continue to feed children when they are ill.
5. Prepare, cook and store food correctly: the '10 golden rules'.
6. Avoid harmful and inappropriate foods.

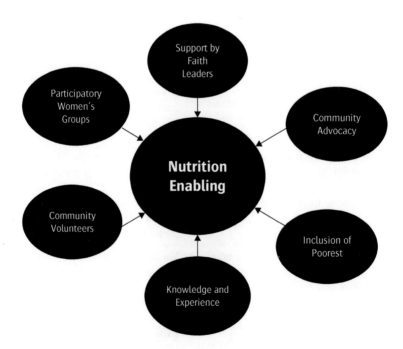

Figure 14.9 Nutrition enabling and nutrition resourcing.

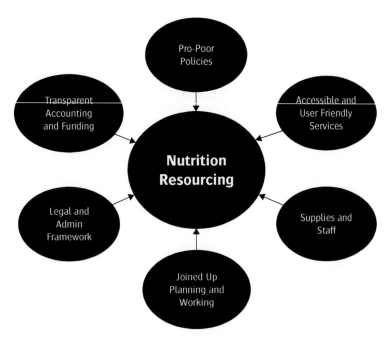

Figure 14.10 Nutrition enabling and nutrition resourcing.

Rule 1. Ensure pregnant mothers have adequate nutrition

The baby's weight at birth and during the first few weeks of life depends mainly on the health and nutritional state of the mother.

In order to achieve adequate nutrition for the child at the time of birth:

1. Encourage adequate weight gain in pregnancy.

Mothers should ideally gain about five to eight kilograms during pregnancy. This depends on:

- Eating sufficient, well-balanced food, with plenty of fluids throughout pregnancy.
- Taking enough rest and helping other family members to recognize and support this.

2. Prevent and treat anaemia.

Prevention of anaemia should start pre-conception: adolescent girls after starting menstruation, and all women of child-bearing age should eat iron-rich foods, such as green leafy vegetables, eggs, and meat where locally available and acceptable.

- Daily iron-folate tablets should be given in pregnancy. For example, it has been shown in Nepal

that the children of mothers who take iron, folic acid and vitamin A supplements in pregnancy perform better than children whose mothers did not take these supplements[17] (but see note below regarding vitamin A).[18]

- Prevent and treat malaria (see Chapter 17), hookworm, and schistosomiasis (bilharzia), ideally before becoming pregnant.

3. Prevent and treat vitamin A deficiency in mothers and infants.

- The mother should eat foods rich in vitamin A—green leafy vegetables; orange, red, or yellow fruits or vegetables; fish; red palm oil in small quantities.
- Mothers are only recommended to take vitamin A supplements if the prevalence of night blindness is higher than 5 per cent or more. It should then be given for the 12 weeks before delivery either as a capsule of 10,000 units per day or 25,000 IU per week. Mothers are not otherwise recommended to take vitamin A supplements.[18]

4. Prevent and treat iodine deficiency.

WHO and UNICEF recommend iodine supplements for pregnant and lactating women in countries where less than 20 per cent of households have access to iodized salt.[19] As mentioned, this salt needs to be reliably iodized in areas where there is iodine deficiency. Communities can be taught how to test this and take action through advocacy if legalized levels are not reached.

Children under six months should receive their iodine through breastmilk but will need extra iodine supplements between six and 24 months. We should follow specific national guidelines as to how this is best done at community level. Where goitre is commonly observed and in many mountainous areas, iodine supplements are especially important unless mothers are regularly using iodized salt (see Figure 14.11). If salt is not reliably iodized they can take a capsule of iodized poppy-seed oil.

5. Discourage smoking, alcohol, and drug-abuse.

If the mother smokes or drinks alcohol during pregnancy, the baby is often born smaller and weaker and is more likely to die in the first months of life. Mothers should not drink alcohol nor smoke during pregnancy.

6. Treat and prevent serious illness.

Tuberculosis, sexually transmitted infections, HIV/AIDS and other chronic illnesses can all seriously affect the baby's health.

7. Ensure regular antenatal care (see Chapter 17).

Teaching pregnant women about nutrition is much more effective if we also encourage husbands and other family members to support them in this.

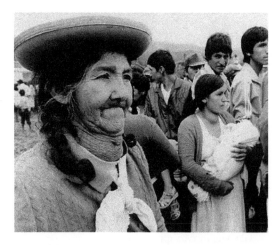

Figure 14.11 Iodine deficiency affecting three generations in the Bolivian Andes.

Rule 2. Promote breastfeeding

If a new vaccine became available that could prevent almost one million child deaths per year, was cheap, safe, could be given orally, had no side effects and needed no cold chain, it would be a public health triumph. Interestingly, if every child was breastfed within an hour of birth, was given only breast milk for their first six months of life, and continued to breastfeed up to the age of two years, about 800,000 child lives would be saved every year.[20, 21]

Many mothers today are being wrongly persuaded to use the bottle instead of the breast. They may listen to the advertising of artificial milk manufacturers, or think that wealthy, fashionable women use infant formula. They may start thinking that breastfeeding is dirty or old-fashioned. What often happens is that a mother tries to combine breastfeeding and formula, then finds her supply of breast milk reduces until she becomes dependant on formula to feed her baby.

Bottle-fed babies are much more likely to die than breastfed babies. Our job is to make sure that our teaching in favour of breastfeeding is more powerful than the pressures on mothers to adopt bottle feeding.

Breast is best because:

1. It is the natural food for babies, having the perfect balance of nutrients and providing natural protection against illness.

2. It is free and easily available.

3. It is clean, so the breastfed baby is far less likely to die from diarrhoea than bottle-fed babies. Washing and sterilizing bottles is tiresome and expensive.

4. Skin-to-skin contact between mother and baby has added benefits, including boosting the child's immunity

5. Breastfeeding is best for the mother. It reduces risks of breast and ovarian cancer, type 2 diabetes, and postpartum depression. It strengthens the bond between mother and child.

6. Breastfeeding, if regular and frequent, acts as a contraceptive and so helps child spacing.

7. Adolescents and adults who were breastfed as babies are less likely to be overweight or obese. They are less prone to type 2 diabetes and perform better in intelligence tests.

Help mothers to understand:

1. Be imaginative.

When helping mothers understand why breast is best, e.g. discuss the money aspect. Families sometimes spend up to one quarter of their income on infant formula.

2. Colostrum is good!

The milk produced in the first few days is not 'bad milk', but full of nutrients and valuable antibodies that the child really needs.

In many communities, children are only breastfed on the second or third day. Patiently encourage mothers to start breastfeeding straight after delivery or within hours of birth.

3. WHO now recommends exclusive breastfeeding until six months.

Exclusive means breast milk alone—no water, teas or anything else.

4. Breastfeeding should be continued where possible for at least two years.

Breastfeeding is usually possible but it has to be learned and many women encounter difficulties at the beginning. To provide support for mothers and newborns, there are 'baby-friendly' facilities in about 152 countries thanks to the WHO-UNICEF Baby-friendly Hospital Initiative.[22]

One method that can help mothers to follow exclusive breastfeeding for the first six months is through peer counsellors. For example, in Burkina Faso and Uganda well-trained peer counsellors visit mothers once before delivery and four times after delivery to encourage exclusive breastfeeding. This has proved inexpensive and effective.[23]

In situations where mothers have to go out to work while still breastfeeding, we need to help families and employers to understand just how important this is.

Mothers often incorrectly believe they cannot make enough milk. Where this is the case encourage them:

- to allow the baby to suckle often, both day and night.
- to drink more fluids.

The more the baby suckles, the more milk is produced. This is especially important in the few days after birth when milk may not flow easily (See Figure 14.12).

The author is currently observing from his own daughter that establishing breastfeeding is not always easy. We need to give imaginative support and encouragement to mothers who are struggling. One helpful website is La Leche League International at www.llli.org.

Strong advocacy remains essential to promote breastfeeding against strong pressures. If the mother has tried breastfeeding and despite her best efforts it does not work, perhaps because of her lifestyle or work patterns,

we should avoid being coercive and instead make sure she uses infant formula correctly with very careful hygiene precautions.

Rules for breast milk substitutes—mothers should use these only if:

- she finds it impossible to breastfeed despite her best efforts;
- the formula milk is very safely prepared and is used at the correct strength and with careful hygiene precautions.

If the mother is not able to breastfeed, one solution to consider is to find a healthy, HIV-negative 'wet nurse' in the community (both Moses and Muhammad were reputedly fed in this way). Other mothers in the family, even grandmothers, may be able to provide breast milk, but this is acceptable only in some communities.

Note on breastfeeding and HIV

The following details are current best-practice at the time of writing but advice changes quite frequently, so we should check any guidelines being used in our country or district.

Women known to be HIV-positive have a significant risk of passing on HIV infection to their infants through breastfeeding, especially if they have become infected

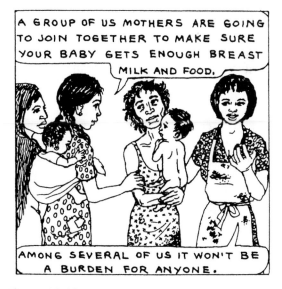

Figure 14.12 Members of a women's club help a recently widowed mother.

during pregnancy or breastfeeding or if they have symptoms of AIDS. This risk is greatly reduced if they use anti-retroviral therapy (ART).

Research shows that partial breastfeeding is more likely than exclusive breastfeeding to cause mothers to pass on HIV to their children. Current advice is that, wherever possible, an HIV-positive mother should receive ART during pregnancy, delivery, and lactation, and that exclusive breastfeeding should be continued for six months. The HIV-positive mother should use ART life-long but from the child's viewpoint she must continue therapy for at least twelve months.

If ART is not available the preferred option is infant formula. However, it is important that there should be a reliable supply of infant formula, and the mother has been carefully instructed how to use it hygienically.[24] If this is not possible, exclusive breastfeeding is still recommended. The mother should be given the opportunity of making the choice herself, after the options have been carefully explained to her. In areas where HIV is common, encouraging mothers to go for voluntary counselling and testing (VCT) is extremely important. In some areas there are visiting teams who can do this testing in homes or in the community (see Chapter 20). Antenatal clinics are also an ideal location. Testing before the twenty-eighth week of pregnancy is crucial in order to draw up the best action plan for mother and baby.

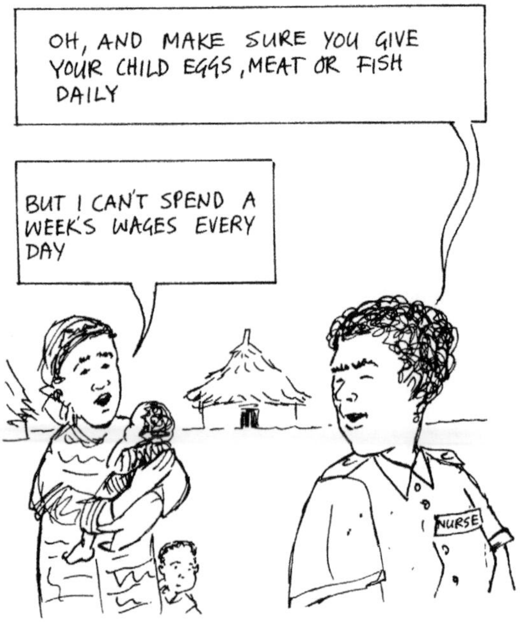

Rule 3. Introduce complementary feeding at six months

This is a summary of advice from the World Health Organization. In order to meet the growing nutritional needs of babies at six months of age, mashed solid foods should be introduced as a complement to continued breastfeeding. Foods for the baby can be specially prepared or modified from family meals. The WHO notes that breastfeeding should not be decreased when starting on solids; food should be given with a spoon or cup, not in a bottle; food should be clean and safe; and young children should be given ample time to learn to eat.[25]

> It is better not to use the term weaning as this means different things to different people. Instead we should use the term 'complementary feeding', which is defined as the process of starting other foods and liquids alongside breast milk, when breast milk alone is no longer sufficient for an infant's nutritional requirements. Complementary feeding lasts from six months to 24 months or whenever breastfeeding is discontinued. This is a critical period of growth, when malnutrition is most commonly seen. It is therefore a danger period for children in resource-poor areas.

Figure 14.13 Make sure that health workers encourage only the use of foods that are available locally and are affordable.

Follow these guidelines:

1. Find out about local food.

Make sure that health workers recommend only foods that are locally available and affordable to all, not the foods they are used to eating, from a different part of the country (see Figure 14.13).

2. Encourage appropriate foods.

Such foods should be:

- easy to prepare;
- rich in energy content, protein and micronutrients
- not too watery;
- soft and easy for the child to eat, such as mashed fruits and vegetables;
- clean and safe;
- without added salt or spice;
- free from hard pieces or bones that cause choking.
- Use correct foods for different ages.

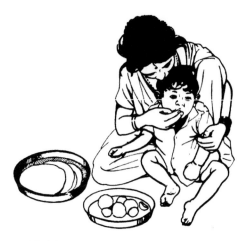

Figure 14.14 Until nutrition workers have experienced the cranky child who refuses to eat what the mother has prepared, they have not come to grips with the most essential element of applied nutrition.

From 6 to 12 months:

- Feed a little at a time, twice a day, to start with, building up to at least four times a day.
- Foods should be soft and easy to swallow and digest.
- Include soft fruits and thick porridge mixes with milk if available.
- Introduce new foods one at a time. Wait until the child is used to one food before offering it another. A good rule is to start a new food about every two weeks.

- From about eight months children enjoy holding small pieces of food (finger food), but wash their hands first.
- Feed the child gently, never using force (Figure 14.14)
- Give mixtures of mashed foods: include such foods as legumes, potatoes, roots such as cassava and yam, eggs, finely chopped meat or fish, as well as cereals and fruit. These can be prepared according to local custom.

The use of flour porridge or *super-flour porridge* started in Nepal and has become increasingly popular. It is especially helpful for feeding children whose growth is faltering on the growth chart, who are recovering from illness, and in areas of food insecurity. Box 14.1 provides a recipe and information for super-flour porridge.

From 12 months upwards:

- The child can eat 'from the family pot'.

Children can eat the same food as adults, but they should have their own plate to make sure they get their fair share. By the age of one year children are eating about half the amount per day that their mothers eat.

- Feed four to six times a day.

Young children will not be able to manage on the one to three main meals a day that adults eat. They have small stomachs and 'like chickens should often be pecking' (see Table 14.2).

Rule 4. Continue to feed sick children

The belief that food should not be given to sick children is a dangerous one, and many children die as a result. Illness leads to malnutrition and malnutrition to illness.

Box 14.1 Recipe for super-flour porridge

Ingredients:
- Two parts pulses—soybeans are best, but others such as peas or lentils be used.
- One part whole grain cereal, such as maize or rice.
- One part another whole grain cereal, such as wheat, millet, or buckwheat.
  1. Clean the pulses and grains.
  2. Roast them separately, and then grind them into fine flour (separately or together). The flour can then be stored in an airtight container for one to three months.
  3. The flour is stirred into boiling water and cooked for a short time. The proper amount and consistency of the porridge will depend on the age and condition of the child.

NB: Salt should not be added.

The exact make-up of the porridge can be varied according to the lentils or cereals available locally.

Table 14.2 **A final point: suggested snacks for young children**

Snacks for young children
Fruits such as mango, pawpaw, banana, avocado.
Boiled egg.
Boiled, pasteurized, or soured animal milk.
Chapati or bread with groundnut paste/peanut butter, or margarine, or dipped in milk.
Small pieces of boiled or fried cassava, plantain, or yam.
Sweet potatoes (orange coloured).

Mothers should continue breastfeeding when children are ill, as much and as often as the child can manage. A child who has started complementary feeding should be gently encouraged to eat, even if not very hungry. We should give soft foods especially if the mouth and throat are sore, and we must give extra fluids if the child has a fever or diarrhoea. Sick children will have small appetites; they should therefore eat their favourite soft foods in small quantities as often as they like.

After an illness there will be catching up to do. Children will need to eat more often than usual, with extra oil or super-flour porridge, until they have regained any weight lost. Children with diarrhoea should also continue to be fed. Oral rehydration can be done with home-prepared liquid foods such as rice water instead of salt-sugar solution (see Chapter 16). We must ensure that sick children eat enough so they can fight any infection successfully.

Rule 5. Prepare, cook and store food correctly

This section is adapted from the WHO Golden Rules of Food Preparation.[26]

Clean or process food appropriately

While many foods, such as fruits and vegetables, are best in their natural state, others are not safe unless they have been processed. For example, always buy pasteurized milk.

Cook food thoroughly

Many raw foods, most notably poultry, meats, eggs, and unpasteurized milk, may be contaminated with disease-causing organisms. Thorough cooking will kill the germs but it must reach all parts of the food.

Eat cooked foods immediately

When cooked foods cool to room temperature, germs start to multiply. To be on the safe side, eat cooked foods as soon as they come off the heat, and always within two hours.

Store cooked foods carefully

If foods are prepared in advance or leftovers are kept, they must be stored in hot (near or above 60 °C) or cool (near or below 10 °C) conditions. This is very important if foods are to be stored for more than four or five hours.

Reheat cooked foods thoroughly

This is the best protection against germs that may have developed during storage. All parts of the food must be thoroughly recooked, in other words, reach at least 70 °C.

Avoid contact between raw foods and cooked foods

Safely cooked food can become contaminated through any contact with raw food. For example, this can happen when raw meat comes into contact with cooked foods, or the same surface and knife are used to cut both raw and cooked food.

Wash hands repeatedly

Wash hands thoroughly before starting to prepare food and after every interruption—especially after cleaning the baby, going to the toilet, or touching animals. Any sores on hands should be covered before cooking. Fingernails should be kept short. Teach children to wash their hands regularly, and always before eating.

Keep all surfaces meticulously clean where food is prepared

Cloths that come into contact with dishes and utensils should be changed and washed frequently. Use separate cloths for cleaning the floor and any surfaces where food is prepared. Avoid feeding infants with a bottle, as bottles and teats are very difficult to clean. Use a cup and spoon instead. Never use containers that have contained chemicals or pesticides for food. Bury or burn any rubbish.

Protect foods from insects, rodents, and other animals

Animals frequently carry germs which cause foodborne disease. Storing foods in closed containers is the best protection. Keep poultry and animals away from the kitchen.

Use safe water

Safe water is just as important for food preparation as for drinking. Wash fruit and vegetables using the cleanest water available, or peel them instead. Be especially careful with any water used to prepare an infant's meal.

Rule 6. Avoid harmful and unnecessary foods

Harmful foods include spoiled or mouldy cereals, beans, and groundnuts, and food that has been inadequately recooked, or stored in containers that have held pesticides, fuels, or chemicals.

The use of unnecessary foods is becoming common in developing countries. Overweight children are fed on 'junk foods' such as artificial milk, tinned baby foods, tonics, bottled drinks, excessive sweets, biscuits, or other fashionable products seen on TV. The money could have been spent to buy healthy, nutritious foods.

Malinche was a Mexican woman who helped the foreign soldier Cortes invade Mexico and conquer the country. Beware the 'Curse of Malinche', which is the belief that anything foreign or western is good and must be better than things made in our own country. We need to help families use foods from their own communities, or only to buy healthy and nutritious food from outside. We also need to be aware of the growing problem of childhood obesity, present in many resource-poor countries as well as richer nations.

Tackle nutritional deficiencies

Sometimes it may be appropriate to consider tackling specific deficiencies with supplementation. Some examples are:

Iron: a study in Zanzibar found that children aged between one and four years given a small iron supplement daily had improved language and motor skills development.[27]

Vitamin A: Current WHO guidelines recommend infants 6–11 months of age should receive 100,000 IU once and children 12–59 months of age should receive 200,000 IU every four to six months as an oral liquid oil-based preparation, or as a capsule in settings where vitamin A deficiency is a public health problem.[28] Vitamin A has often been distributed at the time of polio vaccination Where this vaccination is no longer given, other routes for giving regular Vitamin A need to be set up.[29]

Zinc: There is evidence that regular zinc supplements can reduce pneumonia and mortality in young children.[30] One project in an Indian slum community found that daily zinc supplementation using 10 mg elemental zinc for infants and 20 mg for children reduced the number of children between six months and three years catching pneumonia, especially if they were also receiving vitamin A.

Consider special feeding programmes

Sometimes more serious levels of malnutrition in a community mean that 'The Six Rules' alone are inadequate. We need to assess with the community whether this is a short-term local shortage that the community and programme can manage together, or whether this is a more serious problem that requires specialist outside help.

Feeding programmes are described in some detail due to the periods of food insecurity or famine that are affecting more areas especially in Saharan and sub-Saharan Africa. We always need to be aware of the food security situation in our area and estimates from the best sources about whether a deterioration is likely.

Local/short-term food shortages

In community-based health care (CBHC) we should only start a feeding programme if:

1. There is evidence of worsening food security, i.e. food shortage with increasing evidence of malnutrition.

Early warning signs may be more children with growth faltering or weight loss on the growth chart, or more children with low MUACs. There may be a regional alert, or warnings and instructions from the government or from the World Food Programme or UNICEF.

2. The community is able to share responsibility and take action.

This can be through a health committee, or a church, temple, mosque, school or social committee. It can be a single enthusiastic CHW supported by motivated community volunteers.

3. There is available food from sources fairly close to the community.

We should use the most local and familiar foods available.

How to run a feeding programme

We can help the volunteers, CHW or committee do the following:

1. Select a suitable time and place for feeding.

For example, midday or evening in the CHW's house; morning outside the clinic.

2. Collect and prepare suitable food.

This must be well-balanced and high in energy, protein, and micronutrients. A 'super-porridge' may be appropriate (see Box 14.1). Where available, at least some food should be supplied by the community. Wealthier members can be encouraged to contribute. Volunteers should cook the food themselves in their own homes or communally.

3. Assemble the children, feed them, and keep order.

4. Teach and motivate the parents.

This is an excellent time to teach good nutrition, weigh children with parents' help, and distribute vitamin A and worm medicine if needed. The village health committee or an experienced CHW will usually be the organizer and the motivator, but feeding will always be done in partnership with the community and often as part of a district or regional government programme (see 'Widespread, longer-term food shortages').

For example, in Jamkhed, India, special feeding was needed when the programme first started. Young Farmers' clubs were formed whose members would help to collect the food, assemble the children, and motivate the community. They were careful always to give the same advice and teaching as the CHW. In this way the programme achieved quick results and could then be discontinued.

Some Dos and Don'ts:

Do:

1. Run the programme for a short time only.

As soon as food supplies improve, discontinue, but follow up vulnerable children.

2. Include children with moderate acute malnutrition (MAM).

Choose a cut-off point on the growth chart or the yellow zone on MUAC. Explain eligibility criteria clearly to the community, otherwise envy or mistrust can easily develop. Where malnutrition is widespread and severe, one option is to include all children under five at the start.

3. Follow up each child at home through the CHW or family folder system.

When the feeding programme ends, make sure that each child receives appropriate food at home and continues to gain weight.

Don't:

4. Run the programme for the people.

It should be community-run with our help.

5. Give out free supplies through clinics.

Free supplies should only be given when no food is available and a relief situation applies. Otherwise, we can create dependence and can even make malnutrition worse

6. Start a community feeding programme unless the need for it is confirmed by someone with expert knowledge on nutrition.

It is much easier to start programmes than to stop them, as communities quickly become dependent.

Widespread, longer-term food shortages

If food security is confirmed by experts as deteriorating, we must call on outside help, be in touch with government agencies, and make sure we and the community are involved in an effective response that is co-ordinated with any official national response.

In this situation, relief and aid agencies typically start to arrive, often saving lives but sometimes bypassing or disempowering the community in the process. A good model for us to consider is Community Based Management of Acute Malnutrition (CMAM). Originally known as CTC—community-based therapeutic care—it was originally pioneered in the early 2000s, focusing on emergency settings. It is now widely used in food emergencies. Adequate resources and training are needed for its success.[31]

CMAM is based on building the capacity of local communities and existing structures to respond as effectively as possible.

Its *core* operating principles include:

Maximum coverage and access.

Programmes should be designed to achieve the greatest possible coverage. CMAM aims to reach the entire severely malnourished population.

Timeliness.

Programmes should catch the majority of cases of acute malnutrition before additional medical complications occur. In humanitarian situations, CMAM programmes aim to start case-finding and treatment before the prevalence of malnutrition escalates.

Appropriate care.

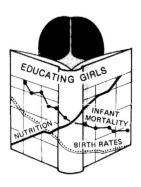

The education of girls is closely associated with a falling infant mortality and birth rate and improved nutrition.

Figure 14.15 Adult female literacy and schooling for girls leads to improved family nutrition.

Reproduced courtesy of David Gifford. This image is distributed under the terms of the Creative Commons Attribution Non-Commercial 4.0 International licence (CC-BY-NC), a copy of which is available at http://creativecommons.org/licenses/by-nc/4.0/.

Programmes should provide simple, effective outpatient care for those who can be treated at home and inpatient care for those who require inpatient treatment for survival.

Care for as long as it is needed.

Programmes should be designed so that people can stay in the programme until they have recovered. CMAM aims to ensure that appropriate services continue for as long as acute malnutrition is present in the population (Figure 14.15).

Here is one example on how this can work in practice.

In discussion with the community, those implementing CMAM will define three levels of care.

1) Supplementary feeding.

This is extra food for children with moderate wasting. Guidelines are available that can be adapted.[32] Usually specially formulated foods are used.

2) Outpatient therapeutic care.

This is needed when a child has uncomplicated severe acute malnutrition, i.e. the child is clinically stable (i.e., alert, no IMCI 'danger signs') and has an adequate appetite (passes the appetite test by being able to eat a set amount of Ready-to-Use Therapeutic Food, RUTF).

3) Inpatient care for a child who has 'complicated SAM.'

This is when a child loses its appetite, is unwell with fever, has dehydration, other danger signs, or complex underlying problems needing admission for more specialized care and investigation. Admission may also be needed if the home situation is difficult and carers cannot adequately look after the child at home.

If a child is admitted, it is for 'stabilization care'—feeding with specially formulated therapeutic milks and treatment of associated clinical problems. As soon as the clinical condition improves, the child may be discharged back to the community to complete treatment at home under the outpatient treatment programme.

In CMAM programmes SAM is treated with specially formulated RUTF. Originally and still most commonly, this is based on a fortified peanut paste (one brand is called Plumpy-Nut), but versions based on other ingredients also exist. RUTF is a nutrient-dense, micronutrient-enriched, easy-to-digest food. It is easy to use at community level.

SAM, whether complicated or not, should be seen as a clinical priority, if not a clinical emergency, and treated accordingly. These are very vulnerable children with high case fatality, hence the need to use WHO-specified RUTF.[33]

In areas of severe food shortage, it is essential that community-based health programmes work alongside respected agencies such as the World Food Programme, UNICEF, and official government programmes.

At the same time, however, we should encourage as much community involvement as possible so that outsiders do not overrule the abilities and wishes of the community. But the community needs to engage with the key principles of treating SAM, using the CMAM principles outlined.

Address root causes: encourage micro-enterprise

As mentioned earlier, poverty is often the root cause of chronic malnutrition. This means that helping a community to generate income can be the most useful way to address the problem. Also increasing female literacy (See Figure 14.15). Ask an expert for help before rushing into this, or collaborate with another CSO that specializes in income generation or micro-enterprise (see Chapter 12).

Many income generation programmes find it helpful to work with women's groups (see Chapter 2) as the cash earned by women tends to go towards feeding the family, rather than alcohol or cigarettes. The two diagrams in Figures 14.9 and 14.10 give further higher-level ideas which can help our health programmes to think 'upstream' about useful actions we can take, including advocacy.

Address food supply: set up kitchen gardens

Kitchen, or home food gardens, can be planted almost anywhere, including urban areas where crops can be grown in buckets or old tyres, near the house, or on ledges or roofs. In many rural areas fewer traditional foods are being grown for family consumption, wild fruit and berries are more difficult to find, and money is often spent on buying less nutritious, 'fashionable' food. This makes it very useful to grow a few highly nutritious foods near the home especially for the benefit of children. Therefore, we can use the following guidelines to address food supply:

1. Assess what crops are most suitable.

If protein is in short supply, beans and lentils can be grown. If there is Vitamin A deficiency, grow green leafy vegetables, and carrots. Pawpaw (papaya) or mango trees can be planted.

2. Choose crops that are easy to grow.

They will ideally need a short growing season and a long cropping season, should be familiar to the community, popular with children, and not prone to disease and pests.

3. Make sure there is sufficient water throughout the growing season.

This can be household waste water providing it is not toxic, or rainwater can be collected from roofs.

4. Feed the soil.

For example, use compost. If on a slope, protect the soil from being washed away, using stones or fixed contours.

5. Involve children in the project or delegate the care of the garden to children.

6. Consider planting trees, especially native ones, that provide nutritious leaves or fruit.

For example, The San Lucas Association in Peru discussed home gardens in village meetings, owing to high rates of malnutrition and because few vegetables were grown locally. They started with a gardening project in four schools, and then many families started to set up their own. Then women's groups started to co-ordinate these gardens in nearby villages. Childhood nutrition improved and sometimes surpluses could be sold for family income.

Consider mass deworming

Although some recent research has cast doubt on the policy of mass deworming, it is still recommended by the WHO and other experts as a valuable and cost-effective

public health measure. We should therefore consider setting up a programme, and work closely with any government programmes which may be present.

Children often have very high intestinal worm (Helminth) levels. Roundworms (*Ascaris*) reduce absorption of food and worsen malnutrition. Hookworm (*Ancylostoma* and *Necator*), whipworm (*Trichuris*), and schistosomiasis (bilharzia) reduce iron levels and can cause anaemia. Often, two or more of these helminths are found together. Regular deworming therefore improves nutrition, reduces anaemia, and enables children to have more energy and, according to many parents, learn more quickly (although this is unconfirmed). Well-run programmes are considered to be cost-effective.

The WHO recommends periodic treatment with anthelminthic (deworming) medicines of all at-risk people living in endemic areas. People at risk include preschool-age children, school-age children, women of childbearing age (particularly pregnant women in the second and third trimesters) and breastfeeding women.

There are various things we can do (and not do!) to make deworming programmes a success in schools.

Do's:

- Make deworming an integral component of a school health programme. Combine deworming with providing iron and other micronutrient supplements when there are known shortages in the children's diet.
- Identify the different roles of teachers and health providers and ensure they work together at all stages of the programme.
- Help teachers understand the benefits of deworming, so that they are supportive and recognize that the investment of time is a useful contribution to education.
- Make careful plans to manage possible side effects. Side effects are uncommon but failure to manage them can ruin the programme's future.
- Make sure that treatment is provided both for intestinal worms as well as for schistosomiasis where needed.
- Make sure that a regular ongoing plan is followed.
- Protect children's development by starting treatment early and continuing throughout primary school.
- Reach out to non-enrolled school-age children. This both enhances the public health impact and encourages children, especially girls, to attend school.

Don'ts:

- Waste time and resources trying to examine each school or child. Deworming drugs are safe and can be given to uninfected children.

- Exclude adolescent girls from systematic treatment. The drugs are safe, even in pregnancy.
- Be afraid to give albendazole 400 mg or mebendazole 500 mg, even to small-looking children. The dose is independent of age and weight.
- Hesitate to use a dose pole instead of a scale to decide the appropriate dose of praziquantel for treating bilharzia. It accurately calculates the dosages for school age children.
- Wait for sanitation to improve before starting deworming—regular treatment will help all children.

See the latest WHO factsheet for an overview.[34]

Two deworming drugs are especially useful—mebendazole 500 mg or albendazole 400 mg given as a single dose. Both are largely free of side effects. Albendazole is now favoured by most donation programmes. Seek advice from the district medical officer (DMO) about any national programme and what drugs are being used. Schistosomiasis (bilharzia) has to be treated with a different drug: praziquantel. Height measuring sticks are often available to calculate the dose easily. If weighing is used, the dose is usually 40mg/kg.

Current WHO guidance indicates that mebendazole or albendazole needs to be given yearly when the prevalence of worm infections in the community is over 20 per cent and every six months if it is over 50 per cent. Although neither drug is completely effective, by using them this frequently worm levels are kept so low that they cause little harm. Using the drugs less often allows worm populations to build up and iron levels to fall. We should follow the guidelines used by our District Health Team or Ministry of Health.

Drug distribution depends on the local situation. If school children are being targeted, the health team can arrange distribution within the school. If school age children who do not attend school are being included (which they should be) CHWs or members of the health team can distribute them in the community. The benefits of the programme can be used to persuade families to send their children to school. Some programmes also distribute other medicines. For example, a project in Gujarat, India distributes vitamin A capsules 200 000 IU and iron tablets (60 mg equivalent Fe) at the same time, also making sure that schools use iodized salt for their cooking. Children have become taller, heavier, less anaemic, see better in the dark, and have felt more active than before.

CBHC should never depend purely on medicine distribution to solve a problem. Our aim is always to improve the health of communities so that outside programmes become less necessary. We should start a deworming programme only if at the same time we actively consider three other areas:

- Working with the community to provide safe water for drinking and washing.
- Working with the community to improve sanitation—this may mean promoting latrines.
- Improving personal and community hygiene.

A combination of these programmes is now a worldwide movement known as a water and sanitation programme, or WAter, Sanitation, and Hygiene programme (WASH; https://www.unicef.org/wash).

Evaluate the programme

This is most simply done by seeing how the nutritional status of children changes over a period of time. The percentage of children under five who are underweight on the growth chart or those aged six months to 60 days with MUACs under 125 mm is compared between the start of the programme and a resurvey two, three, or five years later. However, nutritional status varies with seasons and repeat surveys should therefore be done at the same time of year.

The community can be asked to rank how happy they are with the programme, or the nutrition aspect, on a scale of 1 to 5. Regardless, all stages of the evaluation should be done in partnership with the community. Results should be explained carefully as changes in child nutrition may not be obvious and the community may not realize that improvements have occurred unless this is clearly presented to them (see Chapter 9).

The evaluation of a response to an acute food shortage is best done with expert help and as part of a regional programme.

Further reading and resources

Baby Milk Action. Wide ranging resources on promoting breast-feeding. Available from: http://www.babymilkaction.org

Burgess A, Bijlsma M, Ismael C, editors. *Community nutrition: A handbook for health and development workers*. Oxford: Macmillan; 2009.

Carter I. *Healthy Eating: A PILLARS Guide*. Teddington: Tearfund; 2003. Practical advice on making the most of available food. Available from: http://tilz.tearfund.org/~/media/Files/TILZ/Publications/PILLARS/English/PILLARS_Healthy_eating_E.pdf

Collins S. *Community-based therapeutic care: A new paradigm for selective feeding in nutritional crises*. London: Humanitarian Practice Network; 2004. Available from: http://

motherchildnutrition.org/malnutrition-management/pdf/
mcn-ctc-a-new-paradigm.pdf

Food and Agriculture Organization of the United Nations (FAO).
FAO Hunger Map. 2015. Available from: http://www.fao.org/
3/a-i4674e.pdf

Food and Agriculture Organization of the United Nations (FAO)/
EU Facility Project. *Complementary feeding for children aged
6–23 months: A recipe book for mothers and caregivers*. Phnom
Penh: Food and Agriculture Organization of the United
Nations (FAO): 2011. Available from: http://www.fao.org/
docrep/014/am866e/am866e00.pdf

Food and Agriculture Organization of the United Nations (FAO),
Government of Nepal, Government of Spain. *Nutrition handbook for the family*. 2009. Available from: http://www.fao.org/
docrep/012/al302e/al302e00.pdf

Han JC, Lawlor DA, Kimm SYS. Childhood obesity. *The Lancet*.
2010; 375 (9727): 1737–48.

International Zinc Nutrition Consultative Group. Zinc nutrition publications. Available from: http://www.izincg.org/
zinc-nutrition-publications/

The Johns Hopkins Center for Communication Programs (CCP).
How to make superflour for complementary feeding of an infant. Uploaded 13 July 2015. Available from: https://www.
youtube.com/watch?v=2SCxMwnxxdA

Kerac M, Trehan I, Weisz A, Agapova S, Manary M. *Admission
and discharge criteria for the management of severe acute malnutrition in infants aged under 6 months*. Geneva: World Health
Organization; 2012. Available from: http://www.who.int/nu-
trition/publications/guidelines/updates_management_SAM_
infantandchildren_review8.pdf

Liu L, Johnson HL, Cousens S, Perin J, Scott S, et al. Global, regional, and national causes of child mortality: An updated
systematic analysis for 2010 with time trends since 2000. *The
Lancet*. 2012; 379 (9832): 2151–61.

Living Well with HIV/AIDS, A manual on nutritional care and
support of people living with HIV/AIDS, WHO and Food and
Agriculture Organization of the United Nations (FAO), 2002.
Available from: http://www.who.int/nutrition/publications/
hivaids/Y416800/en/

MUAC measuring tapes, child health charts, weight-for-height
charts, etc. Available from TALC.

Sadler K. *Community-based therapeutic care: Treating severe
acute malnutrition in sub-Saharan Africa*. PhD [disserta-
tion]. London: University College London; 2009. Available
from: http://discovery.ucl.ac.uk/16480/1/16480.pdf

Savage King F, Burgess A, Quinn VJ, Osei AK, editors. *Nutrition
for developing countries*. 3rd ed. Oxford: Oxford University
Press; 2016.

UNICEF WASH programme. Available from: https://www.unicef.
org/wash

World Food Programme. Available from: http://www1.wfp.org/

World Health Organization. *Complementary feeding: Family foods
for breastfed children*. Geneva: World Health Organization;
2000. Available from: http://www.who.int/nutrition/publica-
tions/infantfeeding/WHO_NHD_00.1/en/

World Health Organization. Infant and young child feeding
list of publications. a list of resources to access or download.
Available from: http://www.who.int/nutrition/publications/
infantfeeding/en/

References

1. UNICEF. *Undernutrition contributes to nearly half of all deaths in
children under 5 and is widespread in Asia and Africa*. Updated
June 2017. Available from: https://data.unicef.org/topic/nu-
trition/malnutrition/

2. UNICEF; World Health Organization; The World Bank. *Joint
child malnutrition estimates, 2015. Global database on child
growth and malnutrition*. Available from: http://www.who.
int/nutgrowthdb/estimates2014/en/

3. UNICEF India. *Nutrition*. Available from: http://unicef.in/
Story/1124/Nutrition

4. World Health Organization. *The 2016 Global Nutrition
Report*. 2016. Available from: http://www.who.int/nutrition/
globalnutritionreport/en/

5. Galler J, Bryce C, et al, Socioeconomic outcomes in adults
malnourished in the first year of life: A 40-year study.
Pediatrics. 2012; 130 (1). Available at: https://www.ncbi.nlm.
nih.gov/pmc/articles/PMC3382923/

6. Fergusson P, Tomkins A, Kerac M. Improving survival of children with severe acute malnutrition in HIV-prevalent settings. *International Health*. 2009; 1 (1): 10–16.

7. Groce N, Challenger E, et al, Malnutrition and disability:
Unexplored opportunities for collaboration. *Paediatrics and
International Child Health*. 2014; 34 (4): 308–14.

8. World Health Organization. *Nutrition: Severe acute malnutrition*. Available from: http://www.who.int/nutrition/topics/
severe_malnutrition/en/

9. World Health Organizations. *Global strategy on diet, physical
activity, and health. Childhood overweight and obesity*. Available
from: http://www.who.int/dietphysicalactivity/childhood/
en/

10. World Health Organization. *Nutrition topics: Micronutrient
deficiencies*. Available from: http://www.who.int/nutrition/
topics/vad/en/

11. World Health Organization. *Nutrition topics: Micronutrient
deficiencies—Iodine deficiency disorders*. Available from: http://
www.who.int/nutrition/topics/idd/en/index.html

12. Siva N. A sprinkle of salt needed for Nepal's hidden hunger.
The Lancet. 2010; 376 (9742): 673–4.

13. Chen X. Fetus, fasting, and festival: The persistent effects of
in-utero social shocks. *International Journal of Health Policy
Management*. 2014; 3 (4): 165–9.

14. UNICEF. *Levels and trends in child mortality report 2015*.
2015. Available from: http://www.childmortality.org/files_
v20/download/IGME%20Report%202015_9_3%20LR%20
Web.pdf

15. Tutu E, Browne E, Lawson B. Effect of sulphadoxine-
pyrimethamine on neonatal birth weight and perceptions
on its impact on malaria in pregnancy in an intermittent
preventive treatment programme setting in Offinso District,
Ghana. *International Health*. 2011; 3 (3): 206–12.

16. World Health Organization and UNICEF. *WHO child growth
standards and the identification of severe acute malnutrition in infants and children*. 2009. Available from: http://
www.who.int/nutrition/publications/severemalnutrition/
9789241598163/en/

17. Christian P, Murray-Kolb LE, Khatry SK, Katz J, Schaefer
BA, et al. Prenatal micronutrient supplementation and

intellectual and motor function in early school-aged children in Nepal. *Journal of the American Medical Association.* 2010; 304 (24): 2716–23.

18. World Health Organization. *Vitamin A supplementation in pregnancy guidance summary.* 2016. Available from: http://www.who.int/elena/titles/guidance_summaries/vitamina_pregnancy/en/

19. World Health Organization. *Iodine supplementation in pregnant and lactating women.* 2017. Available from: http://www.who.int/elena/titles/iodine_pregnancy/en/

20. Victora C, Bahl R, Barros AJ, França GV, Horton S, et al. Breastfeeding in the 21st century: Epidemiology, mechanisms, and lifelong effect. *The Lancet.* 2016; 387 (10017): 475–90.

21. Rollins N, Bhandari N, Hajeebhoy N, Horton S, Lutter CK, et al. Why invest, and what it will take to improve breastfeeding practices? *The Lancet.* 2016; 387 (10017): 491–504.

22. UNICEF. *Baby-friendly hospital initiative.* Available from: https://www.unicef.org/programme/breastfeeding/baby.htm

23. Tylleskär T, Jackson D, Meda N, Engebretsen IM, Chopra M, et al. Exclusive breastfeeding promotion by peer counsellors in sub-Saharan Africa (PROMISE-EBF): A cluster-randomised trial. *The Lancet.* 2011; 378 (9787): 420–7.

24. World Health Organization. *Infant feeding for the prevention of mother-to-child transmission of HIV.* 2017. Available from: http://www.who.int/elena/titles/hiv_infant_feeding/en/

25. Pan American Health Organization; World Health Organization. *Guiding principles for complementary feeding of the breastfed child.* 2001. Available from: http://www.who.int/nutrition/publications/guiding_principles_compfeeding_breastfed.pdf

26. World Health Organization. *The WHO 'golden rules' for safe food preparation.* Available from: http://www.paho.org/disasters/index.php?option=com_content&view=article&id=552%3Awho-%22golden-rules%22-for-safe-food-preparation&Itemid=663&lang=en

27. Stoltzfus R, Kvalsvig J, Chwaya HM, Montresor A, Albonico M, et al. Effects of iron supplementation and anthelmintic treatment on motor and language development of preschool children in Zanzibar: Double blind, placebo-controlled study. *British Medical Journal.* 2001; 323 (7326): 1389–93.

28. World Health Organization. *Guideline: Vitamin A supplementation in infants and children 6–59 months of age.* 2011. Available from: http://apps.who.int/iris/bitstream/10665/44664/1/9789241501767_eng.pdf?ua=1&ua=1

29. UNICEF. *Coverage at a crossroads: new directions for Vitamin A supplementation Progammes.* 2018. Available from: https://data.unicef.org/resources/vitamin-a-coverage/

30. Shrimpton R., Zinc Deficiency: what are the most appropriate interventions? *British Medical Journal.* 2005; 330: 347.

31. Collins S, Sadler K, Dent N, Khara T, Guerrero S, et al. Key issues in the success of community-based management of severe malnutrition. *Food and Nutrition Bulletin.* 2006; 27 (3 Suppl): S49–82.

32. World Health Organization. *Guideline: updates on the management of severe acute malnutrition in infants and children.* 2013. Available from: http://www.who.int/nutrition/publications/guidelines/updates_management_SAM_infantandchildren/en/index.html

33. World Health Organization; The World Food Programme; The United Nations System Standing Committee on Nutrition and the United Nations Children's Fund. *A joint statement: Community-based management of severe acute malnutrition.* 2007. Available from: http://www.who.int/nutrition/topics/statement_commbased_malnutrition/en/index.html.

34. World Health Organization. *Fact Sheet: Soil-transmitted helminth infections.* 2017. Available from: http://www.who.int/mediacentre/factsheets/fs366/en/

CHAPTER 15

Setting up a childhood immunization programme

Ted Lankester

What we need to know

Why childhood immunization is important

Immunization saves lives. Smallpox used to cause one in seven deaths, but has been eradicated through immunization. At the time of writing polio has been eliminated from nearly all countries. The World Health Organization (WHO) issued the following statement:

Immunization averts 2 to 3 million deaths annually; however, an additional 1.5 million deaths could be avoided if global vaccination coverage improves. Today, an estimated 18.7 million infants—nearly one in five children—worldwide are still missing routine immunizations for preventable diseases, such as diphtheria, pertussis, and tetanus.[1]

Measles vaccination is a current priority. In 2015, there were 134,200 measles deaths globally—about 367 deaths every day or fifteen deaths every hour.[2] These lives could be saved if this effective, inexpensive vaccine was given in two doses to all children.

Apart from death, many millions more suffer disability, bereavement, and loss of earnings from vaccine-preventable diseases. In terms of community-based health care, making sure all community members are immunized according to national schedules must always be one of our top priorities (Figure 15.1).

The terms immunization and vaccination are used interchangeably in this chapter.

Global strategies: EPI, GAVI, and the Global Vaccine Action Plan

It is helpful to know about the terms we may come across in setting up a programme as they can be confusing and change quite frequently.

The Expanded Programme on Immunization (EPI) was started by WHO and UNICEF in 1974 to implement and organize worldwide immunization, originally against six vaccine-preventable diseases.

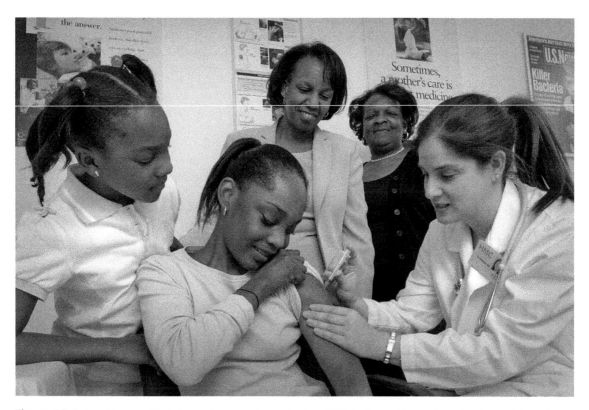

Figure 15.1 An adolescent girl receives an intramuscular vaccination while her sister, mother, and grandmother watch from the background.

The Global Alliance for Vaccines and Immunization (GAVI), set up in the 1990s, is a public-private partnership of UN agencies, donors, the pharmaceutical industry and CSOs, which is driving forwards universal immunization. It aims to improve access, expand the use of vaccines, accelerate research, and support national programmes.

The Global Vaccine Action Plan (GVAP) is an important, forward-looking document.[3] It is a framework to prevent millions of deaths by 2020 and beyond by making essential vaccines available to all children and introducing new vaccines that are being developed. It also emphasizes the integration of vaccination programmes into other aspects of development and community-based healthcare. In addition, GVAP aims to strengthen routine immunization programmes, accelerate control of vaccine-preventable diseases, with polio eradication as the first milestone, and spur research and development for the next generation of vaccines and technologies.

Additionally, UNICEF Supply Division, based in Copenhagen, negotiates with vaccine manufacturers to buy the vaccines most needed in developing countries in bulk and sells to those countries at lower prices.[4] Furthermore, the WHO pre-qualification section assesses all vaccines available through UNICEF to ensure they meet international standards for safety and suitability. This is an important service for countries who do not have the resources to conduct such testing themselves.[5]

One of our main priorities will be to follow and work with the national immunization programme of the countries where we are working. There are likely to be many gaps in coverage which we can help to fill. We may be able to strengthen and deliver immunization services, and engage the community in immunization in new ways.

Recommended vaccines

The summary tables published by WHO give details of the current vaccines recommended worldwide.[6] Each country makes adaptations to this. Six diseases were originally included in the EPI: diphtheria, pertussis, tetanus (DPT vaccine), measles, polio (OPV), and tuberculosis (BCG vaccine).

National immunization schedules now include other diseases depending on the country's resources and how important the diseases are for public health. An example of this is the Indian Academy of Pediatrics (IAP) Recommended Immunization Schedule.[7] Capacity is being increased continually by huge donations and technical support.

Table 15.1 shows the WHO vaccine recommendations for all countries. Recent changes made are shown in Table 15.2.

The full tables from the WHO[6] also give details of specific vaccines for high-risk populations or high-risk areas. These include:

- *cholera* vaccine, which is used in prevention and control measures during cholera outbreaks;

- *meningococcal* vaccine, which is of special value in Saharan and sub-Saharan African countries known as the meningitis belt;

- *yellow fever* vaccine, which is recommended in affected areas of South America and Africa and is rolled out as an emergency during periodic outbreaks of yellow fever;

- *Japanese encephalitis* vaccine, which is used in China and surrounding countries under separate national programmes;

- *typhoid* vaccine, which has been added to the Indian vaccination schedule because this disease is dangerous and prevalent in South Asia.

As the number of vaccines increases, a major challenge is to combine vaccines together so as to reduce the number of injections children and others receive. For example, a pentavalent vaccine against diphtheria, tetanus, pertussis, hepatitis B, and Hib has been introduced in India. Trials are underway to develop vaccines against malaria, and a dengue vaccine is now available, although at the time of writing, it is very expensive. Apart from the specific protective effects of measles and BCG vaccine, there is evidence that these live vaccines boost general immunity, which leads to a decrease in child mortality.[11]

Immunization schedules

Because immunization schedules have become so complex and there is great variation between countries, we should follow the current guidelines of the country where we work. The WHO recommendations for routine immunization (Table 15.1) are intended for use by health ministries to guide national policy. Having adopted one nationally approved schedule, we should be slow to change to another, as this can cause confusion at community level.

Here are further details on some important schedules.

Polio

At the time of writing this is still found in only two countries but outbreaks of the wild virus can still occur unpredictably. To speed up eradication, two strategies have proved useful: National or Subnational (i.e. part of a country) Immunization Days (NIDs, SNIDs). Where NIDs or SNIDs are held we can advertise these and encourage families to attend.

Similar to these are supplementary immunization activities (SIAs) which are extra efforts to deliver polio vaccination to every household. The final eradication of smallpox in 1980 used similar strategies. In community-based healthcare, we are well placed to know which families have not completed their vaccinations. Polio immunization must be continued worldwide until such time as WHO confirms polio is fully eradicated. Consult the WHO and Global Polio Eradication Initiative websites for updated information.[12, 13]

Measles

Measles cannot be fully eradicated until about 96 per cent of children are immunized, otherwise outbreaks can still occur. Reaching this coverage level is very difficult, but building a two-dose schedule into a national programme is a useful strategy. In addition, SIA campaigns can be arranged to revaccinate all children between one and sixteen years of age, regardless of measles immunization.

An alternative to immunization days is to target special approaches at high-risk areas such as poor urban communities where measles immunization rates are below 80 per cent.

In CBHC we should know both vaccination coverage of our target area and the number of measles cases. We can use this information to discuss plans with the district medical officer (DMO) and work alongside district and national programmes. Follow government guidelines on when and how to vaccinate against measles. For example, Measles-Rubella Vaccine (MR) or Mumps, Measles, and Rubella Vaccine (MMR) can be used instead.

Hepatitis B

Most cases of hepatitis B in Asia are transmitted at the time of birth. In Africa, the majority are infected during

Table 15.1 Summary of WHO position papers—recommendations for routine immunization

Antigen		Children		Adolescents	Adults	Considerations
Recommendations for all Immunization programmes						
BCG		One dose				Birth dose and HIV; Universal vs selective vaccination; Co-administration; Vaccination of older age groups
						Pregnancy
Hepatitis B[8]		Three to four doses (see footnote for schedule options)		Three doses (for high-risk groups not previously immunized) (see footnote)		Birth dose
						Premature and low birth weight
						Co-administration and combination vaccine Definition high-risk
Polio		Three to four doses (at least one dose of IPV) with DTPCV				bOPV birth dose
						Type of vaccine
						Transmission and importation risk criteria
DTP-containing vaccine (DTPCV)		Three doses	Two Boosters 12–23 months (DTPCV) and 4–7 years (Td)	One Booster 9–15 years (Td)		Delayed/interrupted schedule
						Combination vaccine
						Maternal immunization
Haemophilus Influenzae type b	Option 1	Three doses, with DTPCV				Single dose if > 12 months of age
	Option 2	Two or Three doses, with booster at least 6 months after last dose				Not recommended for children > 5 years old.
						Delayed/interrupted schedule
						Co-administration and combination vaccine
Pneumococcal (Conjugate)	Option 1	Three doses, with DTPCV				Vaccine options
	Option 2	Two doses before 6 months of age, plus booster dose at 9–15 months of age				Initiate before 6 months of age
						Co-administration
						HIV + and preterm neonates booster
Rotavirus		Rotarix: Two doses with DTPCV. RotaTeq: Three doses with DTPCV.				Vaccine options
						Not recommended if > 24 months old
Measles		Two doses				Combination vaccine;
						HIV early vaccination;
						Pregnancy
Rubella		One dose (see footnote)		One dose (adolescent girls and/or child-bearing aged women if not previously vaccinated; see footnote)		Achieve and sustain 80 per cent coverage
						Combination vaccine and co-administration Pregnancy
HPV				Two doses (females)		Target 9–14-year-old girls; Multi-age cohort vaccination; Pregnancy
						Older age groups ≥ 15 years three doses
						HIV and immunocompromised

Table 15.2 Recent vaccines and their benefits

Vaccine	Benefits
Hepatitis B	257 million people are chronically infected and in 2015, 887,000 died as a result of hepatitis B infection, mostly from liver cancer and cirrhosis. The hepatitis B vaccine has been adopted by most countries and is 95 per cent effective.[8]
Hib vaccine	Protects against the *Haemophilus influenzae* type b bacterium, which causes millions of serious cases of pneumonia and meningitis each year.[9]
Rotavirus vaccine	Protects against the family of viruses, which is the most common cause of death from diarrhoea in children. It causes over half a million deaths of under-fives each year. The introduction of this vaccine has been a major event in global heath.[10]
Conjugate pneumococcal vaccine	Prevents illness and death from pneumococcal infections (*Streptococcus pneumoniae*) which cause a severe form of meningitis, pneumonia, and a variety of other less serious illnesses.
HPV vaccine	Protects against human papilloma virus, which is the main cause of cervical cancer. Along with hepatitis B vaccine, this is an example of a vaccine which prevents death in older age groups.

the second or third year of life. We must always check the policy for the country we are working in. However, the first dose is ideally given within 24 hours of birth, meaning that whoever attends deliveries should usually be responsible for making sure it is given. The latest WHO recommendation recognizes that the birth-dose should be given within 24 hours for best effect, but later doses still have some effect in interrupting transmission from mother to baby. Therefore, in any country that has a 'birth-dose' of hepatitis B vaccine it is now recommended that even if the first 24-hour window is missed, a birth-dose be given at the first opportunity.

Equipment needed

In considering the equipment needed we must remember our twin priorities of maximizing coverage and safety. Success will depend mainly on good organization ensuring that the right equipment, vaccines and supplies are at the right place, e.g. base, clinic or field, at the right time. Government immunization teams may be operating in our area and will usually be responsible for equipment and supplies. We should find out about their programme and work alongside, giving support at community level so that as many children as possible are reached.

The most detailed on-line guidance and resources list for vaccination programmes is found on the WHO website.[14] Vaccination programmes will need the following equipment.

Needles and syringes

There are still some areas of the world where needles and syringes are reused and sterilized, but this is no longer acceptable in EPI programmes, even though in the remotest areas it may still be the only option until we can access sterile supplies as soon as possible.

Before the wider use of disposable needles and syringes, nearly one-third of hepatitis B, 42 per cent of hepatitis C, and 2 per cent of new HIV infections in developing countries were caused by unsafe injections—a total of over 20 million cases. This indicates how important it is to use disposable needles and syringes unless they are impossible to obtain (See Box 15.1).

There are three types of vaccine syringe:

1. Auto-destruct or auto-disable (AD) syringes.

These are used once only, after which the plunger jams. They must be burned after use. AD syringes are the best type, and are rapidly becoming the syringe of choice, although they are more expensive (See Box 15.1).

2. Non-sterilizable syringes.

These are also designed for single use, but in practice if they are not incinerated they may be picked up and reused by someone. Disposable syringes are sometimes prefilled with the vaccine dose.

3. Sterilizable (reusable) glass or plastic syringes with stainless steel needles.

These should only be used if no disposable supplies are available. Their use is not recommended by the WHO. They have to be taken apart, cleaned, and steam-sterilized for 20 minutes at 121–126°C in an autoclave or pressure cooker (see Chapter 5). Sterilization is often done inadequately (or not at all). If this system is used, temperature spot indicators must be attached to the items being sterilized. See also WHO best practice guidelines for injections.[15]

There is also a high risk of needlestick injuries when reusable needles and syringes are being used. For more

Box 15.1 **Best infection control practices for injections**

These best practices are evidence-based and follow the advice of experts.

1. Use sterile injection equipment

- Use a sterile syringe and needle for each injection and to reconstitute each unit of vaccine.[a]
- Ideally, use a new, single-use syringe and needle. Discard a needle or syringe if the package has been punctured, torn, or damaged.[b]
- If single-use syringes and needles are not available, use equipment designed for steam sterilization. Sterilize equipment according to WHO recommendations and document the quality of the sterilization process using time, steam, temperature (TST) spot indicators.[b]

2. Prevent contamination of injection equipment and medication

- Prepare each injection in a clean designated area, where contamination from blood or body-fluid is unlikely.
- Use single-dose vials rather than multi-dose vials.[c] If multi-dose vials must be used, always pierce the septum with a sterile needle.[a]
- Avoid leaving a needle in place in the stopper of the vial.[c]
- Select pop-open ampoules rather than ampoules that need to be opened by using a metal file. If an ampoule that requires a metal file is used, protect fingers with a clean barrier (e.g. small gauze pad) when opening the ampoule.[c]
- Inspect for and discard medications with visible contamination, cracks or leaks.[b] Follow product specific recommendations for use, storage and handling.[b] Discard a needle that has touched any non-sterile surface.[b]

3. Prevent needle-stick injuries to the provider

- Anticipate and take measures to prevent sudden movement of patient during and after injection.[c]
- Avoid recapping of needles and other hand manipulations of needles. If recapping is necessary, use a single-handed scoop technique.[a]

- Collect used syringes and needles at the point of use in an enclosed sharps container that is puncture proof and leak proof and that is sealed before it is completely full.[c]

4. Prevent access to used needles

- Seal sharps containers for transport to a secure area in preparation for disposal. After closing and sealing sharps containers, do not open, empty, reuse, or sell them.[c]
- Manage sharps waste in an efficient, safe and environment-friendly way to protect people from exposure to used injection equipment.[c]

5. All devices

- *Avoid needle-stick.* Whenever possible, use devices that have been designed to prevent needle-stick injury that have been shown to be effective for patients and providers, e.g. AD syringes.
- *Hand hygiene and skin integrity of provider.* Perform hand hygiene (i.e. wash or disinfect hands, e.g. with alcohol) before preparing injection material and giving injections. The need for hand hygiene between each injection will vary depending on the setting and whether there was contact with soil, blood, or body fluids.
- *Gloves.* Gloves are not needed for injections. Single-use gloves may be indicated if excessive bleeding is anticipated.
- *Swabbing vial tops or ampoules.* Swabbing of clean vials tops or ampoules with an antiseptic or disinfectant is unnecessary.
- *Skin preparation of patient before injection.* Wash skin that is visibly soiled or dirty. Swabbing of the clean skin before giving an injection is unnecessary. If swabbing with an antiseptic, use a clean, single-use swab. Do not use cotton balls stored wet in a multi-use container.

a Category I: Strongly recommended and strongly supported by well-designed experimental or epidemiological studies.

b Category III: recommended on the basis of expert consensus and theoretical rationale.

c Category II: recommended on the basis of theoretical rationale and suggestive, descriptive evidence.

details and a temperature chart for sterilization see Chapter 5. If we don't use AD devices we should follow specific advice regarding sizes of needles and syringes.

> *Needles:*
> - 10 mm, 26 gauge for intradermal (used for BCG, usually with a one-dose BCG syringe).
> - 30 mm, 22 gauge for intramuscular and subcutaneous injections (used for most other immunizations).
> - 18 gauge for mixing or reconstituting.
>
> *Syringes:*
> 0.05 or 0.1 ml for BCG.
> 0.5, 1 ml, or 2 ml for other injections.
> 5 or 10 ml for adding diluent.

Vials

These come either as multidose vials usually containing 20, 10, 6, or 2 doses, but commonly 10. These can be used for both liquid vaccine and those that need to be reconstituted, such as BCG.

Single dose vials can be standard design or prefilled AD devices. Multidose vials can also be used as they are more cost-effective but we need to be careful to use these according to the latest WHO policy.[16]

Safety boxes (sharps containers)

These should be used for all autodestruct or disposable needles and syringes. They should be made of tough material, not cardboard—otherwise disposable needles can pierce through them. Place supplies in them immediately after giving the injection without recapping, in order to avoid needlestick injuries. After the immunization session this box should be destroyed, ideally by burning. Special incinerators can be built.[17]

WHO/UNICEF introduced the idea of 'bundling'. A 'bundle' comprises vaccines, AD syringes, and safety boxes. Ideally these three components should always be considered together.

Other field supplies needed

- A tray for placing syringes ready for use.
- Forceps for fixing needles on to syringes, if using reusable needles.
- Spirit for cleaning.
- File for opening ampoules.
- Cold box (or cup with ice) for vaccines currently being used.
- Bowl and disinfectant if reusable syringes and needles used, otherwise a safety box.

- Rubbish bag or bin.
- Equipment for washing hands: alcohol gel or wipes for more frequent cleaning of hands.
- Supply of clean water.
- Adrenalin (epinephrine) and an antihistamine for emergency use.
- A vaccine carrier with ice packs.
- A kit bag in which to pack all supplies.
- Records, registers or means of digital recording.
- A supply of vaccines.
- Paracetamol and other simple medicines.
- A transportable table.

Maintaining the cold chain

The cold chain refers to the proper storage and transportation of vaccines, from the moment of manufacture to the time of injection. The aim is to keep vaccines between 2°C and 8°C. If the cold chain is broken, a vaccine may become useless. However, some vaccines are more sensitive to heat than others.

We should also be aware of the controlled temperature chain, where specific vaccines can be taken outside the cold chain under controlled conditions for special campaigns, such as for meningococcal vaccination in sub-Saharan Africa. Unless vaccines are kept at the right temperature (not too hot and not too cold), they lose their effectiveness (Figure 15.2).

Millions of doses are spoilt and lives lost because vaccines are allowed to warm up or (with some vaccines) freeze. We can help to maintain the cold chain by taking careful precautions at each link:

1. The source.

Identify a reliable source as near as possible to the point of manufacture or import. Only use sources known to be kept cold. If supplies are obtained from the district medical officer, a government hospital, or a private pharmacy, we should check the fridge is working when we collect supplies. Where possible use EPI/GAVI-approved sources.

2. Source to base.

On collection, we should place supplies immediately in a vaccine carrier, usually with ice packs, but freezing the vaccine must be avoided. Before use, ice packs should be 'conditioned', that is: allowed to thaw until there is a small amount of liquid in them, so they do not accidentally freeze vaccines that they come into contact with, On returning to base, we place the vaccines immediately

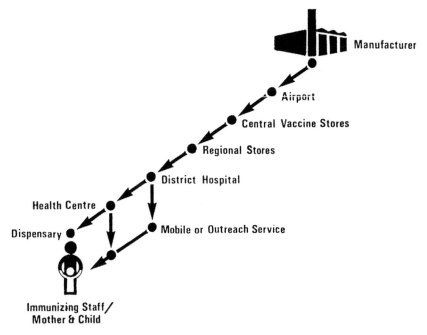

Figure 15.2 Maintaining the cold chain is vital.

in the refrigerator. If the vehicle breaks down, the vaccine carrier is placed in the shade, outside the vehicle while repairs are being made.

3. Base.

Supplies should be kept in a designated refrigerator.

- Place supplies in the back of the main part of the fridge. The door compartment gets too warm, and the cold box gets too cold, especially for DPT-tetanus-hepatitis B pentavalent.
- Do not put food or drink in the vaccine fridge.
- Place any vaccine brought back from the field in a separate place in front of other supplies, where it can be used first.
- Expired vaccines should be thrown away as should those that have warmed up.
- Keep a thermometer with the vaccines to check the temperature. Keep a twice-daily chart. Vaccine vial monitors (VVMs) are strongly recommended for all vaccine supplies. If in any doubt that the cold chain has been broken at any stage check the VVM.
- Maintain the fridge in good working order.
- If the fridge works on electricity, set up an alternative store in case of power cuts, keeping

a good supply of ice in the fridge in case this happens.

- Defrost the fridge regularly and while doing so place the vaccines with ice in the vaccine carrier, or in a second fridge.
- Check the temperature in the fridge twice daily so as to reduce the risk of the fridge overheating and supplies being spoiled.
- Do not open the fridge unnecessarily; check the rubber door seal regularly; seal the electric plug into the socket with tape to avoid accidental disconnection.
- Ensure the vaccines do not freeze, being aware of the heat stability of vaccines.[18]

This chapter provides a few examples,[19] but see the WHO website for a complete list.[20]

1. *The most heat stable*: Hepatitis B, tetanus toxoid, diphtheria/tetanus; Use VVM 30.
2. *Moderately stable*: DPT vaccines; Use VMM 14.
3. *Unstable*: Oral polio, unreconstituted measles, and BCG.
4. *Base to field*: Place vaccines within a box in the vaccine carrier, usually with an ice pack.

5. *Field*: Keep the vaccine carrier in the shade with the lid tightly closed. Take out supplies as they are needed, keeping any supplies being used in a table cold box or bowl filled with ice. Discard any unused reconstituted vaccine at the end of the session.

Using Vaccine Vial Monitors

VVMs (Figure 15.3) are an essential part of monitoring the cold chain and ensuring the vaccines we use have not been spoiled during transit. These are markers made of heat-sensitive material placed on the outside of vaccine vials.

They respond to heat over a period of time and change colour when a vaccine is no longer safe to use because of warming. VVMs therefore tell us if a vaccine has been exposed to too much heat. If there has been an accidental breach in the cold chain, then it is important to check the VVMs to see if the vaccines have been heat-damaged. VVMs usually consist of a square within a circle. Providing the square is lighter than the circle, the vaccine is safe to use. If it matches the circle or becomes darker we should throw the vaccine away.

We should also dispose of any vaccine if it has passed its expiry date, regardless of the VVM. Read all instructions carefully.

Checking for freeze damage

Some vaccine formulations, especially aluminium-based vaccines against diphtheria, pertussis, tetanus, hepatitis B and Hib, alone or in combination, should not be frozen. A survey showed between 14–35 per cent of transport systems caused freezing which can destroy vaccines.[21]

If we are concerned this may have happened we can use the shake test. Do this by taking two vials. Freeze one as the control, then allow it to thaw completely. Label it FROZEN. Take the frozen vial and the vial to be tested—labelled SUSPECT—in the same hand and shake both thoroughly. The vials will look cloudy. Observe the vials side by side. If the sediments settle at the same rate, the suspect vial has been frozen. If the suspect vial sediments more slowly, it has not been frozen.[22] Recent studies have confirmed this is a sensitive and specific test.[23]

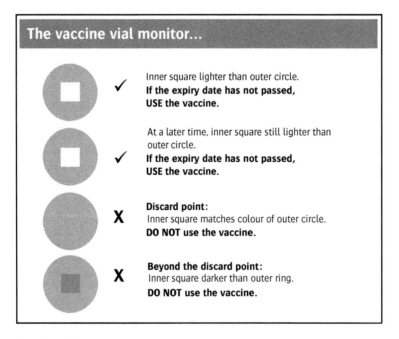

Figure 15.3 Vaccine vial monitors.

What we need to do

Assess needs for immunization in the programme area

There has been a huge uptake of vaccines worldwide. But many of the remotest and most vulnerable communities have very poor uptake. We must remember the world population is increasing by 80 million per year, which brings a vast challenge for vaccine coverage. Recent estimates suggest that 200,000 people move to cities each day, many of them children, so reaching mobile populations is a huge task. This means in practice that our programme needs to maximize vaccine coverage for all children where we are working.

When starting a programme, we need to find out:

1. An accurate record of births, informal or formal.

This may come from birth registration, baptism records, or other records of migration in or out. CBHC can play an important role in ensuring that births are recorded so that health services can register children for vaccinations.

2. Past immunization coverage in the area we are monitoring.

We can find this out most accurately from the community survey. If we are using a family folder system, the immunization status of each child is recorded on the front of the folder. There may be other reliable records we can use.

3. Programmes currently being carried out by government or voluntary organizations.

Some areas will already have effective programmes. In others, there may be good plans on paper but little being done in practice. Sometimes there is a difference between the coverage claimed by the government and actual numbers of immunized children. In many areas, especially countries affected by war or civil conflict, effective programmes have been set up in the past, but have been allowed to lapse. Often it is easy to count the number of vaccines given, but not easy to count the number of children missing out. Community-based health programmes can help identify the total population of under-ones and other eligible children needing immunization, to make coverage figures more accurate.

Discuss plans with the government and support local microplanning

We should make contact with the DMO or person responsible for implementing the national immunization programme in our project area. As well as building good working relationships we will need to find out:

- if government or other teams are already effectively covering our area. If they are not, we can discuss plans to increase coverage by carrying out immunizations and sending returns to the government.
- what schedules are used nationally or locally, for which vaccines, and at what ages.
- where to obtain vaccines, and details of the cold chain being used.
- records needed by the government and how our own records can be used with minimum change and duplication.
- ways of working together so we can reach the community most effectively.
- details of any mass campaigns or supplementary immunization activities (SIAs) that we can promote and support them.

CBHC programmes can also be proactive in supporting micro-planning, in line with the Reach Every District and Reach Every Community strategies, especially to help update records of where children are living, offer non-government infrastructure to help with outreach, and to look at whether immunization services or immunization communications can be integrated with other community activities.[24]

Set targets

Often areas will be covered or partly covered by existing programmes, in which case will we need to collaborate with existing targets and coverage plans. In an unreached area, we might aim for 90 per cent of children under five in our area to be fully immunized within three to five years, or to increase uptake of measles immunization, e.g. from 50 per cent to 80 per cent within three years. We will then need to set yearly targets appropriate for the area and enter these in our logframe (see Chapter 7).

We can work out the total number of children needing immunizations and hence the number of injections we will need to give each year. These figures can be obtained from the family folder or other records, including official or government records. In most developing countries the number of children needing to start immunizations each year will be approximately 2–3 per cent of the population.

Reaching targets may not be difficult where people are educated or where parents have been made aware through radio and television. In poorer areas or scattered communities, it may be a major challenge. Current "fake news" about the danger of vaccines is becoming an increasing hindrance.

Train the team

We may be working alongside trained government teams in which case they can advise on the correct procedures. Our team will still need to be well-trained and reliable in all aspects of vaccinations.

Motivation

Encourage all those involved in the programme to help set targets and contribute to planning. Let them enjoy the results of successful programmes and make suggestions to improve coverage. The more team and community feel this is their programme, the stronger their motivation will be. Any supervisor appointed must be fully involved in giving the immunizations (Figure 15.4).

Information

All team members will need to know why each immunization is needed, and how each immunization is given. They must also be able to give helpful explanations to parents and family members, especially if there are unfounded rumours about the reason vaccines are being given or the dangers they may cause.

It is also important that all team members know how a clinic station and how an outreach session are organized. This will include knowing how to :

- prepare all the equipment in plenty of time using a checklist;
- maintain the cold chain and use cold boxes and refrigerators correctly;
- give injections safely and effectively, especially if using informally trained staff;
- dispose of needles and syringes using any safety box;
- avoid needlestick injuries;
- clean and sterilize supplies if no disposable syringes or AD devices are available; and
- incinerate used supplies safely and thoroughly.

Furthermore, they must be able to identify which children should *not* be given immunizations. Broadly these are as follows (there are more specific contraindications for each vaccine):[25]

- any child who is seriously ill or with a high fever;
- any child who has previously had a serious reaction to a vaccine or is known to be allergic to the vaccine;

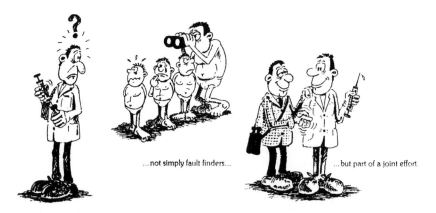

...not simply fault finders...   ...but part of a joint effort.

Figure 15.4 Supervisors must be involved fully in giving immunizations.

- any child whose family refuses permission after careful explanation;
- children with symptomatic HIV infection should not be given BCG or yellow fever (otherwise HIV-positive children can be given all immunizations); and
- children with active TB should not be given BCG.

Safety

We need to be aware of any threats or harm being caused to vaccine workers. There are several countries where communities are suspicious of both vaccines and vaccinators. In some situations, this has led to immunization teams being attacked or killed. We must have adequate safeguards to protect team members in unsafe areas, and follow any official government advice.

Prepare the community

Preparing the community for immunization is a crucial part of any immunization programme. Module 7 of *Immunization in Practice* (see 'Further reading') gives valuable information on this. High-level agencies and government often call this 'community engagement', a useful term for nearly all our work in CBHC. Put another way: 'Nothing about us without us.'

For immunization programmes with all their complexity, close partnership with the community is especially important. Although most communities are now familiar with immunization programmes and willingly join in, there are still many remote areas or family groups who are resistant and suspicious. It is also easy for a programme to become unpopular or for a wrong idea to take hold. We often have to work hard to gain, or regain, the community's co-operation.

Health committee members or CHWs can help to plan and organize any vaccination session. They can help to raise awareness among parents—and among older family members who may oppose the programme. First, however, health workers will need to spend time patiently raising community awareness (Figure 15.5). The programme should only start when parents are ready. It is unacceptable when eager health workers force immunizations on unwilling people. Also, parents, especially in remote communities, may find it strange that we refuse to give penicillin injections when their children have colds and coughs, but give a series of injections when their children are completely well.

In raising awareness for any Community Health activity there are two distinct stages.

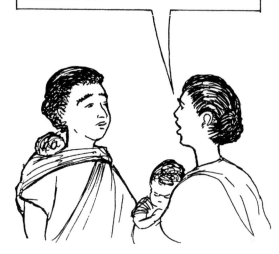

Figure 15.5 Motivation is a key to high immunization coverage

Answering fears and objections

Each individual and each community will have its own ideas about immunization. Common examples of what people may be thinking:

- They don't understand why children need these injections.
- They believe that these diseases don't happen in their area.
- The centre is too far away for them to reach.
- A child in the village died shortly after an injection and the community is suspicious and afraid.
- Rumours persist that injections are a secret form of sterilization.
- They can't afford to lose half a day's wages to bring children to be immunized.
- Waiting times are long and there is no shade to sit in.
- They have had a previous bad experience at the clinic (staff shouting, nurse rude).
- They are afraid of making the spirits angry.

Provide appropriate teaching

After discovering common objections, we can now give appropriate teaching. In doing this we will use a variety of methods, places, and people. Useful methods of teaching include drama, puppetry, question and answer, flash cards, billboards and radio. Suitable places for teaching include individual homes, the clinic, a community meeting place, the CHW's home or veranda, or a temple, church, mosque, or school. Appropriate teachers are the CHWs and health committee members, mothers who have completed immunizations, women's groups, youth and adolescent groups, young farmers' clubs, priests, imams, teachers, and older children. Mobile phones and text messages can be used as reminders. Finally, community members themselves are often more effective than health workers in motivating parents to bring their children for immunizations.

Successful immunization methods

1. Special immunization drives

Mass campaigns are often successful, and we should promote these and join in where possible, we can also organize special immunization drives. We can arrange an annual 'Pulse Strategy'. Each year at a convenient time, the health team working with community leaders arranges, well in advance and with careful publicity, three successive immunization days at monthly intervals. Some programmes that have had poor results with weekly or monthly visits have found this very successful, achieving almost 100 per cent coverage.

2. 'Full-uptake' families get special recognition.

Some programmes give special status to mothers whose children have completed immunizations. They may be given a flag to fly from their home, a badge to wear, a reduction in fees at the clinic or hospital, or bonus points in the next baby competition.

3. House-to-house preparation

For example, one successful programme taught each household about immunizations at the time of the first community survey, giving a time and place the following week where immunizations could be obtained. Many villages in that project reported 80 per cent of their under-fives completing immunizations within one year of the project starting.

4. Use religious leaders to promote immunization.

For example, UNICEF reminds us there is hardly any community without a place of worship, even though many have no school or health facility. A two-year collaboration between UNICEF and Christian and Muslim leaders in Sierra Leone increased immunization coverage of children under one year of age from 6 per cent to 75 per cent.[26] Community and faith leaders can set an example by "publicly" immunizing their families.

Immunization in the community

Immunizations must happen at a place that is convenient for the mother and the child, ideally within the community itself, and they should be carried out at a time of day that is easy for the family (Figure 15.6). Depending on the community, this may be an evening, a mid-day break from the fields, or a full day planned well ahead. It should also be at a time of year convenient for the community. For example, in rural communities, it should not be during harvest, sowing, or other busy times in the fields. It should not be just before major festivals, when mothers are busy, or just after them, when the community is recovering. In cities, timing should avoid major festivals, strikes, or large rallies.

In many areas, immunization sessions will be arranged by the district medical team, and we can cooperate and work alongside them. There are various procedures that can work well for community members. They can be used by mobile vaccination teams from the government, the project, or a combination of both. A team of three or four is adequate for most community-based sessions, but this depends on the size of the community and the expected uptake.

If the programme is doing immunizations without the government's mobile vaccination team, a nurse from the programme should be present to lead the session, backed up by well-trained team members and responsible community leaders.

Motivated community members can organize the mothers and children, keep records, help to maintain order, and explain to people what is happening. Generally, immunizations should be given only by trained and accredited health workers, otherwise in case of accidents or side effects there may be legal problems.

Traditionally, immunization has been done by special teams who visit and carry out immunizations in clinics or the community. There is now a move towards more integrated approaches, e.g. combining preventive services such as growth monitoring, nutrition, bed nets, and even family planning with immunization. There is some evidence that integrating immunization with growth monitoring improves both. This can only be done if it is within the capacity of the health team, but two points can be made. First, we could consider setting

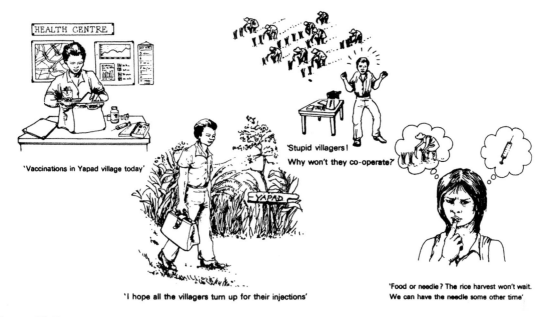

Figure 15.6 Immunization sessions should be convenient for the community.

up or joining multi-function health teams with other appropriate partners or with the government. Second, for programmes with less capacity, we could supply the non-vaccinator component of such teams—either as educators or as community-based organizers.

If we are either following a traditional community immunization approach or using a multi-function team, children or family members will often have health problems they wish to have seen at the same time. Usually, it is better to encourage mothers and children to see their CHW first or to come to the next clinic. However, it can be helpful to keep one member of the team free to deal with cases of minor illness, as this will increase community satisfaction with the mobile team's visit, as long as this does not detract from the main purpose of the day—immunizing as many children as possible.

How to run immunization sessions

This will be a joint venture with the community, which on each successive occasion should take increasing responsibility for setting up the session. Before the programme, the community must know in plenty of time when and where the session will be held. It will also need to know what equipment it should provide (tables, chairs, a room, etc.), what helpers will be needed, and its responsibility in gathering children and informing parents. Reminders or information about new or important vaccines can be sent by text to family or community leaders.

For example, in Pakistan in 2010, an SMS-based service was provided that enabled parents to send a free text message to report areas missed by the national polio control programme. A polio immunization team would then be dispatched.[27] In addition, text messages about the polio campaign were sent to more than 8 million mobile phone subscribers to raise awareness, especially in high-risk areas. Mobile phones are increasingly used to help the uptake of other vaccines.

Before the start of the programme, the team must prepare its supplies. By the time the programme begins (and before parents arrive), the team should have set up its equipment.

1. All team members should know their exact function.
2. Parents and children should wait in an orderly way out of the sun and rain, coming forward one at a time (often easier said than done!).
3. Health teaching should be given to waiting mothers and other family members. This is a good chance for weighing children—'weights can be done during waits'. Figure 15.7 provides an example of how to set up the flow of the programme.

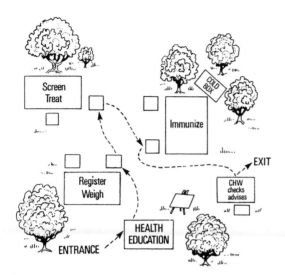

Figure 15.7 Plan for an outside immunization session, making good use of available shade

Reproduced with permission from Hall, DMB., and Elliman, D. 2006. *Health for all Children*. Oxford, UK: OUP. Copyright © 2006 OUP. This image is distributed under the terms of the Creative Commons Attribution Non-Commercial 4.0 International licence (CC-BY-NC), a copy of which is available at http://creativecommons.org/licenses/by-nc/4.0/.

4. Ensure CHWs are ready to visit and advise any parent worried about side effects.

5. Welcoming and informative communication during each encounter is important.

At the start, greet the caregiver in a friendly manner, and ask if they have any questions or concerns, and answer them politely.

6. Write the date of the vaccination(s) being given on the immunization card and explain the disease(s) protected against in simple terms.

7. Mention simply possible adverse events and explain how to handle them.

8. Explain the need for the child to return for each jab in the schedule in order to be fully protected.

9. Write the date for the next vaccination on the immunization card and tell the caregiver.

If appropriate, associate the date with a holiday or seasonal event, to help them remember. Always ask the caregiver to repeat the date back to you.

10. Explain what to do if the child cannot come on the return date, and remind the caregiver to bring the immunization card at every visit.

11. Proceed with vaccination, including explanation of positioning. After vaccination, remind the caregiver when to return with the infant.

12. Record the vaccination both on the childs self-retained record card and on the programme computer or register.

Box 15.2 provides some tips on giving immunizations to children.

In the event of any vaccine being out of stock, inform the caregiver where and when to return for the next doses. While you have your captive audience, remind the caregiver about other services given during immunization sessions, as per national policy, e.g. vitamin A supplementation or tetanus toxoid for women. Inform the caregiver about any immunization campaigns in the coming months.[28]

• After the programme, the team should carefully gather up supplies.

• If reusable or non-AD devices are used, check that none are left behind.

• If drug addiction is a problem in the community, a careful watch must be kept to ensure that syringes are not stolen.

• Fix the time and place of the next immunization session.

• Encourage community members to spread the word. This can be confirmed by text later to avoid confusion.

Immunizations in the clinic

Most of the details described in the previous section also apply to clinic sessions. In most countries, immunizations are available in government hospitals and in primary health centres where they are able to maintain the cold chain. If our programme is running a clinic, it is important to offer vaccines. Many parents may be reluctant to come for immunizations alone, but may accept them if a visit to the clinic is needed for other reasons.

Keeping records

We should use a system that is accurate, simple to use, has minimum duplication, works for our own programme, and provides information the government needs. We can record information by using the government recording system, unless it is too clumsy or complicated. We can also record immunizations as they are given on the child's own self-retained health record. For example, in Indonesia it was found that children who had their own self-retained records had far higher immunization coverage than those who didn't (70.9 per cent versus 42.9 per cent).[29]

Box 15.2 Twelve suggestions for giving immunizations to children

1. Children awaiting immunizations should not watch other children being injected, as this can cause alarm.
2. Prepare the injection without the child seeing it.
3. Use the smallest needle possible:
   a. 26 gauge for intradermal.
   b. 22 for intramuscular or subcutaneous.
   c. If reused, it should be neither blunt nor barbed.
4. Ask the parent about serious reactions. If the child has ever collapsed or been seriously ill after a previous injection, consult the doctor before the immunization.
5. Clean the skin with soap and water if visibly dirty. Otherwise, cleaning is not necessary.
6. Explain to the mother what the immunization is for, what side effects she might expect, and when to bring the child back.
7. Show the mother how to hold her child in a comfortable position.
   a. Injections should be given in the correct part of the body.
   b. For intramuscular injections this should be in the upper outer thigh, but not the bottom.
   c. For subcutaneous and intradermal injections use the upper outer arm.
8. In the case of reusable syringes, place the needle and syringe immediately into a bowl with chlorine solution with no recapping.
9. In the case of AD and disposable syringes, place needle and syringe directly into the safety or sharps container, with no recapping.
10. Make sure that everyone knows procedures to be followed in case of severe reactions, that adrenalin is ready, and that all team members know how to use it.
11. Both the parent and child should ideally wait for fifteen minutes after the immunization.
12. Paracetamol should not be routinely given as it has been shown that this makes some immunizations less effective.[30] NB: *children should never be given aspirin.*

Going family by family, record all children under five beforehand in the register, leaving space for newborn family members to be added. Note each immunization as it is given. Handheld electronic devices can be used to enter details directly into any computerized recording system. Wherever possible, and to save time, standard national forms used for recording immunizations are used alone, sent to the DMO, or immunization officer, with copies being kept by the project. GAVI has its own recommended reporting systems.

Evaluate the programme

Programme evaluation should be done with the community, and results should be explained to all community members.

Each year we can calculate the total numbers of each injection given, first, second, third, fourth, etc., for each community. From this we can calculate the percentage of children under five who have completed each immunization, the percentage who have partially completed, and the percentage of children who remain unimmunized.

If coverage is poor we can design a questionnaire to find out why parents are not bringing their children. Alternatively, this can be the subject of a community meeting where worries, concerns, or wrong perceptions can be discussed and corrected. We can arrange exit interviews for client satisfaction.

Every two or three years we can work out whether the target diseases are becoming less common. We can compare these to district or national averages where these are available and reliable. When working with government teams we should follow and participate in their monitoring of vaccine coverage. Some estimates show that official immunization rates are often over-recorded by as much as 20 per cent. If we record our programme figures carefully, these are likely to be more accurate than official figures.

Further reading and resources

World Health Organization. *Immunization in practice: a practical guide for health staff.* 2015. Available from: http://apps.who.int/iris/bitstream/10665/193412/1/9789241549097_eng.pdf This is the definitive source on all aspects of immunization and needs to be consulted and followed by all health programmes carrying out even the smallest immunization programme.

The State of Vaccine Confidence: 2016, The Vaccine Confidence Project, London School of Hygiene and Tropical Medicine, 2016. Available at: http://www.vaccineconfidence.org/research/the-state-of-vaccine-confidence-2016/

World Health Organization. Immunization, Vaccines and Biologicals: IVB resources. This section of the website has a comprehensive resources section. Available from: http://www.who.int/immunization/documents/en/

Pan American Health Organization. Immunization Newsletter and other useful guides. Available from: http://www2.paho.org/hq/index.php?option=com_content&view=article&id=278&Itemid=2032

References

1. World Health Organization. *News Release—World Immunization Week 2016: Immunization game-changers should be the norm worldwide.* 21 April 2016. Available from: http://www.who.int/mediacentre/news/releases/2016/world-immunization-week/en/
2. World Health Organization. *Measles Fact Sheet.* 2017. Available from: http://www.who.int/mediacentre/factsheets/fs286/en/
3. World Health Organization. *Global Vaccine Action Plan 2011-2020.* Available from: http://www.who.int/immunization/global_vaccine_action_plan/en/
4. UNICEF. Available from: www.unicef.org
5. World Health Organization. *A system for the prequalification of vaccines for UN supply.* 2017. Available from: http://www.who.int/immunization_standards/vaccine_quality/pq_system/en/
6. World Health Organization. *WHO recommendations for routine immunization—summary tables.* Available from: http://www.who.int/immunization/policy/immunization_tables/en/
7. Vashishtha VMV, Choudhury P, Kalra A, Bose A, Thacker N, et al, Indian Academy of Pediatrics (IAP) recommended immunization schedule for children aged 0 through 18 years—India, 2014 and updates on immunization. *Indian Pediatrics.* 2014; 51: 785–800. Available from: http://www.indianpediatrics.net/oct2014/785.pdf
8. World Health Organization. *Hepatitis B Fact Sheet.* Updated April 2017. Available from: http://www.who.int/mediacentre/factsheets/fs204/en/
9. World Health Organization. *Haemophilus influenzae type b (Hib).* 1 May 2017. Available from: http://www.who.int/immunization/diseases/hib/en/
10. World Health Organization. *Rotavirus.* 12 April 2010. Available from: http://www.who.int/immunization/topics/rotavirus/en/
11. Aaby P, Whittle H, Stebell Benn C. Why vaccine programmes can no longer ignore non-specific effects, *British Medical Journal.* 2012; 345 (7864): 25–8. Available from: http://www.bmj.com/bmj/section-pdf/187577?path=/bmj/345/7864/Analysis.full.pdf
12. World Health Organization. *Poliomyelitis Fact Sheet.* April 2017. Available from: http://www.who.int/mediacentre/factsheets/fs114/en/
13. Polio Global Eradication Initiative. Polio Now. Available from: http://polioeradication.org/polio-today/polio-now/
14. World Health Organization. *Immunization, Vaccines and Biologicals—Service Delivery.* Available from: http://www.who.int/immunization/programmes_systems/service_delivery/en/
15. World Health Organization. *Best practices for injections and related procedures toolkit.* 2010. Available from: http://apps.who.int/iris/bitstream/10665/44298/1/9789241599252_eng.pdf
16. World Health Organization. *WHO policy on the use of opened multi-dose vaccine vials (2014 Revision).* 2014. Available from: http://www.who.int/immunization/documents/general/WHO_IVB_14.07/en/
17. Practical Action. *Low-Cost Medical Waste Incinerator Technical Guide.* 2000. Available from: http://sustain.pata.org/wp-content/uploads/2015/02/PRACTICAL-ACTION_medical_waste_incinerator.pdf
18. World Health Organization. *Aide-memoire for prevention of freeze damage to vaccines.* 2009. Available from: http://apps.who.int/iris/bitstream/10665/69673/1/WHO_IVB_07.09_eng.pdf
19. Nelson C, Wibisono H, Purwanto H, Mansyur I, Moniaga V, et al. Hepatitis B vaccine freezing in the Indonesian cold chain: Evidence and solutions. *Bulletin of the World Health Organization,* 2004, 82 (2), 99–103.
20. World Health Organization and PATH. *Temperature Sensitivity of Vaccines.* 2014. Available from: http://www.who.int/immunization/programmes_systems/supply_chain/resources/VaccineStability_EN.pdf
21. Matthias D, Robertson J, Garrison MM, Newland S, Nelson C. Freezing temperatures in the vaccine cold chain: A systematic literature review. *Vaccine.* 2007; 25 (20): 3980–6.
22. Pan American Health Organization. How to perform the 'Shake Test'. *Pan American Health Organization Immunization Newsletter.* 2010; 23 (2): 7. Available from: http://www.paho.org/immunization/toolkit/resources/paho-publication/job-aids/How-to-perform-the-Shake-Test.pdf?ua=1
23. Kartoglu Ü, Özgüler N, Wolfson LJ, Kurzatkowski W. Validation of the shake test for detecting freeze damage to adsorbed vaccines. *Bulletin of the World Health Organization.* 2010; 88 (8): 624–31.
24. World Health Organization. *Immunization in Practice: a practical guide for health staff.* 2015. Modules 4 and 6. Available from: http://apps.who.int/iris/bitstream/10665/193412/1/9789241549097_eng.pdf
25. Centers for Disease Control and Prevention. *Contraindications and Precautions, Best Practices Guidance of the Advisory Committee on Immunization Practices (ACIP).* 2017. Available from: https://www.cdc.gov/vaccines/hcp/acip-recs/general-recs/contraindications.html
26. UNICEF. *Building Trust in Immunization: Partnering with Religious Leaders and Groups.* 2004. Available from: https://www.unicef.org/ceecis/building_trust_immunization.pdf
27. Kazi A, Jafri L. The use of mobile phones in polio eradication. *Bulletin of the World Health Organization.* 2016; 94 (2): 153–4.
28. World Health Organization. *Immunization in practice: A practical guide for health staff.* Module 5: 13. 2015. Available from: http://apps.who.int/iris/bitstream/10665/193412/1/9789241549097_eng.pdf
29. Osaki K, Hattori T, Kosen S, Singgih B. Investment in home-based maternal, newborn and child health records improves immunization coverage in Indonesia. *Transactions of the Royal Society of Tropical Medicine and Hygiene.* 2009; 103 (8): 846–8.
30. Prymula R, Siegrist C, Chlibek R, Zemlickova H, Vackova M, et al. Effect of prophylactic paracetamol administration at time of vaccination on febrile reactions and antibody responses in children: Two open-label, randomised control trials. *The Lancet.* 2009; 374(9698): 1339–50.

CHAPTER 16

Dealing with childhood illnesses

Diarrhoea, acute respiratory infection, and malaria

Ted Lankester

Introduction

In 2017, 5.4 million children died before the age of five years.[1] Children in sub-Saharan Africa are fourteen times more likely to die under the age of five than children in more developed countries.[2] The leading causes of death (excluding perinatal and neonatal causes) were pneumonia (16 per cent), diarrhoea (8 per cent), and malaria (5 per cent); these three diseases are the focus of this chapter. Malnourished children are far more likely to die of these illnesses—45 per cent of deaths in under-five children were attributable to undernutrition.[3]

There has been good progress in reducing under-five death rates in most countries. Increasingly, child deaths are more concentrated in low-income countries and the poorest areas of those countries. Children are at greatest risk in areas where factors such as civil conflict, poor governance, climate change, and high birth rates put health systems under severe strain.

Sustainable Development Goal (SDG) No. 3 includes a target to end preventable deaths of newborns and children under five, and Article 24 of the Convention on the Rights of the Child states that it is a child's right to enjoy the highest attainable standards of health and to have access to health services.[4]

Two causes of death in children are often ignored or forgotten. More than one quarter of a million children die as a result of road traffic accidents each year.[5] Drowning is also a major cause of death; in Bangladesh drowning accounts for 43 per cent of all deaths in children aged one to four.[6] Thus, our child health programmes must also include teaching about how to reduce road traffic and other unintentional injuries.[7]

Integrated Management of Childhood Illness (IMCI)

The Integrated Management of Childhood Illness (IMCI) pioneered by the World Health Organization (WHO) and UNICEF since 1995 is an important worldwide strategy forming the basis of child health programmes in nearly all developing countries.[8] IMCI looks at the commonest causes of death and disability in children and seeks to prevent and cure these by an integrated or horizontal approach (Chapter 1). When well managed, IMCI proves effective in reducing under-five death rates and improving children's health.

IMCI has three related aims:

1. To improve the case management skills of health workers through training, using locally adapted guidelines.
2. To improve health systems, including ensuring availability of essential drugs.
3. To train families and communities how to prevent illness and to know how and when to seek medical help.

As IMCI is introduced in each country, pilot projects are used to write locally adapted guidelines. IMCI is then scaled up. The success of IMCI depends largely on how effectively health workers are trained to recognize serious illnesses, treat them correctly, and refer very sick children.

IMCI has one focus on the use of health facilities. It has another on how children can be cared for in the community and the home setting. Here, it helps communities learn how to seek appropriate care, concentrates on good nutrition, and gives guidance on treatment of important childhood illnesses. Recent evaluations in many countries show that, where IMCI programmes are working well, children become healthier and fewer die. In the poorest communities, setting up IMCI programmes can be challenging. However, IMCI is a useful model and resource for us, with a strong emphasis on prevention and empowerment of communities to treat common illnesses and to seek higher level care when needed.

Other programmes for childhood illness

Many countries have specific programmes targeting common or endemic diseases. More than one billion people, including many children, are affected by diseases known as neglected tropical diseases (NTDs) (Box 16.1). In fact, many of these have been given high priority recently, and so 'neglected' is not always an accurate description. We should check what is present in our community and follow any government programmes. These diseases are prevented by public health measures, often alongside regular medication, which needs to be distributed throughout the community. Community-based health care (CBHC) programmes are ideally placed to link with these vertical programmes and to make sure they are integrated and effective at community level.

Box 16.1 List of neglected tropical diseases (NDTs)

Buruli ulcer and Mycetoma

Chagas disease

Dengue and chikungunya

Dracunculiasis (guinea-worm disease) (now almost eradicated)

Echinococcosis

Foodborne trematodiases

Human African trypanosomiasis (sleeping sickness)

Leishmaniasis

Leprosy (Hansen's disease)

Lymphatic filariasis

Onchocerciasis (river blindness)

Rabies

Schistosomiasis (bilharzia)

Soil-transmitted helminthiases

Taeniasis/Cysticercosis

Trachoma

Yaws (Endemic)

Source: data from World Health Organization, 2016. This box is distributed under the terms of the Creative Commons Attribution Non Commercial 4.0 International licence (CC-BY-NC), a copy of which is available at http://creativecommons.org/licenses/by-nc/4.0/

A note on adolescents

The needs of adolescents—those who are between childhood and adulthood—have been hugely overlooked but are now being given greater priority both by the WHO and others. An excellent summary on needs, challenges, and opportunities can be found in the 2016 Lancet Commission.[9] The leading causes of adolescent deaths in 2012 were road injury, HIV, suicide, lower respiratory infections, and interpersonal violence.[10] Other key issues in these age groups are alcohol and substance abuse, sexually transmitted infections, and childhood pregnancy, all of which are covered elsewhere in this book.

The needs of "tweens and teens" i.e. pre-adolescents and adolescents is nicely summarised by Dr. Ban Ki-Moon, former UN Secretary-general writes:

Adolescents can be key driving forces in building a future of dignity for all. If we can make a positive difference in the lives of 10-year-old girls and boys today, and expand their opportunities and capabilities over the next 15 years, we can ensure the success of the SDGs. For me, the acronym 'SDG' also stands for 'Sustainable Development Generation', and sustainability means engaging future generations today.[11]

Diarrhoea: what we need to know

Why treating diarrhoea is important

Diarrhoea kills over half a million children per year.[12] If we set up effective programmes, most of these deaths can be prevented. Diarrhoea has several deadly effects. It weakens children so they become more likely to become seriously ill from other infectious diseases. It causes them to lose weight and undermines their nutrition. But its primary danger is dehydration—the main reason children die from diarrhoea (Figure 16.1).

Different forms of diarrhoea

The WHO defines diarrhoea as the passage of loose or watery stools at least three times in a 24-hour period. There are different types of diarrhoea and WHO's IMCI approach suggests these categories:

- *Acute watery diarrhoea*—lasting fourteen days or fewer, usually starting suddenly and normally caused by infections.
- *Persistent or chronic diarrhoea*—lasting more than fourteen days and often present because of other factors, e.g. malnutrition, AIDS.
- *Dysentery*—diarrhoea with blood, with or without fever.
- *Diarrhoea with severe malnutrition (marasmus or kwashiorkor)*—the main dangers are severe systemic infection, vitamin and mineral deficiency, dehydration, and heart failure.

Many different germs cause diarrhoea. In developing countries, more than half of the cases are caused by rotavirus infections. Rotavirus is the commonest cause worldwide in children under two years of age, and increasing use of rotavirus vaccine is having an impact. Shigella is the most commonly isolated pathogen in children aged two to five years.

All forms of diarrhoea are treated with oral rehydration solution (ORS) or home-prepared liquid foods, ideally also with zinc supplements, to reduce dehydration. In addition, for persistent diarrhoea, we should try to find a cause, e.g. *Campylobacter*, Amoeba, or *Giardia*, and treat this. For dysentery we should usually use antibiotics.

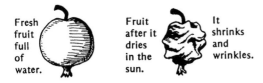

Fresh fruit full of water.   Fruit after it dries in the sun.   It shrinks and wrinkles.

Figure 16.1 If the child with diarrhoea is not given water, he will dry out like fruit in the sun.

ORS and ORT

ORT stands for oral rehydration therapy. This is a treatment for dehydration where packaged oral rehydration salts (ORS) are mixed with water and given to those with

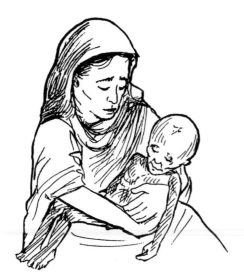

Figure 16.2 This child is dying from dehydration. The nearest clinic is closed. The mother does not know how to make a rehydration drink.

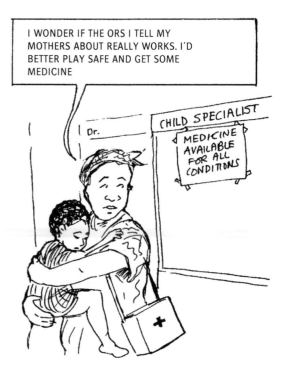

Figure 16.3 Test of a successful ORT programme: does the CHW trust oral rehydration alone when her own child is at risk?

diarrhoea. ORS can also stand for oral rehydration solution, which is water with added sugar/starch and salt; it is life-saving.[13]

Added sugar helps water and salts to be absorbed from the stomach and also gives energy. The use of salt-sugar solution in treating diarrhoea has been described as one of the greatest medical discoveries of the twentieth century.[14] Nearly all cases of dehydration could be prevented and hundreds of thousands of lives saved per year if parents worldwide knew how to make it and give it. Many lives are already being saved by those who do know. It has been calculated that on average it takes a health worker 30 minutes per person to teach the effective use of ORS (See Figure 16.2).

Despite being taught how to use ORS and why it is life-saving, it is puzzling that so many families still fail to use it. Bringing about behavioural change is one of the biggest challenges in community health. Seeking injections and courses of medicine is the first reaction of most parents when any illness strikes. Through patience and persistence, we can instil our life-saving message. One measure of success is that our community health workers (CHWs) not only teach the community about ORS, but also will reliably use it themselves for their own sick children (Figure 16.3). Chapter 4 provides more details on behavioural change.

The dangers of diarrhoea

Diarrhoea is primarily dangerous because it causes death from dehydration, but it also leads to malnutrition if prolonged. It can be highly infectious, spreading rapidly especially where there is poverty and overcrowding, or after man-made or natural disasters, when cholera often also becomes a threat. Sadly, treatment of diarrhoea is still commonly inappropriate and dangerous.

As mentioned, many health workers and families still believe that diarrhoea should be treated by medicines and injections. They may give intravenous (IV) fluids even though the patient is able to drink. One reason why people continue to use medicine is because it appears to cure diarrhoea. However, diarrhoea is usually self-limiting and would have stopped anyway.

Medicines for diarrhoea may be dangerous in themselves, but the greatest danger is the delay they can cause. Instead of starting home-based ORS at once, parents will waste valuable hours seeking ineffective medicines from a clinic or pharmacy.

Table 16.1 **Danger signs of dehydration and when to refer**

Action		Plan A	Plan B	Plan C
1. *Look at:*	*Condition*	Well, alert	Restless, irritable	Lethargic or unconscious; floppy
	Eyes	Normal	Sunken	Very sunken and dry
	Tears	Present	Absent	Absent
	Mouth and tongue	Moist	Dry	Very dry
	Thirst	Drinks normally; not thirsty.	Thirsty, drinks eagerly.	Drinks poorly or unable to drink.
2. *Feel:*	*Skin pinch*	Goes back quickly.	Goes back slowly.	Goes back very slowly.
3. *Decide:*		Patient has *no signs* of dehydration.	If patient has two or more signs, including at least one sign, there is *some* dehydration.	If patient has two or more signs, including at least one sign, there is *severe* dehydration.

Adapted with permission from World Health Organization. 1993. The Management and Prevention of Diarrhoea: practical guidelines, 3rd Ed. Geneva, Switzerland: WHO. Copyright © 1993 WHO. This table is distributed under the terms of the Creative Commons Attribution Non Commercial 4.0 International licence (CC-BY-NC), a copy of which is available at http://creativecommons.org/licenses/by-nc/4.0/

Although ORS potentially can save many lives the incorrect use of ORS may be dangerous. *Too much salt* can be given, which occasionally causes convulsions, and ORS needs careful measurement and the solution must always be tasted before it is given. This is especially the case with diarrhoea caused by rotavirus, as less sodium is usually lost in the stools than diarrhoea from other causes. In practice, this means it is safer to err on the side of over-diluting the ORS rather than risking making it too concentrated.

Too little ORS may be given so it fails to treat dehydration rapidly enough. It may be fed too fast or impatiently, causing vomiting or refusal in the child. Or, the water used for ORS may be contaminated with germs. Ideally, boiled water should be used or, if this is not possible, water from the cleanest possible source.

Certain types of diarrhoea are dangerous. Dysentery caused by shigella or other organisms usually needs antibiotics. Persistent diarrhoea (lasting more than fourteen days) needs diagnosis and further treatment. Serious epidemic forms of diarrhoea, e.g. cholera and typhoid (enteric fever), need a co-ordinated community approach. Regardless of cause, some children may need IV treatment and referral to hospital. Health workers need to train parents to be alert to danger signs of dehydration and to know when referral is needed (see Table 16.1).

Diarrhoea: what we need to do

Setting aims and targets for treatment

Ultimately, we must aim to make sure that every family member in our programme area knows how to make and use homemade ORS, or will reliably obtain ORS packets at an affordable price, with some kept at home. We must also make sure that every child with diarrhoea does actually receive ORS, or a food-based equivalent. In an area where ORS is little used, our targets could be for 50 per cent of parents to understand and use ORS after one year, and 90 per cent after two years. In areas where ORS is known about but little used, our target will be to increase the proportion of families who use it at the first sign of diarrhoea.

For example, a recent unpublished study of 225 mothers in Garhwal, North India showed only 18 per cent recognized an ORS packet or knew how to use it, and only 6 per cent knew how to prepare and administer it. After face-to-face education, 86 per cent knew how to use ORS packets and 80 per cent how to prepare homemade solutions. However, the real test is whether mothers translate this knowledge into practice and are actually using ORS six months later. This was not checked in this study.

Choosing suitable community approaches

Maintaining our approach from the start will make our task much easier. We can follow these guidelines:

1. Decide which overall method is most suitable for the community.

If we consult with the members of the community, we can discover which containers and measurers are commonly used at home. We can find out if ORS packets are available locally, and what liquid foods are fed to children. Ask for suggestions. As many countries now have national programmes, we should familiarize ourselves with them and follow guidelines where possible. Even if there is no national programme, there may still be a method in use in our district or project area. Consult with the DMO and any other programmes nearby.

2. Decide whether to use packet or homemade ORS.

Unless packets are cheap, easy to obtain, and always available, families should learn how to prepare their own ORS at home. They can still use packets when available, but their children will not die when supplies of the packets run out.

Packet ORS along with zinc supplements is becoming more widely available and where families can easily and reliably access these packets, they are the treatment of choice.

Homemade ORS can either be a salt-sugar solution or traditional liquid food, e.g. rice water, soups, gruels, fruit juices, dilute tea, potato water, carrot juice or coconut milk with salt added. Liquid foods have various advantages: they are easily available, children are familiar with them, most reduce stool volume, and they provide food as well as fluid.

3. Decide on containers in which to make up the solution.

Containers used should be known by everyone, be available in the homes, and be always the same size. They should also be carefully washed out with clean water before use. Ideally, it should also be easy for them to be covered after the solution is made. Examples include:

- Beer bottles holding 1 litre or soft drink bottles holding 0.75 litre.

- Medium-sized glasses or cups holding 0.25 litre.
- In south Asia a 'lota' usually holding 0.5 litre *unless this is also used for washing after defaecation.*

4. Decide on measuring devices for the amounts of salt-sugar.

Again, measuring devices for both the salt and sugar must be widely known, easily available, standard size, and simple to use so that mistakes are not made in the amounts measured out. Examples include:

- A 5 ml small spoon (teaspoon)
- Using a four-finger human fistful of sugar and a thumb-and-two-fingers pinch of salt (see below). Although less accurate, this remains an important method in resource-poor communities.
- A TALC (Google this to see availability) or similar measuring device, either bought or homemade.
- A bottle top.

Preparing ORS appropriately

Having decided what is most appropriate in terms of container, measurers, packets, or homemade preparations, we can then prepare the solution.

1. Homemade sugar-salt solution (see Figure 16.4)

To make one litre (as currently recommended by the WHO), add six level small spoons (5 ml teaspoons; plus half a teaspoon of salt to one litre of clean water. Mix

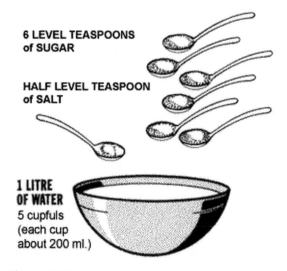

6 LEVEL TEASPOONS of SUGAR

HALF LEVEL TEASPOON of SALT

1 LITRE OF WATER
5 cupfuls
(each cup
about 200 ml.)

Figure 16.4 Homemade salt-sugar solution.

carefully and feed. (*NB: some programmes still incorrectly use eight teaspoons*).

To make a half-litre, either halve the above amounts or, if teaspoons are not available, add one fistful (four-finger scoop) of sugar plus one pinch (thumb-and-two-fingers) of salt to half a litre of clean water. To each of the above we can squeeze in lime, lemon, or orange, if available, to give taste and provide potassium. After adding the salt, it is traditional to taste it to make sure it is not saltier than tears—not always easy to do. If too salty, it can be harmful to the child.

2. Home-prepared liquid foods

Do not use these in children under six months of age, who, if being breastfed, simply need more breastmilk. To make one litre of rice water, grind any sort of ground rice into powder. Then take two to three large level tablespoons of the rice powder (total 50–80 g) and add this to one litre of water. Add two pinches of salt, boil and stir for five to seven minutes, cool, and feed.

Ground dried wheat, sorghum, millet, maize, or potato can be prepared in similar ways. Coconut juice can be given with two pinches of salt added per litre. Do not add any potassium. Weak tea can be used to which are added salt and sugar in the same amounts as in preparing a salt-sugar solution.

3. Packaged ORS

The new standard WHO-recommended packet should contain the following ingredients measured in mmol/L (note change from original WHO ORS packet):

Sodium: 75

Chloride: 65

Glucose, anhydrous: 75

Potassium: 20

Citrate: 10

Total osmolarity: 245

We should make sure that any packets used or recommended contain the substances in the correct proportions, are not overpriced, and have instructions in a language that is easily understood by the local people. Those with only written instructions will be unsafe for use by illiterate members of the community. Pictorial instructions are often useful.

Zinc supplementation has been found to reduce the duration and severity of diarrhoeal episodes and likelihood of subsequent infections for 2–3 months (15–18). Zinc supplements are generally accepted by both children and caregivers and are effective regardless of the type of common zinc salt used (zinc sulphate, zinc acetate, or zinc gluconate).

Routine use of zinc supplementation is at a dosage for 10–14 days of 20 mg per day for children older than six months, or 10 mg per day in those younger than six months (see. http://www.who.int/elena/titles/bbc/zinc_diarrhoea/en/). We should obtain zinc supplements when we can. They are not normally added to the current WHO ORS packets but that may change.

Feeding ORS correctly

- Feed young children from a spoon, giving one teaspoon every 1–2 minutes, or as often as they will take it. Give older children frequent sips from a cup.
- If the child vomits, wait 5–10 minutes, then try again more slowly. ORS, if given slowly, often helps to reduce the feeling of nausea in a child.
- Breastfed children should continue to be breastfed. Children under six months being exclusively breastfed should not be given ORS unless, for any reason, the mother is unable to produce sufficient breast milk, e.g. if she has severe diarrhoea herself.
- As soon as possible, start giving soft foods that are easy to digest in small amounts, e.g. bananas and cereals. As soon as the child has recovered from diarrhoea, give extra food, with a small amount of added vegetable oil.

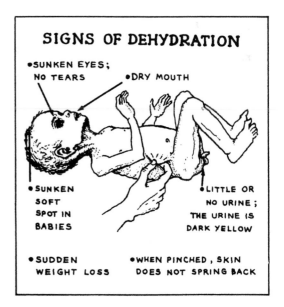

Figure 16.5 Signs of dehydration.

How much ORS to feed

1. Use Table 16.1 and Figure 16.5 to assess the level of dehydration.

2. All children with diarrhoea need to drink ORS or be given a suitable semi-liquid food after each stool. A child aged two years or more needs 100–200 ml after each stool. Children under two need 50–100 ml. If the child has some dehydration (Table 16.1) they need a catch-up phase, e.g. doubling the amount per stool for about four hours (See Figure 16.6).

Do not wait for each stool to give ORS. It must be given frequently or continuously when a child has diarrhoea. If the child has *severe dehydration* they will usually need a nasogastric tube for feeding and /or referral, but before referral also try to give ORS at as high a level as possible if they are still able to drink.

Teach all family members how to use ORS

Our aim is for every community member to know about ORS, and for the use of ORS to enter the folklore of the community. We will need to make sure that every member of every family:

- Knows how to make it.
- Knows how to use it.
- Believes in it so that when diarrhoea occurs ORS is given with confidence straightaway.

Here are some ways of encouraging the community to use ORS:

1. Understand local beliefs about diarrhoea.

Communities are often reluctant to use ORS. We must discover local beliefs about diarrhoea and why people are suspicious of ORS. For example, in parts of Africa and South Asia many people believe that giving fluid makes diarrhoea last longer; therefore, children with diarrhoea are not given fluids. This is quite logical when people believe that diarrhoea, rather than dehydration, kills the child.

Explain to parents that children die, not from the diarrhoea itself but because they dry out (See Figure 16.1). Show them an orange dried out in the sun or a leaky gourd that only keeps holding water if it is continually filled up. Explain also that giving fluid does not necessarily stop the diarrhoea. Mothers know this anyway. In fact, ORS may seem to make diarrhoea worse and children will often pass a stool shortly after receiving ORS. Explain to mothers that this may happen. (It happens less often with liquid food such as rice water).

In another example, people often believe that the only effective treatment for diarrhoea is a medicine, injection or intravenous drip given by doctors. These wrong ideas have to be discussed with the community until they are made aware of the situation. Unless objections are faced up to, people will listen politely, then ignore our advice.

2. Demonstrate the use of ORS in clinics.

Whenever a child comes to the clinic with diarrhoea, a health worker should show the mother or other care-giver how to make and how to feed ORS. Then the mother or caregiver gives ORS to her child on the spot (see Figure 16.6). Clinics can have special rehydration corners with everything ready for demonstration and use.

3. Demonstrate the use of ORS in homes.

This is usually the task of the CHW, who should continue until family members are confident. Make sure that CHWs themselves use ORS in their own families.

4. Help community leaders to know about ORS, to use it themselves and encourage its use in the community.

Teachers, religious leaders, and shopkeepers must all be aware of its value.

5. Teach children and pre-school children.

Older siblings can give it to younger ones. Teaching on ORS should be a central part of school health programmes and any Child-to-Child programme we may be organizing (see Appendix B). Pre-school children can be taught in crèches, and in India, in balwadis.

6. Encourage the community to tune in to radio and TV programmes about ORS.

Other methods to treat diarrhoea

Although using ORS is the most important thing to do, there is other information we need to know.

First, we must also know about and explain the importance of using zinc supplements, which are increasingly available. Details are given in the section 'Prepare ORS appropriately'.

Second, we must also know when to use antibiotics. Antibiotics should not be used routinely for children with diarrhoea. They rarely make any difference and can be dangerous, especially for children under five. Exceptions include dysentery caused by shigella,

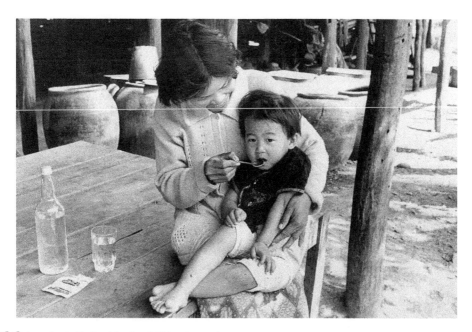

Figure 16.6 A mother in Thailand feeding ORS by glass and spoon.

typhoid and paratyphoid (enteric fever), or amoebiasis and giardiasis, which a lab usually needs to confirm. We should follow national guidelines or IMCI guidance on which antibiotic to use for these.

Third, when cholera is known or likely to be present (epidemic or endemic), the WHO recommends the oral cholera vaccine as part of a cholera control programme. We need to be aware of any control programmes, and also understand cholera diagnosis and treatment. Watery diarrhoea of three or more stools per day of recent onset (24–48 hours) with dehydration should be treated as cholera (until proven otherwise) using the nationally recommended antibiotic, usually azithromycin, doxycycline, or ciprofloxacin. In most instances, children under the age of two are more likely to have rotavirus infection unless previously immunized.

Lastly, we must know when to refer. We should follow the IMCI guidelines (see also Box 16.1). Usually, children admitted to a health facility need an initial IV or nasogastric bolus to treat their severe dehydration. Then the oral route using ORS should be restarted. If referral is not possible consider using a nasogastric tube to give a bolus if the health team is trained and correct equipment is available in the health centre.

Explaining how to prevent diarrhoea

Diarrhoea prevention and treatment must always be taught together. The worldwide 'WASH' strategy (*WA*ter, *S*anitation, and *H*ygiene) introduced by UNICEF in 2006 is explained more in Chapter 21 and can form the basis of our approach and our teaching.

There are certain key tasks for preventing diarrhoea:

1. Rotavirus vaccination.

In many developing countries about 40 per cent of hospital admissions for childhood diarrhoea are caused by rotavirus.[15] Check if this vaccination is available or is part of the immunization strategy of the country. If so, it should be given to all eligible children. If it is not available we can advocate for its use and introduction.[16]

2. Promote breastfeeding.

We should encourage mothers to breastfeed up to two years and promote no mixed feeding until six months (see Chapter 14)

3. Good personal hygiene.

We must also teach good personal hygiene, especially handwashing. The CHW should promote personal,

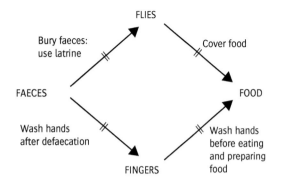

Figure 16.7 Diarrhoea prevention: breaking the '4F cycle'.

food, and water hygiene (See Figure 16.7). Regular hand-washing with soap has been shown to halve the rate of diarrhoea, even if the water is not clean. Infants and children (with help) and those giving and preparing food all need to wash their hands. Families that start using soap and water often gradually stop again, so we must continually reinforce this message, and address any barriers, such as the cost of soap. Establishing behavioural change is one of the biggest wins—and challenges—of community health.

4. Use the cleanest water possible.

We must teach the community to use the cleanest water available for drinking and preparing food. If possible, we can help to improve a community water source (Chapter 21). Where this is not possible, use other methods. Hygienically storing and using water in the home is both important and possible. We can advocate for and work alongside programmes for well-drilling if this is needed in our community or if there is a lack of clean water.[17]

5. Promote the use of latrines or if absolutely not yet possible, burying faeces.

Faeces are often highly infectious—especially children's (see Chapter 21).

6. Design and use fly traps.

7. Set up school teaching programmes on the importance of hygiene and sanitation.

Use Child-to-Child approaches (Appendix B). Make teaching specific, e.g. 'always wash both hands with soap after using the latrine'. See also the WHO's '12 Golden Rules of Food Preparation' (Chapter 14).

Evaluating the programme

After an agreed period, the programme should be evaluated to see if targets are being met:

1. Whether family members are using ORS in practice.

Supervisors can find this out informally by keeping alert, enquiring from community members and CHWs, and by doing spot checks. We can find out more formally by preparing a questionnaire for use on a sample of homes. We could ask:

- 'How often do you use ORS when your child has diarrhoea?' (Always, Frequently, Sometimes, Never).
- 'When your child last had diarrhoea, did you use ORS?'

2. Whether deaths from diarrhoea are decreasing.

We could use our own programme statistics to calculate this by comparing community surveys carried out before and after ORS was introduced, providing our sample is large and our methods are accurate. Alternatively, we could total the various causes of under-five deaths from CHW record books and clinic records. If deaths from diarrhoea have become less common, several factors may be responsible, such as improved nutrition (Chapter 14).

Acute respiratory infection (ARI): what we need to know

A recent combined programme has been set up by WHO and UNICEF known as The Integrated Global Action Plan for the Prevention and Control of Pneumonia and Diarrhoea (GAPPD). This recognizes that the only way to combat these two common, preventable diseases is to fight them together in an integrated approach.[18]

Defining ARI

Infections of the upper respiratory tract (cough, sore throat, and runny nose with or without fever) are very common, especially in children. Most only require care at home, including extra fluids, good nutrition, and

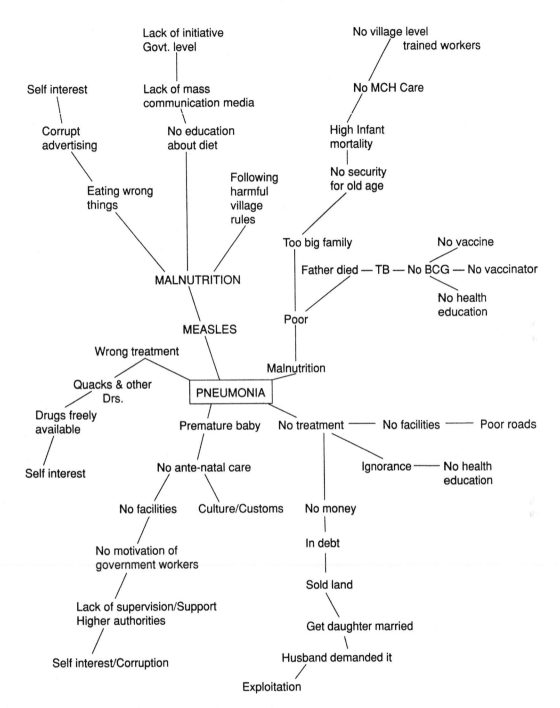

Figure 16.8 Some causes of pneumonia (from a workshop held in Bangladesh).

checking symptoms don't worsen. Acute respiratory infections (ARIs) are where infections reach the lower respiratory tract, causing cough or difficulty breathing.

There is always the risk that a mild upper respiratory tract infection can turn into ARI, most commonly pneumonia, often rapidly and without warning. Children who are weakened by measles, diarrhoea, malaria, or who are malnourished are especially at risk. Pneumonia kills nearly one million children per year.[19]

The two most important symptoms of pneumonia are easy to recognize:

1. Fast respiratory rate.

This is over about fifty breaths per minute in children aged 2–11 months, over about forty in children between 1–5 years of age. (Children under two months have variable breathing rates—two successive counts of 60 or more suggests pneumonia or severe ARI).

2. Lower chest wall in-drawing.

In addition, there may be cough, fever, and blue lips and, when very serious, stridor, drowsiness, and coma.[20]

About one quarter of all cases of pneumonia in under-fives will lead to death in a few days if untreated. This makes quick recognition and immediate treatment essential. Nearly all cases of ARI can be prevented and treated at community level without the need for a doctor.

Causes of ARI

Most cases of pneumonia in developing countries are caused by bacteria—in Africa, it is considered to be about four out of five. Most other cases are caused by viruses. Pneumococcus (*Streptococcus pneumoniae*) and *Haemophilus influenzae* type b (Hib) are two common bacterial causes and there are immunizations against both on the recommended WHO list for all countries. They are being rapidly added to national vaccination schedules and, along with measles and pertussis vaccines (as part of DPT), will save a huge number of lives.

Many fatal cases follow measles or milder infections in children with moderate or severe malnutrition. Untreated or incompletely treated TB increases the risk, as does advanced HIV infection where antiretrovirals are not available, or where cotrimoxazole is not being used as a prophylaxis.

Deaths from ARI occur mainly in poor, remote, or crowded conditions, or where there is a breakdown in civil society or in the aftermath of a disaster.

However, ARI is a risk in all resource-poor areas. Some of the factors leading to pneumonia in a village setting were recorded in a health workshop in Bangladesh. They are shown in the 'spider chart' in Figure 16.8 We can make a similar chart for our own area.

Acute respiratory infection (ARI): what we need to do

Preventing ARI

At community level we can reduce the risk of children dying from pneumonia in a number of ways.

Firstly, we can correct malnutrition (Chapter 14) and monitor children's weight using growth charts. They should be given extra amounts of nutritious food, with added oil, after any illness. Children who are malnourished should be given vitamin A and zinc supplements (especially after a diarrhoeal illness), and those who are anaemic should be given iron supplements.

Secondly, all children should be immunized. Check that all children are fully immunized against DPT, polio, TB, measles, Rotavirus and, where possible, Hib and Pneumococcus (Chapter 15).

Thirdly, we must educate about reducing indoor smoke. Indoor air pollution from cooking fires and tobacco, or environmental pollution affects the ability of the lungs to clear infection. If cooking is done inside with poor ventilation, the community can be encouraged to install chimneys or cook outside (Chapter 21).

Fourthly, tobacco smoking must be strongly discouraged. We can explain that smoke causes serious lung (and eye) disease in children and that smoking in the household puts children at risk through passive smoking (Figure 16.9). It is estimated that passive smoking, i.e. inhaling cigarette smoke from others, contributes to the death of 600,000 people each year.[21] Pollution in cities can also increase the risk of pneumonia and other forms of lung disease, e.g. asthma. All these forms of air pollution are often present together in crowded, stressful, urban conditions.

Figure 16.8 gives a wider picture of "up-stream" actions that can be taken.

Recognizing and treating ARI

Box 16.2 gives overall guidance on caring for those with ARI.

Plan A: Simple cough or cold, and no pneumonia

A simple cough and cold may present with or without fever and a breathing rate less than fifty per minute in infants aged two to eleven months, less than forty

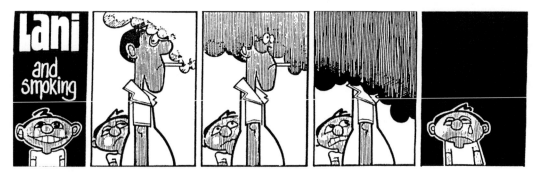

Figure 16.9 Smoking kills smokers, children, and all others who breathe in the smoke.

in children over one year old and no lower chest in-drawing. In this instance, give supportive treatment only (see 'Supportive treatment and feeding'). Antibiotics are not needed. Check regularly to make sure the child does not deteriorate. If he/she does, follow Plan B.

Plan B: Non-severe pneumonia

Non-severe pneumonia presents with a cough with breathing rate more than fifty breaths per minute in infants between two and eleven months, and more than forty per minute in children over one year old, but there is no visible indrawing of the lower chest wall. Here we should provide supportive treatment plus antibiotics, and treat at home. Be vigilant for any deterioration, which may be sudden. If deterioration occurs, follow Plan C.

Plan C: Severe pneumonia

A child presenting with severe pneumonia will be seriously ill with breathing rates faster than fifty per minute in infants 2–11 months, and more than forty per minute in children over one year old. This will be accompanied by indrawing of the ribs plus either vomiting, blue lips, stridor (noisy breathing), drowsiness, or coma. In this situation, give antibiotics (by injection if possible) and refer immediately, accompanying the mother and child or arranging escort. If injection is not possible attempt giving antibiotics by mouth, especially in a poor community where there is no place to refer or it is too far to go. Research shows that high-dose oral amoxicillin is as effective as injectable penicillin even in severe pneumonia, providing the child can swallow it.[22]

Saving lives in ARI depends on the recognition of symptoms early, having antibiotics always available in the community, and treating cases without delay.

Types of antibiotic use in ARI

The choice of antibiotic will depend on cost, availability, and local and national guidelines. There are various possible choices.

1. Amoxicillin three times daily.

This is suitable for all children except those allergic to penicillin. For those too young to swallow pills, the tablet can be crushed or the capsule opened, added to milk or other suitable liquid, and fed at the correct dose. Research suggests that taking amoxicillin for just three rather than five days is just as effective in non-severe pneumonia (but not severe pneumonia) providing no doses are missed.[23]

2. Cotrimoxazole given twice daily for five to seven days.

This approach is suitable for all children over six weeks of age except those who are allergic to sulfa drugs. It is cheaper than amoxicillin.

3. Benzyl penicillin injection once daily for five to seven days.

This approach can be used in clinics for children who are seriously ill and unable to take medicine by mouth. When using injectable penicillin, ask the parent if the child has ever had any reaction or rash following a previous injection or medicine. If they have, do not give it.

More details on treating children with pneumonia are given in the WHO Evidence Summaries.[24]

It is important that we remember that antibiotics should not be used for ordinary coughs and colds. They are unnecessary and their use increases antibiotic resistance so that these life-saving drugs become less effective. It is worth noting there is often confusion about antibiotic resistance and we may need to explain that it is the *disease-causing organisms* that may become resistant

> ### Box 16.2 **Supportive treatment and feeding in ARI**
>
> **Teach family caregivers to carry out the following in all cases of ARI:**
>
> 1. Give plenty of fluids—dehydration leads to death in pneumonia as well as diarrhoea.
> 2. Reduce fever by removing extra clothes and giving paracetamol, but not aspirin.
> 3. Give frequent energy-rich drinks, e.g. fruit juices, soups, etc.
> 4. Children being breastfed should continue, even if their noses seem blocked.
> 5. Continue giving extra foods until children have regained their original weight.
> 6. Babies in cots and cradles should be taken out and unswaddled so they can cough freely.
> 7. Reduce indoor smoke pollution, and ensure no one smokes tobacco inside the house or anywhere near the child.
> 8. Watch for any sign of deterioration and take immediate action as described.

to antibiotics, and not the people who are ill. Box 16.2 provides information about supportive treatment and feeding in ARI.

ARI: the role of the CHW

There is now strong evidence on the effectiveness of CHWs in the treatment of ARI. A large study by Save the Children in Pakistan compared CHWs treating children with pneumonia by using oral antibiotics with referring such children to hospital following existing guidelines. Treatment failures occurred 50 per cent less often in the CHW treatment group.[25] With such compelling evidence we now need good reasons NOT to train CHWs in the careful case management of children with ARI.[26] CHWs have the advantage of living in the community, being easily available, and being able to start treatment early before the disease has become too serious.

For example, BRAC, Bangladesh gave three days of intensive training to community health volunteers in the recognition and treatment of children with ARI. These volunteers were mainly poor, middle-aged women with just five years of schooling. Each was assigned 100–120 households. The volunteers identified children with pneumonia and treated them at household level, referring severe cases. They proved to be almost as accurate, and more cost-effective, than physicians in identifying and treating ARI, provided they were carefully trained and managed.[27]

Most of the nearly one million deaths caused by ARI in the world today could be prevented if each community had an effective, well-trained CHW, with a reliable supply of antibiotics. Furthermore, we could extend this model and consider giving parents the antibiotics to use at home when signs of severe ARI develop. Often, for a variety of reasons, CHWs are not available or families live in remote locations. This approach would need very careful teaching of parents, reliable supplies of antibiotics, CHWs who are already treating ARI effectively, and excellent management (See Figure 16.10).[28]

Teaching

The CHW will teach her community how to prevent and treat ARI, its dangers, and its warning signs. She will demonstrate to parents and older siblings that a fast breathing rate or chest indrawing spells danger and that the child must be brought to her at once. It is not necessary for the parent to be able to read a watch, or to count to 50. With practice, nearly everyone can learn to recognize fast breathing by careful observation alone. The CHW will make sure that all community members understand the two golden rules: children with simple coughs and colds need no antibiotics, and children with fast breathing rates and/or with chest indrawing need to start antibiotics with supportive treatment without delay.

Encouraging immunization of children

The CHW needs to ensure that the vaccines mentioned earlier are taken up. By using a family folder and insert system, or an electronic record system that reveals 'gaps' in coverage, the CHW can focus her time on encouraging the families of defaulting children. Often these are the most vulnerable because of poverty, remoteness, or lack of education.

Supplying antibiotics

The CHW will ideally keep a supply of antibiotics. If this is part of what the community knows and expects, this supply must NEVER run out (Figure 16.10). Community members will only reliably trust and use their CHW if they can be confident she always has the correct

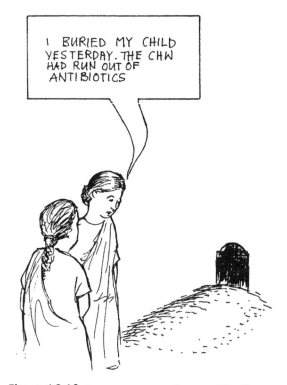

Figure 16.10 Home treatment may have saved her life.

medicines available for those illnesses she is expected to treat. If the community perceives that the CHW cannot be relied upon, children will continue to be taken on long, unnecessary journeys to distant clinics and doctors. The CHW should use the correct antibiotic at the correct dose for the correct length of time, taking care that the parent knows how to use it, and knows how to finish the course. The CHW will record details in her book.

Referring seriously ill children

The CHW must be able to refer seriously ill children. Ideally, she will recognize a child needing referral, start the child on antibiotics at once (if the child can still swallow), and send or accompany the child and parent to the nearest reliable referral centre without delay. NB: we must remember that many children especially in sub-Saharan Africa, do not have access to healthcare and referral is not an option.

Follow-up on children with ARI

The CHW will follow up all children with ARI until they have completely recovered, regained their weight, and resumed growth. She will refer any child who has a persistent cough for more than three weeks (some guidance suggests two weeks) to the clinic or doctor to check for TB, or another cause of persistent cough, e.g. asthma.

As part of the follow-up, the CHW will try to identify preventable risk factors in the home. She will encourage immunizations, good nutrition, and breastfeeding, and discourage smoking. Regular handwashing with soap, for both children and caregivers, has been shown to reduce the likelihood of children getting pneumonia.[28] She will give zinc supplements if available, and if the child is not receiving regular vitamin A supplements these should also be given (Chapter 14). Finally, the use of long-term cotrimoxazole in children who are HIV-positive prolongs their lives. In many programmes, the CHW will be the most appropriate person, either singly or as part of a home care team, to make sure such children receive regular supplies and take them daily.

Malaria: what we need to know

About 3.2 billion people in 95 countries live in areas where malaria is present, and about 1.2 billion live in high-transmission areas. Around half a million people die of malaria annually and an estimated 90 per cent of these deaths are in sub-Saharan Africa. More than two-thirds of malarial deaths occur in children under five.[29] Where malaria is endemic (present all the year round) children are at greatest risk between six months (when immunity inherited from the mother fades) and about five years (when their own immunity increases).

Malaria is becoming less common in some countries and is tending to concentrate in hot spots of high transmission. It is also spreading to some new areas, partly because of global warming and partly where control programmes are difficult to carry out, e.g. South Sudan. The 2018 World Malaria Report gives worrying increases and inadequate coverage (see World Malaria Map Figure 16. 11).[30]

Malaria control efforts appeared to work well during the 1970s but malaria deaths started to increase from

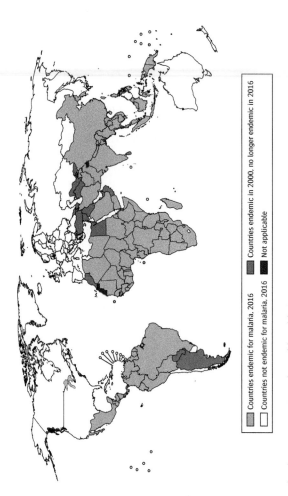

Figure 16.11 Global distribution of malaria transmission risk. World Health Organization, 2016.

Legend:
- Countries endemic for malaria, 2016
- Countries not endemic for malaria, 2016
- Countries endemic in 2000, no longer endemic in 2016
- Not applicable

1980, reaching a peak in 2004, and dropping by 2010,[31] owing to enhanced control measures and priority from donors, especially the Global Fund. Three measures have made a big difference: the use of long-lasting insecticide-treated bed nets, an increase in the use of artemisinin-based drugs, and greater coverage from insecticide spraying. At the same time, the spread of resistance to antimalarial medicines continues to be a threat and finding an effective malaria vaccine is taking longer than many had hoped. Currently the RTS,S vaccine against falciparum malaria is due to be piloted in sub-Saharan Africa.[32]

The Roll Back Malaria (RBM) programme was started in 1998 by four agencies working together: the WHO, UNICEF, The World Bank, and the United Nations Development Programme. RBM consists of regional and national strategies to reduce malaria through governments, health workers, and communities working together in partnership.[33]

The control and treatment of malaria has become more stable but there are still changes and developments about which we should enquire in the country where we are working. We need to know details of any control programme in our area, and work in association with them. Within a national malaria control programme, community-based healthcare can greatly reduce the incidence of malaria in a target population.

Malaria: what we need to do

Preventing malaria

Malaria is caused by the *Plasmodium* parasite carried by the *Anopheles* mosquito. People are infected when a *Plasmodium*-carrying female bites them, thereby injecting *Plasmodium* into their bloodstream. Non-carrier mosquitoes that bite people with malaria become carriers themselves and so the infection continues. Mosquitoes can breed in very small amounts of water, such as water-filled wheel ruts and hoof prints. All sources of standing water need to be identified and dealt with. These measures are also effective against Aedes mosquitoes that carry dengue fever, chikungunya, and Zika.

Ways to reduce breeding mosquitoes

1. Remove or fill areas near houses where mosquitoes breed, such as holes, ditches, the tops of bamboo canes, old cans, and tyres.
2. Drain areas where water collects, such as near boreholes or around standpipes.
3. Build soakage pits for disposal of household waste water.[30]
4. Cover wells and drains.
5. Plan any new building or development programmes with care so that new breeding sites are not created.
6. Clear away vegetation from the banks of streams so that water flows more quickly.
7. Introduce larva-eating fish, e.g. guppy, into areas where mosquitoes breed, e.g. rice paddies and small reservoirs.

8. Add polystyrene beads to pit latrines and septic tanks.
9. Pour petroleum oil onto the surface of small amounts of standing water that cannot easily be drained.

Kill adult mosquitoes

Spraying insecticides was the main form of malaria control until the 1970s. Now it remains one important aspect of control programmes. It is now often known as insecticide residual spraying (IRS). Four classes of insecticide can be used. The best and safest are pyrethroids, although mosquito resistance to these is developing. Others include organochlorines, e.g. DDT, organophosphates, and carbamates.

For *personal protection* spray pyrethroid insecticides into rooms before going to bed.

For *community protection* work alongside any teams that spray residual (persistent) insecticides on the walls of houses.

DDT is effective for this and its careful use is approved by RBM, although at the time of writing there is debate about its widespread re-introduction and other alternatives are being actively sought.[34] Health committee members can accompany any spraying team to explain why it is being done.

Prevent mosquitoes from biting people

This is becoming an increasingly important part of malaria control.

1. Use bed nets.

Long-lasting insecticide impregnated bed nets (LLINs) have now become the most effective way of reducing insect bites and the incidence of malaria, as *Anopheles* mosquitoes mainly bite at night and early morning and late evening. Priority groups are children under the age of five and pregnant women, but it is ideal if all family members use them. In many countries, bed nets for priority groups are distributed free. They use safe pyrethroid insecticides, which work well in most areas; however, resistance to pyrethroids is increasing. Where this occurs a more effective bed net known as a PBO LLIN can be used and is being introduced by SHO. The most effective LLINs can be used for at least three years with repeated washing. Wherever bed nets are widely used malaria becomes less common and fewer children die. Even nets that are not treated with insecticide give some protection.

2. Hang insecticide-treated netting in windows and curtains in doorways if the house design is appropriate.

This reduces malaria but is less effective than bed-nets.

3. Apply insect repellent (e.g. containing DEET) or burn mosquito coils.

These are useful for protecting those especially at risk, or for use in the evening before climbing under bed-nets. Many poorer families cannot afford these.

4. Where local house design makes this possible screen windows and doors to prevent mosquitoes entering the house, and keep doors and windows closed from an hour before sunset until well after sunrise.

The malaria community control programme

For the most effective malaria control, each district selects a variety of measures appropriate for local circumstances. These alter from time to time owing to changes in best practice and changing community and country-wide priorities.

Example 1: Indonesia has had success using a combination of case finding and treatment, indoor insecticide spraying, breeding larvicidal fish, tree-planting in marshy areas, and the use of bed nets.

Example 2: Parts of Tanzania have been experimenting with robust health promotion and social marketing of bed nets.

Example 3: In Pakistan, sponging of cattle (on which mosquitoes feed and rest) with deltamethrin insecticide has proved effective.

Example 4: Vietnam has been very successful distributing bed nets to all households, with biannual re-treatment, training staff in health posts to diagnose malaria using microscopes, and facilitating early diagnosis and treatment. There is a reliable drug supply, and a programme of community involvement and health education. Central to all stages is active partnership between the health programme, the community and national malaria control strategies.

If we are working in an area where malaria is a major cause of death and illness we can follow steps to control malaria within the community.

Step 1. Meet with the district medical officer (DMO)

At an early stage we need to meet with the DMO or other official responsible for any RBM or IMCI programme. This is to learn about national control programmes, discover any district or local strategies, and discuss ways in which the programme can tie in with any government plans. It is very important that everyone works together.

Step 2. Assess the local malarial situation

Before making any plans, we need to find out how common malaria is, and if it is considered an important health problem by the community. Questions we can ask include:

- How common is malaria?
- Is malaria considered an important health problem in the community?
- Which ages are most affected?
- How many (ideally what percentage) of children under five die from malaria?
- Is malaria seasonal or irregular (epidemic), or present the whole year round (endemic)?
- Where/what are the main malaria breeding sites?
- What malaria treatment is recommended for our area or our country?
- Is insecticide residual spraying (IRS) being carried out in our area?
- Is intermittent preventative treatment (IPT) recommended for either pregnant women, infants, or both?
- Are there local beliefs and practices that affect treatment?
- Where and how do community members currently receive treatment?

- What treatments do community members receive, if any?
- Do community members buy treatment and self-treat at home?
- Is malaria either overtreated or undertreated?
- Are mosquito nets distributed free or easily available?
  - Are they treated with long-lasting insecticide?
  - Are they actually used? If not, why not?

Step 3. Assessing community resources

- How much community understanding is there?
- How much community commitment to action is present?
- What control measures are already in place?
- Does the community have resources to buy bed nets or effective treatments?

This information—on both the local malarial situation and resources of the community—can be discovered from:

- A community survey, Participatory Appraisal or discussion with community leaders, teachers and CHWs. This also gives us a chance to discuss how we can work on a programme together.
- The DMO or malaria control officials, such as those working in association with RBM or with the latest district or national initiative.
- Records from the nearest hospital or clinic.
- Our own personal observation.

Knowing answers to these questions will help us select effective control strategies that are acceptable to the community, usually a combination of community-wide measures and personal protection.

Depending on one form of control alone will be insufficient.

Step 4. Plan with community and government

During these sessions we can match up the most effective control strategies with their acceptability to the community. We can liaise between community and government. We can then draw up an action plan for adopting each control measure.

Step 5. Train the CHW and health committee

We may wish to carry out a pilot project, before we introduce any community-wide programme, such as distributing LLINs.

The CHW will have a key role in the care and treatment of malaria, backed up by the health team. She will have a reliable supply of the nationally recommended drug for treatment and know how to use it. Sometimes a specially trained volunteer will be dedicated to the work in a malaria control programme. For example, in Uganda a man named Steven was one of a number of farmers trained as volunteers in a government programme of home-based management. He kept antimalarials and was available constantly for anyone in his village needing treatment. Mothers in this community no longer have to walk miles to the nearest clinic.

- Health committee members or a specially trained malaria action group can work on community-wide prevention.

For example, they can mobilize the community to clear malarial breeding sites, or plant trees in marshy areas for drainage. They can work with the health team and experts to set up fish-breeding ponds from which larva-eating fish can be distributed. They can liaise with government spraying team.

Step 6. Organize a community bed net programme

This is an effective way of reducing malaria, and saving children's lives. These are some guidelines:

1. We become involved only if malaria is a serious problem in the community, and a common cause for children dying. We can this find out as described above.
2. The community should be fully involved and interested in working with the programme and the government. Where malaria is a strong felt need this usually happens easily.
3. Careful training needs to be given to health committee members, women's groups or others involved in management.
4. LLINs must be available at a price most people can afford.

Encourage people to obtain free nets, or to seek out reduced price nets through subsidised sources. If these are not available, the community and programme can advocate for nets to be supplied at affordable prices, or free.

5. The programme must be sustainable after any initial subsidy or donation is no longer available.
6. A pilot programme should be run first, to to discover and solve any problems that come to light.

For example, in hot climates bed nets may be unpleasant to sleep under, and children may take time to get used to sleeping under a net.

A question to think about: Giving out free bed-nets sounds appealing and can lead to quick reductions in the number of malaria cases in children. The question we need to ask is: *When the funding stops and no free nets are available, will families be willing to buy their own nets?*

An observation to make: If nets have been distributed in the community where we work, how many are being used correctly, with children, in particular, sleeping under them, and how many are being used inappropriately, as fishing nets, for storage, or resold as a source of cash?

If LLINs are not available we can organize a programme to soak regular bed nets to make them extra effective against mosquitos. Box 16.3 shows how to organize a programme to soak bed nets.

Advantages of using treated nets:

- They kill mosquitoes and reduce their numbers.
- Bed nets protect from other insects, snakes, and scorpions.
- Bed net users usually sleep better and have fewer skin infections.
- Children are more likely to survive, and pregnant mothers are less likely to become seriously ill or to miscarry.

NB: even nets that have holes or are incorrectly tucked in to beds still give protection (but nets should still be mended and tucked in carefully).

Managing and treating malaria

The problem

Malaria is dangerous and can kill rapidly. It also mimics other diseases, making diagnosis difficult. The malaria parasite is developing resistance to many commonly used, relatively cheap types of malaria treatment, such as chloroquine and in south East Asia, mefloquine. Effective new treatments are increasingly available at subsidized rates. However, they are still too expensive or unavailable for many families, especially those in poorer or more remote areas. In sub-Saharan Africa, the WHO now recommends as first choice artemisinin-combined therapy (ACT) which comes in several formulations: artemether/lumefantrine (Coartem) is one of the most commonly used. It is safe and effective, but unless

---

> ### Box 16.3 **How to organize a programme to soak bed nets**
>
> 1. Fix a day when members of all community households will come to soak their nets.
> 2. Prepare the site.
>   a. An open-air site is safest.
>   b. Have long rubber gloves and bowls available.
> 3. Wash and dry used nets before treatment.
> 4. Make up the solution needed and store it in clean drums or tubs.
>   a. Different substances are used—permethrin is the most common.
>   b. Different nets are used, which absorb different amounts of solution.
>   c. Follow instructions carefully and calculate the amount of solution needed according to the type of insecticide, type and size of net and total number to be soaked.
> 5. Dip the nets.
>   a. Soak thoroughly, then wring out over the container.
>   b. Nets should be dry and clean before soaking.
> 6. Dry the nets.
>   a. Either hang them up, or better still lie them flat.
>   b. A plastic bag will be needed to take the wet net home.
> 7. Clear up and clean up.
>   a. Unused solution should be kept.
>   b. No permethrin or other insecticide should be disposed of near lakes, river or water, as it kills fish and invertebrates.
> 8. Use the opportunity to teach families about other key aspects of childcare such as the use of ORS.

---

heavily subsidized, it is too expensive for most families. At the same time, many of the most vulnerable people live too far from any clinic. Pregnant women and children under five are at greatest risk and they find it even harder to reach treatment.

Recognizing malaria

We must learn about the pattern of malaria in the programme area: how common it is, what time of year it occurs (usually during and just after the rainy season), the symptoms most commonly seen, and other diseases that mimic it. We must also be able to recognize cases of malaria.

Mild malaria

Mild malaria is characterized by fever above 37.5 °C plus one or more of the following: headache, shivering, sweating, vomiting, cough, or diarrhoea. Ask about and observe other symptoms, as there may be another obvious cause, such as ARI or measles, especially where malaria is relatively uncommon. Typhoid fever, acute schistosomiasis (bilharzia), and a range of viral infections, e.g. dengue and chikungunya, can all mimic malaria. To check for fever, use a clinical thermometer, a new crystal thermometer, or estimate with the back of the hand. Studies show that many mothers can estimate fever in their child reliably, but may find it hard to understand—or afford—a thermometer.

Severe malaria

Any or all the symptoms of mild malaria will be present in severe cases, but they will also include one or more of the following: very high fever (39 °C or above), drowsiness, coma, rapid deep breathing, convulsions, very pale mucous membranes, yellow whites of eyes, or cold clammy skin with weak pulse. Many of these severe cases will be in children under five years of age. Where malaria is common, treatment should usually be based on symptoms and unless reliable diagnostic facilities are available locally, not depend on blood slide examinations (which are often not available, cause delay, and may be inaccurate).

Confirming and treating malaria

Rapid diagnostic tests (RDTs) are increasingly available and can be used alongside or instead of malaria slides. CHWs can often be trained how to use RDTs to make diagnosis and treatment more accurate.

Roles and facilities

Mothers and care-givers: in remote, seriously affected areas, mothers can be trained to identify malaria and hold treatment supplies.

CHWs must be carefully trained to recognize and treat where possible with a reliable supply of medicines, and know how and when to refer.

Health centres are where severe cases should be referred and treated without delay. This is important because without accurate diagnosis malaria can be overtreated, especially where medicines are held at home. Other serious diseases can be missed when it is assumed that every case of fever is malaria.

Reliable transport systems are needed so people with suspected malaria are able to reach the nearest reliable centre for diagnosis and treatment. All easier said than done, but an ideal project for a VHC to work on with creative solutions.

Recommended treatments

When recommending treatment, we should follow national guidelines to make sure the medicines we use are the most effective for the area in which we are working. There are wide variations between Africa and affected countries in Asia, the Pacific, and Central and South America. Using dual therapy (two medicines together) is often most effective and helps to slow the spread of resistance. Ideally, this means using ACT where it is available and affordable.

Artesunate suppositories are an underused method of saving lives in remote areas. Transfer to a reliable referral centre, if available, should still be done, but the child is less likely to die in transit if treated by suppository first.

Pregnant women

- Those in their first pregnancy are especially prone to malaria. It can be dangerous for mother and child.
- Make sure infected women are treated promptly, take their full course of medicine and are reassured that the medicine is not harmful to them or their child—on the contrary, is lifesaving.
- Provide them with iron and folic acid tablets.
- To reduce the likelihood or severity of malaria in pregnancy we should also give Intermittent Preventive Treatment in pregnancy (IPTp).

The WHO recommends IPTp with sulfadoxine-pyrimethamine (IPTp-SP, aka Fansidar) in all areas in Africa with moderate to high malaria transmission. This should be given to all pregnant women at each scheduled antenatal visit, starting at the beginning of the second trimester (NB: *not during the first trimester*). Ideally, there should be at least four antenatal care visits (Chapter 17). A recent study in Ghana showed that IPTp in pregnancy can also improve birth weights and reduce neonatal mortality.[35]

Infants

Use intermittent preventative treatment in infants (IPTi), which is a full course of antimalarial medicine delivered to infants through routine immunization services, regardless of whether the child is infected with malaria. The WHO recommends IPTi-SP in most areas of sub-Saharan Africa with moderate to high malaria transmission as it reduces anaemia and malaria frequency and severity.

For example, in one Tanzanian programme, sulfadoxine/pyrimethamine (SP) was given as a single dose at two, three, and nine months, with expanded programme on immunization rounds. This reduced childhood malarial attacks by nearly two-thirds and halved severe malarial anaemia.[36]

Evaluating the programme

Evaluation may partly be done by malaria control experts, under the RBM programme, using RBM evaluation methods. However, community-based monitoring and evaluation is useful to show how effective our programme is. We can find out, for example, the levels of community satisfaction with the malaria programme (rank 1 to 5). We can also determine how much the amount of standing water has been reduced in the community, what proportion of under-fives and pregnant women regularly sleep under an LLIN, how numbers of patients with suspected malaria attending the CHW or health post have changed, as well as changes in the number and percentage of children dying from malaria.

Further reading and resources

Kellerman R, Bope E. *Conn's Current Therapy 2018*. London: Elsevier; 2017.

Sabot O, Schroder K, Yamey G, Montagu D. Scaling up oral rehydration salts and zinc for the treatment of diarrhoea. *British Medical Journal*. 2012; 344; e940.

UNICEF. *One is too many: Ending child deaths from pneumonia and diarrhoea*. 2016. https://data.unicef.org/wp-content/uploads/2016/11/UNICEF-Pneumonia-Diarrhoea-report2016-web-version_final.pdf

Wardlaw T, Salama P, Brocklehurst C, Chopra M, Mason E. Diarrhoea: Why children are still dying and what can be done. *The Lancet*. 2009; 375 (9718): 870–2.

World Health Organization. *Caring for the sick child in the community*. Geneva: World Health Organization; 2011. Available from: http://www.who.int/maternal_child_adolescent/documents/imci_community_care/en/index.htm.

World Health Organization. *Management of severe malaria: A practical handbook*. 3rd ed. Geneva: World Health Organization; 2012. Available from: http://apps.who.int/iris/bitstream/10665/79317/1/9789241548526_eng.pdf

World Health Organization. *The treatment of diarrhoea: A manual for physicians and other senior health workers*. Geneva: World Health Organization; 2005. Available from: http://www.who.int/maternal_child_adolescent/documents/9241593180/en/

World Health Organization. *Treatment of diarrhoea*. Geneva: World Health Organization; 2005. Available from: http://www.who.int/maternal_child_adolescent/documents/9241593180/en/ This is the current standard WHO guidebook.

World Health Organization. *IMCI chart booklet*. Geneva: World Health Organization; 2014. Available from: http://apps.who.int/iris/bitstream/10665/104772/16/9789241506823_Chartbook_eng.pdf

World Health Organization. *World Malaria Report*. 2018. Available from: https://www.who.int/malaria/publications/world-malaria-report-2018/en/

Websites

Integrated Management of Childhood Illness (IMCI). Available from: http://www.who.int/maternal_child_adolescent/documents/imci/en/

Rehydration Project. Available from: http://rehydrate.org/solutions/index.html Resources on homemade and packaged oral rehydration solution.

Roll Back Malaria Partnership. Available from: http://www.rbm.who.int.

World Health Organization. Maternal, newborn, child and adolescent health document centre. Available from: http://www.who.int/maternal_child_adolescent/documents/en/ Especially useful is the document giving protocols for care of childhood illnesses by CHWs. Available from: http://www.who.int/maternal_child_adolescent/documents/9789241548045-2.pdf

References

1. UNICEF/World Health Organization. *Levels and trends in child mortality*. 2018. Available from: https://www.unicef.org/publications/index_103264.html

2. World Health Organization. *Factsheet: Children—reducing mortality*. 2018. Available from: https://www.who.int/news-room/fact-sheets/detail/children-reducing-mortality

3. United Nations. Convention on the Rights of the Child. 1989. Available from: http://www.ohchr.org/EN/ProfessionalInterest/Pages/CRC.aspx

4. World Health Organization/UNICEF. *Children and road traffic injury*. 2004. Available from: http://www.who.int/violence_injury_prevention/child/injury/world_report/Road_traffic_injuries_english.pdf

5. World Health Organization. *Factsheet: Drowning*. 2017. Available from: http://www.who.int/mediacentre/factsheets/fs347/en/

6. Hyder A, Lunnen J. Reduction of childhood mortality through millennium development goal 4 will not be maximised unless injury prevention is integrated into the overall plan. *British Medical Journal*. 2011; 342: d357.

7. The World Health Organization. *Integrated Management of Childhood Illness*. 2017. Available from: http://www.who.int/maternal_child_adolescent/topics/child/imci/en/

8. Patton G, Sawyer SM, Santelli JS, Ross DA, Afifi R, Allen NB, et al. Our future: A Lancet commission on adolescent health and wellbeing. *The Lancet*. 2016, 387 (10036): 2423–78.

9. World Health Organization. *Adolescent health epidemiology*. 2017. Available from: http://www.who.int/maternal_child_adolescent/epidemiology/adolescence/en/

10. Ki-Moon B. Sustainability—engaging future generations now. *The Lancet*. 2016; 387 (10036): 2356–58.

11. UNICEF. *One is too many: Ending child deaths from pneumonia and diarrhoea*. 2016. Available from: https://data.unicef.org/wp-content/uploads/2016/11/UNICEF-Pneumonia-Diarrhoea-report2016-web-version_final.pdf

12. Rehydration Project. *Oral rehydration solutions: Made at home*. 2014. Available from: rehydrate.org/solutions/homemade.htm

13. Water with sugar and salt. *The Lancet*. 1978; 2 (8084): 300–01.

14. Ramani S, Kang G. Viruses causing childhood diarrhoea in the developing world. *Current Opinion in Infectious Diseases*. 2009; 22 (5): 477–82.

15. Isanaka, S, Guindo, O, Langendorf, C, Seck, AM, Plikaytis, B, Sayinzoga-Makombe, N, et al. Efficacy of a Low-Cost, Heat-Stable Oral Rotavirus Vaccine in Niger. *New English Journal of Medicine*. 2017; 376: 1121–1130.

16. Escamilla V, Wagner B, et al. Effect of deep tube well use on childhood diarrhoea in Bangladesh. *Bulletin of the World Health Organization*. 2011; 89 (7): 521–7.

17. World Health Organization. *GAPPD: Ending preventable child deaths from pneumonia and diarrhoea by 2025*. 2013. Available from: http://www.who.int/woman_child_accountability/news/gappd_2013/en/index1.html

18. World Health Organization. *Slideset—Acute respiratory infections*. Available from: http://www.who.int/maternal_child_adolescent/documents/pdfs/cah_01_10_tsslides_ari.pdf

19. Öberg M, Jaakkola M, Woodward A, Peruga A, Prüss-Ustün A. Worldwide burden of disease from exposure to second-hand smoke: A retrospective analysis of data from 192 countries. *The Lancet*. 2011; 377 (9760): 139–46.

20. Addo-Yobo E, Chisaka N, Hassan M, Hibberd P, Lozano JM, Jeena P, et al. Oral amoxicillin versus injectable penicillin for severe pneumonia in children aged 3 to 59 months: A randomised multicentre equivalency study. *The Lancet*. 2004; 364 (9440): 1141–8.

21. Agarwal G, Aswathi S, Kabra SK, Kaul A, Singhi S, Walter SD, et al. Three day versus five day treatment with amoxicillin for non-severe pneumonia in young children: A multicentre randomised controlled trial. *British Medical Journal*. 2004; 328 (7477): 791.

22. World Health Organization. *Revised WHO classification and treatment of childhood pneumonia at health facilities: Evidence Summaries*. 2014. Available from: http://apps.who.int/iris/bitstream/10665/137319/1/9789241507813_eng.pdf

23. Bari A, Sadruddin S, Khan A, Khan I, Khan A, Lehri IA, et al. Community case management of severe pneumonia with oral amoxicillin in children aged 2–59 months in Haripur district Pakistan: A cluster randomized trial. *The Lancet*. 2011; 378 (9805): 1796–1803.

24. Molyneux E, Graham S. Community management of severe pneumonia in children, Editorial. *The Lancet*. 2011; 378 (9805): 1762–4.

25. Hadi A. Management of acute respiratory infections by community health volunteers: experience of Bangladesh Rural Advancement Committee (BRAC). *Bulletin of the World Health Organization*. 2003; 81 (3): 183–9.

26. Hazir T, Fox LM, Bin Nisar Y, Fox MP, Pervaiz Ashraf Y, Macleod WB, et al. Ambulatory short-course high dose oral amoxicillin for treatment of severe pneumonia in children: A randomized equivalency trial. *The Lancet*. 2008, 371 (9606): 45–56.

27. Luby S, Agboatwalla M, Feikin DR, Painter J, Billhimer W, Altaf A, et al. Effect of handwashing on child health: A randomised controlled trial. *The Lancet*. 2005; 366 (9481): 225–33.

28. World Health Organization. *Global Health Observatory (GHO) Data: Malaria*. 2015. Available from: http://www.who.int/gho/malaria/en/

29. Murray CJL, Rosenfeld LC, Lim SS, Andrews KG, Foreman KJ, Haring D, et al. Global malaria mortality between 1980 and 2010: A systematic analysis. *The Lancet*. 2012; 379 (9814): 413–31.

30. World Health Organization. *News Release—WHO welcomes global health funding for malaria vaccine*. 2016. Available from: http://www.who.int/mediacentre/news/releases/2016/funding-malaria-vaccine/en/

31. Roll Back Malaria Partnership. 2017. Available from: http://www.rollbackmalaria.org

32. Soakage pit for proper disposal of waste water. In *Environmentally Sound Technologies for Women in Agriculture*. Silang: IIRR; 1996. Available from: http://collections.infocollections.org/ukedu/en/d/Jii01ee/9.6.html

33. Bouwman H, van den Berg H, Kylin H. DDT and malaria prevention: Addressing the paradox. *Environmental Health Perspectives*. 2011; 119 (6): 744–7.

34. Protopopo N, Mosha J, Lukole E, Charlwood J, Wright A, Mwalimu C, et al. Effectiveness of a long-lasting piperonyl butoxide-treated insecticidal net and indoor residual spray interventions, separately and together, against malaria transmitted by pyrethroid-resistant mosquitoes: a cluster, randomised controlled, two-by-two factorial design trial. *The Lancet*. 2018; 391: 1577–88.

35. Tutu E, Browne E, Lawson B. Effect of sulphadoxine-pyrimethamine on neonatal birth weight and perceptions on its impact on malaria in pregnancy in an intermittent preventive treatment programme setting in Offinso District, Ghana. *International Health*. 2011; 3 (3): 206–12.

36. Hutton G, Schellenberg J, Tediosi F, Macete E, Kahigwa E, Sigauque B, et al. Cost-effectiveness of malaria intermittent preventive treatment in infants (IPTi) in Mozambique and the United Republic of Tanzania. *Bulletin of the World Health Organization*. 2009; 87 (2): 123–9.

CHAPTER 17

Setting up a maternal and newborn health programme

Ted Lankester

What we need to know

Why maternity care is important

The first reason is to prevent unnecessary deaths of mothers during pregnancy and childbirth, and long-term complications afterwards.

The third Sustainable Development goal has this target: By 2030, reduce the overall global maternal mortality ratio to less than 70 per 100,000 live births.[1]

At the time of writing (2016) about 300,000 women die annually in pregnancy or while giving birth, that's about 830 each day. 99% of these occur in developing countries which indicates what a huge priority maternal health will be in the communities where we are working. The maternal mortality ratio in some developing countries in 2015 was 239 per 100,000 live births versus 12 per 100,000 live births in high-income countries. There are huge differences between countries, but also within countries, between women with high and low incomes and between women living in rural and urban areas.[2]

Millions of women worldwide suffer from long-term complications of childbirth, including obstetric fistulae causing leakage of urine or faeces from the birth canal, leading to social rejection. Approximately 30 times more women develop complications than die in childbirth.[3]

The second reason is to reduce the numbers of babies dying around the time of birth (perinatal period), and in the four weeks after birth (the neonatal period) and reduce disability caused by adverse events. (The World Health Organization (WHO) defines the perinatal period as the time between 22 completed weeks (154 days) of gestation and seven completed days after birth. The neonatal period begins with birth and ends 28 complete days after birth).

Forty-five per cent of deaths in children under five occur in the neonatal period. Five million babies are born prematurely each year. Each year there are about two and half million stillbirths, caused largely by the same underlying causes that kill mothers.[4]

At the time of writing, more than half of all women in Africa and south Asia give birth at home without a skilled attendant.

In community-based health care (CBHC) we can play a very important role in helping communities understand and act on the underlying causes behind these alarming statistics. And we can carry out specific tasks that will reduce the numbers of mothers and newborn babies that die unnecessarily.[5]

As we do this, we will be building the capacity of the health care system to bring in more effective long-term solutions. This will include helping to increase the number of skilled attendants and the proportion of mothers giving birth in health facilities, both of which are known to have a major impact on maternal and neonatal death rates.

There are a variety of international initiatives and organizations which we should be aware of (new plans, strategies and initiatives are being set up all the time, frequently changing, or being superseded). The first was the Safe Motherhood Initiative in the 1980s. We should know about the Integrated Management of Pregnancy and Childbirth (IMPAC),[6] the Partnership for Maternal, Newborn and Child Health,[7] and also the Integrated Management of Neonatal and Childhood Illness (IMNCI)—an expanded version of the Integrated Management of Childhood Illness (IMCI). We should also be aware of the Every Newborn Action Plan and Movement. This looks at evidence-based ways to reduce the number of deaths in newborns and stillbirths.[8] The Ending Preventable Maternal Mortality Programme (EPMM) is another recent collaboration.[9]

However, in CBHC, we should always look beyond health activities. For example, in urban areas of east Africa evidence shows that the level of education of the household head relates directly to maternal death rates.[10] So, by linking with programmes that help to improve male and female education, we can save the lives of mothers and newborns. The most recent is the Every Woman Every Child (EWEC) Global Strategy for Women's, Children's and Adolescent's Health (2016–2030). https://www.everywomaneverychild.org/

Why mothers and newborn babies die

The commonest causes, which account for nearly 80 per cent of maternal deaths, are, in order:

1. Haemorrhage during birth or shortly afterwards.

To prevent deaths, we must start emergency treatment within two hours, ideally at a health facility, but misoprostol used in the home can also save lives.[11]

Tranexamic acid given intravenously as soon as bleeding starts reduces bleeding and can be lifesaving.

2. Infection or sepsis.

Usually from unsterile procedures during delivery or from prolonged labour. This requires antibiotics, which can be given at community level.

3. Unsafe abortion.

This results from procedures performed by unqualified practitioners, using unsterile instruments, in unhygienic conditions.

4. Eclampsia.

Eclampsia leads to seizures and, unless carefully treated, to death. This condition can often be recognized and treated through good antenatal care. Magnesium sulphate injections can be given at home and be lifesaving.

5. Obstructed labour and other complications at delivery.

This can cause womb ruptures, which can kill the mother, or the mother may die from exhaustion. Antenatal care can help to predict the likelihood of this occurring by timely referral for a facility-based delivery.

In addition, nearly 20 per cent of deaths in mothers occur from diseases that are made worse during pregnancy and delivery, including malaria and tuberculosis. Areas with a high level of HIV/AIDS have higher maternal mortality rates.[12] Mothers suffering from anaemia are more likely to die in childbirth; malaria and iron deficiency are the commonest causes of anaemia in tropical Africa.[13] Adolescent mothers are twice as likely to die from childbirth as women in their twenties.

Newborn babies die for various reasons, but the three major causes of neonatal deaths worldwide are infections (about 36 per cent), which include sepsis/pneumonia, tetanus, and diarrhoea, pre-term complications (29 per cent), and birth asphyxia (about 23 per cent).[14]

There are various underlying causes for these deaths:

1. Maternal malnutrition and illness during pregnancy.

This can lead to low birthweight babies. Even small increases in average birth weight, e.g. 100g, greatly reduce neonatal mortality. Good nutrition and supplements for malnourished mothers are important.[15]

2. Births of twins or triplets.

Multiple births increase complications during delivery, including maternal haemorrhage, infection, eclampsia and obstructed labour.

3. Lack of care by skilled attendants during and after birth.

4. Unmet need for family planning (see Chapter 18).

Studies have shown that additional contraceptive use could reduce maternal deaths by 50 per cent through a variety of mechanisms. Many babies are 'not wanted' or are conceived earlier than planned.[16]

5. Poverty is closely linked with maternal and perinatal mortality (Figure 17.1).

Nurses, midwives, and doctors are largely out of reach of the poor majority because they are too expensive, and for the rural poor because they are too distant. Even where health care is available, it is often not used. The majority of women in the poorest areas, especially rural areas, do not access facilities.

There are many reasons why women in poorer areas do not access facilities available to them during pregnancy. Pregnancy is frequently considered a natural process that does not require health care professionals and clinics, and TBAs and local remedies are preferred. Additionally, many women are busy, with jobs in home, field, or factory considered a greater priority than spending half of a day visiting a clinic.

Additionally, customs may not allow women to travel when pregnant, nor to see a male doctor, and transport is often inadequate. For example, a hospital in the Kenyan Rift valley recently researched deliveries of women living in a village four kilometres from the hospital. Only one in four delivered in the hospital. The remainder delivered at home, with their main reason being that they couldn't afford bus fares to the hospital.[17] Finally, clinics are disliked because they are too far away, too crowded, too frightening, and too expensive. Also, health care staff often treat women poorly. Around 30 per cent of women report experiencing disrespect and abuse from doctors and nurses when they give birth.

Reducing deaths in mothers and newborns

We know from evidence that the following activities will help to reduce mother and newborn mortality.

1. Train and deploy skilled birth attendants.[18]

Skilled attendants are defined as people with midwifery skills (e.g. midwives, doctors, and nurses) who have been trained to manage normal deliveries and diagnose or treat complications of childbirth. Skilled attendants are higher level workers than TBAs, though there is some overlap. The wider use of skilled attendants is ideal but in practice many of the neediest communities will rely on using TBAs for many years to come. The training of skilled attendants goes beyond the scope of this book.

2. Increase access to good-quality services.

This is perhaps the biggest challenge of all in the neediest communities where death rates are highest. It calls for careful preparation so that, wherever possible, deliveries are preplanned to take place in a health facility with a skilled attendant. This strategy will have the biggest effect when families trust the quality of the health service. They are then more likely to overcome financial and distance barriers.

3. Encourage pregnant women to develop a birth plan.

We should help pregnant women draw up a plan and to discuss it at home with decision makers such as husband and mother-in-law. Together they need to decide where the birth is to take place, what transport to use for an emergency, or for a planned referral to a health centre if this is advised. They will need to set aside costs for

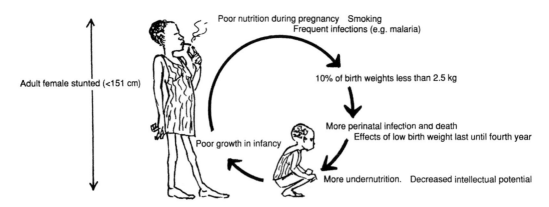

Figure 17.1 Effects of poverty on mothers and infants.

Reproduced courtesy of David Gifford. This image is distributed under the terms of the Creative Commons Attribution Non-Commercial 4.0 International licence (CC-BY-NC), a copy of which is available at http://creativecommons.org/licenses/by-nc/4.0/.

transport and other expenses. When pregnant women and their families decide these matters in advance, it reduces delays and uncertainty at or near delivery. This saves lives.

4. Develop the skills and understanding of women, families, and the community through health promotion and education.

This makes it more likely that women will seek out health care both for pregnancy and delivery. Encouraging and giving guidance on health-seeking behaviour is at the heart of our CBHC programme. Once families understand that every pregnancy can have a life-threatening complication, they will be more willing to reduce that risk by seeking quality services and delivery at a health facility, even if it means travelling further. Nearly everyone knows stories of complicated births and these stories can be powerful ways to talk about safe delivery without causing undue fear.

5. Link maternity services with other aspects of primary care programmes.

These links can be informed by the IMNCI. We should also link with programmes for control of sexually transmitted illness, family planning, immunization, and HIV/AIDS. Effective community-based programmes can significantly reduce deaths of mothers and newborns. The effectiveness of this depends on excellent training and good management, helped by the use of new drugs and technologies that are appropriate at community level. For example, a study in rural India showed a 62 per cent reduction in neonatal mortality through a community-based approach that included training TBAs and local women to treat sick newborns at home.[19]

What we need to do

Prepare the community

Care of the mother during pregnancy is often not a strongly felt need in poor communities. We must help people understand that having healthy mothers and babies will benefit the whole family, including the partner or husband. The key to this will be raising awareness of health issues connected with childbirth, and the actions that families and communities can see in Figure 17.2.

Awareness will also grow after the programme begins. As community health workers (CHWs) are trained and clinics provide mother and child health care, families will start using them, providing user fees are absent, or easily affordable.

Set aims and targets

Our overall aim will be to reduce the number of maternal, perinatal, and neonatal deaths in the target population. We will have various targets.

1. Antenatal care.

We must aim to increase the proportion of women receiving at least eight check-ups during pregnancy, The guidelines were changed by the WHO in November 2016 from the original four visits, and now include antenatal ultrasound.[20] Of course, in many remote areas this remains out of reach, but in terms of helping to strengthen health systems, it should be a main aim of our health programmes.

2. Delivery care.

We must also increase the proportion of deliveries accompanied by a skilled attendant in an adequate health facility. Where this is not practical for a community, we can aim to increase the proportion of deliveries attended by a carefully trained TBA or CHW in the mother's home. We must also ensure that whoever attends the delivery uses a sterile delivery kit.

3. Care after birth.

Basic essential obstetric care services at the health centre level should include at least the following:[21]

- parenteral (i.e. intramuscular or intravenous) antibiotics for severe infection;
- parenteral drugs to cause the uterus to contract, including oxytocin and misoprostol;
- parenteral sedatives for eclampsia (to prevent and treat seizures);
- manual removal of placenta; and
- manual removal of retained products.

Comprehensive essential obstetric care services at the district hospital level (first referral level) should include all the above plus capabilities for surgery, anaesthesia, and blood transfusion.

4. Postnatal care.

Finally, we must work to increase the number of women having a visit at home from a skilled health worker within 48 hours of delivery, and ideally from a skilled attendant at and immediately after birth to ensure at least the correct temperature of the baby, the use of hygienic practices, and support for breastfeeding. Specific targets for each of these aspects must be realistic for the populations we are serving. An example might be for 50 per cent of mothers to attend four (or more) antenatal appointments within three years of starting the programme, and 80 per cent to attend eight appointments within five years. We should add these into our logframe (see Chapter 7).

Train and use traditional birth attendants (TBAs)

TBAs live in or near the community and are usually available when needed. They are usually older women, often of low social status, although in many communities they are well-respected, and their skills are traditional, learned from other TBAs (often their mothers or mothers-in-law). They are usually rewarded by gifts or small cash payments.

Traditionally, TBAs carry out little antenatal care and have poor understanding of hygiene. They assist at births by giving advice (often strongly expressed) and through various interventions, some of which may be inappropriate or harmful. They may be reluctant to transfer women when there are problems in labour because of fear of criticism.

There continues to be controversy about the use of TBAs after studies showed that their use did not improve perinatal mortality. More recent reviews look more promising. As further research is carried out, it is likely that TBAs or CHWs who are taught specific skills and work in well-managed programmes will have increased success in saving lives of both mothers and infants.

According to the latest statement from the WHO, TBA training may be the only means to optimize the use of community-level health workers for maternal and newborn health in settings where there are insufficient numbers of skilled birth attendants or limited access to health facilities. Additionally, many women prefer TBAs.[22]

However, it is also clear that using skilled attendants and facility-based births are more effective than home deliveries in reducing deaths in mothers and babies at the time of birth. Chinese government programmes have encouraged this approach with some success.[23] However, China is a country where facilities and training are being

improved, and this degree of investment is not available in many poor countries.

It is a fact that many of the poorest communities do not have the option of using skilled attendants or health facilities, nor will they for the foreseeable future. Annually, about 40 million women are thought to deliver without a skilled attendant.[24] These women have three choices: deliver with a trained TBA, deliver with an untrained attendant, or deliver alone.

Although maternity waiting homes may be an attractive answer, a study from Timor-Leste showed that only women living within five kilometres of the waiting home were prepared to use it.[25]

Anecdotal evidence suggests that the stress for many mothers giving birth away from home, in unknown surroundings, often with unfriendly staff, at least partly undoes the value of giving birth in a facility.

There is encouraging evidence[26] that fewer mothers and children die if well-trained TBAs and CHWs carry out defined, evidence-based tasks, such as cleaning the umbilicus with chlorhexidine. For example, female health workers in Pakistan are trained in a variety of simple interventions which can reduce neonatal deaths, providing the programme is well managed.[27]

As more skilled attendants are trained and functioning near or in communities, the role of the TBA is likely to gradually change from being the main frontline worker to more of a support role in the community. For example, in Indonesia evidence has shown TBAs can play a vital role if they work in harmony with skilled attendants.[28]

However, in the poorest communities it will be many years before this transition is complete. In the meantime, lives will be lost if TBAs are not trained in specific skills that reduce the death rates of mothers and neonates. Training TBAs often encourages them to refer women and accompany them to health facilities. In many settings, integrating the TBAs with the formal health services can make a profound difference—enabling women to have the support of a trusted TBA, but to deliver in a facility where emergency care is available if a complication occurs. Many countries have banned TBAs. While women may continue to use them, it means that many organizations no longer train TBAs to provide safe and clean deliveries.

Some functions of trained TBAs

Ideally, TBAs will assist and work alongside skilled attendants. However, in many situations they will continue to be the only people who can give antenatal and postnatal care and assist at the delivery. Where this is allowed and appropriate for the setting. We should encourage village

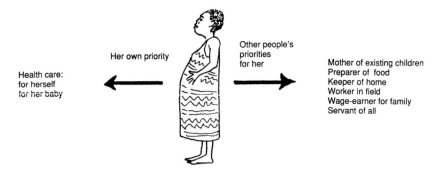

Figure 17.2 Many women from the poorest homes are not free or able to attend antenatal clinics or to have a facility-based delivery.

health committees (VHCs) and women's groups to work with and support the work of TBAs.

In practice, TBAs may carry out or assist skilled attendants in:

1. Antenatal examinations
2. Deliveries in order to:
   a) encourage and instruct the mother;
   b) recognize danger signs early and refer quickly;
   c) assist the delivery of the baby;
   d) assist the delivery of the placenta and check it is complete;
   e) cut the cord using a sterile blade, and tie with a clean cord tie; and
   f) apply chlorhexidine to the neonate's umbilical cord.
3. Care for the newborn by:
   a) immediate drying, keeping warm, and giving any necessary first aid;
   b) putting the baby to the mother's breast within the first 30 minutes to take colostrum; helping to establish breastfeeding;
   c) simple resuscitation measures;
   d) when appropriately trained, offer HIV prevention services and help with antiretroviral prophylaxis for HIV positive mothers and their infants.
4. Care for the mother by:
   a) making sure she is comfortable; and
   b) making sure the bleeding is controlled.
   In carrying out these activities she will use the sterile delivery kit and ensure she:
   a) has clean hands—washed with soap and water after taking off all rings;
   b) performs clean cutting and tying of the umbilical cord; and
   c) has clean surfaces—she will place clean cloths under the mother and baby.
5. Carry out postnatal care.

What TBAs should be taught

We will need to check the government's policy on the use, training, legality and accreditation of TBAs, and make sure we are working within any important national guidelines. Teaching should cover all the listed functions as well as basic delivery techniques where this is allowed by national governments. Training manuals are available in many countries and should be adapted and used, and there are WHO guidelines detailing what topics should be taught (See Figure 17.3).[29]

How TBAs should be trained

The trainer can be a nurse, midwife, skilled attendant, or any appropriately qualified member of the health team with practical experience in delivering babies. Doctors can be called in to teach selected lessons. In practice, TBAs will often be taught by the same individuals who teach CHWs. The timing of training should be co-ordinated with the rest of the community health programme, with CHW training programmes normally taking priority. The location should be the nearest place to the community that has sufficient deliveries to make teaching worthwhile. Often this will be a health centre or small (first-level referral) hospital. Alternatively, basic teaching can be given in the community and extra practical sessions arranged. Community-based visits must always be part of any training programme.

The duration of training might total thirty days. This can either be given in a single thirty-day term, in several separate blocks, or one day per week over a period of time. An alternative is to give seven days together, followed by a weekly training day, until the course is complete. Many TBAs will find it hard to leave their communities for more than a few days at a time. TBAs should be examined and tested thorough verbal examinations, especially in practical procedures and methods of referral, and only then should they be 'accredited' by the project. They will also need continuing development of their skills.

Ways of ensuring successful TBA programmes

Although many TBA programmes work well and reduce mother and child deaths, others have been less successful. As a result, most countries are concentrating on training skilled attendants. If TBAs are also being trained, they should be linked into the health system, and seen as a community-based method of helping people know how and when to seek care in a timely way. This also prevents the TBA being blamed for a complication for which she is not responsible (Figure 17.3).

The following paragraphs provide some suggestions, taken from a variety of projects using TBAs, which may help to make programmes more effective.

First, It is vital to choose appropriate women to be TBAs. As maternity services gradually improve we will need health workers with more education and training than in the past. There is a conflict here because TBAs are deeply embedded in their communities and their roles and skills are often passed down in families. Outsiders should be reluctant to interfere with this and get involved in selection. However, where younger TBAs are available for training, it gives us an opportunity to develop their skills.

For example, Bangladesh's government officially ended TBA training in 1998 and switched to training skilled birth attendants. But most skilled attendants still come from the lower skill bracket and are typically between the ages of 21 and 45 with appropriate levels of education.

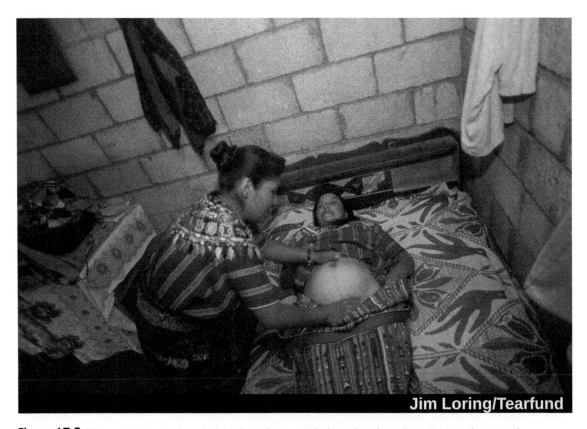

Figure 17.3 TBAs need to be trained to a high level in order to provide the quality of care that is increasingly expected.

Next, the services of trained TBAs must be wanted by the mother and family. The people themselves should request the services of TBAs and be happy with their further training. We can help this process by creating awareness of the TBA's value and how the community will benefit. For example, the largest study to date in terms of asking informed participants about the value of TBAs came from 654 comments and 193 participants. Their conclusions indicated that they supported having trained TBAs as part of pregnancy care. Members noted that TBAs were already frequently used by women because there were no other options. However, a substantial number regarded using TBAs as a threat to the quality of health care. The use of TBAs needs to be specific to each situation according to the need, how much they are accepted locally, and whether safer alternatives are actually used and available.[30]

Next, the relationship between the TBA and the community should be defined. When selecting CHWs whose functions also include working as a TBA, we must make sure the community selects appropriate people, fully understands the real function of a TBA, and agrees about methods of payment or reward.

Next, we must ensure and arrange appropriate training as described above. This needs to be kept simple and practical, with short, interactive training sessions. Many TBAs are illiterate especially when first selected. Becoming literate empowers TBAs, as well as CHWs and mothers, to be more effective carers. However, many TBAs will find literacy training difficult because of their age and background. Training should be given in specific skills known through evidence to have a beneficial impact.

We must guarantee regular and reliable supervision. A trained midwife or skilled attendant (ideally the TBA's trainer) or person of equivalent ability will need to make regular visits, ideally every month and at least every three months, to the TBA in her community. This should be mainly to give training, support, and encouragement. Where this is not possible, TBAs may be willing to travel to the health facility and collect supplies of delivery kits and at the same time to have a regular training update. Programmes that start with enthusiasm often run down, skills are lost, and the community loses interest. We must ensure that the knowledge and skills of TBAs are regularly updated, especially as many will only carry out occasional deliveries and rarely see complications.

Finally, we must ensure support and affirmation from project staff. TBAs must be fully accepted by the health team, treated with dignity and respect, and ideally included in wider health activities.

Teaching TBAs the importance of good record keeping

One of the problems we have is knowing what happens to babies born at home. The TBA is often the best source of information and needs to inform the health facility staff of pregnancies and the outcome of deliveries—whether there were any problems, and whether the newborn remains well. The TBA may need to be trained or helped by a family member or a women's group member to be able to do this accurately and reliably.

Delivery kits for the TBA and skilled attendants

A deliver kit is necessary to reduce birth-related infections as much as possible in the mother and baby. Infection of the mother's birth canal and infection of the baby's umbilicus are common causes of death or illness. A delivery kit should contain the following:

- Soap and a nail brush or nail sticks.
- Sterile gloves.
- Antiseptic solution and cotton wool.
- A small metal or plastic bowl.
- Two clean plastic sheets or towels at least one square metre large—one for the mother to labour on, another for the delivery kit.
- A sterile razor blade for cutting the cord.
- Cord ties (three sterile pieces of cotton).
- Clean gauze to cover the stump.
- String to wrap around the cord dressing.
- Chlorhexidine to apply to the umbilical stump.
- A simple set of pictorial instructions.
- Antibiotics need to be easily available.

For example, in India, Bangladesh, and Nepal research shows that fewer newborn children die when six 'essential cleans' are used: cleaning the cord with antiseptic (chlorhexidine), cutting the cord with a clean blade, tying it with a clean (ideally boiled) thread, cleaning the perineum, and delivering on to a clean sheet. The TBA or attendant must thoroughly clean her hands and her finger nails, in addition to using gloves.[31]

Set up antenatal (prenatal) care

Until recently, the WHO recommended a minimum of four antenatal appointments for women living in resource-poor areas. However, research shows that more mothers and newborns survive if eight antenatal appointments can be arranged. Originally, the WHO specified the exact actions and interventions which should be carried out at each appointment, but at the time of writing there is no detailed guidance on these details and individual countries are likely to draw up a list of actions for their own context.

However, there is a clear overall list which needs to be carried out during the eight appointments.

Box 17.1 shows the WHO's summary of the most significant actions and changes that are now recommended for all pregnancies (see also Figure 17.4).[32]

Here are the key actions to carry out for antenatal care in our clinic or within the community itself:

1. Health promotion

We should provide advice on nutrition and health care, counselling on danger signs in the pregnancy, preparing for a safe delivery and caring for the newborn. We should also promote and encourage breastfeeding.

2. Assessment by health worker

This should include history, examination, and investigation of other warning signs, including raised blood pressure, weight, height, fundal height measurement, blood and Rhesus compatibility, haemoglobin level, and a urine test for infection, protein and diabetes. This assessment should include noticing any signs of significant mental illness, distress, or signs of domestic violence

3. Prevention

We must provide nutritional advice and supplements, including iron and folic acid, and multiple micronutrient supplements where this is national policy (but there is no evidence that vitamin A supplements, sometimes still used, improve the health of the mother or newborn).[34]

We must aim to prevent malaria in high-risk areas, e.g. sub-Saharan Africa with intermittent preventive treatment (IPTp), most commonly sulphadoxine/pyrimethamine (SP) as single doses starting in the second trimester and requiring a total of three doses, given at the antenatal appointment (see Chapter 16). Dihydroartemisin-piperaquine is an alternative. Long-acting insecticide-treated bed-nets (LLITNs) are also needed. We should give tetanus toxoid injections, see Preventing neonatal tetanus (NNT).

4. Treatment

We must treat anaemia and test for and treat sexually transmitted illness, including syphilis cause of stillbirth and other serious conditions. Where HIV is common,

---

> **Box 17.1 Antenatal care model with a minimum of eight contacts recommended to reduce perinatal mortality and improve women's experience of care**
>
> - Counselling about healthy eating and keeping physically active during pregnancy.
> - Daily oral iron and folic acid supplementation with 30 mg to 60 mg of elemental iron and 400 µg (0.4 mg) folic acid for pregnant women to prevent maternal anaemia, puerperal sepsis, low birth weight, and preterm birth.
> - Tetanus toxoid vaccination is recommended for all pregnant women, depending on previous tetanus vaccination exposure, to prevent neonatal mortality from tetanus.
> - One ultrasound scan before 24 weeks' gestation (early ultrasound) is recommended for pregnant women to estimate gestational age, improve detection of foetal anomalies and multiple pregnancies, reduce induction of labour for post-term pregnancy, and improve a woman's pregnancy experience.
> - Health care providers should ask all pregnant women about their use of alcohol and other substances (past and present) as early as possible in the pregnancy and at every antenatal visit.
>
> **2016 WHO ANC model:[33]**
> **First trimester**
> Contact 1: up to 12 weeks
> **Second trimester**
> Contact 2: 20 weeks
> Contact 3: 26 weeks
> **Third trimester**
> Contact 4: 30 weeks
> Contact 5: 34 weeks
> Contact 6: 36 weeks
> Contact 7: 38 weeks
> Contact 8: 40 weeks
>
> Return for delivery at 41 weeks if not given birth.

we must encourage women to come forward for voluntary counselling and testing (VCT) as early as possibe and always by the 28th week and to start antiretroviral therapy when needed to lower the risk of mother-to-child transmission.

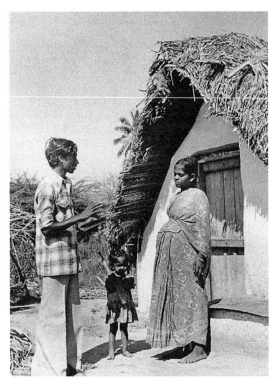

Figure 17.4 A CHW advises a mother on the importance of antenatal care.

Reproduced courtesy of John and Penny Hubley. This image is distributed under the terms of the Creative Commons Attribution Non-Commercial 4.0 International licence (CC-BY-NC), a copy of which is available at http://creativecommons.org/licenses/by-nc/4.0/.

5. Developing a birth plan

The birth plan must include an action plan for those delivering at home, as well as how and when to arrange a facility–based delivery.

6. Discussing future family planning needs and child spacing where relevant

For time-saving and convenience at all antenatal appointments, ensure that pregnant women are able to sit down at each clinic station and that waiting is kept to a minimum. Before the woman sees the health worker or skilled attendant, make sure that her weight, blood pressure, urine and blood tests are taken. There should be no user fees; if this is not possible, fees should be kept as low as possible so that services are affordable by all. Use the time that patients are waiting to deliver health teaching, and mothers have preparations ready for unexpected deliveries. For further details on clinics see Chapter 13.

Identifying patients who will need special care

We will learn from antenatal appointments some of the risks which are likely to lead to difficulties in childbirth. This often becomes more obvious further on in the pregnancy. For example, a Nigerian study showed the value in identifying three particular risks: multiple births, previous perinatal deaths, and Rhesus incompatibility.[35]

However, many problems at the time of birth will occur in women who have not shown any particular risk factors. Therefore, we must be vigilant in the care of our whole maternal population especially near or at the time of delivery, and make sure that each expectant mother has a birth plan.

In many of the poorest communities it is not possible to arrange special or comprehensive obstetric care but we should be as creative as possible in minimizing risks. For example, we can arrange rapid access to well-functioning facilities, whether that is a mobile health unit, a district hospital, or an upgraded maternity centre. And as mentioned, we can ensure that each woman has a birth plan in place. A good option is for expectant mothers with risk factors becoming apparent later in pregnancy to move to a maternity waiting home nearer to a centre which has emergency facilities. Fuller details can be found at http://www.unfpa.org/public/home/mothers/pid/4385.

For example, Cuba, Ethiopia, and Nicaragua were some of the earliest countries to set up networks of maternity waiting homes, located near hospitals; many other countries have followed suit. These waiting homes are for women needing comprehensive obstetric care and who are referred a month before the delivery is due. As labour starts they are easily transferred to the nearby hospital.

Additionally, Malaysia is one of many countries that has set up community birth centres attached to health clinics. At these centres, mothers needing special care wait in units with four to six beds. Centres are staffed by experienced midwives with doctors available. Most deliveries occur in the centre, but those with serious complications can be transferred to a nearby hospital.

Finally, the use of Mother Buddies is proving a helpful addition at community level to help the most vulnerable pregnant women. Known as IMPACT, this was first used in Malawi. Each pregnant woman is visited eight times by trained church volunteers over a twelve- to fifteen-month period (i.e. six to nine months of pregnancy and six months after birth). These volunteers provide targeted assistance including encouragement to attend for antenatal care. They are assisted by a mobile phone system called MiHope, which enables hundreds of chat messages to be sent for the price of a single SMS message. For more information, please see http://tilz.tearfund.org/en/resources/publications/footsteps/footsteps_91-100/footsteps_91/mother_buddies/

Preventing neonatal tetanus (NNT)

The WHO estimates that in 2015, almost 35,000 newborns died from NNT; this is a 96 per cent reduction from the situation in the late 1980s.[36] There is currently a global objective to eliminate maternal and neonatal tetanus.

In NNT, muscles contract so that breathing becomes impossible. Germs enter the body through wounds, and in newborn babies through the umbilical cord. Traditional dressings often contain tetanus germs.

Preventing NNT by tetanus toxoid (TT) injections

Many mothers at greatest risk will not come to antenatal clinics. This means that community health programmes should offer tetanus immunizations to girls and young women of childbearing age at every possible opportunity. NB: It is good practice to shake the vial before giving the vaccine.

For the number of injections needed follow any official national and regional guidelines. If not available or in doubt we can follow the following schedule:

Not previously vaccinated/immunization status unknown: give two doses of TT/Td one month apart before delivery, and a further dose during each pregnancy, up to a total of five.

Previous receipt of 1–4 doses of TT: give one dose of TT/Td before delivery. To give the fullest protection the last dose of tetanus toxoid must be given at least two weeks before delivery.

For more information, see http://www.who.int/immunization/diseases/tetanus/en/

Preventing NNT by other measures

- Maintain clean practices during delivery.
- Cut the umbilical cord with a sterile blade or razor.
- Use a sterile or boiled cord-tie.
- Apply chlorhexidine 5 per cent solution on the umbilical stump at least once.
- Make sure that no traditional dressing, dung, or ash is put on the stump.

These measures together can be very effective.

For example, in Rwanda, NNT has been almost eliminated. This has occurred through the twin approach of high TT coverage and more hygienic delivery practices, including care of the umbilical stump.

Set up delivery (intrapartum) care

Birth is the most dangerous time of life both for mother and child. The purpose of good delivery care is to make birth as safe as possible for both. The WHO recommends a skilled attendant should be present at every birth who can:

- provide continuing good quality care that is hygienic, safe, and sympathetic.
- recognize and manage complications, and carry out life-saving measures for mother and baby.
- refer promptly and safely where necessary and without delay. This involves preplanning quick methods of referral, and making sure each pregnant woman has a birth plan.

There is still a long way to go before skilled attendants can be present at birth in many of the poorest communities. However, this should be our eventual aim because it reduces deaths in mothers and newborns. We should consider advocating for this to be prioritized as a human right for the mother and child. In the meantime, we need to ensure that TBAs, CHWs, women's groups, and VHCs work together to ensure the best possible care is available with the resources that are available We should always aim for women with risk factors to be delivered in health facilities, or to be transferred to maternity waiting homes whenever this is possible.

We also need to recognize that, for example, in South Asia, 90 per cent of women who died of a post-partum haemorrhage had *NO* identifiable risk factors. All women are potentially at risk of a complication and one in seven women need more advanced care.[37] As it is impossible to predict who will need advanced care we need to ensure that all women have a birth plan for emergency facility-based delivery, with a skilled attendant whenever possible. If not reliably possible, the birth plan also needs to include details of how to have the safest possible delivery at home.

There are some specific actions we can take at community level to help reduce deaths. It is likely these and other simple interventions that can be taught to CHWs and TBAs will become increasingly widely used.

1. Misoprostol to prevent death from postpartum haemorrhage.

Careful training and protocols are needed and ideally a skilled attendant should be on hand in case of complications. However, misoprostol can be taken as a tablet, put under the tongue, or used in suppository form. For example, studies from Afghanistan, Bangladesh, and Nepal have shown that misoprostol taken by mouth by women as soon as their baby is born saves lives. Misoprostol can also be used to help expel the products of conception in incomplete abortion, another life-threatening condition.

2. Magnesium sulphate.

This reduces the likelihood of a seizure during eclampsia, which can cause death or injury to the child. This is given by injection and is ideally done in a health facility, as birth by Caesarean section is often essential, but it can also be used at community level after careful training; again, this must be under carefully drawn up protocols.

3. Delay cutting the umbilical cord for three minutes after delivery.

This delay helps to increase iron reserves in the newborn. It has also been shown to improve motor and social skills in children when tested at the age of four.[38]

4. Chlorhexidine.

This should be applied to the umbilical stump, as it reduces deaths from infection of the stump, including NNT.

Where the birth should take place

1. In the health centre (or referral hospital).

This is the place of choice under the care of a skilled attendant. However, as mentioned, this may not be practical for many of the poorest and most remote communities. Moving nearer to a centre a few weeks before the due date is an option that works for some.

Another option is to use conditional cash transfer (CCT) schemes (usually as a government policy). Money is paid to mothers as an incentive and to help cover the costs of giving birth in a health facility using a skilled attendant. Increasingly, as national governments progress towards universal health coverage, many government-run hospitals are providing free care for maternal health services. In practice, there are always some additional costs for families, and CCT or local savings schemes can assist to prepare for these out-of-pocket expenses.

2. In the mother's home.

This is a less-ideal option, and, where possible, a skilled attendant should be present. It is essential to use a sterile delivery kit.

3. In a TBA delivery unit, upgraded maternity home, or mobile unit.

In some programmes, TBAs conduct deliveries in informal units rather than in the woman's home. For example, in Nigeria children born in traditional maternity homes by trained birth attendants survived as well as those born in hospital.[39] We need to make sure any such site has been checked in advance and we have worked with the TBAs in making conditions as clean and appropriate as possible. In some areas, there are also more advanced midwifery facilities where skilled attendants may be able to attend or visit.

Recording the delivery

The person carrying out the delivery should fill in details on the antenatal card, and on the family folder insert card, register, or other system used by the project, either manual or digital. Many births in resource-poor areas are not adequately recorded or not recorded at all. The health worker responsible for the birth (either present or responsible for the referral to a health facility) must also be trained to take responsibility for recording the birth according to the system used by the health programme. This involves giving the details, e.g. place, date, any complications etc. to the health team using the established record system.

Children who are unregistered can face a variety of difficulties later, and if unrecorded may not be included in the government list of those requiring immunizations and other essential health care.

Set up postnatal and newborn care

This is essential both for the mother and child. Four out of ten of all under-fives that die do so in the first month of life. This amounts every year to about three and a half million babies.[40] Up to two-thirds of these deaths can be prevented by relatively simple interventions that can be carried out at home by health workers.

Table 17.1 gives a detailed list of the tasks that the WHO recommends as the most important. Tasks in the left-hand column and some tasks in the middle column are possible in most community situations.

It is useful to follow this list as far as we can. The suggestions in the main text below give a simplified picture of what can be done by skilled attendants or trained TBAs or CHWs at community level within the home during the first few weeks after the delivery.

Table 17.1 **Health promotion for mother and newborn, including immunization, nutrition, advice on breastfeeding, and safer sex. A suggested plan for community postnatal care**

	Routine care (offered to all women and babies)	Additional care (for women and babies with moderately severe diseases and complications)	Health Specialized—obstetrical and neonatal care (for women and babies with severe diseases and complications)
Postnatal maternal care (up to six weeks) Essential	• Assessment of maternal well-being • Prevention and detection of complications (e.g. infections, bleeding, anaemia) • Anaemia prevention and control (iron and folic acid supplementation) • Information and counselling on nutrition, safe sex, family planning, and provision of some contraceptive methods • Postnatal care planning, advice on danger signs and emergency preparedness • Provision of contraceptive methods	• Treatment of some problems (e.g. mild to moderate anaemia, mild puerperal depression) • Pre-referral treatment of some problems (e.g. severe postpartum bleeding, puerperal sepsis)	• Treatment of all complications - severe anaemia - severe postpartum bleeding - severe postpartum infections - severe postpartum depression • Female sterilization
Situational	• Promotion of LLITN use	• Treatment of uncomplicated malaria	• Treatment of complicated malaria
Newborn care (birth and immediate postnatal) Essential	• Chlorhexidine to umbilical stump Promotion, protection, and support for breastfeeding • Monitoring and assessment of well-being, detection of complications (breathing, infections, prematurity, low birthweight, injury, malformation) • Infection prevention and control, rooming-in • Eye care • Information and counselling on home care, breastfeeding, hygiene • Postnatal care planning, advice on danger signs and emergency preparedness • Immunization according to the national guidelines (BCG, HepB, OPV-0)	• Care if moderately preterm, low birth weight, or twin • Support for breastfeeding, warmth • Frequent assessment of well-being and detection of complications e.g. feeding difficulty, jaundice, other perinatal problems • Kangaroo Mother Care follow-up • Treatment of mild to moderate local infections (cord, skin, eye, thrush) • Birth injuries • Pre-referral management of infants with severe problems: - very preterm babies and/or birth weight very low - severe complications - malformations • Supporting mother if perinatal death	• Management of severe newborn problems—general care for the sick newborn and management of specific problems: - preterm birth - breathing difficulty - sepsis - severe birth trauma and asphyxia - severe jaundice - Kangaroo Mother Care (KMC) • Management of correctable malformations

Table 17.1 **Continued**

	Routine care (offered to all women and babies)	Additional care (for women and babies with moderately severe diseases and complications)	Health Specialized—obstetrical and neonatal care (for women and babies with severe diseases and complications)

Situational	• Promotion of infant's sleeping under LLITN	• Presumptive treatment of congenital syphilis
		• Prevention of mother-to-child transmission of HIV by ART
		• Support for infant feeding of maternal choice
			• Treatment of:
			  - congenital syphilis
			  - neonatal tetanus

Postnatal newborn care
(visit from/ at home)
Essential
	• Assessment of infant's well-being and breastfeeding
	• Detection of complications and responding to maternal concerns
	• Information and counselling on home care
	• Additional follow-up visits for high-risk babies (e.g. preterm, after severe problems, on replacement feeding)
		• Management of minor to moderate problems and feeding difficulties
		• Pre-referral management of severe problems:
		  - convulsions
		  - inability to feed
		• Supporting the family if perinatal death
			• Management of severe newborn problems:
			  - sepsis
			  - other infections
			  - jaundice
			  - failure to thrive

Checking the newborn immediately after birth

The attendant checks the mother. Most importantly, she makes sure the uterus remains well contracted and there is no excessive blood loss. As mentioned, TBAs and CHWs who have been specifically trained can also use misoprostol, which stimulates uterine contractions and can prevent death from postpartum haemorrhage (PPH).

For example, in some parts of Tanzania, TBAs are using 1000 µg rectally to treat PPH; in the Gambia, women are given 600 µg sublingually to prevent haemorrhage; and in Indonesia, women are given misoprostol to self-administer as soon as the baby delivers. The person carrying out the delivery should leave only when she is sure there are no danger signs in mother and baby. She should refer at once if she is concerned, and especially if vaginal bleeding continues.

The attendant checks the newborn, ensuring the newborn is breathing well and is comfortable and warm. The baby should be placed next to the mother and wrapped when not sharing her body heat. She can use the Kangaroo method (see Further reading) in cold climates and when children are very small or born early. She should encourage the mother to put the child to the breast within 30 minutes of delivery, and give useful tips on how to do this. She should also delay bathing for 24 hours.

In addition, all birth attendants should be trained in essential (resuscitation) care for small babies, the special care needed for small or premature babies born in low-resource areas. Birth attendants and mothers learn how to keep them warm by skin-to-skin wrapping and to keep babies nourished with alternative feeding methods. This is likely to be a growing area of importance in low-resource settings. For more information, see https://www.aap.org/en-us/advocacy-and-policy/aap-health-initiatives/helping-babies-survive/Pages/default.aspx

Within the first 24 hours

The attendant should check the newborn for obvious abnormalities such as breathing problems, swelling of the stomach, deformity, or jaundice. All babies should be weighed or have their mid-upper arm circumference (MUAC) measured, and all these details should be recorded on the home-based record card if she is able, or a specially designed chart for illiterate TBAs. Alternatively, details can be recorded in her record book or diary, or any other system used by the health programme. She should then give the first hepatitis B immunization to prevent mother-to-child infection. Where this is national policy she gives or arranges BCG.

The attendant should also check the mother for any fever or continuing blood loss. She should also check for any feeding problems, actively encourage breastfeeding, and give encouragement and appropriate advice if the mother is finding this difficult. She should also discuss any other concerns the mother may have.

Within the first two weeks

Most national governments have commenced a home-based newborn care programme, and our programmes should support those wherever possible. Many advocate for visits on days one, three, and seven after the birth. Our health programmes should integrate with this programme for postnatal care where it exists.

During this two-week period, the attendant pays special attention to fever and any vaginal discharge in the mother, and should continue to monitor any feeding problems, any sign of infection in the baby, and continue to support the mother and listen to any ongoing concerns. She should offer to help with any problems with breastfeeding She should also revisit family planning and, where relevant, safer sex practices and advise on how other immunizations can be given.

If the mother is HIV-positive, the attendant can give guidance on using infant formula or help to ensure exclusive breastfeeding, i.e. whichever method the mother has opted for. If mothers or partners are concerned that they might be HIV-positive, the TBA can explain when and where VCT is available.

If the community has both a TBA and a CHW, now is the time for the TBA to hand over care for the mother and child to the CHW. When the handover happens, we must make sure that the TBA, CHW, or other person who attended the delivery passes full details to the relevant programme health worker. This ensures that health care for mother and newborn can be properly integrated into the programme (Figure 17.5).

Keep records

The following records can be kept:

1. Home-based record card (HRC).

Mothers should keep any HRC and make sure that any health worker who sees her checks it and enters

notes on it. Ideally, we should use any nationally recommended record card used to record details of the delivery and postnatal care of mother and child. A duplicate or summary can be kept in the family folder.

2. Record card with symbols

This is designed for use by illiterate CHWs or TBAs. It needs to be designed for each country and district, and may use symbols that may need explaining or adapting. This card is kept by the mother. It may be used in addition to the HRC.

3. The master register or programme computer.

Details from HRCs, or duplicates kept in the family folder, or from registers or tallies can be entered as convenient.

Evaluate the programme

After an agreed time, we will need to evaluate the programme to see whether the aims and targets set at the beginning are being met. There are some additional ways we can monitor and evaluate the success of our programme.

1. Antenatal coverage: the percentage of pregnant women who have attended for four or more antenatal checks or with trained midwife.
2. Nutritional status of the newborn: the percentage of newborn babies weighing more than 2500 g or having MUACs of 8.7 cm or more.
3. Supervised deliveries: the percentage of births attended by a skilled attendant; the percentage of deliveries where a sterile delivery kit was used.
4. Maternal care and newborn care: the percentage of women who have attended 3+ postnatal visits; the percentage who have used either oxytocin or misoprostol (uterotonics) at birth; the percentage of newborns who have had chlorhexidine applied to the umbilical stump.
5. Maternal mortality rates and perinatal mortality: compare rates at the start of the project with those after three or four years. Only largescale projects will obtain valid statistics.

Because maternity programmes are both complex and important, and donors will expect careful evaluation, some programmes will wish to monitor their progress more consistently. For more information, see also http://www.who.int/maternal_child_adolescent/documents/

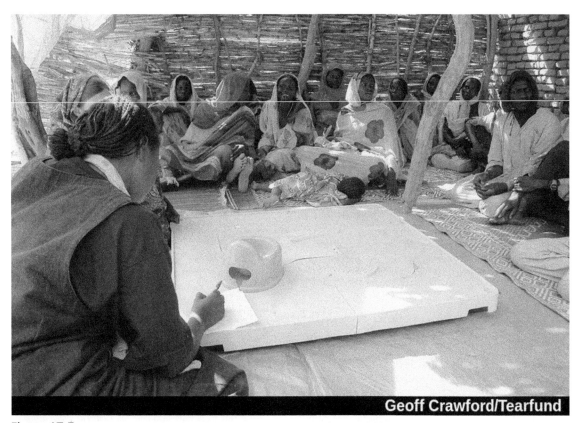

Figure 17.5 Women in Sudan learn about the ongoing care of babies and young children.

improving-maternal-newborn-care-quality/en/ The results of any evaluation should be shared with the community as a basis for joint planning.

Summary

Many millions of mothers and babies die each year from causes related to childbirth. Nearly all such deaths can be prevented through setting up effective, community-based maternity care backed up by a good referral centre. Before starting any programme, we must have detailed discussions with the district medical officer and follow all appropriate national guidelines. Ideally, all deliveries should be carried out by skilled attendants in health facilities and this should be the eventual goal of our programmes. Trained TBAs and CHWs also have a role to play as they work in co-operation with the programme and with health facilities to promote access to antenatal care, delivery and postnatal care. An important tool to co-ordinate the care of pregnant women is the antenatal record card. A birth plan is needed, which ideally includes the mother being within easy distance of a good health facility if an emergency occurs. The postnatal care of the mother and newborn care is an essential part of any programme in order to reduce death and illness. Many deaths are preventable at community level if good procedures and training are set up and well managed.

Further reading and resources

A timely arrival for Born Too Soon: Editorial. *The Lancet.* 2012; 380: p1713; see also *Born too soon: The global action on preterm birth.* Available from: www.who.int/pmnch/media/news/ 2012/preterm_birth_report

Burns A, Lovich R, Maxwell J, Shapiro K. *Where women have no doctor: A health guide for women.* Berkeley, CA: Hesperian Healthguides; 1997. A comprehensive guide to women's health problems and how to prevent and treat them.

Cousens S, Blencowe H, Stanton C, Chou D, Ahmed S, Steinhardt L, et al. National regional and worldwide estimates of still-birth rates in 2009 with trends since 1995: A systematic analysis. *The Lancet.* 2011; 377 (9774): 1319–30. DOI:10:1016/S0140-6736(10)62310-0

Crook B, Robinett D. *Basic Delivery Kit Guide.* Seattle: Program for Appropriate Technology in Health; 2001. Available from: https://path.azureedge.net/media/documents/MCHN_BDKG.pdf A guide for organisations wanting to develop locally based delivery kits.

King M. *Primary mother care and population.* Stamford: Spiegl Press; 2003. Available from: https://www.talcuk.org/books/primary-mother-care-and-population-.htm

Klein S, Miller S, Thomson F. *A book for midwives: Care for pregnancy, birth and women's health.* Berkeley, CA: Hesperian Foundation; 2004. A new edition of this outstanding book on all aspects of maternity care. See Appendix E.

The Lancet. Maternal Survival Series 2016. Available from: http://www.thelancet.com/series/maternal-survival. There is also a *Lancet* series on Maternal Health (2016), some of which is relevant for community-based maternal care. A number of useful slide sets are also available from TALC. See Appendix E.

Networklearning.org. *A TBA Manual and How to Adapt it to Your Local Culture.* 2002. Available from: http://www.networklearning.org/index.php/library/a-tba-manual/76-a-tba-manual-and-how-to-adapt-it-to-your-local-culture-doc

The Safe Motherhood Initiative and Partnership for Safe Motherhood and Newborn Health. Available from: http://www.safemotherhood.org/

The White Ribbon Alliance. Global alliance of reproductive, maternal and newborn health and rights. Available from: http://www.whiteribbonalliance.org

World Health Organization. *Basic Newborn Resuscitation: A Practical Guide.* Geneva: World Health Organization; 1998. Available from: http://apps.who.int/iris/bitstream/handle/10665/63953/WHO_RHT_MSM_98.1.pdf?sequence=1　See also Appendix E.

World Health Organization. *Essential Newborn Care Course.* Geneva: World Health Organization; 2010. Available from: http://www.who.int/maternal_child_adolescent/documents/newborncare_course/en/index.html

World Health Organization. *Home-based maternal records: Guidelines for development, adaptation, and evaluation.* Geneva: World Health Organization; 1994. Available from: http://apps.who.int/iris/bitstream/10665/39355/1/9241544643_eng.pdf. An excellent manual to help guide not only recording systems but the coordination and content of maternity programmes. See also Appendix E.

World Health Organization. *Making pregnancy safer: The critical role of the skilled attendant. A joint statement by WHO, ICM and FIGO.* Geneva: World Health Organization; 2004. Available from: http://www.who.int/maternal_child_adolescent/documents/9241591692/en/. See also see http://www.womendeliver.org

World Health Organization. *Managing Maternal and Child Health Programmes: A Practical Guide.* Geneva: World Health Organization; 1997. Mainly aimed at the District level but with helpful ideas to improve management in larger programmes. Available from: WHO. See Appendix E and from http://www.who.int/reproductivehealth.

World Health Organization. *Safe childbirth check list.* Available from: http://apps.who.int/iris/bitstream/10665/199179/1/WHO_HIS_SDS_2015.26_eng.pdf?ua=1

World Health Organization/Department of Reproductive Health and Research. *Kangaroo mother care: A practical guide.* How mothers can look after their babies, especially those that are low birth weight. Available from: http://www.who.int/maternal_child_adolescent/documents/9241590351/en/

World Health Organization. *Strategy for women's, children's, and adolescent's health (2016–2030).* Available from: http://www.who.int/life-course/partners/global-strategy/en/

References

1. United Nations. Sustainable Development Knowledge Platform. 2016. Available from: https://sustainable-development.un.org/sdg3
2. World Health Organization. *Maternal Mortality Factsheet.* Geneva: World Health Organization; 2016. Available from: http://www.who.int/mediacentre/factsheets/fs348/en/
3. Say L, Chou D, Gemmill A, Tunçalp Ö, Moller A-B, Daniels J, et al. Global causes of maternal death: A WHO systematic analysis. *The Lancet Global Health.* 2014; 2 (6): PE323–33. Available from: http://www.thelancet.com/journals/langlo/article/PIIS2214-109X(14)70227-X/fulltext
4. A timely arrival for Born Too Soon: Editorial. *The Lancet.* 2012; 380: p1713; see also *Born too soon: The global action on preterm birth.* Available from: www.who.int/pmnch/media/news/2012/preterm_birth_report
5. Pattinson R, Kerber K, Buchmann E, Friberg IK, Belizan M, Lansky S, et al. Stillbirths: How can health systems deliver for mothers and babies. *The Lancet.* 2011; 377 (9777):1610–23. DOI:10;1016/S0140-6736(10)62306-9
6. World Health Organization. *Integrated management of pregnancy and childbirth (IMPAC).* Available from: http://www.who.int/maternal_child_adolescent/topics/maternal/impac/en/
7. World Health Organization. Partnership for maternal, newborn and child health. Available from: http://www.who.int/pmnch/en/
8. Health Newborn Network. Every Newborn joint action platform. Available from: http://www.healthynewbornnetwork.org/issue/every-newborn/
9. World Health Organization. *Strategies toward ending preventable maternal mortality (EPMM).* Geneva: World Health Organization; 2015. Available from: http://apps.who.int/iris/bitstream/handle/10665/153544/9789241508483_eng.pdf?sequence=1
10. Mswia R, Lewanga M, Moshiro C, Whiting D, Wolfson L, Hemed Y, et al. Community-based monitoring of safe motherhood in the United Republic of Tanzania. *Bulletin of the World Health Organization.* 2003; 81 (2):87–94. Available from: http://www.who.int/bulletin/volumes/81/2/Mswia0203.pdf

11. Potts M, Prata N, Sahin-Hodoglugil NN. Maternal mortality: One death every 7 min. *The Lancet*. 2010; 375 (9728):1762–3.
12. World Health Organization. *Tuberculosis in women factsheet*. 2015. Available from: http://www.who.int/tb/publications/tb_women_factsheet_251013.pdf
13. Schantz-Dunn J, Nour NM. Malaria and pregnancy: A global health perspective. *Reviews in Obstetrics and Gynecology*. 2009; 2 (3): 186–92.
14. World Health Organization/Partnership for Maternal, Newborn & Child Health. *Newborn death and illness: Millennium Development Goal (MDG) 4*. 2011. Available from: http://www.who.int/pmnch/media/press_materials/fs/fs_newborndealth_illness/en/
15. Shankar AH, Jahari AB, Sebayang SK, Aditiawarman, Apriatni M, Harefa B, et al., Supplementation with Multiple Micronutrients Intervention Trial (SUMMIT) Study Group, et al. Effect of maternal multiple micronutrient supplementation of fetal loss and infant death in Indonesia: A double blind randomized controlled trial. *The Lancet*. 2008; 371 (9608): 215–27.
16. UN Economic and Social Council: Commission on the status of women. Resolution 56/3. Eliminating maternal mortality and morbidity through the empowerment of women. New York: United Nations; 2012.
17. Kitui J, Lewis S, Davey G. Factors influencing place of delivery for women in Kenya: An analysis of the Kenya demographic and health survey, 2008/2009. *BMC Pregnancy and Childbirth*. 2013; 13:40. DOI: 10.1186/1471-2393-13-40
18. Sibley LM, Sipe TA, Barry D. Traditional birth attendant training for improving health behaviours and pregnancy outcomes. *Cochrane Database of Systematic Reviews*. DOI: 10.1002/14651858.CD005460.pub3
19. Costello A, Osrin D, Manandhar D. Reducing maternal and neonatal mortality in the poorest communities. *British Medical Journal*. 2004; 329 (7475): 1166–8.
20. World Health Organization. *Guidelines on antenatal care*. Available from: http://apps.who.int/iris/bitstream/10665/250796/1/9789241549912-eng.pdf?ua=1
21. World Health Organization. *Essential Obstetric Care factsheet*. Available from: http://www.who.int/mediacentre/factsheets/fs245/en/
22. World Health Organization. *Summary: Traditional birth attendant (TBA) training for improving health behaviours and pregnancy outcomes*. Available from: https://extranet.who.int/rhl/topics/pregnancy-and-childbirth/antenatal-care/traditional-birth-attendant-tba-training-improving-health-behaviours-and-pregnancy-outcomes
23. Feng XL, Guo S, Hipgrave D, Zhu J, Zhang L, Song L, et al. China's facility-based strategy and neonatal mortality: A population-based epidemiological study. *The Lancet*. 2011; 378 (9801): 1493–500.
24. UNICEF Data: Monitoring the Situation of Children and Women. *Delivery care*. Updated June 2018. Available from: https://data.unicef.org/topic/maternal-health/delivery-care/
25. Wild K, Barclay L, Kelly P, Martins N. The tyranny of distance: Maternity waiting homes and access to birthing facilities in rural Timor-Leste. *Bulletin of the World Health Organization*. 2012; 90 (2):97–103. DOI:10.2471/BLT.11.088955
26. Wilson A, Gallos ID, Plana N, Lissauer D, Khan KS, Zamora J, et al. Effectiveness of strategies incorporating training and support of traditional birth attendants on perinatal and maternal mortality: Meta-analysis. *British Medical Journal*. 2011; 343:d7102. DOI 10.1136/bmj.d7102
27. Bhutta ZA, Soofi S, Cousens S, Mohammad S, Memon ZA, Ali I, et al. Improvement of perinatal and newborn care in rural Pakistan through community-based strategies: A cluster-randomized effectiveness trial. *The Lancet*. 2011; 377 (9763): 403–12. DOI:10:1016/S0140-6736(10)62274-X
28. UNICEF. Traditional birth attendants and midwives partner for women's health in Indonesia. At a glance: Indonesia. UNICEF Newsline; 9 April 2008. Available from: https://www.unicef.org/infobycountry/indonesia_43515.html
29. World Health Organization. Antenatal care. The WHO Reproductive Health Library; 2018. Available from: https://extranet.who.int/rhl/topics/preconception-pregnancy-childbirth-and-postpartum-care/antenatal-care
30. Owolabi OO, Glenton C, Lewin S, Pakenham-Walsh N. Stakeholder views on the incorporation of traditional birth attendants into the formal health systems of low-and middle-income countries: A qualitative analysis of the HIFA2015 and CHILD2015 email discussion forums. *BMC Pregnancy and Childbirth*. 2014; 14: 118. DOI:10.1186/1471-2393-14-118
31. Seward N, Osrin D, Li L, Costello A, Pulkki-Brännström A-M, Houweling TAJ, et al. Association between clean delivery kit use, clean delivery practices, and neonatal survival: Pooled analysis of data from three sites in South Asia. *PloS Med*. 2012; 9 (2): e1001180.
32. World Health Organization. http://apps.who.int/iris/bitstream/10665/250796/1/9789241549912-eng.pdf?ua=1
33. World Health Organization. Current WHO Ideal times for antenatal contacts http://apps.who.int/iris/bitstream/10665/250796/1/9789241549912-eng.pdf?ua=1 Page 105
34. Costello A, Osrin D. Vitamin A supplementation and maternal mortality. *The Lancet*. 2010; 375 (9727): 1675–7. DOI:10.1016/S0140-6736(10)60443-6
35. Aniebue UU, Aniebue PN. A risk assessment for pregnancy using the World Health Organization classifying form in primary health-care facilities in Enugu, Nigeria. *Tropical Doctor*. 2008; 38 (3). DOI: 10.1258/td.2007.070039
36. World Health Organization. Maternal and neonatal tetanus elimination (MNTE). Updated 27 January 2017. Available from: http://www.who.int/immunization/diseases/MNTE_initiative/en/
37. World Health Organization, UNICEF, UNFPA and The World Bank. *Trends in maternal mortality: 1990 to 2008. Estimates developed by WHO, UNICEF, UNFPA and The World Bank*. Geneva: World Health Organization; 2010.
38. Andersson O, Lindquist B, Lindgren M, Stjernqvist K, Domellöf M, Hellström-Westas L. Effect of delayed cord clamping on neurodevelopment at 4 years of age: A randomized clinical trial. *JAMA Pediatrics*. 2015; 69 (7): 631–8.
39. Olusanya BO, Inam VA, Abosede OA. Infants delivered in maternity homes run by traditional birth attendants in

urban Nigeria: A community-based study. *Health Care for Women International*. 2011; 32: 474–91.

40. You D, Hug L, Chen Y, Newby H, Wardlaw T. *Levels and trends in child mortality: Report 2014—Estimates developed by the UN Interagency Group for child Mortality Estimation (UN-IGME)*. New York: United Nations Children's Fund; 2014. Available from: http://documents.worldbank.org/curated/en/953551468153557611/Levels-and-trends-in-child-mortality-estimates-developed-by-the-UN-Inter-agency-Group-for-child-Mortality-Estimation-IGME-report-2014

CHAPTER 18

Setting up a family planning and reproductive health programme

Clare Goodhart, Ted Lankester, and Claire Thomas

According to the Bill and Melinda Gates Foundation, each dollar spent on family planning can save governments up to six dollars, which then can be spent on improving health, housing, water, sanitation, and other public services.[1]

In recent years, international aid has been focused on stemming the HIV epidemic. Researchers have found a potential saving of twenty-five US dollars for every one US dollar spent on family planning at HIV/AIDs care and treatment facilities,[2] but the opportunity to address the huge unmet need for contraception has been missed.

Family planning and sexual health are topics we need to include in our community health programmes (CHP) at an early stage. They are not add-on extras, even in those societies and cultures where there are objections and taboos. We need to ensure (in ways appropriate to community culture) that these services are available to as many families as possible, and to women of reproductive age, whether single, partnered, or married. The unmet need for contraceptive services is currently estimated to be over 225 million people.[3] In Africa, only about one eligible woman in three uses contraception.

The 2012 London Family Planning Summit gave rise to FP2020, a global initiative to increase access to contraception by 120 million women by 2020.

A key target for the third Sustainable Development Goal (SDG) is universal access by 2030 to sexual and reproductive health care services, including for family planning, information, and education. Modern contraception, however, contributes to the SDGs in many different ways, directly by contributing to a reduction in maternal and infant mortality, but also indirectly by reducing poverty (SDG1) and hunger (SDG2), increasing availability of education (SDG4), contributing to gender equality (SDG 5), the sustainability of cities (SDG 11), and impacting on climate change (SDG 13).

The World Health Organization (WHO) has adopted a strategy on reproductive health that includes antenatal, delivery, and postpartum care, high-quality services for family planning, eliminating unsafe abortion, and combating sexually transmitted infections (STIs), including HIV. This has come about because such a high burden of illness among women in their child-bearing years is directly related to sex and reproduction.[4]

What we need to know

Family planning (FP) saves lives

At least one woman dies every minute from causes related to pregnancy. In developing countries, a woman's lifetime risk of dying is almost 100 times higher than the risk for a woman in more developed countries—1 in 75 compared to 1 in 7,300.[5]

Family planning could prevent up to one-third of maternal deaths by allowing women to delay motherhood, space births, avoid unwanted pregnancies and unsafe abortions, and stop having children when they have reached their desired family size.[6] An estimated 20 million unsafe abortions are performed each year, resulting in 67,000 deaths annually, mostly in developing countries.[7]

Women aged 15 to 19 are twice as likely to die from maternal causes as older women; many adolescents are physically immature, which increases their risk of suffering obstetric complications.[8] Each year 2.5 million teenagers in developing countries undergo abortions, many of which are performed unsafely.[9]

Births close together result in higher infant mortality. International survey data shows that babies born less than two years after their next oldest sibling are twice as likely to die in the first year as those born after an interval of three years.[10] Recent research also shows that a short interval between pregnancies makes premature delivery and neonatal death more likely.[11] Child spacing leads to healthier children because there is more milk, more food, more love, and by the time the next child is born, the next youngest has passed the most vulnerable age for malnutrition and associated illness (Figure 18.1) Healthier children do better in school and become better educated adults who, in turn, will provide more successfully for their children.

FP reduces population growth and poverty

Our world is overcrowded. Currently, world population stands at over 7.4 billion people, and it is growing by 1.18 per cent, or 83 million people per year—more than the population of the United Kingdom. It will therefore double in about 58 years, unless urgent action is taken to slow it down. Clearly, the planet will not be able to sustain this huge population.[12]

In India alone, about 14 million people are added to the population each year, giving an equivalent need for over 120,000 new primary schools to educate the extra

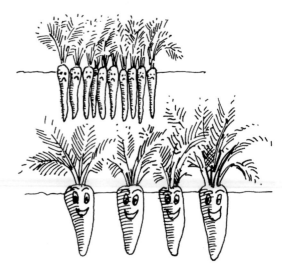

Figure 18.1 Well-spaced children, like well-spaced carrots, grow better.

Reproduced with permission from Morley, D. (1986). My Name is Today. London, UK: Macmillan Education. Copyright © 1986 Macmillan. This image is distributed under the terms of the Creative Commons Attribution Non-Commercial 4.0 International licence (CC-BY-NC), a copy of which is available at http://creativecommons.org/licenses/by-nc/4.0/.

children (Figure 18.2). By 2020, the population of India is expected to exceed that of China.[13]

In 2002, former UN Secretary-General Kofi Annan said that 'the eradication of extreme poverty and hunger cannot be achieved until questions of population and reproductive health are squarely addressed. And that means stronger efforts to promote women's rights, and greater investment in education and health, including reproductive health and family planning'.[14] Those words are even truer today, as in many developing countries women who complete secondary education have on average at least one child fewer than women who complete only primary education.[15]

When a population is either too large or increasing too fast, the following problems arise:

1. Poverty. There is less money, less food, less water, and less living space for the poor. The rich remain largely unaffected.

2. Disease. Overcrowding increases the spread of infection. Health services cannot cope with numbers of patients.

3. Urbanization. Cities grow rapidly, far outstripping resources. Overcrowding, lack of sanitation, water

**Results of a 3% population growth rate on a village of 10 houses
The population will double every 20 years**

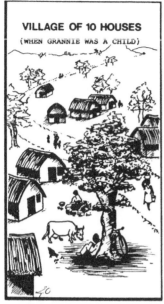

VILLAGE OF 10 HOUSES
(WHEN GRANNIE WAS A CHILD)

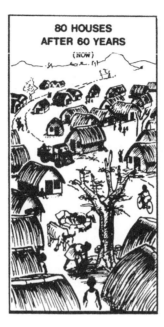

80 HOUSES
AFTER 60 YEARS
(NOW)

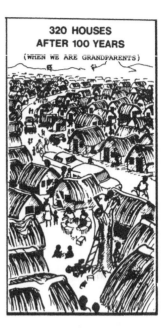

320 HOUSES
AFTER 100 YEARS
(WHEN WE ARE GRANDPARENTS)

Figure 18.2 Expanding villages.

Reproduced with permission from Morley, D. (1973). Paediatric Priorities in Developing Countries. Cambridge, UK: Butterworths. Copyright © 1973 TALC. This image is distributed under the terms of the Creative Commons Attribution Non-Commercial 4.0 International licence (CC-BY-NC), a copy of which is available at http://creativecommons.org/licenses/by-nc/4.0/.

pollution and shortage, drug abuse, and sexual exploitation become more widespread. The number of homeless people and street children increases.

4. Social breakdown. Lack of resources triggers exploitation, unequal distribution of wealth, injustice, civil disturbance, and may contribute to war within countries and between countries.

Common obstacles to FP

National objections

Some governments disapprove of FP, perhaps because they perceive themselves as having relatively low populations, or for political or religious reasons. Other governments may support FP, but fail to back this up with properly stocked contraceptive services.

Family objections

Children are needed to assist on the farm and at home; earn money, especially if living in cities; look after and provide for parents and older relatives; give the family status in the community; and carry on the family name,

farm or business (Figure 18.3). In many cultures, boys are valued more than girls, meaning families will increase in size until two or three sons reach maturity.

Personal objections

There are many common (often moral) objections to FP:

- Is it permitted by my religion?
- What happens if my children die?
- Will my FP method be reversible?
- Will I lose my manhood or womanhood?
- What will happen to my periods?
- Will my sex life be affected?
- Will there be side effects?
- Will my husband be suspicious?
- Will my partner agree to use FP methods?
- Will the government force me to use FP?
- Will it be difficult to get good advice and obtain regular supplies?

Each country, community, and couple will have its own questions and objections. Sometimes several minor

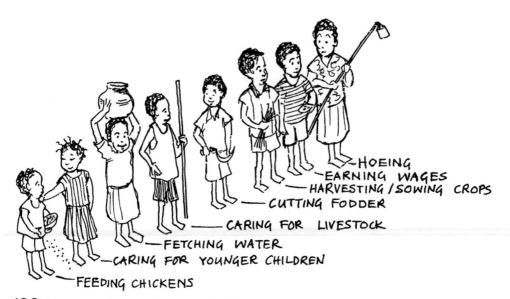

HOEING
EARNING WAGES
HARVESTING / SOWING CROPS
CUTTING FODDER
CARING FOR LIVESTOCK
FETCHING WATER
CARING FOR YOUNGER CHILDREN
FEEDING CHICKENS

Figure 18.3 The poor person's question: 'How can I afford not to have a large family?'

fears, combined with a reluctance to discuss FP, may prevent a couple from seeking advice. We will need to discover and meet these objections. For example, in Bangladesh, family planning workers have discovered people's real objections by setting up focus groups. These comprise eight to ten people of similar background, with a facilitator who encourages the people to share their ideas and fears. Objections are discovered and ways of overcoming them are suggested by the community.

In Jordan, family planning uptake has been increased by engaging the support of religious leaders from both Muslim and Christian communities. These leaders have helped to educate their congregations about the value of using reproductive health services.[16]

Reasons why birth rates fall

Often, birth rates decline as a result of decreasing poverty and increasing education. In turn, the age of marriage increases, as do delays in when couples start having children. Because children are more likely to survive, there is less of a need to have a large family. Because family income increases, fewer children are needed to carry out household tasks, bring in extra money, or act as financial security for old age. This means that, in the long term, tackling poverty reduces population growth.

Additionally, birth rates drop via increased use of FP methods. Our programmes should aim to increase both the choice and availability of family planning methods.

Available family planning methods

Full details of each of these methods, along with their relative advantages and disadvantages,[17] can be found in the summary of methods in Table 18.1. The WHO also provides counselling flip charts and medical eligibility criteria wheels for easy reference to which methods are suitable for which women.[18]

1. Permanent methods

Permanent FP methods include vasectomy for men and tubectomy (tubal ligation) for women. These can be used when no more children are wanted. Couples are only likely to accept these types of methods if there is a high chance that all their existing children will survive to adulthood, and where little stigma is attached to them. As a rule, permanent methods are only appropriate in very stable relationships and when both partners agree. Many experts argue that too much emphasis is given to these methods, and uptake is low (Figure 18.4).

2. Long-acting reversible contraceptive methods (LARCs)

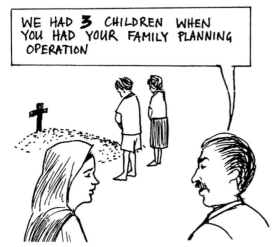

WE HAD 3 CHILDREN WHEN YOU HAD YOUR FAMILY PLANNING OPERATION

Figure 18.4 Permanent FP methods are appropriate only if the couple has at least three healthy children likely to survive into adult life.

LARCs include implants and intrauterine devices. These last from three to twelve years, depending on type and method. Both methods can be offered immediately postpartum, which is a huge advantage for women in remote areas. They are appropriate for women who want to delay starting a family, space their children, or who have completed their families. Experts believe we should be giving more emphasis to these methods.

The contraceptive implant, a progestogen rod inserted by a health professional into the upper arm, e.g. Norplant (lasts three years) and Jadelle (lasts five years). An intra-uterine device (IUD) lasts twelve years, and is also known as the coil. It contains copper and is inserted into the womb by a health professional. There are various brands. Some religious groups are particularly concerned with avoiding any contraceptive method, e.g. IUD, that is perceived to interfere with implantation of the fertilized egg, although the main mode of action is that the copper interferes with sperm motility prior to fertilization.

Finally, the intra-uterine system (IUS) lasts five years, and contains progestogen. It is a good option because it reduces menstrual bleeding, but the cost prohibits its use in many developing countries. Examples are Mirena and Jadess.

3. Short-acting hormonal methods

These methods are used mainly to delay starting a family, for child spacing or to prevent conception in more casual relationships. Injectable contraceptives contain progestogen, and usually last thirteen weeks, depending on the make. These include Depo-Provera, Sayana (designed for self-injection), and Noristerat (eight-week duration). Injectables are popular in sub-Saharan Africa, partly because they can be used without the knowledge of the male partner. The combined contraceptive pill, i.e. 'The Pill', contains an oestrogen and a progesterone, and is typically taken for three weeks followed by a one week gap (or placebo tablets). It can alternatively be taken using the "continuous pill taking method". Other combined hormonal methods remain too expensive for use in developing countries, e.g. the vaginal ring (the NuvaRing is inserted by the user into the vagina), and patches (Evra patches can be used for three weeks followed by a one-week gap).

4. Barrier methods

Condoms are enormously valuable, in that they provide dual protection against unplanned pregnancy and STIs, including Hepatitis B and HIV/AIDS. Female condoms are actively promoted by WHO but uptake is poor. Diaphragms or cervical cap, inserted at the time of sex, are alternative barrier methods with relatively low efficacy, but this can be increased by using spermicides with them.

5. Emergency contraceptives

These are considered safe and should be taken as soon as possible after unprotected sex, but they can still be effective up to five days later.[19] They work primarily by preventing or delaying the release of the egg. There are several specific products taken as single doses (e.g. Levonelle—1.5mg levonorgestrel, or EllaOne—3mg ulipristal). If these are not available, taking two doses twelve hours apart of four combined oral contraceptives, e.g. Microgynon, or a single 40- or 50-tablet dose of a progestin-only pill such as Micronor is almost as effective (see Figure 18.5).

The most effective method of emergency contraception is to insert the copper IUD within five days of unprotected sexual intercourse. This has the advantage of providing *ongoing* contraception, which is an important consideration after any emergency contraception.

All women and girls at risk of an unintended pregnancy have a right to access emergency contraception

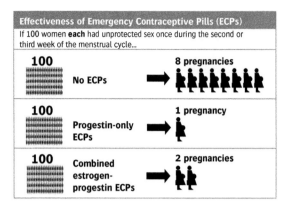

Effectiveness of Emergency Contraceptive Pills (ECPs)
If 100 women **each** had unprotected sex once during the second or third week of the menstrual cycle...

100 No ECPs	**8 pregnancies**
100 Progestin-only ECPs	**1 pregnancy**
100 Combined estrogen-progestin ECPs	**2 pregnancies**

Figure 18.5 Effectiveness of emergency contraception pills.

and these methods should be routinely included within all national FP programmes. Moreover, emergency contraception should be integrated into health care services for populations most at risk of exposure to unprotected sex, including post-rape care and services for women and girls in emergency and disaster settings.

6. Traditional methods

In many societies and religious groups, traditional methods remain an important way of preventing unwanted pregnancies. They are only successful if both partners are committed. The rhythm or standard days method depends on avoiding having sex during the fertile days before and after ovulation. 'Moon beads' and CycleBeads are useful aids for this method.[20]

Exclusive breastfeeding for six months results in lactational amenorrhea (LAM), which reduces the likelihood of conceiving, especially if breastfeeding is regular throughout the 24-hour period. A woman can rely on LAM for contraception if she is engaging in exclusive, regular breastfeeding of a child and has had no return of menses.

Coitus interruptus is when the man withdraws his penis before ejaculation; this has a high failure rate (see Table 18.1 and Figure 18.6).

Method	If method is used consistently and correctly (perfect use):	If method is occasionally used incorrectly or not used (typical use):
Implants	less than 🤰	less than 🤰
IUD	less than 🤰	less than 🤰
Male and female Sterilization	less than 🤰	less than 🤰
Injectables	less than 🤰	🤰🤰🤰🤰🤰🤰
Pills	less than 🤰	🤰🤰🤰🤰🤰🤰🤰🤰
Male condoms	🤰🤰	🤰🤰🤰🤰🤰🤰🤰🤰🤰🤰🤰🤰🤰🤰🤰🤰🤰🤰
Standard Days Method	🤰🤰🤰🤰🤰	🤰🤰🤰🤰🤰🤰🤰🤰🤰🤰🤰🤰
Female condoms	🤰🤰🤰🤰🤰	🤰🤰🤰🤰🤰🤰🤰🤰🤰🤰🤰🤰🤰🤰🤰🤰🤰🤰🤰🤰🤰
Diaphragm	🤰🤰🤰🤰🤰🤰	🤰🤰🤰🤰🤰🤰🤰🤰🤰🤰🤰🤰
Withdrawal	🤰🤰🤰🤰	🤰🤰🤰🤰🤰🤰🤰🤰🤰🤰🤰🤰🤰🤰🤰🤰🤰🤰🤰🤰🤰🤰
Spermicides	🤰🤰🤰🤰🤰🤰🤰🤰🤰🤰🤰🤰🤰🤰🤰🤰🤰🤰	🤰🤰🤰🤰🤰🤰🤰🤰🤰🤰🤰🤰🤰🤰🤰🤰🤰🤰🤰🤰🤰🤰🤰🤰🤰🤰🤰🤰

If 100 Women Use a Method for One Year How Many Will Become Pregnant?

Figure 18.6 Comparative effectiveness of contraceptives. Note: The lactational amenorrhea method (LAM) is a highly effective, temporary method with one to two pregnancies per 100 women in the first six months after childbirth.

Table 18.1 Summary of contraceptive methods

Method	Method of use	How long does it last?	Advantages	Disadvantages	How long does it take to work?	When can it be used after birth?	When does fertility return after stopping/removal?
IUD (copper coil)	Insertion into uterus using aseptic technique.	5–10 years	• Long lasting • No hormonal side effects • Doesn't interfere with sex.	• Can cause serious pain for several weeks/months. • Doesn't protect against STIs.	Immediately	Six weeks or within 48 hours postpartum.	Immediately
Implanon	Small rod-like implant under skin in upper arm.	Three years	• Long lasting. • Doesn't interfere with sex. • Periods irregular or stop altogether.	Can cause tender breasts, spots, headaches, bleeding irregularities.	Immediately if inserted on first day of cycle, otherwise use condoms for a week also.	Immediately	Immediately
Depo-Provera injection	IM injection every three months in the thigh/buttock/arm.	Three months	• Man doesn't need to know. • Doesn't interfere with sex. • Can ease painful periods.	• Weight gain. • Menstrual disturbance (irregular/amenorrhoea). • Decreased bone density with prolonged use leading to osteoporosis.	Immediately on day 1–5, otherwise use condoms for a week also.	Immediately except for exclusively lactating mothers—wait six weeks.	Can take up to a year.
COCP (21-day packs or 28-day packs with the last seven days as a placebo).	One pill at same time every day.	• Advised not to take over age 35 if high risk factors (obesity/smoker). • Not to be taken over age of 45.	• Man doesn't need to know • Doesn't interfere with sex. • Lighter, less painful, more regular periods.	• Doesn't protect against STIs. • If you miss one, take immediately and use condoms for a week. • Cannot take with rifampicin (TB drug) • Breakthrough bleeding.	Immediately if started on first day of cycle, otherwise use condoms for a week also.	After six months	Immediately
POP	One pill at same time every day.	As long as needed.	• Man doesn't need to know. • Doesn't interfere with sex.	• Doesn't protect against STIs. • If you miss one, take and immediately use condoms for a week. • Menstrual disturbance, e.g. irregularity/amenorrhoea. • Headaches, mood swings, breast tenderness (usually subside after few months).	Immediately if started on first day of cycle, otherwise use condoms for a week also.	Immediately	Can take up to six months but can often return immediately.

(continued)

Table 18.1 Continued

Method	Method of use	How long does it last?	Advantages	Disadvantages	How long does it take to work?	When can it be used after birth?	When does fertility return after stopping/removal?
Condoms	• Male rubber condom covers the erect penis. Squeeze air from the top as roll down. Check expiry date. • Female condoms to be inserted in the vagina and cover the external genitalia.	For the duration of sex.	Protects against unwanted pregnancy and STIs/HIV.	Many men don't want to use them.	Immediately	Immediately	Immediately
Moon Beads	• Beads on a string, one bead for each day of 28-day cycle. • Different colours for safe and unsafe days. • Shouldn't be able to get pregnant ('safe days') between days 1–7 and 22–28.		• Natural. No hormones.	• Only works if the cycle is regular. • Easy to make mistakes as hormones can easily fluctuate and alter the cycle.		As soon as your periods start again properly.	
Withdrawal method	Man withdraws penis before climax.			Not a reliable method if you definitely don't want to get pregnant.			Immediately

						Fertility begins when your menstrual cycle restarts.
Lactational	Exclusive and frequent breastfeeding of baby.	Until periods begin +/or until you begin to introduce other feed/drink and weaning.	Cheap, no hormones involved, no side effects.	You can still get pregnant unless you are *exclusively feeding, and frequently.*	Immediately	The first six weeks after birth are the safest.
Bilateral Tubal Ligation (BTL)	The fallopian tubes are occluded by clips under general anaesthesia.	Permanent	No further interventions needed.	Woman may regret it.	• Up to a month. • Make sure woman knows that extra contraception must be used until next menstrual period starts.	Six weeks is the recommended wait.
Vasectomy	Tubes that carry sperm from a man's testicles to the penis are cut, blocked, or sealed.	Permanent	• Man can take responsibility. • Reversal is possible but with reducing success rates.	Most Ugandan men don't want them because they feel it emasculates them.	• Two months. • Need to use extra contraception for two months after operation.	

Protecting against sexually transmitted infections (STIs)

Key facts from the WHO:[21]

- More than one million sexually transmitted infections (STIs) are acquired every day worldwide.
- Each year, there are an estimated 357 million new infections either chlamydia, gonorrhoea, syphilis or trichomoniasis.
- More than 500 million people are estimated to have genital infection with herpes simplex virus (HSV).
- More than 290 million women have human papillomavirus (HPV) infection.
- The majority of STIs have no symptoms or only mild symptoms that may not be recognized as an STI.
- STIs such as HSV type 2 and syphilis can increase the risk of acquiring HIV.
- Over 900,000 pregnant women were infected with syphilis resulting in approximately 350,000 adverse birth outcomes, including stillbirth, in 2012.
- Both hepatitis B and HIV infection are spread through sex, but also by other means. Hepatitis B is between 50 and 100 times more infectious than HIV.
- STIs can have serious long-term health consequences, such as infertility or mother-to-child transmission.

The ABC approach for protection against STIs is promoted by governments and religious groups:

- *Abstinence*
- *Be* faithful
- *Condoms*

While these principles will keep many people safe, the reality is that most young people become sexually active before the age of 18. The US has spent more than $1.4 billion since 2004 telling young people in Africa to abstain from sex before marriage and then commit to a single partner. That funding didn't influence the number of sex partners people had, the age at which they started having sex, or teenage pregnancy rates.[22]

Evaluations of comprehensive sex education programmes show that they can help youth delay onset of sexual activity, reduce the frequency of sexual activity, reduce the number of sexual partners, and increase condom and contraceptive use. Importantly, the evidence shows youth who receive comprehensive sex education are *NOT* more likely to become sexually active, increase sexual activity, or experience negative sexual health outcomes.[23] Effective programmes exist for youth from a variety of racial, cultural, and socio-economic backgrounds. Young people need honest, effective sex education—not ineffective, shame-based, abstinence-only programmes.

What we need to do

Deciding to develop an FP programme

To help us decide to develop an FP programme, we must first answer a few questions.

1. Is FP allowed or encouraged by government?

Usually, developing FP services is encouraged by government, but there may be variations due to specific religious or cultural objections. Where this is the case, we should act with care, but still do all we can to make services available. Equally, we must not coerce families into using FP.

Furthermore, it is important to build a good understanding of the political and social will to develop FP services. Do the people, government, and social bodies want it? Have they asked us to provide it? If not, we need first to focus preliminary efforts on creating awareness, tackling any misconceptions, and thus generating greater demand.

2. Is it a felt need in our target area?

Increasingly, couples are aware of FP, but there remains a large unmet need. Although most communities will have some couples using some form of contraception, very few will be aware of the range available. In some communities, there will be a lack of services of any kind. Unmet need is defined as the proportion of the population of reproductive age who wish to delay or avoid having a child but are not currently using any family planning. By understanding the proportion of the population who are eligible for family planning but have an unmet need we can determine the potential need for family planning services.

We can assess unmet need of FP by asking the following questions:

- Are they of reproductive age and eligible for family planning?

Consider *excluding* those who are post-menopausal, have had a hysterectomy, or are currently pregnant.

● Do they wish to have a child in the next two years?

This question identifies the need for contraception. Those who do not wish to have a child in the next two years have *need*.

● If a need is established, are they using any FP method?

If they are not, this determines they have a need which is *unmet*.

3. Use comparative family size evaluation to determine demand.

Another useful assessment is to survey how many children families/women wish to have, compared with the Total Fertility Rate or average family size. For example, in Uganda, where most women desire to have 4.8 children, the average family size is 6.7.[24] This shows that women are having at least two more children than they desire. This helps us identify potential demand for FP services in the area.

4. Is there a need related to STIs?

Dual contraceptive methods (combining barrier methods with a hormonal or non-hormonal method) are the gold standard for preventing both unwanted pregnancy and STIs. This means it is important to find out more about prevalence (percentage of a population affected with a particular disease at a given time) and incidence (the number of new cases of a disease in a population over a period of time) of both HIV and other key STIs. Is incidence increasing or decreasing? How aware is the community of STIs and their dangers? What proportion of the population might be using barrier contraception?

5. Consider teenage pregnancies and termination rates.

Teenage pregnancy and unwanted pregnancies are useful markers of need. If the data is available, it is useful for building a case for family planning services and awareness building.

6. Consider maternal death rates.

Finally, we should also consider the maternal death rates. High maternal death rates can be linked to unwanted pregnancies and to poorly spaced births, both of which can be prevented by effective family planning services.

7. Is the programme sustainable?

It is absolutely vital to work closely with local, regional, and national health service infrastructure to sustain an FP programme. We need the ownership and buy-in of local institutions to ensure any FP programme is effective and sustainable. This includes engaging with key cultural and religious institutions. Without them, it is unlikely a programme will work and there may be opposition.

For FP to be sustained, it is also important that we integrate it with other key programme areas. Family planning should never be a stand-alone or vertical programme, but rather a valuable, recognized part of health and community-based services. It forms special linkages with:

● HIV services;
● STI services;
● Outpatient clinics;
● Community clinics;
● Child health services/immunization programmes;
● Maternal health services (antenatal for building awareness and postnatal to start or restart family planning services); and
● Mental health services.

Ideally, family planning education, training, and services should be provided in our community health programme. If this is not possible to start with, we should concentrate on the key areas of STIs, including HIV, postnatal care and child immunization programmes.

We will need trained staff, reliable supplies, efficient planning, long-term commitment and effective community partnership if the programme is to continue. Finance, too, is needed in order to provide good, reliable, local and affordable supplies.

Set aims and targets

Programme aims and targets will vary according to the communities we work with. An eventual aim, if this ties in with the community's wishes, is to develop a family norm of three children, spaced three or more years apart. This change in community behaviour will often take many years to achieve.

Another useful aim is to reduce the unmet need for FP. This is a valuable community-led aim as the couple/woman defines their own need. As mentioned, increasing the number of couples who space their children by three or more years is a valuable target. Again, we can set targets depending on the circumstances of the communities we are working in. Box 18.1 suggests some specific targets for a community with low uptake.

A further valuable aim is to increase the contraceptive prevalence rate—defined as the percentage of

---

Box 18.1 Specific target suggestions for a community with low FP uptake

Years 0 to 3:

- Create awareness so that an increasing number of couples wish to use FP services and protection against STIs.
- Provide FP when requested.
- Set up an effective mother and child programme that will help to stimulate demand.
- Educate and train providers at a community level
- Develop a screening programme for unmet needs and subsequent provision of services
- Build relationships with key community stakeholders (i.e. religious and cultural leaders, school heads, etc.).

Year 3 onwards:

- Promote FP actively through community-level education programmes.
- Create community-level advocates through local stakeholders/institutions (i.e. schools, religious organizations, village health volunteers).
- Develop a youth-friendly service in local health institutions (see 'Youth outreach' section for further detail).
- Set outcome targets for the project area, e.g. reduce unmet need (defined in 'Deciding to develop an FP programme') for FP and teenage pregnancy rates by 50 per cent at three years and 80 per cent at five years.

---

women who are practising, or whose sexual partners are practising, any form of contraception. It is usually measured for 'in-union' women ages 15 to 49. Depending on the rate in our community (which requires trust and tact to discover) we could aim to increase this by perhaps 10 per cent per year for three years, i.e. a community with 40 per cent contraceptive prevalence could increase to 70 per cent after three years.

In all areas of the world, we need to maximize the use of condoms as dual protection against unwanted pregnancy and STIs. A key target therefore will be to see annual increases in the use of condoms. All these targets are usually incorporated into the logframe (see Chapter 7).

Prepare the community

An interest in FP will usually develop when families know that their children are likely to survive. FP tends to grow naturally as primary health care takes effect. As women realize there are ways of controlling their fertility and protecting themselves from unplanned pregnancies, they will develop a strong interest in using services to gain control over their lives. But services need to be available or their desire cannot be met. A motto commonly used is 'Choice, not Chance'.

We can increase interest and uptake in the following ways:

- meeting objections, lack of understanding and questions through discussion in clinics and in the community;

- working through religious groups, priests, imams, or other leaders and encouraging them to support family planning;
- teaching on family planning through women's clubs, youth clubs, co-operatives, and schools;
- training TBAs and CHWs to be FP motivators and suppliers;
- using national publicity campaigns, in particular, radio broadcasts, details of which can be passed on to the community;
- including FP as a subject in literacy courses;
- HIV and STI awareness campaigns; and
- the use of local HIV/AIDS support groups or home-care teams.

Methods used for teaching must be appropriate for the culture, remove fears, answer questions and underline the benefits of contraception.

Benefits may include: more money, food and space for the family; no more worries about unwanted pregnancies; a better sex life; more peace and quiet at home; fewer dowries to pay.

Cascade training and community outreach

A useful method for helping the community to engage with FP is through cascade training.[25] Cascade training integrates basic teaching and public speaking skills into FP training, so that trainees can pass on, or 'cascade', their training to colleagues and the wider community This helps health workers to feel more confident and motivated to engage in community outreach work, deliver health talks, and run educational activities at a community level. For this to work effectively, health institutions/NGOs need to provide funding and motivation to build community outreach work into health workers' job plans. The training can be integrated with other important public health topics such as HIV/AIDs awareness, vaccination, hygiene and sanitation.

For example, the USHAPE project in South West Uganda[26] adopted a 'whole institution approach' to FP training, where all staff at local community hospitals were given a basic level of training to increase awareness and tackle misconceptions. Then, selected clinical staff, such as midwives, nurses, and clinical officers were given more intensive training to develop skills as counsellors, method providers and community health educators

Community health workers (CHWs) in cascade training

CHWs or village health teams are a vital resource in cascading correct and accurate information about FP into the community. Programmes should hold regular events to update CHWs' FP and sexual health knowledge, advise them of the available services, and encourage them to screen and refer those with unmet needs. Their unique access to the heart of communities enables them to be trusted advocates of positive FP messages, which can go a long way to achieving cultural and behavioural change.

Men's engagement

We must always remember how important it is for men to be involved in FP, both at the family and community (leadership) level. Our programmes must focus on their needs and their responsibilities as well.

Screening, counselling, and education of men should be an integral part of any FP programme. Men are often put off from attending clinics, which are often viewed as focusing on women, especially when located in hospitals. Planning community outreach targeted at men, in locations and with events of special interest to them, is important. We should consider where men normally congregate and what interests they have, such as sporting events and local gathering spots. We must listen to their concerns and reservations, so that they feel engaged. Tackling men's myths and misconceptions about FP often increases women's access, uptake, and continuing use of services. Above all, we want to encourage and empower men to use barrier methods against unwanted pregnancy and to minimize the spread of infections.

Youth outreach

Young people are another important and underserved target group for any FP programme. We will need to do careful preparatory work with religious and educational groups before starting a youth outreach programme. One place to start is to demonstrate the number of teenage pregnancies and the social challenges they cause. A youth-targeted programme can combine abstinence messages with comprehensive sex and relationship education and teaching about contraception. This combined approach—education, services, preventing teenage and unwanted pregnancies, and improving sexual health—can be a winning combination and may help to reassure those who are traditionally opposed to anything beyond teaching sexual abstinence.

Using systems of anonymous questions and feedback are helpful to tailor the programme to the specific needs of youth and to discover areas of ignorance and fear. UNFPA advocates 'youth-friendly corners' and services in local health clinics as a means of engaging young people in a comfortable, confidential environment.[27]

> The UNFPA advises that youth-friendly services should include:
>
> Universal access to *accurate* sexual and reproductive health information;
>
> A range of *safe* and *affordable* contraceptive methods;
>
> *Sensitive* counselling;
>
> *Quality* obstetric and antenatal care for *all* pregnant women and girls;
>
> The *prevention* and *management* of sexually transmitted infections, including HIV.

Young people can also be reached through local youth groups or schools. Working through youth groups and schools can break down barriers between young people and health facilities and encourage them to access services in the future. But these approaches must be sensitive to the way young people behave and think in their community or circle, and should be based on friendship and shared understanding, not fear and coercion. These activities can also (dare we say it?) be fun.

Ensure supplies

It is better not to start a programme at all than to start and run out of supplies (Figure 18.7). Community members must have confidence that supplies are always available. Nothing destroys a promising FP programme so successfully as running out of supplies.

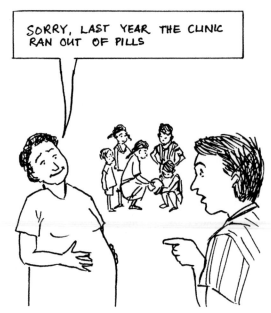

SORRY, LAST YEAR THE CLINIC RAN OUT OF PILLS

Figure 18.7 It is better not to start a programme at all than to start and run out of supplies.

Reproduced courtesy of David Gifford. This image is distributed under the terms of the Creative Commons Attribution Non-Commercial 4.0 International licence (CC-BY-NC), a copy of which is available at http://creativecommons.org/licenses/by-nc/4.0/.

To ensure supplies:
1. Identify two or more sources for each type needed.
2. Obtain adequate initial stocks.
3. Order well ahead of need.
4. Protect supplies, especially condoms, pills, and injections from spoiling in storage.
5. Set up a reliable system for moving supplies from central stores to clinics and other outlets.
6. Encourage couples to use locally available, good-quality supplies; these are often available through schemes set up by NGOs, e.g. Marie Stopes International.

We must ensure dependable supplies are available locally at a reasonable price. We must also ensure we have medicines to treat the STIs that are found in the areas where we are working.

Affordability is essential for the success of any FP programme. The health programme with the community can help to lobby for funds to enable services to be free or nearly free. Without the community knowing that supplies are likely to continue to be free, the programme is unlikely to work. Many governments are now providing free FP supplies, but experience on the ground does not always reflect national policy. We therefore need to monitor costs and access to FP supplies, as part of our programme monitoring.

Organize an FP clinic

Although some activities, including distribution, take place in the community, the clinic usually remains the focal point of an FP programme. While we could set up a separate family planning clinic, there are advantages of FP being part of a general clinic:

1. All health needs are met together, at the same time and place. This is especially convenient for patients who travel a long distance.
2. It reduces project time and resources if FP uptake is low.
3. It enables confidential advice to be given to women who may wish to keep their interest secret, especially when stigma or suspicion surrounds this area of personal need (generally couples, not individuals, should be counselled.)
4. When patients who may be eligible for FP come for other reasons, the need for FP can be raised with them, so increasing uptake.

However, there are also advantages of running separate FP clinics (which should always offer sexual health and STI services):

1. Staff can concentrate on FP rather than trying to provide a range of mother/child health (MCH) services as well.
2. FP can be given priority. In a combined clinic, FP can easily get squeezed out or forgotten because of more immediate needs.
3. Waiting time may be shorter.
4. Mutual support can be gained from fellow clients, thus encouraging uptake.
5. It may give an opportunity to help diagnose and treat STIs more easily and confidentially than in a general clinic.

When a health centre first starts, a room can be set aside exclusively for FP activities during an MCH or general clinic. As clinics develop and numbers increase, separate reproductive health, i.e. FP plus STI clinics, can be considered.

Who is involved in an FP clinic?

The Family Planning Provider (FPP), often a nurse, will usually manage the programme. There are various names used for this role, e.g. community reproductive health worker, which better describes a wider role they develop when more fully trained. Assistants such as TBAs, CHWs, or responsible community members will also be involved. There will also be a visiting doctor, whose tasks may include tubectomies and vasectomies on prearranged days, either at the referral hospital or the clinic if this has adequate facilities, and inserting IUDs and IUSs and contraceptive implants. A doctor can advise on difficult cases and give training and supervision. He/she will oversee the treatment of STIs.

In one central African country, guidelines were drawn up about how an FPP should be selected, trained, and used:

1. A member of the health team, usually a woman, is selected and sent for special FP training.
2. The person chosen is acceptable to the community being served, in terms of gender, age, and personality.
3. The training takes place within a well-functioning FP clinic, so that the trainee becomes familiar with all techniques and advice.
4. On her return, the FPP carries out FP sessions at set times each week, during which she is not diverted into other primary health activities. Times of FP sessions are posted outside the clinic and made known to the community.
5. As soon as possible, the FPP starts training another health team member, to share her work and substitute when she is absent.
6. She avoids being rushed, allowing about ten minutes per patient.

Men should be encouraged to attend with their partners, and programmes should ensure a welcoming and open environment for men to engage. (see 'Men's engagement').

Instruction sheets for the *provider* on each FP method should be used. The WHO has several useful resources and counselling aids that can be used. At a minimum, instruction sheets should include the following:

- indications for use;
- method of use;
- any absolute reasons they should not be used;
- any serious side effects;
- duration and effectiveness;
- instructions to patient;
- type of examination needed if any;
- follow-up; and
- treatment of any minor disease or infection discovered.

Instruction sheets for the guidance of the *client* will also be needed, in the local language and with clear illustrations. We must ensure we do not put unnecessary medical barriers against family planning methods because of rare dangers or side effects (see Further reading and resources below).

Medicines to treat STIs will need to be available in any clinic we set up. If our clinic provides voluntary counselling and testing for HIV, we must always have the nationally recommended, antiretroviral therapy (ART) available, or know where they can easily, reliably and affordably be obtained.

Keeping FP records

These could include:

1. Person's own self-retained card. Record the method (and number if OC pill used). Also record the treatment of any STI.
2. Family folder insert card, if used. Record type, amount, and date for review.
3. FP register or computerized record (see Figure 18.8).
4. Some programmes with a strong FP emphasis can give each client a special FP record card.

There will be rare occasions when no record should be made in order to protect confidentiality.

Community-based distribution of FP supplies

Community-based distribution (CBD) refers to using ordinary members of the community as providers of FP supplies. CBD is especially useful where contraceptive use is low, clinics are difficult to reach (or intimidating), and where there are few qualified health workers.

Social marketing, though overlapping with CBD, has important differences. It refers to the commercial but subsidized sale of pills, injections, and condoms with small profits made by a middle man. This means that users need to pay a small amount. Doctors may be involved in helping to set this up, but care must be taken to ensure supplies are easily affordable

Keys to successful CBD

There are three sets of factors for successful CBD (see Table 18.2).

1. Support from three sources: the organizing health programme, the suppliers and the community.

This will come about as we raise awareness, involve the community, respond to their suggestions, and identify and train suppliers. Every task we do, or change that we bring about, must be largely acceptable to the community and within the laws of the country. A range of people can become suppliers: shopkeepers, pharmacies, trained TBAs and traditional healers, village health committee

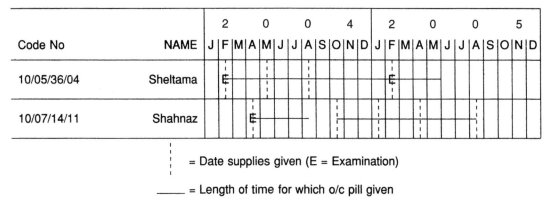

Figure 18.8 Sample page from oral contraceptive pill section of FP register used in one project.

members, factory supervisors or workers, barbers and locally respected community members or religious leaders. For example, in Afghanistan, women have nearly a one in eight chance of dying as a result of pregnancy and delivery, contraceptive use is known to be 300 times safer than pregnancy, and the Quran promotes two years of breastfeeding. This is the backdrop to a programme that increased the contraceptive prevalence rate by 25 per cent in just eight months, due to government support, encouragement from religious leaders (mullahs), and the use of community health workers.[28]

There can also be an overlap with those who act as directly observed treatment (DOT) supervisors in tuberculosis (TB) programmes and for ART in people living with HIV, as antiretrovirals become more widely used and available (see Chapter 20). However, levels of confidentiality and community confidence have to be strong to allow mixed roles such as these.

Table 18.2 Factors affecting the success of CBD programmes

Support	Accessibility	Quality
Strong commitment of the sponsoring institution.	Services offered at popular locations.	Sponsoring institution adheres to standards and protocols for contraceptive distribution.
Participation of members of the community.	Dependable supply of contraceptive methods.	Adequate training for personnel.
Adequate numbers of dedicated distributors.	Travel time and cost required to reach service points kept to a minimum.	Users receive all the necessary information to permit them to make informed choices.
CBD is acceptable within legal, ethical and cultural norms.	Waiting time to receive services kept to a minimum.	Contraceptives are medically approved, have not reached their expiry dates, and are locally known and trusted.
Financial and material support from the sponsoring institution, the community, and donor agencies.	Services affordable to all potential users, including those on a low income.	Client-provider confidentiality is respected.
Plans in place to ensure the sustainability of the CBD programme.	Referrals offered for other family planning services.	A follow-up system exists to maintain contact with users.

2. Accessibility and acceptability of services and supplies (i.e. easy use and do not cause offence).

CBD can include contraceptive pills, injections (by pharmacists or even storekeepers who have been adequately trained), condoms, spermicides, plus referrals for IUDs, IUSs, implants or permanent FP methods to the nearest clinic or hospital. For example, in sub-Saharan Africa, injectables are often the most popular form of contraception. CBD workers in Madagascar learned to inject successfully, counsel and manage clients' questions. This increased contraceptive use, with 1,662 women accepting injectables from a CBD worker. Of these, 41 per cent were new FP users. Nearly all clients interviewed said they intended to return to the CBD worker for re-injection and would recommend this service to a friend.[29]

3. Quality of the services, including medical backup.

Services must be well managed to ensure quality, reliability of supply, training of suppliers, follow-up and maintenance of ethical standards. Our community health programme can provide checklists and protocols to guide suppliers about medical backup or referral. We can provide simple, illustrated client leaflets to explain options.

A summary of FP stages

FP provision has four stages:

1. Motivation.

Motivation includes various levels and aspects around FP. We must help the couple or individual to understand their need for FP so they actively request it. Motivation can come from the community, clinic, advice over the radio, the Internet, or mobile phone. However, friends, other family members, CHWs, TBAs, skilled attendants, other health workers, teachers, members of women's clubs, religious leaders, store-keepers, film and sports stars (see Figure 18.9) can all also be helpful in increasing uptake of FP.

2. Counselling

We must provide a general explanation about different FP methods to help the couple or individual choose the best method for them. Detailed explanations about the method chosen, including how to use it, its failure rate, any side effects and necessary follow-up should be part of the conversation (Figure 18.10). The counsellor must be ready to answer questions, and depending on the literacy of the client, be able to supply written or visual back-up material. Counselling can happen in the clinic, the hospital, the community, or in private homes, and can be given by a health worker, nurse, skilled attendant,

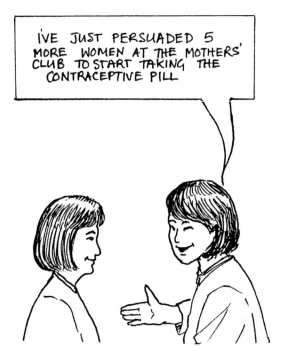

Figure 18.9 Satisfied customers make effective family planning promoters.

Reproduced courtesy of David Gifford. This image is distributed under the terms of the Creative Commons Attribution Non-Commercial 4.0 International licence (CC-BY-NC), a copy of which is available at http://creativecommons.org/licenses/by-nc/4.0/.

TBA, or the FPP. Additionally, the community distributor or sometimes store-keeper in the case of pills, injections, condoms and spermicides may also help.

We may wish to train providers to use the counselling tool for family planning, a four-stage technique for effective counselling (Box 18.2):

Box 18.2 4 stage FP counselling tool

Step 1: Establish rapport and assess client's needs and concerns.

Step 2: Provide information to address client's identified needs or concerns.

Step 3: Help client make an informed decision or address a problem.

Step 4: Help carry out client's decision.

Source: data from World Health Organization, the Population Council, and the United States Agency for International DevelopmentTechnical Consultation on Community Counselling. New Delhi, India: WHO. Copyright 2011 © WHO. This table is distributed under the terms of the Creative Commons Attribution Non Commercial 4.0 International licence (CC-BY-NC), a copy of which is available at http://creativecommons.org/licenses/by-nc/4.0/

This counselling tool was developed as a collaborative effort during the Technical Consultation on Community Counseling, convened by the WHO, the Population Council and the United States Agency for International Development, which took place 25–29 July 2011 in New Delhi, India.

3. Providing the service

Initial FP provision, including giving the first supplies, injection, or insertion, should happen in the clinic for IUDs, IUSs, injectables, implants, as well as for transdermal patches, the vaginal ring, and sometimes for the first pack of pills. FP provision can be given in the community or clinic for condoms, further pills and short-acting methods. Any surgical procedures should take place in the clinic or hospital.

FPPs or nurses can insert IUDs, give injections, and sometimes provide the first pack of pills; other health workers or community distributors can issue condoms and repeat supplies of pills. Doctors should be seen for any operations, medical back-up, and referrals.

4. Follow-up

We must provide follow up after any operations or surgical procedures, and check for wound infections or other side effects, and answer any questions. IUDs should be checked at least once after insertion and then follow an 'open-house' policy with no set return dates until replacement, which needs considering every ten or more years.

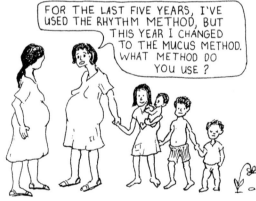

Figure 18.10 Encourage couples to use the most reliable methods.

Injections should be repeated at the prescribed intervals, and for implants no set follow-up is necessary, but women are free to return at any time, especially if there are bleeding problems. Finally, for those taking pills, we should carry out yearly checks.

All methods benefit from an open-house policy. We must guarantee that everyone knows they can return with any problems or questions, at any time. All follow up should be done at the clinic or community, and by the least qualified health worker able to do it competently.

Include facilities for controlling STIs

At the outset, we need to be especially aware of the overwhelming sexual health needs of young people. Over one-third of the world, i.e. about 1.8 billion people, are adolescents or children.[30] They are, or soon will be, sexually active.

These young people arrive in huge numbers in the cities of the developing world, where sexual health services are almost completely absent. They will probably be unable to access FP advice. If they develop an STI they will not know where to get treatment. Many will have virtually no knowledge about how to avoid STIs, including HIV/AIDS.

Their real-life situation will often mean they fail to apply the information they do have. An increasing number, including children, drift into commercial sex work for want of other work or are victims of trafficking. Migration to cities with no reproductive health services is fuelling an epidemic of STIs, backstreet abortions and increased spread of HIV/AIDS. In addition, large numbers of babies are born to teenage mothers in urban situations with virtually no facilities or backup (see Further reading and resources).

This is a situation where CHPs need to find creative solutions and work alongside any government-led services for adolescents that may have been drawn up, but perhaps imperfectly implemented. In urban areas in particular, we need to be aware of gender violence, the abuse of young girls and boys, and other sexual practices which undermine the long-term physical and mental health of those who have been abused (see Chapter 27). This may lead us into areas such as advocacy.

To set up facilities for the control of STIs, we need to consider firstly prevention, and secondly treatment (see Box 18.3).

Box 18.3 *The Five Cs of STI Control:*

Counselling: educate about sexual health and transmission of STIs.

Condoms: educate about usage and provide easy access.

Confidentiality: ensure that staff understand the importance of confidentiality.

Compliance: ensure that patients complete their antibiotic course.

Contact tracing: gain patient's trust and understanding; be sensitive, but persistent in tracking down contacts.

Adapted with permission from Booth, B. et al. Urban Health and Development. Copyright © Macmillan, TALC and Tearfund. This box is distributed under the terms of the Creative Commons Attribution Non Commercial 4.0 International licence (CC-BY-NC), a copy of which is available at http://creativecommons.org/licenses/by-nc/4.0/.

Preventing STIs

In our programmes we should include the prevention of STIs as a normal part of our health teaching in home, community, and clinic. Because this is sometimes a very sensitive area, we should make sure that our approach is culturally aware and that the community knows that any personal counselling given will be completely confidential. Furthermore, the prevention of STIs will tie in with many parts of our health programme and needs to be integrated with it. This will include any HIV/AIDS programme we are involved with, including VCT and providing ART; antenatal care; CHW training and the teaching by CHWs in the community; curative care in our clinics; our FP programme; school health teaching; and involvement in podcasts, other Internet and SMS technology, social media, radio, and television.

We have already looked at the classic ABC approach, which on its own is fairly ineffective, compared with sexual health education programmes. The adapted ABC approach, and the CNN approach, are both currently in widespread use:

A: *A*bstain from sex or delay first sex for as long as possible.

B: *B*e faithful to one partner or minimize the number of sexual partners.

C: *C*orrect and *c*onsistent *c*ondom use—both male and, where appropriate, female condoms.

The CNN approach provides guidance in harm reduction for high-risk groups:

C: *C*ondom use.

N: Clean *n*eedles, especially among IV drug users.

N: *N*egotiation, especially by women who are not in stable relationships, e.g. commercial sex workers, to increase the likelihood of safer sex.

Both approaches, which arose out of attempts to control the HIV pandemic, have their critics and their supporters. We should decide what approaches and what forms of advice and supplies will be most acceptable and effective in our communities. In both cases we need to set up comprehensive sexual health education programmes, which can be used alongside either of the approaches above.

Finally, we should be aware of the future use of microbicides. These are substances that kill organisms which cause STIs.[31] They will be largely used in association with condoms, mainly as intravaginal gels or creams. One that is currently being trialled is an impregnated vaginal ring. Microbicides have been slow to live up to their original promise. NB: microbicides must not be confused with spermicides such as nonoxynol-9, which kills sperm and therefore acts as a partial contraceptive, but have no effect on disease-causing organisms.

Treating STIs

We will need to decide how much we are able to diagnose and treat STIs in our clinic and how much we will refer them to other centres. In practice, there are three reasons we should include STIs in our health programme.

Firstly, STIs are common, dangerous, and unless treated can have serious effects on past, present and future partners, such as infertility and the risk of an ectopic pregnancy (pregnancy outside the uterus).

Secondly, there will often be no other practical options for treatment, especially in rural areas.

Lastly, we can use what is known as the syndromic approach. This is a relatively easy way of treating symptoms or groups of symptoms with particular drugs, without needing to use a laboratory. Typical examples would be the appropriate antibiotic treatment for urethral discharge, genital ulcer or vaginal discharge. The WHO provides guidelines which are updated every few years as the common STI organisms develop resistance to treatment.[32]

Evaluate the programme

At regular intervals we should evaluate the effectiveness of our FP programme and our diagnosis and treatment of STIs. This will require baseline information before starting, which should include the Contraceptive

Prevalence Rate (CPR) and the Total Fertility Rate (TFR). CPR is described under Set aims and targets, and is most easily remembered as:

$$\frac{\begin{array}{c}Number\ of\ women\ aged\ 15\text{--}49\\ (or\ partners)\ using\ contraception\end{array}}{Total\ number\ of\ women\ aged\ 15\text{--}49}\times100$$

The TFR is the average total number of children to which women have given birth by the end of their reproductive period. Both these figures can be calculated for communities from information on the family folder obtained at the time of the community survey. For information on use of contraceptives to calculate CPR, we may need to postpone asking questions until we have the full confidence of the people.

One option would be to do a specific survey one year after a community survey or do a small sample survey to obtain a baseline CPR. Every three to five years we could resurvey the community and compare the new CPR to the baseline. Every five to ten years we could in addition calculate the new TFR—the chief outcome indicator—which takes longer to show changes.

Unmet needs can be monitored routinely by implementing a screening programme in local clinics or hospitals. This helps to monitor the community's response to the actions we are taking and also measures screening coverage as a marker of how effectively the health workers have engaged with the community. Routine screening programmes can be cross-referenced periodically to assess whether progress in meeting unmet needs compares favourably with other programmes in the country.

In addition, it is always useful to monitor the acceptability of our programme to different groups of users. We can devise questions and rank answers from 1 to 5. We can evaluate using these and other areas we have prioritized in our programme aims, such as teenage pregnancy rates, maternal death rates and termination rates.

Further reading and resources

Bateson D, McNamee K, Briggs P. Newer non-oral hormonal contraception. *British Medical Journal*. 2013; 346 (7898).

Brown R, Brown J. *The family planning clinic in Africa*. 3rd edn. New York: Macmillan; 1998.

Counselling tool for family planning. https://www.fptraining. org/resources/counseling-tool-family-planning-flip-chart Flannelgraph on Family Planning STDs and AIDS. Available from: TALC.

The Lancet Series on Sexual and Reproductive Health. 2006. Available from: http://www.thelancet.com/series/sexual-and-reproductive-health

MacGregor EA, Guillebaud J. The 7-day contraceptive hormone free interval should be consigned to history. *BMJ Sex Reprod Health*. 2018; 44: 214–220.

Macmillan A, Scott GR. *Sexually transmitted infections*. New York: Churchill Livingstone; 2000.

United Nations Population Fund. Adolescent reproductive health. Available from: http://www.unfpa.org/resources/adolescent-sexual-and-reproductive-health

World Health Organization. *Community-based distribution of contraceptives*. Geneva: World Health Organization; 1995.

World Health Organization. *Family planning: A Global Handbook for providers*. 2018. Available from: www.fphandbook.org

World Health Organization. *Medical eligibility criteria wheel for contraceptive use*. 2015. Available from: http://srhr.org/mecwheel/

World Health Organization. *WHO Selected Practice Recommendations*. 3rd edn. Geneva: World Health Organization; *Selected practice recommendations for contraceptive use*. 2016. Available from: http://apps.who.int/iris/handle/10665/252267.

Websites

Family Planning 2020. Available from: http://www.familyplanning2020.org

Family Planning Handbook. Available from: www.fphandbook.org

Marie Stopes International. Available from: http://www.mariestopes.org.uk

Training Resource Package. Available from: https://www.fptraining.org

Ugandan Sexual Health and Pastoral Education (USHAPE). Available from: http://www.ushape.org.uk

United Nations Population Fund. Available from: http://www.unfpa.org.

References

1. Bill & Melinda Gates Foundation. Family planning strategy overview. Available from: http://www.gatesfoundation.org/What-We-Do/Global-Development/Family-Planning

2. World Health Organization. *Contraception factsheet*. 2014. Available from: http://apps.who.int/iris/bitstream/10665/112319/1/WHO_RHR_14.07_eng.pdf

3. World Health Organization. *Family planning/contraception factsheet*. Updated 2016. Available from: http://www.who.int/mediacentre/factsheets/fs351/en/

4. World Health Organization. Progress report. Reproductive health strategy: To accelerate progress towards the attainment of international development goals and targets. 2010. Available from: http://www.who.int/reproductivehealth/publications/general/rhr_10_14/en/

5. Ahmed S, Li Q, Liu L, Tsui AO. Maternal deaths averted by contraceptive use: An analysis of 172 countries. *The Lancet*. 2012; 380 (9837): 111–25.

6. Carr B, Gates MF, Mitchell A, Shah R. Giving women the power to plan their families. *The Lancet*. 2012; 380 (9837): 80–2.

7. Grimes D, Benson J, Singh S, Romero M, Genatra B, Okonofua FE, et al. Unsafe abortion: The preventable

pandemic. *The Lancet*. 2006; 368 (9550): 1908–19. Available from: http://www.thelancet.com/journals/lancet/article/PIIS 0140-6736(06)69481-6/abstract

8. Akhter S. Complications of adolescent pregnancy and its prevention. *The Daily Star*. 28 July 2013. Available from: http://www.thedailystar.net/news/complications-of-adolescent-pregnancy-and-its-prevention

9. World Health Organization. *Adolescent pregnancy: Maternal, newborn, child and adolescent health*. Available from: http://www.who.int/maternal_child_adolescent/topics/maternal/adolescent_pregnancy/en/

10. Kozuki N, Walker N. Exploring the association between short/long preceding birth intervals and child mortality: Using reference birth interval children of the same mother as comparison. *BMC Public Health*. 2013; 13(Suppl 3): S6. Available from: https://www.ncbi.nlm.nih.gov/pmc/articles/PMC3847658/

11. Williams E, Hossain M, Sharma RK, Kumar V, Pandey CM, Baqui AH. Birth interval and risk of stillbirth or neonatal death: Findings from rural north India. *Journal of Tropical Pediatrics*. 2008; 54(5): 321–7.

12. Population Media Center. *Global Population*. Available from: http://www.populationmedia.org/issues/population/

13. The United Nations. *2015 Revision of World Population Prospects*. New York: United Nations: 2015. Available from: https://esa.un.org/unpd/wpp/

14. United Nations Population Fund. *Statement—population and reproductive health: Key to the achievement of the MDGs*. New York: UNFPA; 2005. Available from: http://www.unfpa.org/press/population-and-reproductive-health-key-achievement-mdgs

15. Cohen J. Make secondary education universal. *Nature*. 2008; 456 (7222): 572–3.

16. Gavlak D. Family planning gains ground. *Bulletin of the World Health Organization*. 2011; 89 (11): 782–3.

17. World Health Organization. *Family planning: A global handbook for providers*. Geneva: World Health Organization; 2018. Available from: http://apps.who.int/iris/bitstream/10665/44028/1/9780978856373_eng.pdf

18. World Health Organization. *Medical eligibility criteria wheel for contraceptive use*. 2015. Available from: http://srhr.org/mecwheel/

19. World Health Organization. *Emergency contraception factsheet*. Updated 2017. Geneva: World Health Organization; 2017. Available from: http://who.int/mediacentre/factsheets/fs244/en/

20. CycleBeads. *Plan or prevent pregnancy naturally*. Available from: https://www.cyclebeads.com/

21. World Health Organization. *Sexually transmitted infections (STIs) Fact sheet*. Updated 2016. Available from: http://www.who.int/mediacentre/factsheets/fs110/en/

22. Lo N, Lowe A, Bendavid E. Abstinence funding was not associated with reductions in HIV risk behavior in sub-Saharan Africa. *Health Affairs*. 2016; 35 (5). DOI: 10.1377/hlthaff.2015.0828

23. Advocates for Youth. *Comprehensive sex education: Research and results*. 2009. Available from: http://www.advocatesforyouth.org/publications/1487

24. Uganda Bureau of Statistics (UBOS) and ICF. *Uganda demographic and health survey 2016*. Kampala, Uganda/Rockville, MD: UBOS and ICF; 2018. Available from: https://dhsprogram.com/pubs/pdf/FR333/FR333.pdf

25. Stanback J, Griffey S, Lynam P, Ruto C, Cummings S. Improving adherence to family planning guidelines in Kenya: An experiment. *International Journal for Quality in Health Care*. 2007; 19 (2): 68–73.

26. USHAPE. *Uganda Sexual Health and Pastoral Education*. Available from: https://ushape.org.uk/

27. United Nations Population Fund. *Adolescent sexual and reproductive health*. 2014. Available from: http://www.unfpa.org/resources/adolescent-sexual-and-reproductive-health

28. Huber D, Saeedi N, Khalil Samadi A. Achieving success with family planning in rural Afghanistan. *Bulletin of the World Health Organization*. 2010; 88 (3): 161–240.

29. Hoke T, Wheeler S, Lynd K, Green MS, Razafindravony BH, Rasamihajamanana E, et al. Community-based provision of injectable contraceptives in Madagascar: 'task shifting' to expand access to injectable contraceptives. *Health Policy and Planning*. 2011; 27 (1): 52–9. Available from: http://heapol.oxfordjournals.org/content/early/2011/01/20/heapol.czr003.full

30. United Nations Population Fund. *The power of 1.8 billion: Adolescents, youth and the transformation of the future*. State of world population 2014. New York: UNFPA; 2014. Available from: https://www.unfpa.org/sites/default/files/pub-pdf/EN-SWOP14-Report_FINAL-web.pdf

31. World Health Organization. *Microbicides*. Available from: http://www.who.int/hiv/topics/microbicides/microbicides/en/

32. World Health Organization. *Growing antibiotic resistance forces updates to recommended treatment for sexually transmitted infections*. News release. 30 August 2016. Available from: www.who.int/mediacentre/news/releases/2016/antibiotics-sexual-infections

CHAPTER 19

Setting up a community tuberculosis (TB) programme

Ted Lankester

What we need to know

What is TB?

Tuberculosis (TB) is a life-threatening disease that normally affects the lungs but can involve almost any part of the body, in which case it is called extra-pulmonary TB. The typical symptoms of TB are weight loss, chronic ill health and fever. Lung (pulmonary) TB also causes cough, often with sputum, sometimes with blood. Chest pain is commonly present. TB can mimic a wide variety of illnesses. Where AIDS is common the two diseases are often found together.

The cause of TB is a bacterium called *Mycobacterium tuberculosis* (also known as the acid-fast bacillus—AFB). Overcrowding, poor health and malnutrition make infection with an AFB more likely and more serious, as does HIV infection. TB is largely a disease of poverty.

TB starts as germs enter the lungs, commonly in childhood, and multiply to form a nodular patch or granuloma, with nearby swollen lymph nodes, together known as a primary complex, or a Ghon focus/complex. At this stage, germs may enter the blood and spread to other organs. If the person is in weak health or has low immunity at the time of infection, the complex may enlarge at once to give active (primary) TB. If the newly infected person is in good health, the disease may spread no further. This is known as latent TB, which is present in one-third of the world's population. There is always the danger that later in life, especially during a time of stress, illness, poor diet, or HIV, the latent infection will become active; this can lead on to fully developed (post-primary) TB. This happens to about one person in ten who has latent TB.[1]

TB is spread by people with active pulmonary TB through coughing, sneezing, talking, or spitting. The bacilli are then inhaled by others, who can become infected.

A less-common form of TB, *Mycobacterium bovis*, is found mainly in Africa, especially among herdsmen, and is caused by ingesting infected milk. *M. bovis* should probably be categorized as a neglected tropical disease (NTD, see Chapter 16).

TB as a serious global disease

TB is one of the top 10 causes of death worldwide. Ending the TB epidemic by 2030 is among the health targets of the Sustainable Development Goals.[2]

HIV/AIDS is the most important reason why TB is increasing. People living with HIV are more than 30 times more likely to become infected with TB than those without HIV. Other diseases, especially non-communicable diseases, along with malnutrition, smoking, and the misuse of drugs and alcohol increase the likelihood of latent TB becoming active.

Travel spreads TB, especially through refugees, economic migrants, and displaced people.[3] Multidrug-resistant TB (MDR-TB) is increasing globally at a rapid rate. Poorly managed programmes and incorrect or incomplete treatment makes the spread of resistance more likely.

Poverty is a major cause or social determinant of TB. For example, a Ugandan study from a poor urban area in Kampala showed that there were 9.2 new cases per 1000 population per year compared with an expected rate of two new cases per 1000. This finding suggests that urban TB also may be much higher than expected elsewhere, especially where HIV/AIDS is common.[4]

Loss of health personnel is becoming a major problem, especially where HIV/AIDS is common. WHO has warned that a TB workforce crisis is becoming a major problem in TB control.

National tuberculosis programmes (NTPs) set up guidelines, plans and resources relevant to each country. Any TB programme we set up should liaise closely with the NTP and follow any guidelines they produce.

- In 2017, 10 million people fell ill with TB and 1.6 million died from the disease (including 0.3 million among people with HIV).
- TB is a killer in HIV-positive people: in 2015, 35 per cent of HIV deaths were due to TB.
- Over 95 per cent of TB deaths occur in low- and middle-income countries.
- Six countries account for 60 per cent of the total, with India leading the count, followed by Indonesia, China, Nigeria, Pakistan, and South Africa.
- In 2017, an estimated one million children became ill with TB and 230,000 children died of TB (including children with HIV-associated TB).

- Globally in 2015, an estimated 480,000 people developed MDR-TB.
- Globally, TB incidence is falling at about 2% per year. This rate must become a 4–5 per cent annual decline to reach the 2020 milestones of the 'End TB Strategy'.
- An estimated 54 million lives were saved through TB diagnosis and treatment between 2000 and 2017.

Methods being used to control TB

The 'End TB Strategy', adopted by the WHO in 2014 is a roadmap to speed up the end of the TB epidemic, which is one of the targets under the third SDG. The strategy aims to reduce TB deaths by 90 per cent, to cut new cases by 80 per cent by 2030, and to ensure no family is burdened with catastrophic costs due to TB.[5] The WHO has gone one step further and set a 2035 target of 95 per cent reduction in deaths and a 90 per cent decline in TB incidence—similar to current levels in low TB incidence countries today.

We should also be aware of the Stop TB Partnership, which is a global consortium of countries, organizations and the private sector,[6] and of The Global Fund to fight AIDS, TB, and Malaria, which is a major contributor through funds and expertise.[7]

WHO's ENGAGE-TB approach[8] is committed to integrating community-based TB activities into the work of non-governmental and civil society organizations. It aims to help set up partnerships between the NTPs and NGOs for community-based action in TB response.

Any community programme we set up will need to be aware of these three global strategies as well as the national guidelines adopted by each NTP.

As mentioned TB control is made more difficult and more important by the worldwide rise of resistance to commonly used TB medicines, especially isoniazid and rifampicin. TB that is resistant to at least these two medicines is known as MDR-TB. Treatment regimens for MDR-TB include two or more drugs to which the particular strain of TB is sensitive. Total treatment often lasts for 18–24 months, but a cheaper 9–12-month regimen is currently being introduced by the WHO. It is still far more expensive to treat MDR-TB than non-resistant TB.

Extensively drug-resistant TB (XDR-TB) is a rarer type of MDR-TB that is resistant to other TB medicines as well as isoniazid and rifampin. Resistance to medicines underlines the huge importance of treating TB effectively so that MDR-TB is less likely to develop.

Two keys to all successful programmes are case-finding and assuring that the full course of TB treatment is taken by patients.

Case-finding can be done both through passive case-finding (self-referral) and active case-finding through systematic screening in high-risk groups to discover as many as possible of the infectious TB patients in the area where we are working.

As regards *TB treatment*, we should aim for full treatment and cure rates of at least 90 per cent for rifampicin-containing regimens. Using DOTS (Directly Observed Treatment-short course) is the WHO-recommended strategy underpinning End TB (see below).

New ways are continually being identified to scale up TB control. These include the development of a more effective vaccine, the introduction of new TB medicines,[9] a prospective shortening of the first standard treatment phase to four months, more effective case-finding, and quicker, more accurate testing using the Xpert MTB/RIF test (where available). Also important is the greater use and co-ordination of private and voluntary providers, including pharmacists, into national control programmes. Community health programmes have a great opportunity to be actively involved.[10]

Integrated, patient-centred care and prevention (the expanded DOTS programme) consists of five components:

1. Standardized treatment schedules with support and supervision.

For patients taking treatment, support is essential to make sure that they take the correct medicines in the correct doses at the correct intervals. This is most effectively done through engagement of trained health care professionals or community health workers (CHWs) and volunteers.

2. Diagnostic services.

Trained microscopists diagnose sputum-positive cases as near to the patient's home as possible. The ability to detect drug resistance is made as universal as possible using the Xpert MTB/RIF test.

3. Medicine supplies.

Medicines must be high quality, accessible, and always available, following NTP guidelines. Ideally some or all of these should be available as combined preparations. This reduces the large number of tablets that patients have to swallow and increases compliance.

4. Monitoring and recording.

Tracking the progress of each patient and therefore the impact of the programme as a whole.

5. Political will.

The commitment of the country and its national—and local—leadership to make this programme a priority and to give it public and financial backing is vital for our success.[11]

Global strategy focuses on

(a) providing universal access to TB care, and prevention, with greater attention to vulnerable and hard-to-reach populations.

(b) Systematic screening of contacts and selected groups and preventive treatment of selected groups are integral.

(c) The importance of infection control measures to prevent the spread of TB is highlighted.

(d) The WHO promotes an integrated approach in collaboration with other public health programmes. This includes linking with HIV, maternal and child health, nutritional care, diabetes care, lung health and mental health services.

(e) Digital health tools are being recommended to help all aspects of implementing programmes so they can be more effective.[12]

In summary, from the CBHC perspective. The treatment of MDR-TB and XDR-TB is complex, so it is essential we follow the regimens recommended in our national TB programme and ensure that any programme we are involved with is as effective as possible. Poor compliance and inadequate programme management can worsen the TB problem by increasing resistance and the expense of treatment. One other thing is clear. We should never start a TB programme 'on our own', without fully integrating with our NTP (see below).

What we need to do

Deciding whether to participate in a TB programme

TB is usually a curable disease, but is difficult to treat and requires considerable time and commitment. It can be expensive unless there is reliable subsidy or free medicines.

Following NTP guidelines can be complicated, especially in areas where HIV/AIDS is common or there is a high proportion of MDR-TB. This means we should only participate in a programme after careful consideration. We must also remember that the End TB Strategy is a worldwide initiative and we must work alongside any national programme and follow its guidelines carefully.

However, there are still many areas without an effective TB programme and civil society organizations (CSOs) can make a valuable contribution. Treating TB inadequately is worse than not treating it at all, because germs will develop resistance, making TB in the target area much harder to cure in the future.

We will need to ask certain questions when deciding to participate in a programme.

1. Does the community want a programme?

Will people work in partnership with us? Are they prepared to take on increasing responsibility for helping to manage the programme?

2. Is TB common in our programme area?

We can usually discover the incidence of TB in our area from national or official figures and annual rates of infection. Alternatively, we could consider starting a programme, e.g. if more than 1 per cent of people in our community survey had possible TB.

3. Is TB already being adequately treated in the area?

Although the NTP may be functioning and private doctors may be treating patients, effective programmes may not be present in the neediest areas, such as urban slums, remote mountain, or island communities. For example, on the island of Malaita in the Solomon Islands, some areas had no community-based programme and relied on a hospital for diagnosis and treatment. All treatment was done by admission to a TB ward. Few patients attended the hospital and there was a low detection and treatment completion rate. A community-based research programme enabled residents to suggest their own solutions for improving TB care and the best ways of setting up a community programme.[13]

As well as finding out who is involved in TB control, we need to discover how much they are actually doing. Is there an effective and comprehensive programme that includes the neediest members of the community?

Part of our assessment will be through meeting the district medical officer (DMO) or TB Officer, and directors of any other programmes involved in TB treatment in our area. It is essential we work alongside and strengthen existing programmes rather than setting up alternatives. However, in areas with no effective treatment, we should be ready to set up TB services following NTP guidelines and in agreement with local health authorities, providing we have the long-term capacity.

4. Have we the resources to set up a TB programme?

We will need:

-   An experienced doctor to plan, advise, give clinical care and liaise with the NTP;
-   Health workers to identify cases, organize treatment and ensure follow-up;
-   A reliable, subsidized supply of drugs (often difficult);
-   Money, unless free supplies are available and guaranteed from the government, a donor, or an agency; and
-   A referral system for diagnosis and treatment of other conditions linked to TB, especially for complex cases, MDR-TB, or those with TB and HIV.

5. Is our project likely to be long term or permanent?

Because it takes many years for a TB programme to be effective, we will need to guarantee that our programme can continue for a number of years.

In summary, can we provide excellent, reliable, and sustainable management of the programme?

Deciding which aspects of TB control to set up

A comprehensive TB programme

A comprehensive programme involves both the programme *and* the community taking full responsibility for case-finding, treatment, follow-up and evaluation in close association with, or as part of, the national TB programme (see Figure 19.1). If this approach is decided, we may wish to start TB control at the same time as setting up clinics. Alternatively, we can set up a community health programme first, with health posts or mobile clinics, and add a TB component later. Unless we already have experienced TB-trained health workers, it is usually better to build our own capacity first.

A selective TB programme

If a local programme already exists, we should work in co-operation with it, or take over responsibility for selected parts of the programme. For example, the government (DMO) is usually responsible for the overall planning of programmes and the supply of drugs. However, coverage may be inadequate at the

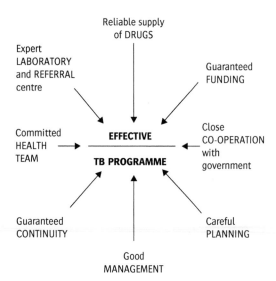

Figure 19.1 The essential ingredients in an effective TB programme.

Reproduced courtesy of Ted Lankester. This image is distributed under the terms of the Creative Commons Attribution Non-Commercial 4.0 International licence (CC-BY-NC), a copy of which is available at http://creativecommons.org/licenses/by-nc/4.0/.

> ### Box 19.1 **What we can contribute to a selective TB programme**
>
> - Awareness-raising, behaviour change, communication and community mobilization.
> - Reducing stigma and discrimination.
> - Screening and testing for TB and TB-related illness (e.g. HIV counselling and testing; diabetes screening) including through home visits.
> - Facilitating access to diagnostic services (e.g. sputum or specimen collection and transport).
> - Initiation and provision of TB prevention measures (e.g. isoniazid preventive therapy, TB infection control, BCG vaccination).
> - Referral of community members for diagnosis of TB and related diseases.
> - Treatment initiation, provision and observation for TB and co-morbidities.
> - Treatment adherence support through peer support and education and individual follow-up.
> - Social and livelihood support (e.g. food supplementation, income-generation activities).
> - Home-based palliative care for TB and related diseases.
> - Community-led local advocacy activities

community level, giving CSO programmes an opportunity to contribute. A variety of specific tasks we can be involved with are given in Box 19.1.

Setting aims and targets

Our indicators will be in line with the End TB Strategy and our own NTP. This will include both the percentage of notified TB patients identified through community referrals, and the treatment success of patients who received community treatment support. More information on tracking these indicators[14] is found under 'Evaluate the programme'. The DMO or TB officer should help us set realistic targets and ways to monitor our work. NB: we must use the same categorizations as the NTP. Success in our 'quantitative' targets will be largely measured from the annual returns we send in.

Creating awareness in the community

Creating awareness is one of the key factors in eradicating TB. Once community members recognize their illness, believe it can be cured and ask for treatment, our programme is more likely to succeed. In order to do this, we will need to understand local beliefs and customs, and the difficulties especially faced by the poor in getting diagnosed and completing treatment (Figure 19.7).

Local beliefs and customs vary from place to place but common fears include:[13]

- TB can't be cured (this is true in the experience of some).
- Only the poor, low castes, or those under a curse get TB.
- TB patients are unclean and should be kept away from their families or communities.
- TB is inherited.
- If you have TB it means you have AIDS (especially where HIV/AIDS is common).

In practice, patients may face discrimination, be excluded by their community, and barred from marriage. Stigma may increase in areas where people assume that if you have TB you also have AIDS.

The poor also face greater difficulties; imagine a poor villager or slum-dweller who starts to cough up blood. A frightening sequence of thoughts may occur (see also Figure 19.2):

→ 'Now I've caught the disease that killed my close friends'

→ 'I don't have the energy to chase after a cure'

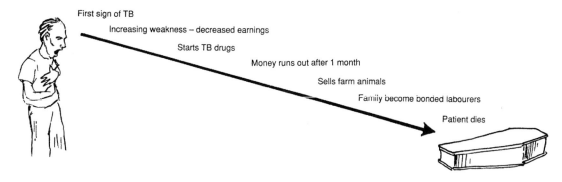

Figure 19.2 TB in practice. Within one year this TB patient died and his family lost their farm, their money, their independence, their dignity, and their future.

→ 'Can I trust the doctor or will I be cheated?'

→ 'I've only enough money for four weeks of medicine: how can I afford six months?'

→ 'I don't know who will take me to the clinic or pay for the journey'

→ 'I'm worried I will get AIDS if I have to have injections: per-haps I've caught it already'

→ 'If I can't go to work my family will starve and my children may die.'

In the case of a woman with TB, these problems are multiplied. Often her family may be unwilling or unable to spend money on her treatment. They may prevent her from attending a clinic when she should be busy at home, collecting firewood or water, or earning money. Recent research from the Gambia has shown how essen-tial it is for health workers to understand why patients with TB do not seek treatment or discontinue treatment early. When we discover what the reasons are in our community, we can help people overcome these obs-tacles (see Figure 19.3).

Health workers often talk about health-seeking be-haviour. This refers to the action people take (or don't take) when they become ill. Many people with symp-toms of TB first seek out private practitioners. Usually the diagnosis and treatment they receive is inadequate and they may be charged high fees. Up to 50 per cent of TB patients in some Asian countries first see a private practitioner, so appropriate NTP-based treatment is dan-gerously delayed.

One practical solution is to include and train pri-vate practitioners in any programme with which we are involved. Some may be unwilling and many will need big shifts in attitude. However, by including this huge group of 'unofficial' health workers we can help reduce treatment delays and the use of wrong drugs. It

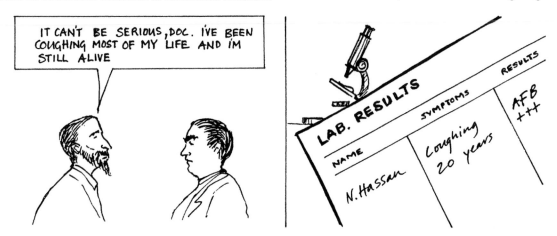

Figure 19.3 An elderly villager or slum dweller with a chronic cough. TB or COPD? Sputum testing is essential to differentiate.

may also help solve the shortage of trained health care workers in our programme area. However, while the use of public-private partnerships, i.e. a public-private mix, is becoming more widespread, we need to check the quality and how easily the poorest communities can access services before getting involved.

Non-governmental and faith-based organizations can participate helpfully in TB programmes. Nearly every community has a priest or imam who can be taught how to encourage members of their congregation to come for diagnosis, and to complete treatment. They can also tackle stigma.

Teachers can help children of all ages to understand TB and to have enlightened attitudes. The children can then influence other family members, including parents, to change unhelpful beliefs and ideas, so that they come to understand more about the disease and how it can be cured. This can be part of a child-to-child programme.

Identifying TB cases (case-finding)

There are two main ways in which we discover people who have infectious TB. *Passive case-finding* (or self-referral) refers to diagnosing patients who report symptoms, for example, to a health centre, hospital, private practitioner, clinic, or CHW. *Active case-finding* refers to a search for cases in the community. These can either be those with symptoms or those who may be smear-positive but have no significant symptoms. In some cities in high-income countries, e.g. in the north of England, there are programmes for identifying latent TB in high-risk groups.

TB programmes in the past were based largely on passive case-finding and only when cure rates reached levels of at least 85 per cent was active case-finding encouraged. However, current evidence suggests that active case-finding should be practised, especially among certain population groups: everyone living in the same household as a TB patient, everyone known to be HIV-positive, slum residents, prisoners and people addicted to tobacco, drugs, or alcohol. Household contacts of those diagnosed with MDR-TB and XDR-TB should be followed up with particular care.[15]

New, innovative ways can be used to identify and treat TB cases. For example, in Harare, a mobile van using a loudspeaker was found to be more effective at identifying undiagnosed TB patients than knocking on doors. This approach led to a lower incidence of TB in the populations of the 46 suburbs covered.[16]

New guidelines on active case-finding are available from WHO.[17] There is a form of case-finding midway between active and passive, although it is not currently part of WHO strategy. We can call this opportunistic case-finding. It refers to discovering patients who are in contact with a clinic or health programme for reasons other than TB–related symptoms. For example, an elderly man might attend a clinic with severe toothache and be found to have a chronic cough, or our community survey might uncover community members with symptoms suggestive of possible TB. In remote areas or where TB patients are highly stigmatized, this can be a useful way of discovering cases at little extra cost.

Symptoms that suggest infectious TB:

1. In adults and older children.

Anyone with a *cough* and *sputum* for more than two weeks (three weeks is often still taken as a more practical alternative) is considered a 'TB suspect' or 'possible TB case'. We use the latter term, as the word 'suspect' may reinforce stigma. We must remember that chronic obstructive pulmonary disease (COPD), often caused by smoking, can mimic TB and needs very different treatment (Figure 19.3). Also, these symptoms are common aspects of the common cold leading to secondary chest infections or may be caused by severe air pollution.

Weight loss, fever (especially night sweats), *chest pain*, or *haemoptysis* (the coughing up of blood or blood-stained sputum) makes the diagnosis more likely. Furthermore, often symptoms have a gradual onset. AIDS can accompany or mimic many of these symptoms.

NB: there are other forms of TB that affect different organs in the body. These patients should still be treated but usually, being non-infectious, are a lower priority in terms of community control.

2. In younger children.

The diagnosis of TB in children is more difficult than adults and has until recently been given less priority. The reason for both these facts is the same: children rarely cough up sputum. This means they are more difficult to diagnose but are also less of a public health priority.

The key is always to consider the diagnosis of TB in any child who remains ill and fails to gain weight. Common symptoms include any of those found in adults. NB: children usually swallow any sputum they cough up. Further symptoms include:

- Weight loss or failure to gain weight for ≥ 4 weeks with no obvious cause.
- Unexplained fever or night sweats with negative malaria smear or no response to malaria treatment.

- Large painless lymph nodes, most commonly in the neck, with or without discharge to the skin. This is sometimes known as 'scrofula' or TB adenitis, but other conditions can mimic this.

Making a diagnosis

Although the information given here gives a broad picture of diagnosing TB, it is important for programmes to follow the specific NTP guidelines on diagnosing TB.

1. In adults and older children.

First, we must carry out a sputum test by staining a slide and using a microscope. Wherever possible carry out three tests. If only one is positive, try to confirm with a further test. Although this can confirm cases of TB, many—probably up to half—are missed. Use the Xpert MTB/RIF blood test as it increasingly becomes available. This diagnoses TB and, very significantly, also identifies resistance to rifampicin, a cornerstone drug in TB treatment. At the time of writing this should be our diagnostic test of choice.[18]

In 2016, four new diagnostic tests were recommended by WHO—a rapid molecular test to detect TB at peripheral centres where Xpert MTB/RIF cannot be used, and three tests to detect resistance to first- and second-line TB medicines. Find out if these are being used or are available in your NTP. However, we must remember the value of diagnosing patients in their communities rather than expecting them to travel long distances for slightly more accurate diagnoses. We need to assess the trade-off between these two.

Sputum is most likely to give an accurate result if produced from a deep cough, preferably when first waking in the morning. It should be produced away from other people and placed in a clean, sealed, labelled container and taken or sent as soon as possible to the nearest laboratory accredited to test for TB.

There are two priorities when sputum testing through microscopes. Firstly, tests must be carried out by an accredited lab, with lab workers who have been adequately trained and continue to carry out a sufficient number of tests for their skills to be maintained.

The second priority is to carry out the test in as convenient a location as possible for the patient, e.g. at the health post, clinic or primary health centre nearest to the patient's home. The further patients have to travel, the less likely they will be diagnosed and treated.[19] This means that the community-based treatment of TB has enormous advantages over many programmes based in distant clinics and hospitals.

It is sometimes possible for a community worker to collect sputum tests from patients' homes and transport them to a reliable laboratory. With training, the Xpert MTB/RIF is a valuable test for 'near-patient testing' in a well-organized community health clinic, giving almost immediate results.

It is reasonable for us to aim to incorporate sputum testing and/or MTB/RIF testing into the most peripheral centre where standards can be guaranteed. In CBHC, we should aim to include a well-trained and accredited microscopist in our health team so that these tests can be carried out locally. All lab workers need to be well trained, motivated and reliable. False-negative sputum

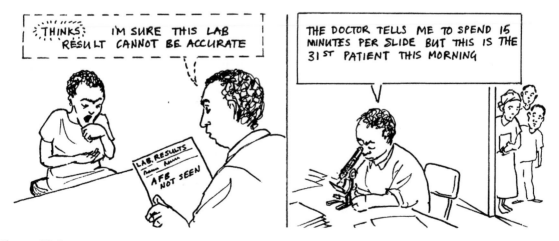

Figure 19.4 Results can be inaccurate if laboratory workers are overworked.

tests results can occur when the microscopist is overworked or poorly motivated (Figure 19.4). False-positive results occur when lab workers record what they think the doctor wants or expects.

Research workers are trying to make the sputum testing quicker and more accurate. One way is to add 5 per cent sodium hypochlorite (NaOCl, bleach) to sputum, according to special instructions. Follow any guidelines from the NTP about this or other improved ways of examining sputum.[20]

X-rays are not generally recommended, although the procedure is widely used and in practice is quite valuable, especially in children. However, it must *not* replace the more accurate ways of testing for sputum-positive TB. Thousands of patients in poor communities have been bankrupted by being treated for TB when there is no evidence that they have it (Figure 19.3).

2. In younger children

In low income countries, children make up 15–20 per cent of all TB cases and many have co-infection with HIV.[21] As mentioned, they are more difficult to diagnose than adults.

Unless they can produce sputum (as opposed to saliva). We will normally have to diagnose according to 'best guess' rather than definite confirmation. If we suspect TB, the following list can help guide us about whether to start treatment:

- A chest X-ray, which may show typical changes.
- A tuberculin or Mantoux test if available—a strongly positive test suggests TB. This is best used where a child has symptoms and a chest X-ray suggesting pulmonary TB; the Mantoux test in such cases adds weight to the TB diagnosis. It is less useful in areas where HIV in children is common.
- In some places, an IGRA blood test is available and helpful.
- Known recent contact with an infectious TB case.
- More controversially, trials of two different antibiotics for one week each. Failure to respond makes TB more likely.
- Monitoring speed and degree of improvement after starting treatment.

Recording TB cases and keeping records of outcomes

In order to have consistent recording systems we should put any patient diagnosed with TB into one of the categories listed in Table 19.1 or the categorization model used in our NTP. Although these categories may seem complex, it is important we follow them. They are based on a scientific system and give an accurate way of monitoring our programme, and comparing it with the findings of others.

Also, for record-keeping to be the same nationwide and globally we should record the outcome for each patient we start on treatment, under one of the categories in Table 19.2.

The exact record forms we use in the programme must tie in with the reporting systems needed by the

Table 19.1 **Registration group by outcome of most recent TB treatment**

Registration category	Outcome of most recent treatment
New patient	Patient has never had treatment, or has had anti-TB drugs for fewer than four weeks.
Relapse	Patient has been declared cured after one full course of treatment and has been diagnosed with TB again.
Treatment after failure	Patient has been treated for TB and their treatment failed at the end of their course of treatment.
Treatment after loss to follow up or defaulter	Patient has previously been treated for TB and was declared lost to follow up at the end of their most recent course of treatment.
Transfer in	Transfer from another district or programme.
Chronic case	Patient remains TB-positive or becomes positive again after completing a fully supervised re-treatment course.

Table 19.2 **Definitions of treatment outcomes**

Recording Category	Definition
Cured	A pulmonary TB patient with bacteriologically confirmed TB at the beginning of treatment who was smear- or culture-negative in the last month of treatment and on at least one previous occasion.
Treatment completed	A TB patient who completed treatment without evidence of failure BUT with no record to show that sputum smear or culture results in the last month of treatment and on at least one previous occasion were negative, either because tests were not done or because results are unavailable.
Treatment failed	A TB patient whose sputum smear or culture is positive at month five or later during treatment.
Died	A TB patient who dies for any reason before starting or during the course of treatment.
Lost to follow-up	A TB patient who did not start treatment or whose treatment was interrupted for two consecutive months or more.
Not evaluated	A TB patient for whom no treatment outcome is assigned. This includes cases 'transferred out' to another treatment unit as well as cases for whom the treatment outcome is unknown to the reporting unit.
Treatment success	The sum of cured and treatment completed.

NTP. We should also record details of treatment on the patient-retained record card, and we can also record data on family folder insert cards, or our own TB register or computer. We should keep records as simple as possible and avoid time-wasting duplication.

Using the End TB Strategy, patient supervision, and support

As mentioned, if we decide to participate in a TB programme, we need to make sure that any component or task we choose to do is accepted and adopted by the community.

Here are some examples from the field:

Example 1: the Bangladesh Rural Advancement Committee (BRAC) is a programme set up by the NGO and uses community health volunteers. The BRAC programme for the same cost cured three patients for every two in the government system. CHWs in each village made the programme more convenient and increased the number of women being cured of TB. This shows that well-managed, community-based programmes using CHWs are cheaper and more convenient than government programmes that bypass community involvement.

Example 2: In many African countries, treatment supporters or community volunteers (CVs) are identified by the community after a new TB case has been diagnosed and referred back to the community. The CVs provide effective support to patients, often for just five minutes a day at no cost (they live nearby and are often neighbours or friends of the TB patient). Ideally, CVs and patients are in regular contact with health facility staff to monitor treatment, and to supply new drugs etc. This approach works in areas where there are no CHWs but still depends on strong partnership with the community.

Example 3: A Chinese programme originally covered a number of provinces in a programme supported by the World Bank. It had cure rates of 95 per cent (but case detection rates were much lower than the 70 per cent target). Keys to high cure rates here included free-of-charge diagnosis and treatment, financial incentives to village doctors (NB: important and possibly unsustainable), signing of contracts between village doctors and patients, the use of blister packs for medicines, and strong political will, management and reporting systems. These last aspects are relatively easy within the Chinese cultural and political system, and enabled

344   **Chapter 19** Tuberculosis

this programme to be replicated successfully in many provinces.

Successful TB programmes are far more difficult in countries where HIV/AIDS is common or where MDR-TB is prevalent. India has successfully expanded its TB programmes and there are several keys to success in areas where this has been achieved: reliable drug supplies, careful appraisal of communities before starting the programme, intensive monitoring and supervision, and expert advice and support, especially in the early phases of the project.

The message for us in CBHC is that well-managed programmes based on participation offer an excellent way of achieving high treatment success rates, providing we work with the NTP and provide creative leadership. This is also the case if we are involved in scaling up existing programmes.

Who should supervise the treatment and support the patient?

The person overseeing treatment (using the DOTS approach) must be trusted by the patient and live nearby. These treatment supporters will need to be trained and helped to see the importance of what they are doing. Different programmes will use different supporters. Examples include CHWs or volunteers, teachers (for school children), shop-keepers, HIV/AIDS home-care providers, priests and other faith leaders, traditional health practitioners and health workers in a nearby health facility, providing they are not overworked or demotivated. They will need to be answerable officially to the health programme, whether civil society or government, and maintain confidentiality. In some cases, they can be given some incentive or reward for the service provided, but many will do this out of goodwill.

The WHO is encouraging the idea of patient support rather than mere observation of treatment. It is important to ensure a system for contacting persons lost to follow up in case they fail to meet with the treatment supporter as agreed.

What treatment regimes should be used?

Medicine regimes used will depend on the NTP, which will have details of drug resistance, cost, availability of supplies, and other factors. We should liaise with the district TB officer, follow NTP guidelines, and work out a system of medicine supply and reporting that ties in with the NTP and works for our programme. In practice, many programmes and private practitioners continue to use medicines that are not in line with national

guidelines. This often contributes to the development of MDR-TB.

Regimes are subject to change, and at the time of writing there are recommendations for changes to several regimes. The details of treatment regimens for non-resistant TB and MDR-TB are beyond the scope of this book. We should follow the guidelines in our NTP, and not stray from their recommendations. For non-resistant TB, a six-month regime using four medicines is commonly used. For MDR-TB, much longer regimes up to two years are used, but shorter regimes of 9–12 months are increasingly recommended. There is a need for new drugs and several are already being introduced.

Confirmation of treatment success

The key to confirming treatment success is repeat sputum tests: if possible, two tests should be carried out. Sputum tests are normally negative by the end of the second month. If they are not, follow NTP guidelines about how or whether to change the regime. Remember that treatment success means both achieving negative sputum tests *and* continuing treatment for the full duration.

Encouraging adherence to treatment (case-holding)

As mentioned, there has been a shift in thinking, from trying to enforce adherence to treatment (compliance) to working in partnership with patients (concordance). Treatment is supervised in a spirit of goodwill and co-operation, and in partnership with the patient. In practice, however, we will still need a mixture of information, encouragement, incentive and discipline to encourage all patients to complete treatment (Figure 19.5).

The CHW can be a very important person in this process. Here are some examples of how she is important.

1. She can ensure medicine is taken regularly.

Taking medication regularly is important throughout the course of treatment and absolutely essential in the initial phase. If patients are unreliable in taking medicines, the CHW can hand them out personally.

2. She can collect supplies from the clinic.

She can do this either for all TB patients in the community or for those too ill to collect medicines themselves.

3. She can be the main point of contact between the senior health worker and the community.

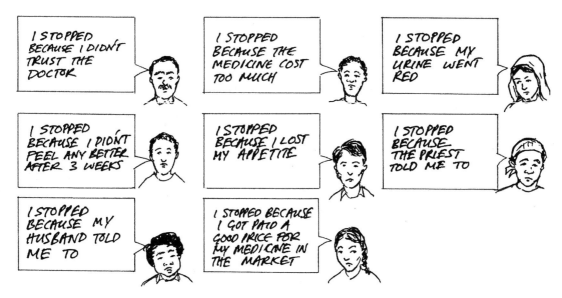

Figure 19.5 Reasons and excuses for poor compliance.

She can let the senior health worker know about any patients who are failing to take treatment.

4. She can encourage known possible cases to have sputum tests.

She can accompany these people to the clinic or take a carefully contained sputum specimen to the clinic for them.

In programmes using trained and motivated CHWs, it can be part of their agreed responsibility to ensure as best as they are able that every TB patient in the community who starts treatment takes medicine regularly until the course is complete. From time to time, a supervisor or other trained health worker can visit TB patients in their homes along with the CHW.

Some ways of improving compliance are listed in Box 19.2. Box 19.3 shows a TB advice sheet used in a Himalayan health programme for patients with TB. We can adapt this for the programme in our area and add appropriate illustrations. Information about treatment supporters can be added.

Understanding links between TB and HIV/AIDS

We must follow some facts and guidelines if we are working in areas where HIV is common. TB and HIV form a dangerous combination, and HIV is an important reason why TB has become increasingly common. Approximately, ten per cent of people with TB have a co-infection with HIV; they need to receive treatment for both with antiretroviral therapy (ART) and with TB drugs.

Without TB treatment, HIV-infected people with TB usually die within months, although they usually respond just as well to TB treatment as those who are HIV-negative. We must therefore ensure that people living with HIV/AIDS have access to TB diagnosis and treatment, and that TB patients have access to voluntary counselling and testing for HIV, and to ART when shown to be HIV-positive (see Chapter 20).

Active case-finding

In people living with HIV/AIDS we need to be strongly proactive in TB case-finding (sometimes called enhanced case-finding) through easily accessible testing and by raising awareness in the community. Xpert MTB/RIF rapid test is recommended as the initial TB diagnostic test for people living with HIV.

When patients are using combined treatment for both TB and HIV, drug regimens are confusing, making careful supervision important. Drug interactions and side effects are common, making good medical management and clear guidelines essential. TB treatment regimes in people living with HIV are generally similar to those for other patients. ART should be given to all TB patients

---

Box 19.2 **Twelve practical suggestions to encourage compliance**

1. Explain about TB carefully, and give written instructions (Figure 19.7). Even if the patient is unable to read, a family member or friend probably can.
2. Understand local beliefs so that advice can be focused and appropriate.
3. If TB treatment is not reliably being supplied free and you have advocated for this with the government, work out with patients how they can pay for the whole course of treatment.
4. Where TB treatment cannot be provided free, consider asking patients for payment of a deposit at the start of treatment, returnable in full or in part on completion, and entitling them to medicines at overall reduced cost.
5. Explain about common side effects so patients will not be worried if they occur, for example, reddening of the urine with rifampicin.
6. Spend extra time with older sputum-positive men and women with chronic cough. They are often highly infectious, less willing to take treatment, and need extra encouragement to be diagnosed and continue treatment.
7. Make sure members of the patient's family understand about treatment so they can support the advice given.
8. Set up a patient supervision and support strategy that is acceptable and accessible for the TB patient, ideally home- or neighbourhood-based.
9. Consider starting a TB support group—a regular meeting of those with TB who, helped by a facilitator, can encourage each other and share concerns and practical solutions.
10. Learn to spot 'hidden defaulters' and those lost to follow-up. These are people who claim to be regular but who forget or are untruthful about treatment, or those who move in and out of urban slums and therefore default from treatment.
11. Make sure health workers are kind, and treat TB patients with dignity and respect.
12. Make sure good quality supplies of the correct scheduled medicines never run out. Have a standby supply of medicines in the community in case bad weather, snow, floods, or civil unrest prevent further supplies arriving.

Box 19.3 **A message about tuberculosis for TB Patients and their families**

The tests we have done have shown that you have TB. This is a very serious illness. If you do not take medicine regularly, the TB may kill you. You will also spread it to others, including children.

But you can be cured of TB if you take your medicine regularly, according to what the doctor tells you. You must not miss even a single dose of medicine. After you have been taking medicine for more than about one month you may start to feel much better and think that you are cured. You must still go on taking medicine for the full length of time. If you stop when you feel better then later the disease will come back much worse and it will be much harder to treat.

Even though the cough might take time to stop even with regular and correct medicine, most people with TB stop being infectious to others after two weeks of treatment. It is very important that you stop smoking and avoid too much alcohol. You should eat good, nourishing food, including green vegetables, lentils, milk, eggs, and meat if these are available. There are no foods that you should stop eating. You should avoid getting too tired but you can continue to work unless you are advised not to. When you cough put a hand or cloth over your mouth. This stops other people from catching your germs. Try not to spit in the house or near other people. If you have to cough up sputum then put it into a cloth or small container and burn or bury it. If you are coughing a lot, try to sleep separately from other members of your family—if possible in a different room during the first two weeks of treatment. This will make it less likely they will catch your germs, especially children. Make sure that you bring any other people in your family or village who have a bad cough to the clinic. We can check them to see if they have TB. You can come back to the clinic or see the CHW any time you want, if you have anything you want to talk or ask about. But remember, the most important thing is to be completely regular with your treatment, and never miss a dose. If you miss treatment or stop taking it, your TB will get worse.

But if you are regular, your TB will get better and you will be cured.

living with HIV, irrespective of their CD4 counts; the most recent recommendations suggest that all patients with confirmed HIV should start on ART. Co-trimoxazole preventive therapy (CPT) should be given to those living with HIV, especially in the later stages of the illness. Once active TB is ruled out, people living with HIV should receive isoniazid preventive therapy (IPT) 300 mg daily, definitely for six months, ideally for longer.

Patterns of infection

In those infected with HIV, pulmonary TB is still the most common form, although a higher number of infected cases are sputum-negative, and TB in other parts of the body occurs more frequently. A classic presentation of TB is more common during early stages of HIV infection: atypical presentations are more common later, when the patient's immune system has been seriously harmed by HIV.

With all the above recommendations we should, as always, follow the NTP guidelines which will vary from time to time according to priorities, supplies and national capacity.

Controlling TB in the community

The best method of reducing TB in a community is to cure infectious TB patients. TB will decline in a community if we succeed in three key objectives over a period of time:

1. Use passive and active case-finding to discover infectious cases.
2. Treat TB patients so that 90 per cent or more are cured.
3. Tackle the underlying causes of poverty.

Most successful TB control programmes will depend on the following:

1. *Staff competence*: Train programme staff in clinical, communication, and management skills.
2. *Management/planning*: Excellent programme management is essential for long-term success.
3. *Long-term commitment*: Find ways in which the programme can be sustained, keeping medicines permanently affordable. This usually means accessing free supplies but advocacy and persistence are often needed for this to happen.
4. *Implementing a TB programme with all five programme components*: (e.g. expanded DOTS' in the section 'Methods being used to control TB') If this is not possible, there are several less-ideal options, including patient supervision

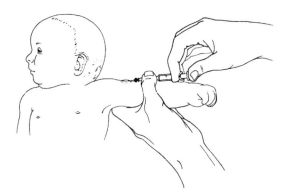

Figure 19.6 Immunization in practice: Giving BCG vaccine.
Reproduced courtesy of Ted Lankester. This image is distributed under the terms of the Creative Commons Attribution Non-Commercial 4.0 International licence (CC-BY-NC), a copy of which is available at http://creativecommons.org/licenses/by-nc/4.0/.

and support through a daily visit to the health centre. If the patient lives a distance from the centre, then simple community-based approaches can be used.

5. *Giving BCG immunization to all infants*: This is best given at birth, or within a month, or within the first year (Figure 19.6). BCG prevents TB meningitis but has only a small impact on reducing the number of TB cases.
6. *Integrating the TB programme into CBHC*: Obtain expert advice and funding to back it up. Try to include (and train) private practitioners who see TB patients.
7. *Following NTP guidelines*: This includes treatment schedules, recommended practices, reporting and ongoing liaison.
8. *Ensuring continuity*: If our programme fails or closes down we must hand over all programme components to others trained and accredited to take this on.
9. *Using fixed-dose combinations of tablets (FDCs)*: This improves compliance.
10. *Integrating the diagnosis and treatment of TB and HIV/AIDS*.
11. *Prioritizing nutrition*: This must be done for the whole community, but especially children and those known to have TB and/or HIV/AIDS.
12. *Promoting literacy*: In addition to adult education, this includes increasing the proportion of children, *particularly girls*, who receive post-primary education.
13. *Reducing air pollution*: This includes tobacco smoke and indoor cooking fires. This requires strong leadership, advocacy and persuasion to reduce the use of tobacco in all its forms. Research has shown that smoking is associated with half the male TB deaths in India.

In practice, TB will only be eradicated from a community if, over a prolonged period, all sputum-positive cases are identified and treated, and overall living

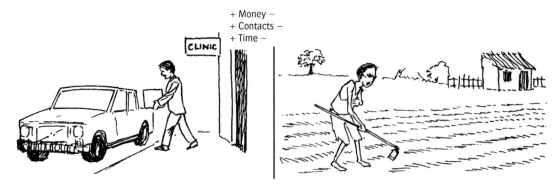

Figure 19.7 In practice TB is often curable for the rich and incurable for the poor.

conditions improve. In addition, a high incidence of AIDS makes eradication extremely difficult. However, TB can be controlled so that the prevalence starts to decline.

As soon as all community members are sputum-negative there will be no local source of infection even though reactivated latent cases may continue to occur for many years. However, migration into the community or displacement of people can re-expose them to infection.

Evaluating the programme

As with any community health activity, we will need to evaluate our programme at regular intervals to see whether we are reaching the targets we set.

Each year we should record (as percentages), using the categories in Table 19.1, the numbers of new patients started on treatment, and, using the categories in Table 19.2, the outcome of patients on treatment. From these figures we can monitor the success of the programme, in particular the number and percentage of newly diagnosed patients in the community, and the percentage cure rate of patients started on treatment. Other evaluations could include:

- BCG vaccination: the proportion of children under one or under five who have a BCG scar.
- Community satisfaction with our service: this might include comments on the side effects of drugs, ease of collecting medicines, whether drugs are affordable, health workers' attitudes, and convenience of TB strategies, especially patient supervision and support. Answers could be ranked for satisfaction from 1 to 5.

Further reading and resources

Falzon D, Jaramillo E, Schünemann HJ, Arentz M, Bauer M, Bayona J, et al. WHO guidelines for the programmatic management of drug-resistant tuberculosis. *European Respiratory Journal*. 2011; 38: 516–28. Available from: erj.ersjournals.com/content/erj/38/3/516.full.pdf

Harries AD, Mahler D. *TB/HIV: A clinical manual*. 2nd edn. Geneva: World Health Organization; 2004. Available from: www.who.int/maternal_child_adolescent/documents/9241546344/en/

World Health Organization. *Implementing the End TB strategy: The essentials*. Geneva: World Health Organization; 2015. Available from: http://www.who.int/tb/publications/2015/end_tb_essential.pdf?ua=1.

World Health Organization. *Treatment of tuberculosis: Guidelines for national programmes*. 4th edn. Geneva: World Health Organization; 2010. Available from: www.who.int/iris/bitstream/10665/44165/1/9789241547833_eng.pdf

Websites

Stop TB Partnership. Available from: http://www.stoptb.org.
World Health Organization. http://www.who.int/tb/en

References

1. Behr M, Edelstein P, Ramakrishnan L. Revisiting the timetable of tuberculosis. *British Medical Journal*. 2018; 362: k2738.
2. World Health Organization. *Tuberculosis Fact Sheet*. Updated 2017. Available from: http://www.who.int/mediacentre/factsheets/fs104/en/
3. World Health Organization. *Tuberculosis and HIV*. 2015. Available from: http://www.who.int/hiv/topics/tb/en/
4. Guwatudde D, Zalwango S, et al. Burden of tuberculosis in Kampala, Uganda. *Bulletin of the World Health Organization*. 2003; 81 (11): 799–805.

5. World Health Organization. *The End TB Strategy*. 2016. Available from: http://www.who.int/tb/post2015_TBstrategy.pdf?ua=1

6. Stop TB Partnership. *Who are our partners*. 2017. Available from: http://www.stoptb.org/about/partners_who.asp

7. The Global Fund to fight AIDS, tuberculosis and malaria. Available from: www.theglobalfund.org/

8. World Health Organization. *About the ENGAGE-TB Approach*. 2017. Available from: www.who.int/tb/areas-of-work/community-engagement/background/en/

9. Diacon A, Dawson R, Floyd K, Lönnroth K, Getahun H, Migliori GB, et al. 14-day bactericidal activity of PA-824, bedaquiline, pyrazinamide, and moxifloxacin combinations: A randomised trial. *The Lancet*. 2012; 380 (9846): 1902–13.

10. Raviglione M, Marais B, et al. Scaling up interventions to achieve global tuberculosis control: Progress and new developments and Stop TB partnership. *The Lancet*. 2012; 379 (9833).

11. World Health Organization. *Pursue high-quality DOTS expansion and enhancement*. 2017. Available from: http://www.who.int/tb/dots/en/

12. World Health Organization. *Implementing the End TB strategy: The essentials*. Geneva: World Health Organization; 2015. Available from: http://www.who.int/tb/publications/2015/end_tb_essential.pdf?ua=1.

13. Massey P, Wakageni J, Kekeubata E, Maena J, Laete'esafi J, Waneagea J, et al. TB questions, East Kwaio answers: Community-based participatory research in a remote area of Solomon Islands. *Rural Remote Health*. 2012; 12 (2139). Available from: http://www.rrh.org.au/articles/subviewnew.asp?ArticleID=2139

14. World Health Organization. *Operational guidance—Integrating community-based tuberculosis activities into the work of nongovernmental and other civil society organizations*. 2012. Available from: http://apps.who.int/iris/bitstream/10665/75997/1/9789241504508_eng.pdf

15. Becerra MC, Appleton SC, Franke MF, Chalco K, Arteaga F, Bayona J, et al. Tuberculosis burden in households of patients with multi-drug-resistant and extensively drug resistant tuberculosis: A retrospective cohort study. *The Lancet*. 2011; 377 (9760): 147–52.

16. Corbett E, Bandason T, Duong T, Dauya E, Makamure B, Churchyard GJ, et al. Comparison of two active case-finding strategies for community-based diagnosis of symptomatic smear-positive tuberculosis and control of infectious tuberculosis in Harare, Zimbabwe (DETECTB): A cluster-randomised trial. *The Lancet*. 2010; 376 (9748): 1244–53.

17. World Health Organization. *Systematic screening for active tuberculosis—Principles and recommendations*. 2013. Available from: http://apps.who.int/iris/bitstream/10665/84971/1/9789241548601_eng.pdf

18. Boehme C, Nicol M, Nabeta P, Michael JS, Gotuzzo E, Tahirli R, et al. Feasibility, diagnostic accuracy and effectiveness of decentralised use of the Xpert MTB/RIF test for diagnosis of tuberculosis and multidrug resistance: A multicentre implementation study. *The Lancet*. 2011; 377 (9776): 1495–1505.

19. Kizito K, Dunkley S, Kingori M, Reid T. Lost to follow up from tuberculosis treatment in an informal settlement (Kibera), Nairobi, Kenya: What are the rates and determinants. *Transactions of the Royal Society of Tropical Medicine and Hygiene*. 2011;105 (1): 52–7.

20. Kaore NM, Date KP, Thombare VR. Increased sensitivity of sputum microscopy with sodium hypochlorite concentration technique: A practical experience at RNTCP center. *Lung India*. 2011; 28 (1): 17–20.

21. World Health Organization. *Roadmap for childhood TB: Toward zero deaths*. 2013. Available from: http://www.who.int/tb/areas-of-work/children/roadmap/en/

CHAPTER 20

A community development approach to HIV care, prevention, and control

Ian D Campbell, Alison Rader Campbell, and Clement Chela

Figure 20.1 shows a community response to HIV.

What we need to know

What are HIV and AIDS?

AIDS stands for the acquired immune deficiency syndrome. This is a disease in which the body's immune system collapses, and which, without treatment, usually leads to death within a few years. It is caused by the human immunodeficiency virus (HIV).

An individual usually becomes HIV-positive within three months of contact, but the time between becoming HIV-positive (seroconversion) and the development of AIDS is variable, ranging from months to a number of years—for many people, between five and ten years. During this latent period, the person living with HIV can be free of symptoms but is infectious to others.

HIV is spread mostly through unprotected sexual contact with an HIV-positive individual. In addition, it can be passed on through infected blood transfusions, infected needles, and breast milk, and crucially from mother to foetus before or during childbirth.

AIDS became generally known in the early 1980s, and HIV spread extremely rapidly, initially in many countries in sub-Saharan Africa and in the Asia-Pacific region. There is now consistent progress in making access to treatment available. Treatment suppresses HIV, so that people with HIV can enjoy a good quality of life. Also, people who are stable on HIV treatments are at very low risk of spreading the virus to others. One of the areas of good progress is in the prevention of HIV transmission from mother to foetus. However, there is still no cure.

Global extent and improvement

HIV has caused much damage to many communities around the world. HIV causes havoc to families, as the

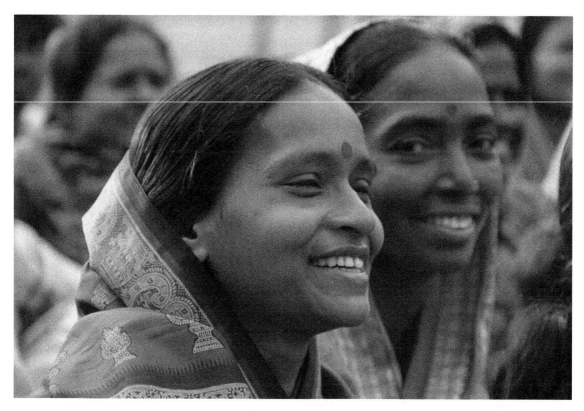

Figure 20.1 Bihar, India. A community responding to HIV, 2012. GLoCon.

sick and dying are primarily in the reproductive age groups. They are also the main breadwinners, leaving behind orphans and aging parents as survivors and sending many into a spiral of poverty and hopelessness.

However, the good news is that more people are *living* with HIV than ever before. This is not because the disease is spreading faster than expected, but because HIV treatment options have expanded dramatically, leading to many with HIV living to their national expected life-spans.

At the time of publication, UNAIDS reports the following figures:[1]

- About 36.9 million people globally were living with HIV in 2017.
- About 21.7 million people were accessing antiretroviral therapy.
- About 15 million were not.
- About 1.8 million people became newly infected with HIV in 2017.

- AIDS-related deaths have been reduced by more than 51% since the peak in 2004.

Effective response

The dramatic increases in the lifespan of people living with HIV and reduction in deaths from the disease are due to effective programmes using powerful drugs known as antiretrovirals (ARVs), which prolong life for many people infected with HIV.

ARVs, or more often known as antiretroviral therapy (ART), is now more generally available for community programmes in low- and middle-income countries. Its cost is still high in many countries, side effects can be severe, and not taking it regularly can make it ineffective. This means, as with medicines treating tuberculosis (Chapter 19), these must be taken reliably and consistently. However, they hold enormous value in treating individuals and restoring hope to communities and have been life-changing even in resource-poor settings. But, at the same time, in every part of the world, there are people who are unaware they have been infected with HIV. It is also true that prevention of new infections through community approaches has sometimes been neglected because of the newer emphasis towards access to treatment.

In many countries, AIDS is still the primary health priority and there is a great and on-going need for community-based HIV/AIDS programmes to be established and maintained. These community programmes can be based in a variety of settings, including hospitals and health centres, clubs and churches, or in homes of the community.

We must also be aware of the persistent increase in HIV with men having sex with men (MSM), among drug users, and some prison populations.

In HIV and AIDS community-based programmes the *three most important responses* will be:

1. Prevention and care promotion.

We need to ensure that all prevention actions are linked with treatment access and practical HIV care in the communities. Families need to take a central role. This will help to reduce stigma which causes discrimination against HIV-positive people and fear that reduces the uptake of treatment. Genuine caring builds trust, which is the key to success. Experience in community counselling shows local communities can make healthy choices about preventing HIV and caring for those with AIDS.[2]

Positive people support groups for People Living with HIV (PLWH) are used in some areas. They include their family members and widen the circle of care to include faith and other community groups. Care is often carried out by relatives, friends, and community members, and is always better done as teams. Home care must also include treatment adherence as well as palliative care for those who need it. When done well, home-based care has the added benefit of influencing prevention in the neighbourhood through people seeing what is being done and building relationships. There are more details in Chapter 28 and see Figure 20.2.

2. Voluntary HIV Counselling and Testing (VCT)

VCT of persons at any risk is vital to reinforce prevention messages and serves as a gateway to early identification of people living with HIV. Crucially, testing—when realistic treatment opportunities are available—helps to obtain treatment early. Community leaders have an

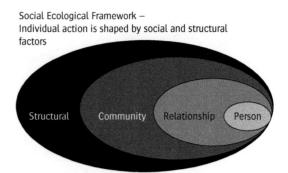

Social Ecological Framework – Individual action is shaped by social and structural factors

Figure 20.2 A social model for prevention.

Reproduced courtesy of Ian D. Campbell. This image is distributed under the terms of the Creative Commons Attribution Non-Commercial 4.0 International licence (CC-BY-NC), a copy of which is available at http://creativecommons.org/licenses/by-nc/4.0/.

important role in advocating for reliable and consistent testing facilities. Church and other faith leaders need to be well informed and supportive, as in many of the most affected communities most people will listen to their advice. Leaders and other opinion shapers have shown the way in some communities by getting themselves tested publicly.

3. Treatment with anti-retroviral therapy (ART).

ART treatment should be the norm but 15 million are not yet accessing it. Access is a key priority for community members to work with and advocate with the government, to make sure it is always available. Empowered communities working with government providers have shown remarkable progress even in places where basic health infrastructure is limited.

These three areas of activity form a continuum of care which builds the capacity of communities to treat and care for those vulnerable to HIV and gives dignity and fullness of life to people living with HIV.

Effective responses to HIV will vary greatly between different communities. They will need to be designed to build on respect, and respond to the beliefs and cultures of programme leaders and community members. We also need to be aware of new responses and approaches.

Our overall aim is to encourage approaches involving both the community and health services. Empowered people can make good choices and work together. Resilient communities can help to reduce levels of HIV infection and suffering caused by AIDS through ongoing learning and by finding and carrying out their own solutions involving local leadership (Figure 20.3) providing they are evidence-based.

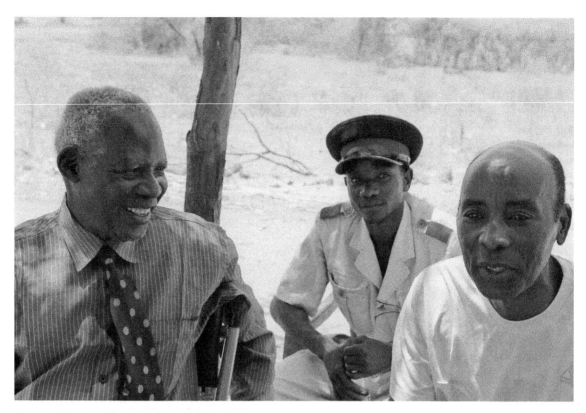

Figure 20.3 Sianyoolo, Zambia: Finding solutions: meeting with chief. (Also the birthplace of community counselling, see section below).

What we need to do

Community appraisal using 'SALT'

HIV is linked to human behaviour which is shaped by culture, knowledge, attitudes, and beliefs. It is not simply a health issue. We must understand these factors in order to work with communities and to help them reduce their vulnerability. Health facilities will need to work with communities, mobilizing them and collaborating to build a joined-up response.

One effective way of doing this is a form of community linkage and empowerment known as SALT[3] (see also Chapter 2), and this approach is valuable in many areas of community-based health care (CBHC). SALT enables the coming together of all actors to build a locally owned, shaped, and driven response.

SALT methodology is especially effective, because a local 'story' about community issues builds trust and

a shared desire to act together. SALT is a word to help us remember the four parts of this approach. They include:

Local STORY,
APPRECIATING human strengths for response,
LISTENING and LEARNING, and
Building TEAM approaches

that can help transfer from one community to other communities. The further use and value of this method is further described as this chapter develops.

The content of our appraisal consists of two main areas: enquiring about concerns and understanding key local strengths. This can be done through a civil society organization (CSO), government, or any other player working alongside the community. Faith-based organizations (FBOs) when well informed and supportive can play a very valuable role. Of course, all activities musts be done with full community partnership. There is more about appraisal in Chapter 6.

Enquire about concerns

Exploring deeply felt concerns is our first priority. HIV may not be an active concern during the first part of any SALT conversation. But wherever HIV is present in a community, HIV easily becomes a focus as families and neighbourhoods talk about challenges and hopes. As trust becomes established we can ask *community members* what they think about HIV/AIDS. Their answers usually include the way they feel as well as the way they think others feel. Box 20.1 shows examples of questions which can be asked. Gathering information with community members will also help people see that answers do exist. This awareness can encourage us and stimulate action by local communities.

Box 20.1 **Examples of questions we can ask *community members* to learn what they think about HIV/AIDS**

What do people *know* about HIV?
- How is HIV transmitted?
- What do we think causes AIDS?
- What are the symptoms and signs?
- How do we talk to a person living with HIV?
- What makes us vulnerable to infection?

What do people *feel* about HIV?
- What do you think people with HIV experience in our community? How do they feel?
- How does the family cope when a family member is living with HIV, i.e. how can the family adjust?
- If community members are HIV-positive or fear they might be, do they feel they must keep this quiet, for fear of what people will think, i.e. is there stigma?

What do people *believe* about the behaviours that allow HIV to be transmitted?
- What behaviours and beliefs increase the risk of HIV?
- How can these behaviours change?
- What beliefs, opinions or strategies can help to reduce spread?
- How can a safer future be formed for the next generation?

Ask *local health workers* from hospitals, clinics, or community-based programmes how they assess the situation. Those involved with VCT will often have a deep understanding of how the community perceives HIV. The presence of VCT also helps clarify what actions are needed. Additionally, we can contact *district and national health authorities* to seek information and guidance, and to explore partnership possibilities.

We need to respond not only to the present concerns and felt needs of the community, but also to the concerns of health authorities, who can see long-term trends, and the solutions that are needed. We can help this process by making sure the voice of the community is clearly heard by the authorities. We can help people express their deep concerns, as some may feel too vulnerable to do this without support.

Because HIV prevalence in the community is often unknown, we need to realize that the existence of even one confirmed person with HIV usually means that many others are HIV-positive. Moreover, once the virus has entered a community the problem will grow. This means that it is usually only a matter of time before the community recognizes the problem of HIV and the need for an appropriate, robust response.

Understand key local strengths

The way a community responds to HIV can be thought of as *four key strengths*, which apply to all programmes. How they are expressed will be different for each programme.

1. *Care.* This is best understood as 'being with' or 'standing alongside' each other, rather than just providing services. It includes sharing and support as well as encouraging prevention.
2. *Community.* This is best understood as 'belonging.' Home, neighbours, and friends become the environment for care, and for reducing stigma and risk.
3. *Change.* Being well informed helps community members clarify choices and act. Attitude and behavioural change are possible in individuals, families, and even whole communities.
4. *Hope.* The experience of hope is to live fully and positively within family, community, culture, and faith. Hope also helps to build confidence for the future and to sustain healthy changes in behaviour.

These four basic concepts are *transferable*. In other words, they are found in all cultures but we have to explore, apply and develop them for our own situations. We can help people show their strengths by asking about their concerns, their hopes, and ways of responding when faced with difficult situations.

Kenya case history[4]

At Kithituni, Kenya, a local church group was concerned about AIDS in the community. They developed action groups with women, youth, men, and children that met every week. After a year, about ten other nearby communities had started to make responses. After seven years, 72 communities had been involved and 15 of those had transferred their ideas and action to other communities. Links to local churches were developed and small amounts of government funding were raised to help communities network and learn from each other's experiences. The Kithituni community today has received many visitors from other communities, governments, and NGOs. Visitors often react with astonishment that through 'coming together' such strength can emerge, which in turn leads on to such effective and sustained change. Figure 20.4 shows community voices changing policy in Kithituni, Kenya.

What resources do we need?

The foundation for a strong community response is a group of committed people, from communities and health centres, who are concerned for individuals and the community. Such a group can make decisions and gather ideas more effectively than people working alone.

In addition, we will need *links to a referral hospital or facility* that does HIV testing, or can pass on samples to a testing centre. It will usually also be a source for ART. Local community members can be trained, supported, and mentored by partner clinics or hospitals. If ART is not available, local communities must be mobilized to demand this as it is a basic right for people with HIV. No one should die today for lack of medication. ART is now the central plank of care, rather than an option.

As soon as HIV testing is known to be available, questions will arise within the community that will need to be answered, and *counselling* will become necessary. Indeed, HIV testing should always be accompanied by VCT. In many parts of the world, community volunteers are selected and trained to do VCT, which, if done sensitively, can improve the community's response to the HIV epidemic. VCT needs to be combined with a follow-up plan that includes care, support, access to ART,

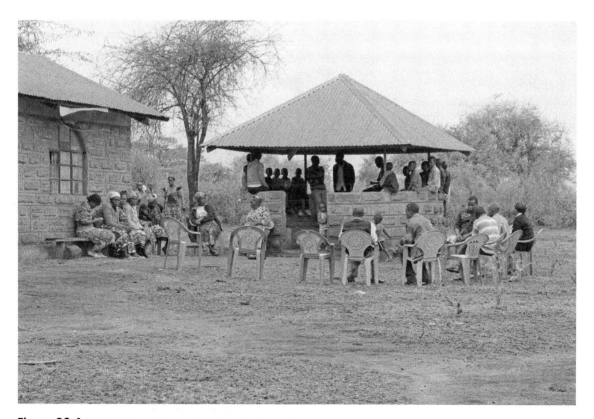

Figure 20.4 Kithituni, Kenya: Community voices changing policy.

and help with ensuring life-long adherence to it. When effective therapy is available, and people with HIV are treated with basic respect and dignity, fear and stigma tend to lessen. As more people come forward for testing and treatment, the whole response to HIV improves, which often leads to lower infection rates.

HIV care ultimately has to be local, as it is for life. People must have ready access to treatment and/or reliable community visits by HIV workers. Many teams find that they can walk, use bicycles or motorbikes, and public transport. At the same time, ensuring that people living with HIV have care facilities close to where they live is an important strategic step when developing long-term treatment programmes.

Take steps to develop a response

Many people who are concerned about HIV and AIDS will have neither formal health qualifications nor existing links with hospitals and clinics. This need not stop local action for care and change. An HIV response can start with even one motivated person. However, we want to build a responsive community so all actions should build on getting a team of committed people together. Faith-based communities have particular strengths here in being able to self-organize and also to reach out beyond their boundaries.

It is helpful at this stage to be aware of the post-2015 concept of SRHR,[5] which is an umbrella term for various issues that affect men and women. It represents four separate areas: sexual health, sexual rights, reproductive health, and reproductive rights. It helps to inform the most effective ways of working with communities in all areas connected with sexuality.

We should also be aware of the concept of mainstreaming. HIV has in the past tended to work largely within it its own world. Now, HIV responses are increasingly linked and 'mainstreamed' into wider health programmes, both those relating to sexuality and also beyond. SRHR and mainstreaming need to be understood as emerging practices as we look at the stages below. The following sections explain the steps to stimulate response.

Step 1: Form a team

An effective team will comprise committed and caring people, drawn from community members and the health team. Employed team members can work on HIV part-time provided their roles are defined and the structure of the team is regularly examined. HIV response needs specific attention, yet it should also be 'mainstreamed' throughout the health system. So, additional staffing, office facilities, and some funding may be needed, but a lot can happen without any extra staff or much expense, at least in the early stages.

As local communities become increasingly active, the tasks of health care providers will change. As community members take on more tasks, the priority will be to facilitate community-to-community transfer, so that HIV response expands and becomes self-sustaining.

Often, community members lack confidence to manage at home and they feel dependent on health services. For this reason, reassurance about support needs to be given at an early stage. Good and reliable home care is crucial, especially in building up strengths and abilities that exist within communities. Promoting hope is also essential. As early as 1987, an AIDS care unit was formed at Chikankata Hospital in the Southern Province of Zambia.[6] This included a home care and prevention team. The decision to shift the emphasis from the hospital to the community was based on identifying community resources and listening to their views. What the community stated then remains true today, and includes:

- other health programmes should continue;
- the family is the greatest long-term strength;
- people prefer to die at home;
- people learn best by talking together; and
- changes in behaviour are best achieved through activating traditional leadership and helping the community to take responsibility for care and prevention.

This work has been sustained for 30 years, and continues.

As health care workers, we may be tempted to oversimplify or impose solutions. It is usually better to discover the community's own beliefs and understand how communities work together and solve problems. From the beginning, any team should demonstrate a willingness to visit local communities simply to learn, appreciate, and understand the capacity of the local community. In an area where an early HIV response is happening, the team's first step could be a SALT visit. Figure 20.5 depicts a support and learning team.

The SALT visit helps team members realize that effective efforts do not need to depend on outsiders. Action in the spheres of home and neighbourhood is as important as action in a health centre. Figure 20.6 depicts a SALT team learning from a local community's story in Rio de Janeiro, Brazil.[7]

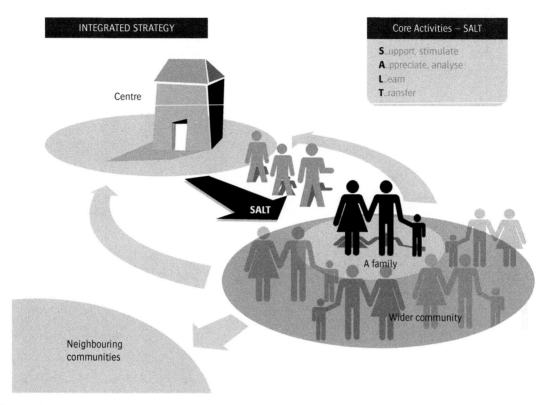

INTEGRATED STRATEGY

Centre

Core Activities – SALT
Support, stimulate
Appreciate, analyse
Learn
Transfer

SALT

A family

Wider community

Neighbouring
communities

Figure 20.5 SALT: Support And Learning Team.

A team learns by visiting homes and neighbourhood. Using the SALT terminology again we can summarize like this:

- *Support* and *Stimulate* the *Story* of home, family, neighbourhood.
- *Appreciate* capacities to care, build community, decide for change, and have hope.
- *Listen, Learn*.
- *Team* approach, *Transfer* vision and action from one person, family, or community to another.

Figure 20.7 shows home and family voices influencing policy in Yunnan, China.

Step 2: Develop community care and counselling

- Action in the spheres of *home* and *neighbourhood* complements action at a *health facility*.

- We can draw on information from our community appraisal (see Chapter 6) and from any other information gathered at the *clinic/hospital*.
- *Care* for patients at home and help family and other local people to do the same.
- Support families, through home visits and family *counselling*.
- Encourage the formation of a *community action group* that may become a community care and prevention team.
- Promote discussion within the wider community, through a *facilitative approach* that helps people to reflect and consult, then to clarify solutions and apply their response.
- *Community counselling* helps to prevent the spread of HIV, by stimulating people in neighbourhood groups and other community settings to sustain their behaviour change.

Figure 20.8 shows the community counselling cycle.

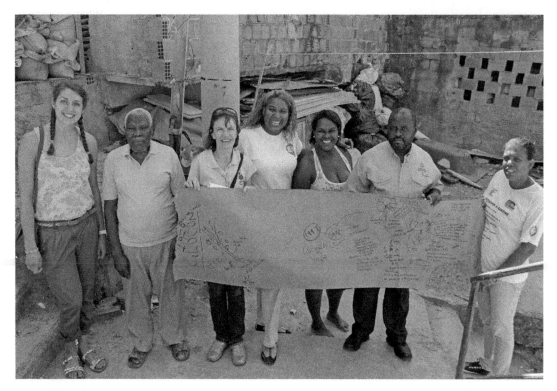

Figure 20.6 Rio de Janeiro, Brazil: SALT team learns from local community story.

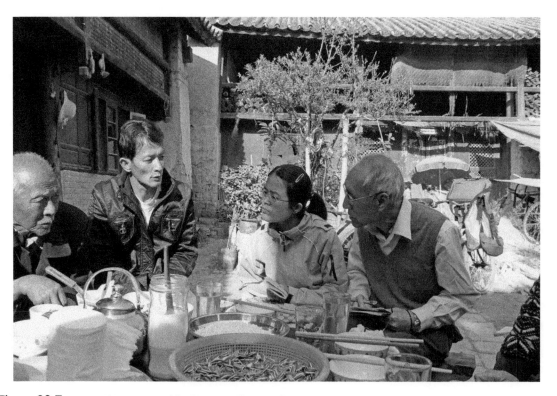

Figure 20.7 Yunnan, China: Home and family voices influence policy.

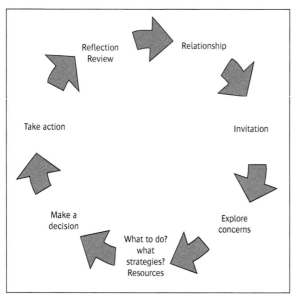

The following are shown within the figure:

- Reflection Review
- Relationship
- Take action
- Invitation
- Make a decision
- What to do? what strategies? Resources
- Explore concerns

• The community counselling cycle aids facilitation as a guideline for how a conversation can develop and progress. it supports a dynamic conversation.
• The facilitators' role is to keep track of where the conversation is at within the cycle, and ask strategic questions that keep it moving forward.
• The cycle is not completed in one conversation. it may take several months or longer to work around.

Figure 20.8 Community counselling cycle.

Step 3: Identify specific risk situations

Many people do not realize that the family and neighbourhood are not the only centres of risk. For example, truck drivers working along transport corridors are in a high-risk situation, which frequently introduces HIV into previously unaffected communities. Each truck driver will have a friend, wife, or partner living somewhere else, and most commercial sex workers also have some form of family life. Specific risk situations may also include boarding-school children, youth culture, men having sex with men (MSM), many prison situations, and cultural norms of sexual behaviour. The challenge for the team is to enter these situations, by invitation.

The pathway to identifying risk is through home and community conversations, in SALT, home-care, and community counselling. Building trust between all those involved is always one key to progress.

In 1990, one community action for change in Southern Province of Zambia was scaled up and transferred to all parts of the country through the action of the traditional leadership Council of Chiefs. In this area, tradition demands that a family member has sexual intercourse with the spouse or partner of the person who has died. In many areas, this has been a major cause of increased HIV infection. By common agreement over a year of community counselling and discussions, thousands of community members have been choosing non-sexual means to address this tradition. Community-based care and prevention teams (CPT) help sustain the change.

Step 4: Help communities and health workers learn together

Communities can help set the pace for HIV response. This includes expansion of home-care, ways of preventing HIV from spreading, and reducing stigma. The health team can give support so the community builds its confidence. Community-to-community visits can be arranged by a facilitation team of health and other staff. Community members can also join—they will learn in the process and speed up the useful learning that emerges.

Health teams and communities learn through SALT and other methods about local concerns, hopes and ways of working. Crucially, they should do an analysis after any community visit, reflect on the strengths they have seen, and how the team has functioned, and plan next steps. The facilitation team is an interface of learning between the hospital/clinic and the community. Figure 20.9 shows learning and analysing through SALT.

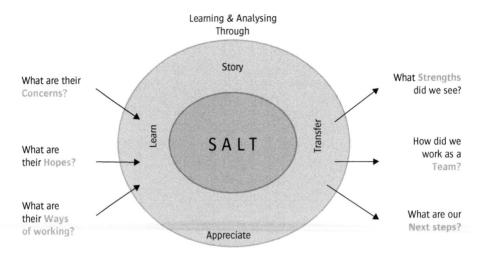

Figure 20.9 Learning and analysing through SALT.

Step 5: Integrate community response with the health facility

We now need to integrate the community's response to HIV with general processes of treatment and management within the hospital or clinic. An integrated response includes:

1. A multidisciplinary approach.

The full HIV response to diagnosis, care and treatment involves staff from medical, nursing, laboratory, education, counselling, administration, and pastoral care. Part of a community-led response will be a link to staff in a hospital or clinic, and these are essential for ART. Where they are not in place, this must become a priority for the team to ensure access to ART.

2. Close co-operation.

This must exist between the community-based organization (e.g. church, mosque, or other support group) the clinic, and community members, as well as from the government District Health Team.

3. A hospital or clinic management plan.

Any plan should include a diagnosis/counselling/treatment regimen; planned discharge, with family involvement; liaison with the home care team, community leaders, and community CPTs, as well as access to hospital or clinic care when required.

Step 6: Obtain additional funds

Although early steps as described can be started with relatively limited funding, we need to make sure that any programme started at community level, including access to treatment, is fully sustained. Wherever possible, we should integrate with government services, which ideally will be able to carry many of the programme costs. Where funding is needed, we will need to discover ways in which donors and government are working on HIV within the region where we work. This may be an integrated programme, such as SRHR as mentioned above, rather than specific HIV programmes. Chapter 5 discusses funding for CBHC programmes in more detail.

Writing an HIV project proposal

In addition to the general requirements for a proposal (see Chapter 5) a proposal for HIV should include several specific elements.

- A description of HIV in the district and its *possible impact on other areas of development*, as background to the project.
- The vision and main goal should emphasise an *expanded community response to HIV*. Action will not be only at a clinic or centre. This justifies activities such as visits by health teams to communities, skills training, and learning between communities.

  Ways in which the HIV programme will be *integrated* into other aspects of community-based care, ideally within the SRHR framework and including maternal and child health, tuberculosis control, and mental health services.

- *Baseline studies* including Knowledge, Attitude, and Practice (KAP) and how the programme will be documented or used for research.
- *The strategy of linking home-care to prevention in a participatory and relational way.* Note that linking care with prevention will also enable ART to reach more people, with access to drugs, monitoring of side effects and compliance given top priority.
- We must indicate how our organization will *network* with district, provincial and national health systems and other providers.
- Clear timelines and *methods of monitoring* will be needed along with plans for regular *evaluation*.

Understand confidentiality in home and neighbourhood

HIV/AIDS can be surrounded by fear, especially when it first appears, and stigma can develop. Communities will often be protective or suspicious of those wishing to discuss the topic. Any team needs invitations to discuss concerns about HIV and AIDS.

Communities are made up of relationships. It is these relationships that will bear the strains caused by HIV. When HIV is discovered in a community, changes begin to take place immediately, through a ripple effect, from the person who is infected, out to his/her closest relatives and friends, then almost invisibly to the surrounding community. Communities become aware of something happening. There is uneasiness, curiosity, anxiety. Information becomes a source of fear and speculation, as ideas become attached to the facts. There is shared secrecy, which produces stigma.

Yet often people in the same neighbourhood, family, or group share and learn together because they know that HIV is everybody's problem. This is what is known as shared confidentiality: when the community knows what is going on inside it, without saying it aloud (Figure 20.10).

Confidential sharing must be based on trust, which comes from establishing a caring relationship. There are many entry points for expressing care. For example, there may be existing programmes in the community for health, teaching, or worship. There may be institutions that have links with the community. Home visits may start as an expression of care for the community.

Households will welcome home visits, which are usually best carried out by a team of two to three people.

When the SALT approach is used, visits help to normalize the situation and encourage people to share their concerns for other community members. Home visits and community counselling together have a greater impact than either alone in the same geographic area, provided they are carried out with sensitivity.

Confidentiality is of great importance. Within the home, conversation is about persons and their HIV status. It is therefore person centred. Within the context of community counselling, confidentiality is more about issues raised and felt, and the community's response to them. This is known as issue-centred confidentiality. Both forms of confidentiality must be respected. Figure 20.10 shows how shared confidentiality works.

Community counselling

Community counselling is a conversation-based activity of local groups and communities, where a counselling team responds to invitations from local community groups. The goal of community counselling is to facilitate care and changes in thinking and behaviour in the community. It can and should involve a wide range of people who are not health staff. It stimulates the whole community to take responsibility for care and change. Community counselling includes:

- Building a relationship of trust, especially between the counselling team and the community group.
- The community identifying problems and exploring solutions.

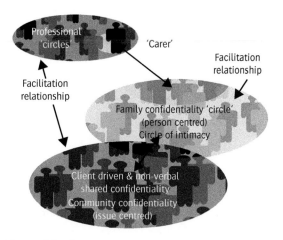

Figure 20.10 How shared confidentiality works.

Reproduced courtesy of Ian D. Campbell. This image is distributed under the terms of the Creative Commons Attribution Non-Commercial 4.0 International licence (CC-BY-NC), a copy of which is available at http://creativecommons.org/licenses/by-nc/4.0/.

- Decision-making by the community, including the planning of strategies.
- Implementing any actions decided upon.
- Evaluating the response together, and exploring any additional problems.

Chapters 2 and 6 give further background to this overall process.

These elements of community counselling must be explored at a pace with which the community feels comfortable. The cycle may be faster or slower than we expect. Our aim is to facilitate the discussion, help to clarify the proposed strategies, reflect back, probe, yet not impose our views. However, the facilitators still need to help move the group towards making decisions and planning strategies. Sometimes this will mean narrowing down a range of options that the community has explored first.

If the facilitator rushes to reach conclusions, some deeper issues may not be faced. So, although each meeting should conclude with the question 'What next?' the answer at times may simply be to meet again.

Community counselling is not very costly financially, but does take a great deal of energy, time and teamwork. It is a key to sustaining and expanding care and prevention.

The role of the community counsellor team is wide-ranging, and includes:

- Opening up *concerns* which will arise during community conversations.
- *Linking* the community and the health services.
- Helping to implement community-specific *strategies*.
- *Referring* patients to hospital when necessary.
- *Helping to initiate and follow up ART* with help from local clinics.
- *Counselling in bereavement.*
- Arranging for *process recording* by a team from within the community and counselling team and sharing this with other communities to develop community resilience. Figure 20.11 is an example.[8]

As community counsellors carry out these functions they will aim to:

- *Involve* every member of the discussion group.
- *Reflect* the discussion back to the group by summarizing at regular intervals what has been discussed or agreed upon.
- Keep the discussion on the agreed *subject*.
- Encourage positive *relationships* between group members.

Community name.. Date...............................

Issues/concerns discussed	Strategies discussed	Decisions made	Action taken	Results	How do they know? (Indicators)
Youth and sexual activity; they seem unaware of risk Men travel for work Lack of local employment	We need to teach our young: • Grandmothers should resume their traditional role in this • Teachers could organize • Talk to youth for their point of view More employment by way of income-generating projects	Talk to the youth: one community counsellor and a group of grandmothers will gather the youth for a discussion	Discussion with youth was held on (put in date)	The youth are very interested (see reports of youth discussion on date)	They want to meet with this group to discuss further They are also forming their own strategies and want to keep meeting themselves

NOTES ON TONE OF MEETING: Several people (put in their names) were trying to shift the discussion to the topic of economic development, saying that nothing could be done without jobs and money. Others in the group, especially (put in their names) strongly challenged this view. After three hours, agreement was reached on the specific action to be taken.

Figure 20.11 An example of 'process recording'.

- Take care to be seen as a *facilitator*, rather than the person in control.

More details on how to follow this type of approach are found in Chapter 4.

In summary, we must remember that helping a community change its behaviour is very different from trying to control behaviour. *Facilitating behaviour change* is the most effective AIDS control measure, and is at the heart of many of our activities in CBHC.

Health teams need to work with community and political leadership so that community counselling is supported. Programmes and communities can work together to advocate for effective support from both politicians and government health departments. Community counselling is a strong foundation for advocacy.

Involve communities in the use of antiretroviral therapy (ART)

ART is now available more widely, at more affordable prices, or free of charge. These drugs delay the development of AIDS. As mentioned, the use of antiretrovirals is now central to HIV treatment and control. ART has been the single most important factor in the rapid decrease in AIDS deaths, remarkable extensions of lifespans for people living with HIV, and even reductions in HIV spread. So successful has the ART rollout been in many areas that some communities, donor agencies, and countries no longer see HIV as the serious problem it still is.

It should be noted, however, that ART treatments must be used in the context of well-managed programmes, with HIV testing and 'DOT' style supervision of treatment (see Chapter 19). ART can prolong life, reduce suffering from secondary infections, and minimize mother-to-child transmission (see Chapter 17). Current advice is that ART should be started in everyone who is HIV-positive, regardless of other measurements such as CD4 count and viral load.

Mother-to-child transmission

Today no child should be born with HIV if their mother has been started on ART and given proper mother-to-child prevention. But in practice, preventing mother-to-child transmission through ART is not 100 per cent sufficient, especially when people are not in stable relationships and regular with their medications, so prevention efforts through other means must be continued.[9] Chapter 17 provides more details about preventing and managing mother-to-child transmission.

Co-infection with TB

Any active HIV treatment programme will also have to address co-infection with TB as most people living with HIV contract TB if TB is prevalent (see also Chapter 19). Anyone who is HIV-positive and has symptoms of TB, especially a cough for more than two or three weeks, must be carefully assessed for TB and started on anti-TB treatment.

The good news is that people with HIV who are co-infected with TB are treatable using standard TB medications. The key is good adherence to medications, which is made more difficult by the additional pill-load of TB medications. Also, past incomplete treatments for TB leading to multi-drug resistant strains (MDR-TB) make co-treatment more challenging. Treatment of co-infection therefore needs regular, skilled support and monitoring.

In all situations, HIV programmes that include family members in supporting treatment have higher rates of compliance. When combined with home care and community counselling, treatment prolongs life, reduces stigma, and helps to control the levels of HIV in a community.

However, poorly managed programmes, where people start and stop treatment without adequate support and monitoring, are likely to cause increasing drug resistance, which will make HIV harder to bring under control. We should be aware that overly centralized programmes that require patients to revisit hospital or clinic constantly, while reducing emphasis on home care and support, have lower rates of compliance. Community-managed treatment should be encouraged, with adequate referral links.

The community management of ART requires clear guidance. In 2005, The Salvation Army developed a field-based multi-country tested guideline,[10] affirming the linked roles of PLWH, family, neighbourhood, faith entity, and local clinic. General guides are useful, yet in our own context, we need to shape our own guidelines, adhering to national and WHO ethical practice standards.

Some important principles for programme design

1. Human resource development.

Communities and health staff need to strengthen skills, activities and systems. The human capacity to care is central, but workload and timetables need to ensure that people are not overloaded, which can lead to discouragement and burn-out. We must make opportunities for people to share problems and griefs, and to gain strength from each other or from specially trained counsellors or mentors.

2. Integration.

The heart of integrated management is the link between two processes: care for people, and change of attitudes and behaviours in the wider community. It requires health staff to attune themselves with local realities by visiting homes and neighbourhoods and being willing to learn from them, as in the SALT method.

3. Partnership between community and government—rights and responsibilities.

To be successful, HIV responses need to be decentralized and grounded in the community. But we will still need to follow national policy, allow our programmes to be supported, make use of VCT, and work to make ART treatment a reality and life-long friend of people living with HIV. Central to all partnerships is the role of PLWH themselves. Where they are given agency and support, the results are encouraging.

As community-based responses to HIV develop, people become aware of the bigger picture. This may lead to advocating for more government support and supplies for our programme. However, we need to remember that bigger is not always better. When community-based organizations are successful, it may be important to protect our particular approach from take-over by other entities (even occasionally, well-meaning government agencies).

The best pathway for advocacy and action both locally and nationally is through PLWH. It is always preferable for PLWH to lead community and team-wide processes of developing responses. Their presence in the process is a powerful advocacy tool and serves to 'normalize' HIV responses in communities.

Since HIV continues to be a disease of shame in most communities, the challenging but wonderfully powerful process of giving PLWH a voice to speak up is vital to real community-based change. When the voices of people suffering from HIV/AIDS are effectively heard, policy changes. Human rights must be strengthened if the challenges of HIV are to be effectively addressed. When human rights are disrespected, our personal humanity and our common life with others are also threatened. Communities addressing the challenges of HIV can also be enriched by this process in areas far beyond HIV.

4. Training and expansion.

Ongoing training of all staff members is important, both to encourage the team and to make sure it is well informed about HIV care and control. ART is complex and all team members will need to know the basic principles, and be able to answer questions from community members.

As experience grows, other groups needing help may visit the health facility or programme. Later, more formal learning programmes can be set up if the numbers of interested visitors grow. Learning themes can include the integration of home care, community counselling, VCT, ART, the roles of the health facility, and systems for team-building, monitoring, and networking.

Monitoring and Evaluation

It is often the actual responses and stories of PLWH, families, neighbourhoods, and other community groups that show us what is really happening in the longer term. For example:

'We found one woman [who] shared that she had had a strong reaction to the medicines, but she persisted for three months and gained full strength. We asked her to share her experience, and she continues to do this in the village.'

'Why do we have to get medicines from the hospital? It is a long distance; we can get them from the clinic, here.'

Figure 20.12 shows types of data that can be collected easily at a health centre or hospital.

We need indicators that are both qualitative and quantitative (see Chapter 9). UNAIDS and WHO have methods for evaluating HIV programmes looking at 'big picture' approaches which are often not appropriate for smaller scale community-based programmes.[11] If we are applying for funds, or receiving donor funds, we will usually be asked to monitor our programme according to their wishes or guidance.

Some examples that may be helpful at community level are:

- Qualitative indicators, e.g. assessing how much the community values the process and outcome of SALT and other approaches we use.

- Process indicators, e.g. the number and range of activities that members of the community, facility, or heath team have carried out.

- A combination of intervention and response types of indicators. Figure 20.12 illustrates the use of both

Administration	• total persons seen • new persons seen • total families seen • new families seen • patients preferring home care to periodic checks at hospital
Clinical care	• number with pre-AIDS • number with AIDS • number asymptomatic • number persons or families/friends with nursing care felt needs
Laboratory	• total contacts tested • number contacts HIV+ • results from all sources (inpatients, outpatients, etc.)
Mortality	• total persons known to have died • number died at home • number died in hospital/readmission

Education	• number of persons (friends, families) applying what they know in
	   – action for prevention (self reported)
	   – involvement in home care
	   – helping others to know what to do for care and prevention

Pastoral care	• number funerals attended • number times pastoral care invited in the form of prayer, scripture, counsel
Counselling	• number children of HIV+ persons • number families with HIV+ primary breadwinner • number families headed by HIV+ single mother • number families with abnormal atmosphere due to disease • number persons, family members, friends, communities acknowledging lifestyle changes in social activity, family life, sexual behaviour
Transfer	• members of PLWH who motivate others to respond • how many others respond (as a result of the influence of a PLWH) • how many families transfer response to other families • how many families are responding as a result of the action of PLWH • how many communities transfer • how many communities are responding as a result of transfer from a community by PLWH

Figure 20.12 Types of data that can be collected easily (health centre or hospital).

categories in health centres or hospitals. Figure 20.13 shows that response indicators are also significant.

• Community response is most easily measured by on-going monitoring in homes and neighbourhoods, or process recording (see Figure 20.11) and categorized by expressions of care, behaviour change, income generation, and transfer of vision and learning from other communities.

When communities act for care and change, self-measure for progress, and transfer to other communities, we know they are competent and confident in their own future.[12] When local response indicators are gathered

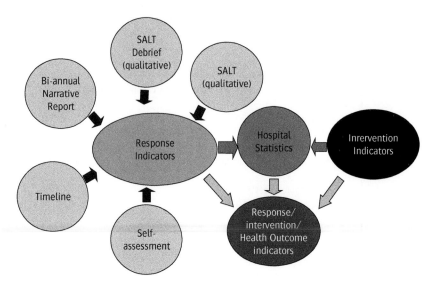

Figure 20.13 Response indicators are also significant.

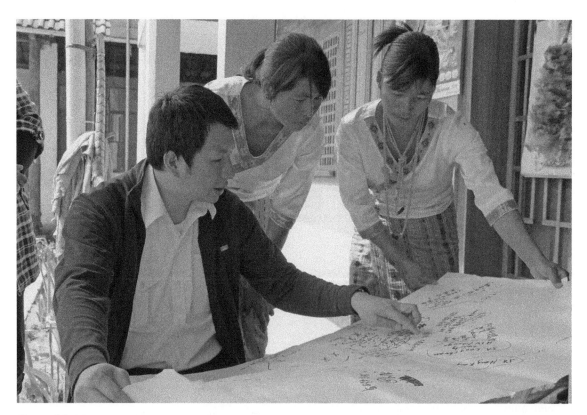

Figure 20.14 Village residents map their influence, after five villages were declared 'drug-free' in 2012, following SALT practice. Longchuan County, Yunnan Province, China

systematically over several years, and shown alongside district intervention indicators, it becomes easier to see how local community response is a very significant influence for sustaining outcomes and impact.

In addition, we also need some quantitative indicators to show the impact of our HIV programme in prevention, prolonging lives and well-being. These include indicators such as the proportion of PLWH who can access ART and the proportion known to take ART regularly (see Chapter 9). We must be sure to choose a comparatively small number of indicators relevant to our programme and make sure that we measure with care and accuracy. Funding for HIV programmes depends a great deal on clear indications of outcomes.

Figure 20.14 shows village residents mapping their influence, after five villages were declared 'drug-free' in 2012, following SALT practice, Longchuan County, Yunnan Province, China.[13]

Acknowledgements

This chapter draws on experiences with communities around the world since original involvement with a response to HIV and AIDS developed in collaboration with the Chikankata Hospital (Zambia) staff and community leaders in 1987. Photographs are from Ian D. Campbell's previously unpublished work with The Salvation Army, Interhealth Worldwide, and Affirm Facilitation Associates. Technical assistance was provided by Robin Rader.

Further resources

Affirm Facilitators. Stories of response from community conversations around the globe (GLoCon), a documentary trailer showing the impact of these conversations over the past twenty-five years, 'Neighbourhood matters most', and other resource documents on building community capacity for care and change. Available from: http://www.affirmfacilitators.org

Avert. Global information and advice on HIV and AIDS. Available from: http://www.avert.org/

UNAIDS. Global AIDS response progress reporting. Reporting overview for 2016. Available from: https://aidsreportingtool.unaids.org/static/docs/GARPR_Guidelines_2016_EN.pdf

NAM Aidsmap. HIV & AIDS—sharing knowledge changing lives. Available from: http://www.aidsmap.com/

References

1. UNAIDS. *Fact Sheet*. 2018. Available from: http://www.unaids.org/en/resources/fact-sheet

2. Campbell ID, Rader AD. HIV counselling in developing countries: The link from individual to community counselling for support and change. *British Journal of Guidance and Counselling*. 1995; 23 (1): 33–43.

3. Affirm Facilitators. *Methodology for SALT team visits (SALT protocol)*. Available from: http://www.affirmfacilitators.org/downloads.html

4. Affirm Facilitators. *Synthesis of community story: Kenya, April 2012*. The Global and Local Community Conversation (GLoCon). Available from: http://tinyurl.com/Kenya-GLoCon

5. The United Nations Universal Access Project. *BRIEFING CARDS: Sexual and reproductive health and rights (SRHR) and the post-2015 development agenda*. 2016. Available from: http://www.unfoundation.org/what-we-do/campaigns-and-initiatives/universal-access-project/briefing-cards-srhr.pdf

6. Chela CM, Campbell ID, Siankanga Z. Clinical care as part of integrated AIDS management in a Zambian rural community. *AIDS Care*. 1989; 1 (3): 319–25.

7. Affirm Facilitators. *Synthesis of community story: Brazil, September 2013*. The Global and Local Community Conversation (GLoCon). Available from: http://tinyurl.com/BrazilGLoCon2013

8. The Salvation Army. *Community counselling: A handbook for facilitating care and change*. 1998. Available at: http://tinyurl.com/CommunityCounsellingCareChange

9. McMahon J, Elliott J, et al. Viral suppression after 12 months of antiretroviral therapy in low- and middle-income countries: A systematic review. *Bulletin of the World Health Organization*. 2013; 91 (5): 377–85E.

10. The Salvation Army International Headquarters. *Guidelines for establishing community-led antiretroviral treatment through a human capacity development approach*. 2005. Available from: http://www1.salvationarmy.org/ihq/documents/ART_100.pdf

11. UNAIDS. *A framework for monitoring and evaluating HIV prevention programmes for most-at-risk populations*. 2008. Available from: http://www.unaids.org/sites/default/files/sub_landing/17_Framework_ME_Prevention_Prog_MARP_E.pdf

12. Campbell I. *Human capacity development for response to HIV*. Plenary presentation at the 2008 Pepfar HIV/AIDS Implementers' Meeting, Kampala, Uganda. Available at: http://www.affirmfacilitators.org/downloads.html

13. Affirm Facilitators. *Synthesis of community story: China, February 2012*. The Global and Local Community Conversation (GLoCon). Available from: http://tinyurl.com/ChinaLongChuan

CHAPTER 21

Setting up environmental health improvements

Ted Lankester

What we need to know

Why environmental health improvements are important

More than one person in five globally has no access to clean water, and nearly one person in three lacks basic sanitation. As healthcare workers and community members one of our priorities will often be to 'cure illness.' This chapter, more than any other in this book, points us to the primary priority of 'turning off the tap of ill health'. By this we mean looking at the causes, or determinants, of ill health, and doing everything we can within our communities to reduce or remove these causes.

This chapter gives a few ideas about how we can help to do this at community level, but also looks at some broader actions we can take. Environmental health is so complex that the community, health programme, national bodies (e.g. water boards), and government services need to work together and mutually recognize each other's role.

Establishing and strengthening the community's links with these actors is one of the most useful roles community leaders can play. More data on water and sanitation are found in Box 21.1.

WAter, Sanitation, and Hygiene (WASH) should be higher than they are on the global health agenda, but, despite progress, they lag behind in terms of government policies and funding. Quite good progress is being made on drinking water. Sanitation is often more difficult to introduce and sustain. Many diseases are caused by water that has been contaminated by human faeces, or by faecal pathogens in the environment. Environmental health measures are directed towards keeping human and animal waste separated from human contact.

Every day, more than 800 children die as a direct result of unsafe water or absence of basic sanitation.[3] Countless more suffer from associated diseases, including diarrhoea, dysentery, typhoid (enteric fever), cholera, hepatitis (A and E only), intestinal worms, trachoma, and bilharzia (schistosomiasis). Many people, especially children, are weakened by repeated such infections, and these also contribute to growth stunting (see Chapter 14). Effective sanitation that safeguards dignity is especially vital for girls of school age. Lack of basic facilities hinders girls from attending school, which causes a serious economic effect on individuals, families, communities, and countries.

WHO estimates that 6.5 million deaths each year are caused by air pollution making this the largest environmental threat to health.

Box 21.1 **Data on water and sanitation**

- In 2015, 71% of the global population (5.2 billion people) used a safely managed drinking-water service – that is, one located on premises, available when needed, and free from contamination.
- 89% of the global population (6.5 billion people) used at least a basic service ie an improved drinking-water source within a round trip of 30 minutes to collect water.
- 844 million people lack even a basic drinking-water service, including 159 million people who are dependent on surface water.

- Globally, at least 2 billion people use a drinking water source contaminated with faeces.
- In 2015, 39% of the global population (2.9 billion people) used a safely managed sanitation service.
- 68% of the world's population (5.0 billion people) used at least a basic sanitation service.
- 2.3 billion people still do not have basic sanitation facilities such as toilets or latrines.
- Of these, 892 million still defecate in the open, for example in street gutters, behind bushes or into open bodies of water.[1,2]

The key importance of improving WASH are spelled out in Sustainable Development Goal 6, which states:

by 2030 we should achieve 'universal and equitable access to safe and affordable drinking water for all',

and

by '2030, we achieve access to adequate and equitable sanitation and hygiene for all and end open defaecation, paying special attention to the needs of women and girls and those in vulnerable situations'.

Success in reaching these targets would enable people to lead healthier and more productive lives and improve the economies of all low-income nations.

Some key actions include improving the quality and availability of water, ensuring the safe disposal of human waste, especially faeces, and improving hygiene at personal, household, school, and community levels. These components have been described as the legs of a three-legged stool. Unless all legs are present, the stool falls over. WASH is an evidence-based worldwide movement and practice that combines the key elements of environmental health and involves a number of key agencies.[3]

This chapter concentrates on water supplies and waste disposal (interested readers are referred to Chapter 16 for ways to improve the hygiene of individuals and communities). Research has shown just how essential this is: regular hand-washing with soap can almost halve diarrhoea, and is thought to be able to save nearly a million lives a year.[4] It can also reduce the spread of respiratory infections and other infections like trachoma.

In community-based health care (CBHC) we can strengthen all three legs of the stool. Community members can adopt and sustain hygiene practices, and they can also use their entrepreneurial skills to make vital improvements in water and sanitation at community level. They can become involved in advocacy with government departments to bring improvements at a higher level. This is especially valuable in slum communities.

For example, in the ASHA project, Delhi, health workers and community members became exasperated by the rubbish accumulating in the streets and the complete lack of any garbage disposal facilities. By advocating to the respective civil authority, regular garbage disposal was arranged and has been sustained with great benefit.

It is worth emphasizing that any technology that is led by government or agencies such as a water board should be understood, accepted, and 'part-owned' by the community. For large-scale, more complex programmes, these agencies have ongoing responsibility to maintain infrastructure, but daily maintenance needs to be carried out by trained community members, especially in more rural settings.

Water sources and supplies

Why clean water is needed

Some health experts believe that the number of water points per 1000 people is a better indicator of health than the number of hospital beds. Water is needed for two main reasons: to drink and to wash. However, many farmers may view watering fields or animals as far more important than human cleanliness and laundry.

Many diarrhoeal diseases, including cholera, are caused by drinking dirty water or eating food contaminated by faeces (Table 21.1). Others, such as scabies and trachoma, are caused by having insufficient water for washing clothes, bodies, and faces. This means that each community will need a small supply of very clean water for drinking (at least two litres a day and more in hot climates) and a much larger supply of adequately clean water for washing. One guide is for communities to have at least 30 litres per person per day of clean water within half a kilometre of the home or settlement.

Surface water (rivers, lakes, ponds, etc.) is often highly contaminated with both germs and chemicals from pesticides and fertilizers. Rainwater, when safely collected and stored, and groundwater (stored in permeable rocks more than 100 metres underground), are usually of higher quality and safe to drink unless poisoned by minerals such as arsenic or fluoride.

It is important to realize that simple improvements at household level make a huge difference. These include regular handwashing with soap and water after defaecation and touching animals and before eating or preparing food (see also the food hygiene measures in Chapter 14).

Handwashing, plus point-of-use disinfection of drinking water, plus safe storage has an even greater effect. When starting an environmental programme it is therefore best to start with household improvements which are easier to sustain and can easily be carried out by community members. For example, many communities cannot afford to use soap regularly. Research from Bangladesh has shown that using water alone can help protect against diarrhoea, even though less effectively than when soap is used. Moreover, handwashing before eating, preparing food, and after using the toilet were shown as being more important than handwashing at other times. This simplifies the message in communities where time and resources are limited and helps to reduce the time taken in handwashing during the day and the amount of water needed.[5]

In summary, in CBHC we should first concentrate on simple improvements at individual and household level, including behavioural change. When basic knowledge and practice is better understood by community members we then have the basis for improving water supplies and building latrines with full community involvement.

Improving existing water sources

Some aspects of improving a water source are within reach of a community health programme. Sometimes government agencies and other experts can be called in for more detailed advice or to make major improvements such as drilling wells. For example, in some African and South Asian settings, it is common to have a district water office (DWO), as well as water and sanitation co-ordination committees that oversee water and sanitation budgeting and programming. When working well, they co-ordinate and use resources more effectively, especially if members of a village health committee (VHC) are also involved.

Improving water sources can raise credibility for our other community-based activities. But health behaviours need to change. And the community needs to learn how to use and maintain any improved system.

Women traditionally do most of the water carrying i.e. the further away the water source, the greater the time and energy spent in carrying. In turn, this means less time is available for looking after children, work in the home and fields, and earning money. A reliable water source near the home therefore has multiple benefits for the family. In addition, women fetching water are often in danger of sexual harassment and

Table 21.1 Bradley Classification of Infective Diseases Related to Water

Category	Example
I. Waterborne	
a) Classical	Typhoid
b) Neoclassical	Infectious
II. Water-washed	
a) Superficial	Trachoma, Scabies
b) Intestinal	Shigella, dysentry
III. Water-based	
a) Water-multiplied percutaneous	Bilharzia
b) Ingested	Guinea worm
IV. Water-related insect vectors	
a) Water-biting	Gambian sleeping sickness
b) Water-breeding	Onchocerciasis

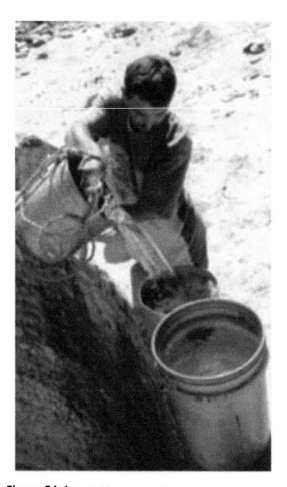

Figure 21.1 A reliable water supply near the home has multiple health benefits for the family.

rape. They can become seriously fatigued, especially if they have young children or are pregnant. Carrying heavy loads such as water can cause injury and accidents (Figure 21.1).

Rainwater harvesting and rainwater tanks

Rainwater is often an underused source of clean water. Even intermittent or seasonal rain can be harvested from roofs and stored in appropriate containers, e.g. ferrocement tanks. Rainwater gives easy access to water and, providing roofs and tanks are big enough, is low-cost, easy to manage, and provides a clean, uncontaminated supply. It should be the first option to consider in many communities, even if there is no tradition of rainwater collection.

Harvesting can be done in a variety of ways depending on the local situation and type of housing. In houses with corrugated iron roofs, a simple gutter can be constructed to run into a tank built next to the house.[6] Plastic sheeting can also be used to collect water. Such sheeting is often distributed in refugee camps. The sheeting can be tethered to four posts in the ground with run-off into a clean, contaminant-free container (Figure 21.6). Sheeting can also be placed over the roofs of thatched huts for clean run-off of water.

Rainwater tanks may quickly become dirty. They can be made safer by:

1. Cleaning the tank and entrance pipe before the rainy season or using a first flush diverter device (see Figure 21.2).

2. Placing a filter or screen where the water enters the tank to keep out insects, leaves, and dirt.

3. Placing a sealed cover over the tank to keep the water clean and to prevent mosquitoes from breeding in it.

4. Ensuring that taps alone are used for withdrawing water.

5. Chlorination, which is often better done nearer the point of use.

Springs

Spring water is usually clean when it emerges from the ground, but it can quickly become contaminated when it pools at source, or is carried and stored.
It can be made safer by:

1. Erecting a fence with a gate around the spring to keep out animals.

2. Building a ditch to allow water to drain away.

3. Building a stone wall or 'box' around the spring itself, through which a pipe runs, or preferably a double pipe (see Figure 21.3).

Wells and boreholes

Wells come in a variety of forms, including step wells, open wells (from which water is collected by rope and bucket), and tubewells (from which water is raised by a hand pump, see Figure 21.4). Open wells may be covered and fitted with hand or mechanical pumps.

Well water can be made safer by:

1. Fixing a removable cover.

2. Building an outward-sloping apron wall around the well, 0.5–1m high.

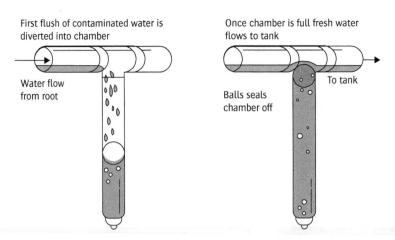

First flush of contaminated water is diverted into chamber

Water flow from root

Once chamber is full fresh water flows to tank

To tank

Balls seals chamber off

Figure 21.2 A first flush diverter.

Reproduced with permission from *Rain Harvesting*. © Copyright 2018 Rain Harvesting Pty Ltd. Available at: http://rainharvesting.com.au/product/downpipe-first-flush-diverters/. This image is distributed under the terms of the Creative Commons Attribution Non Commercial 4.0 International licence (CC-BY-NC), a copy of which is available at http://creativecommons.org/licenses/by-nc/4.0/.

The wall prevents dirty water from running into the well and acts as a shelf where waterpots can be placed. The slope helps water to drain and discourages people from standing on it.

3. Building a concrete drainage channel around the outside of the wall.

4. Providing one container to draw water.

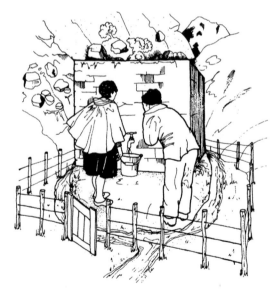

Figure 21.3 A properly protected spring.

Reproduced with permission from World Health Organization. Copyright © 2017 WHO. This image is distributed under the terms of the Creative Commons Attribution Non Commercial 4.0 International licence (CC-BY-NC), a copy of which is available at http://creativecommons.org/licenses/by-nc/4.0/.

This container with its fixed rope is allowed to rest only on the apron wall, never on the ground. Those using the container clean their hands before use and touch only the outside of the container and handle, never the inside.

5. Ensuring that no one uses the well for washing.

6. Encouraging the community to set up its own system for keeping the surrounds clean, repairing the well when needed, and keeping the hand pump in good repair.

7. Chlorinating the well at regular intervals (see 'Water treatment' for constraints in doing this).

8. Ensuring there are no pit latrines within 30 metres, and that the bottom of the pit is at least two metres above the level of groundwater. The area should not be prone to flooding.

In order for these improvements to made and maintained there needs to be excellent community organization as well as understanding and agreement from community members. Maintaining the infrastructure and changing behaviours to ensure the correct use of wells needs time to become embedded in the community's culture.

Arsenic contamination of a water supply is extremely dangerous. In several countries of the world, arsenic contaminates well water, e.g. Bangladesh, where about 80 million people are potentially exposed, and parts of Argentina, Chile, China, India, Mexico, and the United States. Arsenic poisoning leads to skin

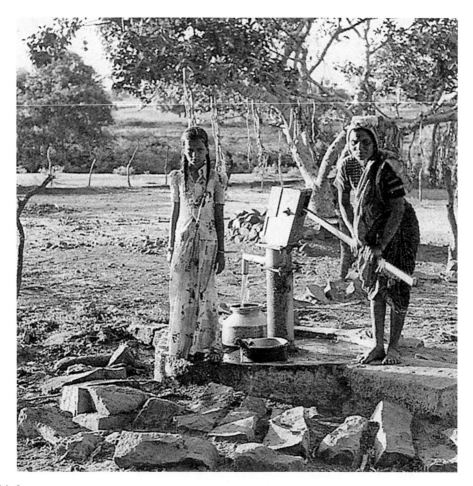

Figure 21.4 A tube well with hand pump, sunk in the low-caste area of a village in western India.

pigmentation, bronchitis, high blood pressure, liver problems, and cancer, with effects taking up to ten years to appear. Research shows that arsenic increases deaths from liver, lung, and bladder cancers, and also from cardiovascular disease, especially when combined with smoking.[7,8]

If we know or suspect arsenic contamination of water in our area, we must call in the government or water authorities to carry out measurements and mark unsafe water points. We then need to find other sources, such as treated surface water or rainwater harvesting. Other techniques are being developed.[9]

Ponds and watering holes

Although widely used, water from these sources is dangerous and can spread a variety of diseases, including bilharzia (schistosomiasis), especially in Africa. Pond water should not be used for drinking unless there is no alternative, in which case it should be boiled or filtered before drinking. Any pond used as a water supply or for washing should not also be used for washing or watering animals. Small ponds can be protected by a fence.

Rivers and streams

Most river water is contaminated. If river water has to be used, we should ensure that:

1. Water is collected from the river above the village, preferably through a sand filter, infiltration gallery, or, in the case of hill communities, a gravity flow system. Of course, if there are other villages upstream this system won't guarantee safer supplies.

2. Bathing, washing, and the watering of animals takes place only below the village (Figure 21.5).

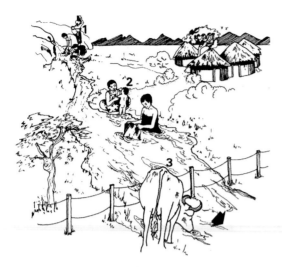

Figure 21.5 River water. 1. Draw water from above the village. 2. Bathe and wash downriver from the village. 3. Exclude animals where possible.

Water from standpipes or other piped systems

Tap water is not always clean. It may come from a dirty source or become contaminated through cracks in the pipes. Tap water can be made safer by:

1. Water treatment if this is available
2. Checking the source is clean.
3. Checking the pipes to make sure there are no leaks or joins.
4. Keeping the surrounds of a standpipe (standpost) clean and well drained.
5. Building a concrete or wooden platform on which to rest buckets.
6. Constructing a fence to keep away animals.
7. Encouraging the community to set up a system for checking source, pipes, tap, and surrounds and keeping them clean and in good repair (see 'Work through a Community Action Group').

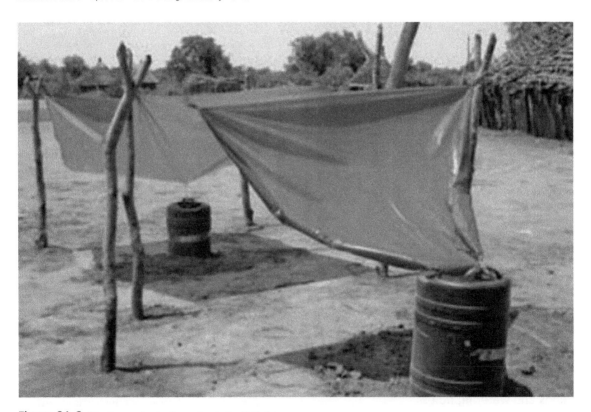

Figure 21.6 Ultra low-cost water harvesting in South Sudan

Developing new water sources

Larger programmes or programmes in areas where improved water is a strongly felt need can help their communities develop new sources or make major improvements in storage or transport. Government, local politicians, and decision-makers are responsible for providing the support and expertise needed.

Examples might include:

- Piping water to suitable sites in the community or into each house
- Drilling tube wells.
- If arsenic in groundwater is suspected, call in government experts to test levels.
- Additionally, hand pumps can be installed in existing wells, and community water tanks can be built.

For example, one rural village in southern Asia with a single spring at an inconvenient site below the village decided to construct a large storage tank with multiple taps within the village itself. Capital costs were obtained from the health project to buy a diesel pump and piping for lifting water from the source into the water tank. The community built the tank and was taught how to maintain it. All members now have easy access to clean water throughout the day. Projects on this scale need careful planning and co-ordination between community, programme director, government departments, and donor agencies.

Water storage

Water may be dirty when collected, or become contaminated in transit or storage, especially in hot climates, crowded conditions, or from distant sources. Storage containers can be made of many different materials. Earthenware or clay pots are suitable but should not be placed on dirty surfaces where germs can leach in. No container should be used that has ever contained pesticides or dangerous chemicals. Storage is improved if containers are kept off the floor and away from animals and children, covered, and cleaned regularly, e.g. with bleaching powder. Even if water is clean at the time of storage it can become contaminated at the point of use, usually by dirty hands or implements being put into the water.

Water storage is made safer if the community can learn to:

- Cover the container with a tight-fitting lid
- Use containers with a tap or spigot.

- 'Tip, don't dip'—tip water into a cup or glass or use a long-handled dipper that is held only at the handle's end and used for pouring, not for drinking from directly.[10]

We need to make sure that improvements at the point of use are familiar to the community or work easily.

For example, one study showed that an improved container proved popular in a refugee camp in Malawi and reduced diarrhoea by one-third in children under five. It holds 20 litres, has a lid with a hole just large enough to fill from a hand pump, a handle, and spout for pouring. For more information on environmental health in emergency situations, see Further reading. It is also worth remembering that the results of one study may not be easily replicated.

Water treatment

There are various ways of reducing the number of germs in water. They include the following:

1. The three pot method (Figure 21.7).
2. Filtration—there are various methods such as charcoal filters (Figure 21.8).
3. Disinfection with chlorine or bleach.

Although this can be done at community level, e.g. in the storage tank or well, it can also be done in each household. One method is to take one cup (about 250ml) of household or laundry bleach and mix it with three cups

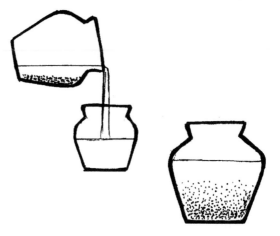

Figure 21.7 The three-pot method .

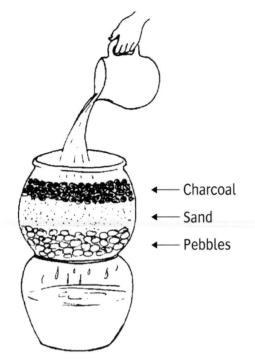

Figure 21.8 Charcoal filter.

Reproduced with permission from PATH, Seattle, Washington, USA; and adapted with permission from Peace Corps Times. This image is distributed under the terms of the Creative Commons Attribution Non Commercial 4.0 International licence (CC-BY-NC), a copy of which is available at http://creativecommons.org/licenses/by-nc/4.0/.

of water to make one litre. Add three drops of this solution to one litre of water and allow it to stand. If the water is badly contaminated, six drops can be used. There are a few drawbacks. Any organic matter in the water inactivates the chlorine. Accurate dosing is needed, and many people dislike the smell and taste of chlorine.

4. Boiling water for one minute will kill most germs.

Boiling drinking water is not usually a practical option. It is only appropriate if there is an adequate supply of fuel and a water source that is highly contaminated. The use of extra fuel can contribute to ill health by adding to indoor smoke inhalation.

5. Exposure to sun—the 'SODIS' (solar disinfection) method.

There is now uncertainty about the effectiveness of this method, and it should only be used if there is no alternative, and according to technical guidance.[11] It involves placing water in transparent containers in the sun. Plastic bottles for soft drinks or bottled water are ideal. Leave them in full sun, e.g. on the roof of the house, for at least five hours. Their lower half can be painted black or they can be placed on black-painted corrugated iron or plastic sheets to aid heat absorption.

In addition to these examples, there are constantly new technologies regularly being tried out and developed.

Methods of waste disposal

It is helpful to think of waste under four headings: liquid waste, solid household waste, human waste, and household smoke. We will look at the first three here, and household smoke later in the chapter.

Liquid waste disposal

Liquid waste is household wastewater, including water used for washing clothes and utensils. It is sometimes known as sullage. Where washing takes place outside, this is usually less of a problem. Where washing takes place inside with an exit pipe, pools of stagnant water quickly form by the house or in the street, especially in urban areas.

Community hygiene can therefore be greatly improved when stagnant wastewater is removed and containers of stagnant water are covered or removed. For example, in one programme in Delhi, India, during a dengue fever outbreak, school-aged children wrote and performed a play within the slum community about mosquito breeding sites. The children then went from house to house pointing out where stagnant water could be removed.

Wastewater can be disposed of in various ways:

1. Through toilet-flushing in pour-flush systems
2. Using it to water vegetables in a kitchen garden, providing there are no harmful chemicals such as bleach in the water.
3. In a soakage pit.

This can be constructed below ground outside each house, by making a cubic hole with sides about 1.5 m, lined with brick or stone. For example, a newsletter of the CRHP programme in Jamkhed, Maharashtra India reported that its 'programme recommends soak pits, which are easy-to-build pits, made from layers of sand, rocks and bricks that filter excess water from each household. Each soak pit is built and implemented by the families in each community with support from the project. This creates knowledge and ownership for each household. As a result, malaria has been eliminated in villages that have fully implemented soak pits. We see an immediate improvement in the lives of children and families'.[12]

4. A simple communal drainage system of covered drains (or pipes).

This is effective if well-constructed and regularly cleaned. It is the method of choice in poor urban areas.

Household solid waste disposal

This can be disposed of in a household or community tip, or in cities by putting pressure on the civic authorities to arrange refuse removal. The disposal of waste and its separation into different components for recycling is becoming increasingly important and systems and advice change frequently. We should make sure we follow any guidance available in our area either from government or from a specialist programme. Commonly, cardboard, paper, food and drink cans, aluminium foil, and plastic bottles and bags can be recycled. The scheme below is a more traditional example often used in rural areas:

1. Material suitable for burning.

These types of materials, e.g. paper, can be incinerated well away from homes at appropriate times.

2. Solid matter for burying.

Each household should dig its own hole at least one metre deep, or the community can make a communal rubbish pit, which must be at least 20 metres from the nearest house. The distance from the nearest water source ideally needs to be guided by an expert as it depends on a number of factors. A figure of 100 metres is sometimes given. Any rubbish tip should be covered with several inches of earth to reduce flies, and protected by a fence or enclosure to keep out animals. Needles, syringes, and other waste from health centres must not be disposed of in this way.

3. Organic (vegetable matter) for composting.

Organic matter, along with animal dung, can be rotted down and used as fertilizer after four to six months. A shallow pit is dug and kept covered by a few inches of soil. Wooden posts can be inserted as 'chimneys' to help take air into the pile, which speeds up the decay.

Human waste disposal

Faeces are highly infectious and remain so for some time. It has been estimated that one gram of faeces can contain ten million viruses (including hepatitis A and E), one million bacteria (e.g. cholera and shigella), and parasite cysts and eggs.[13,14] In urban areas or wherever there is overcrowding, virtually everyone, especially children playing outside, will be affected by faecal contamination. This effect is multiplied when the same open spaces are used for defecation, children's play, agriculture, and communal gatherings. Nearly one billion people (almost one in seven) still practise open defaecation.

Studies have shown that safe disposal of children's faeces can reduce diarrhoeal disease by up to 40 per cent. Since children 'go anywhere, any time,' the whole community needs to be involved in the sanitation programme so that children's faeces are disposed of effectively; of course, the same is true of faeces in general. Safe disposal of faeces prevents flies landing on them, which further reduces the incidence of diarrhoea and similar vector-borne diseases.

For example, trachoma, a severe infectious eye disease affecting many millions of poor people, is spread by a fly called *Musca sorbens*. This fly seeks out human eyes but breeds in human faeces. Latrine use has been shown to reduce trachoma transmission, but regular hand- and face-washing reduces it still further.[15,16] The World Health Organization (WHO) and other international agencies have set up a web-based information service called Sanitation Connection[17] which gives further information.

There are various methods of human waste disposal. Before entering into the weird and wonderful world of trying to change sanitation behaviour, we need to discover existing sanitation schemes in the area, or any government-led plans or campaigns in the pipeline. Many countries already have national sanitation campaigns and it is important to co-ordinate with them to avoid clashes or duplication of approaches.

Traditional open field defaecation.

We must do all we can to establish latrine disposal of faeces, rather than open field use. However, if this really is impossible for the moment, some improvements can be made. The site should be a safe distance from any house, at least ten metres from any water supply, and away from any paths. For example, in many parts of the world, but especially in south Asia, paths are used as the public toilet. This spreads germs throughout the community. The health team, supported by the community health worker (CHW) and health committee, can help the community set up alternative sites. But before simply telling community members to change their practices, we need to ask why people follow a particular custom. For example, the reason for defaecating on village paths in one Himalayan community where the author used to work was unexpected: dirty paths were less likely to be frequented by ghosts at night.

Further improvements to open field defaecation include:

- Wearing shoes. This reduces the risk of hookworm and other infections.
- Digging a small hole with a stick or spade and the faeces placed there and covered with earth. This will help to keep off flies and animals. Sunny areas should be used rather than shady ones, which helps to reduce germs.
- Accompanying young children who use the site.

NB: the open field system is only appropriate in rural areas with relatively low populations, and for communities still unready or unwilling to use latrines.

The simple pit latrine

This is also known as the sealed-lid latrine Figure 21.9. Simple latrine building using local initiatives has taken

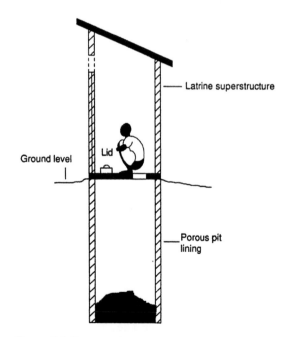

Figure 21.9 The simple pit latrine.

> ### Box 21.2 **Building a pit latrine**
>
> A classic basic latrine design consists of a pit in the ground two to three metres deep, lined by bricks, blocks, concrete rings, or by making use of an old oil drum. If the soil is hard and firm throughout the year, only the top 0.5 to 1 metre needs to be lined.
>
> In all cases, the lower part of the pit should have small holes so liquid can seep out. The pit is covered by a slab, ideally made of concrete at least 80mm thick with 6mm iron bars every 150mm in both directions to prevent it from collapsing. The size of the slab should extend right up to the lined side of the pit, or beyond it if an oil drum is used. The squat hole should be shaped like a key-hole, 400mm long, 100mm wide at the narrow end, 200mm wide at the larger end. This size and design is safe for all but the smallest children. The hole is fitted with a tight-fitting cover with a handle. A wall can be built for privacy, using wattle, grass, mud, or brick. The problems of flies and smell are reduced by replacing the cover after use and by scrubbing the slab regularly with soap and water. However, these problems are more effectively solved by using VIP or water-seal latrines.

a leap forward through a self-help movement known as community-led total sanitation,[18] which aims to eliminate open defaecation. It encourages local people to use simple materials such as bamboo, tin, and jute to build latrines in ways that are most acceptable to the community (Box 21.2). This approach has eliminated open defecation in many areas of Asia and Africa. It often works better than top-down schemes, which are often imposed by governments and programmes on reluctant people. It relies on skilled and persistent facilitators explaining the value of latrines to each household. Usually both men and women facilitators are needed.

One way to raise awareness is community mapping of where members from each household usually defaecate. Mapping is helpful because, in the words of one activist, 'most people see that they are surrounded by shit', which often motivates the community to do something about it! However, we also need to keep in mind that a badly constructed or sited pit latrine can be worse than open defecation—by bringing defecation closer to the home while not safely separating faeces from human contact. Simply building basic latrines as the 'end' goal can add to our problems, since no one wants to use a

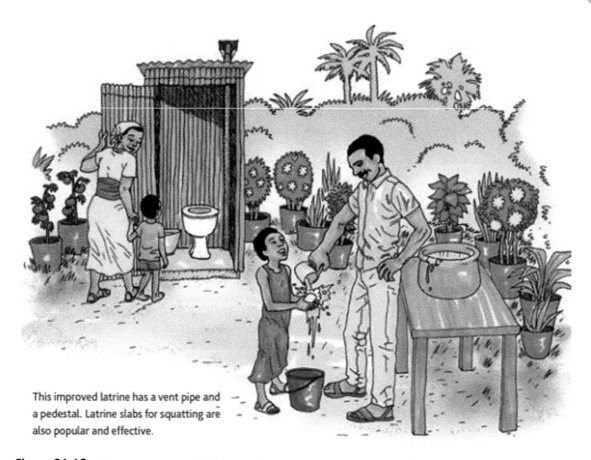

This improved latrine has a vent pipe and a pedestal. Latrine slabs for squatting are also popular and effective.

Figure 21.10 Using a VIP Latrine (Ventilated, Improved, Pit).

smelly, fly-ridden latrine. Latrines must also ensure privacy and safety for women and children. Adults can accompany them for reassurance to start with, and can help with cleaning afterwards.

When children defaecate into a container in the home, the parents should empty this into the latrine, not outside the home. Remember that young children's faeces are often more infectious than adults'. Either make sure that children can use the adult latrine safely, or construct smaller, child-friendly versions where they feel more comfortable.

VIP, or water-seal, latrines are basically the same design as the simple pit latrine, but contain a ventilating pipe, the end of which is screened (Figure 21.10). The pipe must be high enough above the roof to ensure good air flow and be at least 150mm in diameter. It can be painted black and the added heat absorption is thought to help create an updraught. The screen should be made of fibreglass or stainless steel to prevent corrosion. The squat hole should not be covered. The shelter should have no windows and be quite dark. These measures trap flies (which are drawn up the pipe by the light and the updraught), improve ventilation and reduce smell effectively.

The pour-flush latrine

Pour-flush latrines are more expensive. They are appropriate in communities where water is used for anal cleansing, as in much of Asia, or in other areas where there is a demand for them. They need a source of sufficient water. Any latrine used can have either a single pit, or double pit, as shown in Figure 21.11. All latrines must be used and sited correctly. Consider also whether a simple low-cost improvement, e.g. the Sanplat is worth using.

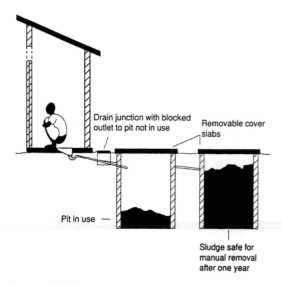

Drain junction with blocked
outlet to pit not in use

Removable cover
slabs

Pit in use —

Sludge safe for
manual removal
after one year

Figure 21.11 Pour-flush latrine with twin pit.

Reproduced courtesy of David Gifford. This image is distributed under the terms of the Creative Commons Attribution Non Commercial 4.0 International licence (CC-BY-NC), a copy of which is available at http://creativecommons.org/licenses/by-nc/4.0/.

The correct position and use of latrines (including the Sanplat)

Latrines are of no value unless they are well maintained and well cleaned, and unless the population, including children, has been carefully taught how to use them. Soap and water must be kept near the latrine for handwashing, and leaves, paper, or water kept in the latrine for anal cleansing according to custom. A good way to spread diarrhoeal diseases is to build public latrines, give no health teaching, forget the soap, and arrange no maintenance. Such buildings quickly become a serious health risk to the entire community. Latrines should be near the home, ideally about six metres away so they can be used in bad weather and, where possible, 30 metres away from and below any water source.[19]

The Sanplat is a specially designed concrete platform that can be installed in existing latrines and supported by a floor of logs and clay. It uses much less concrete than the standard slab, meaning more people can afford it (see Further reading).[20]

What we need to do

It is worth emphasizing here that any community programme should co-ordinate with and where possible be part of any existing public health and WASH programmes. Health outreach and sanitation programmes are now very common in many non-conflict situations. Examples of these include Ethiopia's Health Extension Workers and Health Development Army, Uganda's Village Health Teams, and District Water Offices (DWOs) common in many African and South Asian contexts.

It is also worth quoting from an adapted UN official definition of basic sanitation because hidden among its words (in italics) are principles and objectives that should be central to our programme:

"Basic sanitation is the *lowest-cost option* for securing *sustainable access* to safe and convenient facilities and services that *provide privacy and dignity* while ensuring a *clean and healthful living environment* both at home and in the neighbourhood of users".[21]

Help the community to identify its needs

The community may identify problems with its water supply. These problems may include:

1. Supplies are too distant.

In some communities women and children spend up to two to three hours per day collecting water.

2. Supplies are intermittent.

Water sources may dry up at certain times of year, meaning more distant sources have to be used. In the case of piped supplies, water may only flow once or twice per day (or per week).

3. Supplies are contaminated.

The community may not always fully understand the need for clean water or believe their existing supplies are sufficiently clean.

4. Supplies are only available for the rich, high castes, or the dominant tribal group.

The poor may have to use a more distant or contaminated source. The community, especially women, will already be aware of any need to improve water supplies, in particular the time taken for collection. It will often be a strongly expressed need in our first meetings with the community.

In contrast to water supplies, the community may not see a need to change their attitude towards sanitation practices or existing patterns of waste disposal (Figure 21.12). Often these habits will be strongly tied in with traditions, and we will need to give convincing reasons to persuade people to make changes. Creating awareness is therefore an important part of any sanitation programme, and programmes that are 'demand-led' rather than 'supply-led' tend to work better (Box 21.3). In other words, building latrines and *then* persuading people to use them often fails to work. Promoting latrines as a home improvement or a sign of being educated, rather than for health reasons, can increase demand. This works especially well when we target younger community members.

Whatever the motivation, it is generally better to wait until families are ready to build their own latrine and for them to pay for most of it themselves, rather than constructing the latrine for them free of charge. Revolving loan funds may make this possible for poorer community members (see Chapter 12).

Understand culture and beliefs

In both water and sanitation programmes we need to help the people identify their own needs and suggest their own solutions. Most communities have strong beliefs about waste disposal and traditional rights over water use. The knowledge, attitude, and practice of the community must be understood before any plans are drawn up. In many parts of the world, especially the Middle East, Saharan Africa, and central Asia, there is a severe lack of water. Any increase in water use by one family or community may mean less for another. Local and regional conflicts can develop as a result.

There may also be ingrained gender-based beliefs to do with latrine use. For example, in parts of Latin America it is believed that women who use the same latrines as men may become pregnant, and in parts of east Africa, daughters are forbidden to use the same latrine as their fathers.

Further examples include some communities in Uganda (e.g. dropping children's faeces around the compound is a sign of pride and shows how many children you have) and some south-west African communities (e.g. squatting over a pit can cause a miscarriage or that angry visitors will place bad medicine in a pit to bewitch a family). In the latter example, community latrines became popular in one community once the Tangalamenas (traditional leaders) tried them in their own yards with good results (no bad luck, fewer flies, and less smell).

These stories, and others from around the world, show how important it is to understand local beliefs before we start sanitation programmes. Most commonly of all, however, social embarrassment, especially for young women, is a major community concern.

Box 21.3 Eleven guidelines for planning an improved sanitation programme

1. Aim for a sustainable programme which makes long-term improvements. This will not happen quickly—it may take many years to be achieved.
2. Identify with the community an appropriate latrine design for the area. It should be technically able to provide adequate sanitation, affordable for most people and culturally and socially acceptable.
3. Discuss and involve all plans and actions with the future users of the sanitation—especially the women and community representatives or leaders. Work with people. Don't aim to do the work for them.
4. Don't offer to give people latrines or to subsidise them. The desire to achieve rapid results often leads to serious problems. A credit scheme or revolving loan fund may help many people build a latrine while leaving them fully responsible.
5. Promote latrines so that people desire to have one—don't threaten people that they 'must get a latrine or else …'.
6. Use any means possible to promote improved sanitation. Convince community leaders, local officials, teachers, and primary and community health workers, and encourage them to assist in the promotion work.
7. Either encourage people to build the latrines themselves or privatize the construction of latrines by training local builders.
8. Make sure all latrine construction is backed up with full health and hygiene education and help on how to use and clean the latrine properly.
9. Co-ordinate the work with those aiming to improve the water supplies or other forms of sanitation.
10. Keep the programme costs as low as possible and keep staff numbers low. This will help the programme run for a longer period.
11. Encourage and help schools, churches, clinics and other institutions to improve their sanitation. This has a good demonstration effect on everyone seeing them.

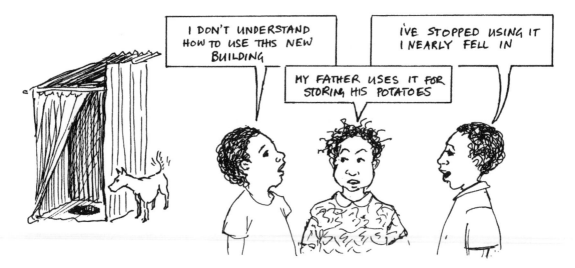

Figure 21.12 Awareness raising, joint planning, and ownership are the keys to successful sanitation.

Assess what resources are available

We will need to ask the community the following questions, while being aware of what support there might be from the government or a voluntary group implementing WASH. However, before we do this, community members will need to be aware and informed so they can answer these questions and make effective choices:

- What is the level of interest?
- How much time will be available to make changes and at what time of year?
- What skills are present, including both technical and managerial skills?
- What materials are available?
- What sources of funds are available?
- What degree of co-operation is possible between the different groups who will need to work together?
- How is the community motivated about using the new facility?

We should encourage the community to contribute its own resources as much as possible.

Choose what improvements to make

This should be done by the community with guidance from the health team (Figure 21.12). Any improvements chosen should be culturally acceptable, and affordable for most people.

In choosing improvements, the following have to be 'matched up':

- The community's priorities.
- Resources available.
- Ability of the community to manage the project and upkeep afterwards.
- Methods used successfully in nearby areas, either by government or other voluntary agencies.
- Government or national guidelines, which should be followed where they exist, and we should seek out funding that may be available.
- The culture of the people, with regards to sanitation, although we will promote the use of latrines if at all possible.
- Traditional water rights, being careful not to cause conflict with neighbouring communities.

In practice, it is wise to start with small, simple schemes such as improving existing systems. For example, The International Committee of the Red Cross carried out a latrine improvement scheme in Kabul, Afghanistan. This included either constructing a new latrine or renovating an existing one to ensure the following: adequate capacity (2.1 cubic metres), an underground soakage pit for urine, venting with a nylon mesh, and a removable door to make emptying the vault easier. These improvements led to a reduction in the deaths of children under eleven years of age and were found to be equally, or more, cost-effective as other programmes targeting children's health.[22]

In another example, the author recently visited a programme in Musoma district, Tanzania, which the community calls 'turning off the tap of ill health by turning on the tap of clean water.' The programme uses an outside agency that specializes in training householders to construct ferrocement tanks and fitting gutters to roofs for rainwater harvesting. The success of storing water for weeks at a time was first demonstrated in the local school, from where the idea spread to surrounding villages. This created a demand for similar modifications to all houses in the community, carried out by household members with training from the programme.

Progressing from smaller projects to larger ones has several advantages, which include a greater likelihood of success. Without this the community will quickly lose confidence and trust. Additionally, useful experience is gained—by the health team and the community, and the community learns how to manage projects within its capacity. It is worth noting that any large-scale improvements should be piloted first.

Work through a Community Action Group (CAG)

The Community Action Group (CAG) is basically a VHC, but it is more likely to get things done if given a dynamic name (see also Chapter 7).

This section also applies to other community groups, such as women's groups, village health clubs and, water user committees. These are ways we can take things forwards.

1. Help to set up, or strengthen, a CAG or other community group.

We can use an existing community group even if they may need further training and encouragement to become effective. We should aim to include at least one CHW, one or two older school children, and a representative of any co-ordinating agency. Above all, women must be strongly represented.

It has often been shown that water and sanitation programmes often work best when women are involved in planning them and carrying them out. The reason for this is quite obvious: water programmes bring greatest benefit to women, who, after implementation, spend much less time in fetching water than before. Additionally, women usually take greater interest and responsibility than men in matters of family hygiene.

2. Ensure that the CAG is informed, motivated, and trained.

We will need to train the group to understand why changes are being made, any benefits it will bring (e.g. convenience, time, money savings, self-respect), how to act as motivators and agents of change, and how to set up and organize the programme. In training the CAG, we can use interactive teaching, visits to other programmes, and discussion with community members to generate ideas. Elders, opinion formers, teachers, religious leaders, traditional healers, and children can all be included.

In our communities, teaching on water and sanitation needs to be given to school children, and school latrines need to be built. The community can help advocate for the government to carry this out, but local people will need to be involved in its management and maintenance. UN and government led-approaches are also important to help programmes to be effective and sustainable. Therefore, we should also learn and help the community learn from the WHO Sanitation safety manual[23] and from the Sphere Handbook 2018, see Further Reading below.

3. Enable the CAG to manage the programme.

This will involve careful forward planning, communicating about all programme stages with the community, involving outside agencies, and co-ordinating the process through an action plan. A simple task analysis sheet from Marakissa in the Gambia in Table 21.2 shows a method used in a small successful latrine-building programme.

4. Empower the CAG to maintain any new community facility. This is a key, permanent function of the CAG.

It has been estimated that in many poorer communities 35–50 per cent of water and sanitation systems break down and become useless after five years. Villages are littered with the wreckage of disused water tanks, broken pumps, and abandoned equipment, which now lie unrepaired and unusable while community members return to their traditional practices. Sometimes this is because the community never wanted a new system in the first place. Often it is also because no one has been given either the training or responsibility for keeping equipment in working order. A combined approach known as PHAST (*P*articipatory *H*ygiene *A*nd *S*anitation *T*ransformation) is proving successful in both rural and urban communities to help address this problem.[24]

Although the upkeep of equipment should ideally become the community's responsibility, this very much depends on the equipment, and our programme context. Even in countries with a large percentage of rural

Table 21.2 **Task analysis sheet from Marakissa in the Gambia showing a method used in a small successful latrine-building programme**

Things to be done	When	By whom
• Meet with village leader re community Health Nurse working in village.	August	M.P.
• Meet with village leader re CHN to do survey of every compound.	Sept/Oct	M.P. & F.C.
• Training for CHN to do survey work – population breakdown, latrines, health education (worm flip chart).		M.P. & F.C.
• Survey of village.	Sept/Oct	CHN
• Meet village leader and heads of compounds re incentives for latrines & de-worming all compounds with latrines.	Nov	F.C
• Analyse results of survey – how many interested in having new latrines?		
• Arrange for Health Dept. to make cement slabs for latrines. Give nos.	Dec	M.P.
• Organise transport of slabs from Banjul to Marakissa.	End Jan	M.P.
• Arrange for Mr Jobe, Health Inspector, to visit Marakissa.	Early Feb	M.P.
• Meet heads of compounds again to discuss details.		M.P.
• Mr Jobe to inspect siting of latrines with reference to well sites.		Mr Jobe
• Arrange for Govt. Info. Office to show film 'How to Dig your Latrine' at the village Independence Celebrations.	Early Feb	M.P.
• Filp chart worm/latrine talk – Primary School, classes 4, 5 & 6.		Fatou
• Showing of film.	Mid Feb	Fatou Film unit
• Latrine construction – holes to be checked before slabs issued.	Feb-May	I.S.& clinic
• Issuing of slabs.		compound man
• Deadline to finish.	May	
• All compounds to be visited.	June	F.C. M.P.
• Inform Mr Jobe of total no. new latrines.		I.S. Fatou
• Contact Mr Fal (Health Dept.) re no. of slabs required after rice harvest for others wanting new latrines.	July	M.P.
• Photograph new latrines with owners.	June-Aug	M.P. F.C
• De-worm compounds with new latrines.		& Fatou

M.P. – Mariyn Pidcock; F.C. – Fansainey Colley, I.S. – Ibrinia Sabally

populations, we have fast-growing peri-urban settings in which local utilities and DWOs play an important (and salaried) role in operating and maintaining equipment. Thus, at community level we need to establish strong connections with local utilities and DWOs for guidance, operational help, and effective lines of advocacy. This is crucial because, especially in urban settings, communities increasingly pay for services through taxation and user/connection fees.

In practice, we need to:

1. Encourage the CAG to take responsibility for upkeep of simple equipment.

The CAG takes charge and in turn can select, arrange training for, supervise and pay an individual to carry out regular maintenance and cleaning.

2. Identify suppliers (ideally more than one) of spare parts and other materials for upkeep.

3. Establish the key connections with government sources, utilities, water boards, etc., mentioned, and ensure that authorities carry out their responsibilities, which may require advocacy.

4. Ensure that training is given by appropriate government or other water and sanitation advisors to those

in the community who are involved in this aspect of community development when interest is high. The CAG should co-ordinate this.

Help the community take action on other environmental hazards including air pollution

There are a variety of other environmental hazards, some of which are shown in Table 21.3. Of these, the most important is probably air pollution, which seriously affects people's health, especially that of children. Nine out of ten people live in areas where pollution exceeds limits set by the WHO,[25] and includes pollution from a variety of sources, including factories, coal-fired power plants, and motor vehicles. Additionally, the impact of dust and sand storms is often underestimated. In some areas traditional burning of crops creating smoke adds to the problem as does excessive use of fireworks during festivals eg Divali in Delhi. However, two of the most important sources, which we can help to reduce at community level are household smoke and cigarette smoking.

Household smoke: the polluting factor is indoor cooking, especially when there is also poor ventilation, e.g. in urban slums or cold weather. Some fuels are especially polluting, e.g. wood, dung, coal, or crop waste. Charcoal is less polluting, but should not be obtained

Table 21.3 **Ideas to tackle a variety of dangers and nuisances in an urban environment.**

Ways of minimising risk from environment hazards	
Solid waste	• Educate community on ways to dispose of household waste and show them what should not be done • Organise a campaign to increase proper disposal of household waste • Install garbage bins that prevent entry by animals • Learn rights and laws about municipal cleaners, garbage bins, and garbage • Press municipality to collect garbage regularly from community collection sites • Hire and supervise street cleaners, ideally from the community, to keep streets and footpaths clean • Consider organising the collection of solid waste into three types: items for recycling, waste that generates fertiliser (composting), and unusable waste • Organise a campaign to remove mosquito breeding sites in the community • Investigate possibility of whether there is chemical pollution from near by industries
Flooding hazards	• Ensure that authorities inform slum when upriver dams are released • Weigh advantage and disadvantage of relocation
Electrical hazards	• Press for legal electrical connections for community households • Monitor existing wiring
Fire hazards	• Press for legal hook-ups to natural gas lines for the community • Check illegal hook ups to gas line for leaks • Monitor homes for flammable chemicals
Vehicular accidents	• Avoid unnecessary risks when travelling on roads • Avoid travel during rush hour • Avoid begging/selling at traffic lights • Travel on less busy streets (unless a security risk)
Workplace hazards	• Avoid drinking alcohol before operating machinery or travelling • Obey safety rules when operating dangerous machinery • Advocate for safe working conditions in factories
Air pollution	• If possible, cook with clean fuel (natural gas or electricity) • If not possible, install smokeless cooking stove/chimney or cook outdoors • If not possible, provide ventilation if cooking indoors • Stop smoking tobacco inside the house and preferably stop completely • Avoid travel during rush hour • Take less travelled streets
Noise pollution	• Encourage setting radios, tape players at low volume • Advocate for ear protectors when working with loud equipment

by cutting down or raiding indigenous forests. Indoor stoves are used by over three-quarters of the rural population in many African and Asian countries.

The WHO estimates (2016) that 4.3 million people a year die prematurely from illness attributable to the household air pollution caused by the inefficient use of solid fuels for cooking. Among these deaths:

- 12 per cent are due to pneumonia;
- 34 per cent from stroke;
- 26 per cent from ischaemic heart disease;
- 22 per cent from chronic obstructive pulmonary disease (COPD); and
- 6 per cent from lung cancer.[26]

At community level, we need to raise awareness of the dangers of cooking on inside hearths and stoves. Most people will be aware of smoke nuisance, but may be unwilling to change age-old practices. We can encourage the use of modified, fuel-efficient stoves with flues or smoke hoods, or less-polluting fuels. We should also consider cooking methods using renewable energy, e.g. solar ovens. Bringing electricity to a community (whether solar, hydro-electric, or other sources) has multiple and obvious benefits including cooking, heating, and lighting.

Cigarette smoking: passive inhaling of other people's smoke, especially family members, is known to have a serious effect on children. About one per cent of deaths worldwide is caused primarily by passive smoking, and over one-quarter of these deaths occur in children.[27]

This is a call for us at community level to prioritize tobacco control programmes, and also to get involved in advocacy against tobacco use where we can (see Chapter 22 for more details). Ideally, this should be a community-wide initiative so that smoking becomes frowned upon and is no longer seen as trendy or 'cool'.

Smoke, from whatever source, makes lung, heart and eye diseases worse. Indoor air pollution increases the danger of TB. But the most important effect is the increased risk of pneumonia in children under five. Exposure to household air pollution is thought to be a factor in about a third of cases. A Guatemalan study showed that building outside chimneys can reduce severe pneumonia in children by a third.[28,29]

Table 21.3 gives various ideas on how we can tackle a variety of dangers and nuisances in an urban environment.

Evaluate the programme

This chapter suggests many actions and improvements that can be applied to environmental health programmes. However, the simplest way to evaluate a programme is to measure the change or extent of any impact from before an intervention was made compared to afterwards. For example, we could check if:

- quality of life has improved, e.g. percentage change of families with clean water source 15 minutes' walk or less from the house;
- use of latrines by family members, specifically women, children, and teenage girls has risen;
- health has improved, especially a reduction in the frequency of diarrhoeal episodes among children and/or improvements in the average weight of children under five. Of course there can be various reasons for these improvements but whatever the cause it is worth noting them.

We should also estimate the community's satisfaction with any major change that has been made. This can be done by questioning and ranking satisfaction from 1 to 5. Evaluations can be carried out by the community, through inspection, questions, and surveys. Often, however, the answers will be obvious and visible and best told by stories or shown by photographs.

Further reading and resources

Adams J, Bartram J, Chartier Y, Sims J. *Water, sanitation and hygiene standards for schools in low cost settings*. Geneva: World Health Organization; 2009. Available from: http://www.who.int/water_sanitation_health/publications/wash_standards_school.pdf

Booth B, Martin K, Lankester T. *Urban health and development: A practical manual for use in developing countries*. Oxford: Macmillan; 2001.

Carter I. *Encouraging good hygiene and sanitation*. Teddington: Tearfund; 2005.

Conant J, Faden, P. *A community guide to environmental health*. Berkeley, CA: Hesperian Health Guides; 2008.

Crofton J, Simpson D. *Tobacco: A global threat*. Oxford: Macmillan; 2002.

Davis J, Garvey G, Wood M. *Developing and managing community water supplies*. London: Oxfam; 1993.

Franceys R, Pickford J, Reed R. *A guide to the development of on-site sanitation*. Geneva: World Health Organization; 1992. See Appendix E.

Global Handwashing Partnership. Available from: http://www.globalhandwashing.org.

Greaves F, Webster L. Sanitation and the Millenium Development Goals. Footsteps. 2007; 73: 1–2. Available from: http://www.tearfund.org/tilz.

GWSI—Global Water and Sanitation Initiative. Available from: http://www.ifrc.org/en/what-we-do/health/water-sanitation-and-hygiene-promotion/global-water-and-sanitation-initiative/

Howard G, Bogh C, Goldstein G, Morgan J, Prüss M, Shaw R, et al. *Healthy villages: A guide for communities and community health*. Geneva: World Health Organization; 2002. Available from: http://apps.who.int/iris/bitstream/10665/42456/1/9241545534.pdf

Pasteur K. *Keeping track: CLTS, monitoring, certification and verification.* Brighton: Community Led Total Sanitation Knowledge Hub; 2017. Available from: http://www.communityledtotalsanitation.org/resource/keeping-track-clts-monitoring-certification-and-verification

Sanitation Connection. Available from: http://www.fastonline.org/CD3WD_40/ASDB_SMARTSAN/Sanitation-Connection.htm

Savage G, Velleman Y, Wicken J. *WASH: The silent weapon against neglected tropical diseases.* Available from: http://www.ntd-ngonetwork.org/sites/default/files/uploaded/WASH%20the%20silent%20weapon%20against%20NTDs%20%282%29.pdf

Simpson-Hebert M, Sawyer R, Clarke L. *The PHAST Initiative: Participatory hygiene and sanitation transformation.* Geneva: World Health Organization; 1997. Available from: http://www.who.int/water_sanitation_health/hygiene/envsan/EOS96-11a.pdf

SODIS: Safe drinking water for all. Available from: http://www.sodis.ch/index_EN

The Lancet Commission on pollution and health. Vol. 391, February 3, 2018, Pages 462–512

The Sphere Handbook. 2018. Sphere – Sphere Standards. Available from: https://www.spherestandards.org/handbook-2018/

Waterlines. Quarterly online journal. Available from: http://www.developmentbookshelf.com/loi/wl

Wisner B, Adams J. *Environmental health in emergencies and disasters: A practical guide.* Geneva: World Health Organization; 2002.

Wood S, Sawyer R, Simpson-Herbert M. *PHAST Step-by-step guide: A participatory approach for the control of diarrhoeal diseases.* Geneva: World Health Organization; 1998. Available from: http://www.who.int/water_sanitation_health/publications/phastep/en/

References

1. World Health Organization. *Sanitation factsheet.* 2018. Available from: https://www.who.int/news-room/fact-sheets/detail/sanitation

2. World Health Organization. *Drinking water factsheet.* 2018. Available from: https://www.who.int/news-room/fact-sheets/detail/drinking-water

3. UNICEF. *Water, sanitation and hygiene.* Available from: https://www.unicef.org/wash/

4. Curtis V, Cairncross S. Effect of washing hands with soap on diarrhoea risk in the community: A systematic review. *The Lancet Infectious Diseases.* 2003; 3 (5): 275–81.

5. Luby SP, Halder AK, Huda T, Unicomb L, Johnston RB. The effect of handwashing at recommended times with water alone and with soap on child diarrhea in rural Bangladesh: An observational study. *PloS Medicine.* 2011; 8 (6): e1001052.

6. Tearfund. Natural Resources. *Footsteps.* 2010; 82. Available from: http://www.tearfund.org/~/media/files/tilz/publications/footsteps/footsteps_81-90/82/fs82.pdf

7. Argos M, Kalra T, Rathaus PJ, Chen Y, Pierce B, Parvez F, et al. Arsenic exposure from drinking water, and all-cause and chronic-disease mortalities in Bangladesh: A prospective cohort study. *The Lancet.* 2010; 376 (9737): 252–8.

8. Chen Y, Graziano JH, Parvez F, Liu M, Slavkovich V, Kalra T, et al. Arsenic exposure from drinking water and mortality from cardiovascular disease in Bangladesh: prospective cohort study. *British Medical Journal.* 2011; 342: d2431.

9. World Health Organization. *Arsenic Factsheet.* 2016. Available from: http://www.who.int/mediacentre/factsheets/fs372/en/

10. World Health Organization. *Safe household water storage.* 2017. Available from: http://www.who.int/household_water/research/safe_storage/en/.

11. SODIS: Safe drinking water for all. Available from: http://www.sodis.ch/index_EN

12. CRHP. 2014. Available from: http://www.jamkhed.org

13. Coombes R. Toiling for toilets. *British Medical Journal.* 2010; 341: c5027.

14. Water Aid and Tearfund. *The Human Waste,* 2002.

15. Montgomery M, Desai M, Elimelech M. Assessment of latrine use and quality and association with risk of trachoma in rural Tanzania. *Transactions of the Royal Society of Tropical Medicine and Hygiene.* 2010; 104 (4): 283–9.

16. Emerson P, Cairncross S, Bailey RL, Mabey DCW. Review of the evidence base for the 'F' and 'E' components of the SAFE strategy for trachoma control. *Tropical Medicine and International Health.* 2000; 5 (8): 515–27.

17. Sanitation connection: An environmental sanitation network. Available from: http://www.fastonline.org/CD3WD_40/ASDB_SMARTSAN/Sanitation-Connection.htm

18. Community-led total sanitation. 2011. Available from: www.communityledtotalsanitation.org

19. World Health Organization. *Simple Pit Latrines.* Available from: http://www.who.int/water_sanitation_health/hygiene/emergencies/fs3_4.pdf

20. SanPlat Latrines. *What is SanPlat?* Available from: http://www.sanplat.com

21. Population-Environment Research Network. Available from: www.populationenvironmentresearch.org

22. Meddings DR, Ronald LA, Marion S, Pinera JF, Oppliger A. Cost effectiveness of a latrine revision programme in Kabul, Afghanistan. *Bulletin of the World Health Organization.* 2004; 82 (4): 281–9.

23. World Health Organization. *WHO Sanitation safety manual.* 2015. Available from: http://www.who.int/water_sanitation_health/publications/ssp-manual/en/

24. World Health Organization. *The PHAST Initiative.* 1997. Available from: http://www.who.int/water_sanitation_health/hygiene/envsan/EOS96-11a.pdf

25. World Health Organization. *Ambient (outdoor) air quality and health factsheet.* 2016. Available from: http://www.who.int/mediacentre/factsheets/fs313/en/

26. World Health Organization. *Household air pollution and health factsheet.* 2016. Available from: http://www.who.int/mediacentre/factsheets/fs292/en/

27. Öberg M, Jaakkola MS, Woodward A, Peruga A, Prüss-Ustün A. Worldwide burden of disease from exposure to second-hand smoke: A retrospective analysis of data from 192 countries. *The Lancet.* 2011; 377 (9760): 139–46.

28. Smith KR, McCracken JP, Weber MW, Hubbard A, Jenny A, Thompson LM, et al. Effect of reduction in household air pollution on childhood pneumonia in Guatemala (RESPIRE): A randomized controlled trial. *The Lancet.* 2011; 378 (9804): 1717–26.

29. Miller R, Agerstrand C. Targeting of household air pollution: Interpretation of RESPIRE. *The Lancet.* 2011; 378 (9804): 1682–4.

CHAPTER 22

Non-communicable and chronic diseases

Nathan Grills

What we need to know

Although non-communicable diseases (NCDs) are now the commonest cause of death worldwide, they have still not been given enough priority. This is especially true at community level, which is where cases need to be prevented, as well as diagnosed and treated. The actions we can take at the community level have not been researched or put into practice to the same extent as those for infectious illness and maternal and child health. This chapter provides the background and importance of NCDs, as well as what can be done relatively easily at the community level to prevent them.

- NCDs kill 40 million people each year, equivalent to seventy per cent of all deaths globally.
- More than three-quarters of NCD deaths—30 million— occur in low- and middle-income countries (LMICs).
- Seventeen million NCD deaths occur before the age of 70; eighty-seven per cent of these 'premature' deaths occurred in LMICs.
- Cardiovascular diseases (CVDs) account for most NCD deaths, or 17.7 million people annually, followed by cancers (8.8 million), respiratory diseases aka Chronic

Obstructive Pulmonary Disease (COPD) (3.9 million), and diabetes (1.6 million).

- These four groups of diseases account for 81 per cent of all NCD deaths.
- Tobacco use, physical inactivity, the harmful use of alcohol, and unhealthy diets all increase the risk of dying from an NCD.[1]

Defining NCDs

NCDs are non-infectious diseases which generally affect adults and continue through old age, leading to serious complications and early death, particularly when left untreated. This is why they are also known as chronic diseases. Many factors contribute to the global pandemic of NCDs (see Figure 22.1), including sedentary lifestyles, poor dietary habits, a huge increase in urban populations, and, above all, more people living longer. NCDs are commonly but less accurately known as chronic diseases. The presence of two or more chronic medical conditions is known as multimorbidity.[2]

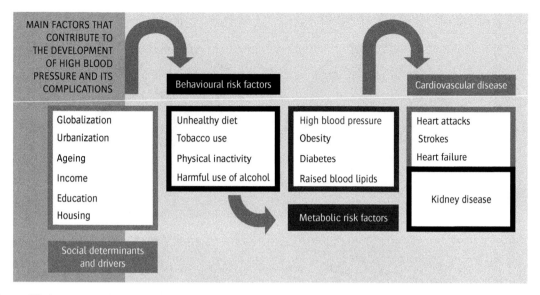

Figure 22.1 Factors contributing to high blood pressure and its complications.

Why our community health programme should respond

NCDs need to be prevented, diagnosed and treated early at the community level.[3] They cause more avoidable deaths than any other group of illnesses, and have replaced infectious diseases as the leading cause of death and disability (see Figure 22.2). Although infectious disease (ID) will continue to be important in community-based healthcare, NCDs overlap with ID in areas such as diabetes–TB, tobacco use–TB and HIV–CVD.

It is a myth that NCDs affect only the rich and affluent. NCDs affect LMICs and high-income countries (HICs) alike. The poorest people in LMICs and HICs are most affected by NCDs.[4]

The UN high-level meeting on NCDs acknowledged 'the vicious cycle whereby non-communicable diseases and their risk factors worsen poverty, while poverty contributes to rising rates of non-communicable diseases, posing a threat to public health and economic and social development'.[5] The World Health Assembly has set a target of reducing premature mortality from NCDs by 25 per cent by 2025.[6] Achieving this requires every level of the health system to respond. NCDs need to be prevented, diagnosed, and treated early. Studies show that community and primary healthcare play an important role.[7]

Where we should focus our attention

We might be inclined to believe that our community programme will be unable to deal with these complicated diseases requiring cardiac bypass, oxygen therapy, sophisticated chemotherapy, and insulin injections. Indeed, community health cannot treat all NCDs, but it can help to prevent the occurrence of:

- eighty per cent of premature heart disease;
- eighty per cent of strokes;
- eighty per cent of type 2 diabetes;
- forty per cent of cancer.[8]

This is because many of these NCDs share common behavioural risk factors (Table 22.1), and reducing these risk factors in the community makes a huge difference. This is a traditional community health role and can be done with limited resources.

Key health messages

Our community health programme is ideally placed to educate communities about NCDs and these four key risk factors. 'PATH' is a useful acronym:

- Physical activity.
- Alcohol moderation.

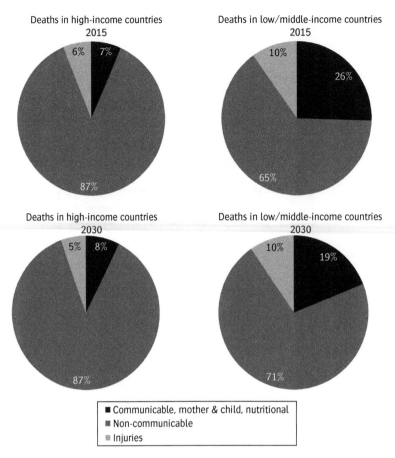

Figure 22.2 Deaths in HICs and LMICs.

Source: data from Murray, CJ. et al. Mortality by cause for eight regions of the world: Global Burden of Disease Study. *The Lancet.* 2017. 349(9061), 1269-76. Copyright © 1997 Elsevier. This image is distributed under the terms of the Creative Commons Attribution Non-Commercial 4.0 International licence (CC-BY-NC), a copy of which is available at http://creativecommons.org/licenses/by-nc/4.0/.

- Tobacco cessation.
- Healthy eating.

Physical activity

The importance of physical activity for health is seriously neglected worldwide, especially in LMICs.[9] Physical inactivity contributes to the risk of colon cancer, breast cancer, type 2 diabetes and heart disease. It is thought to account for six to ten per cent of deaths from major NCDs worldwide.[10]

To promote physical activity, the WHO recommends being physically active every day.[11] The WHO guidelines recommend (Figure 22.3):

Table 22.1 Modifiable risk factor for the four major NCDs.[8]

		Common Risk Factors for NCDs			
		Tobacco use	Unhealthy diets	Physical inactivity	Harmful use of alcohol
NCDs	Heart disease and stroke	X	X	X	X
	Diabetes	X	X	X	X
	Cancer	X	X	X	X
	Chronic lung disease	X			

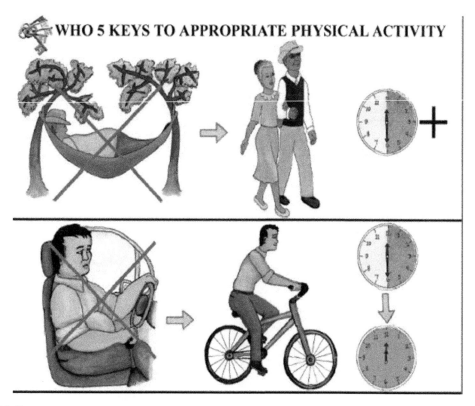

Figure 22.3 Example of education about physical activity.

Reproduced courtesy of Arnold Gorske. This image is distributed under the terms of the Creative Commons Attribution Non-Commercial 4.0 International licence (CC-BY-NC), a copy of which is available at http://creativecommons.org/licenses/by-nc/4.0/.

1. 150 minutes of moderate-intensity activity per week (e.g. 30 minutes on five days/week), or
2. 75 minutes vigorous activity per week, or
3. An equivalent combination of the above.
4. School-aged children should have at least 60 minutes of moderate-to-vigorous physical activity each day.

Evidence on what works can be found in the 2009 report published by the WHO, 'Interventions on diet and physical activity'.[12]

Alcohol

Alcohol is the risk factor ranked third as a cause of morbidity.[13] Figure 22.4 provides further information. Alcohol use contributes to:

- Social and psychological problems;
- Liver cirrhosis and cancer;
- Pancreatic inflammation;
- Brain and heart damage (e.g. stroke, high blood pressure (BP));
- Risky behaviours and suicide;
- Motor vehicle crashes and injuries;

- Breast cancer;
- Birth defects.

Liver disease is responsible for seventy per cent of alcohol-related deaths.[13]

The guidelines established by the WHO indicate that a standard drink is generally between 8 and 12 grams of alcohol. The recommended safe alcohol intake is defined as:

- Less than or equal to two standard drinks per day for women.
- Less than or equal to three standard drinks per day for men.
- Not more than four standard drinks on one occasion.
- There is no safe drinking level for driving.
- Pregnant women should not drink alcohol.[14]

Tobacco

There is *no* safe level of tobacco use. Tobacco is the single greatest cause of avoidable illness and death.[15] There is strong evidence that smoking causes disease in nearly all organs of the body, poor health, and harm to unborn babies.[16]

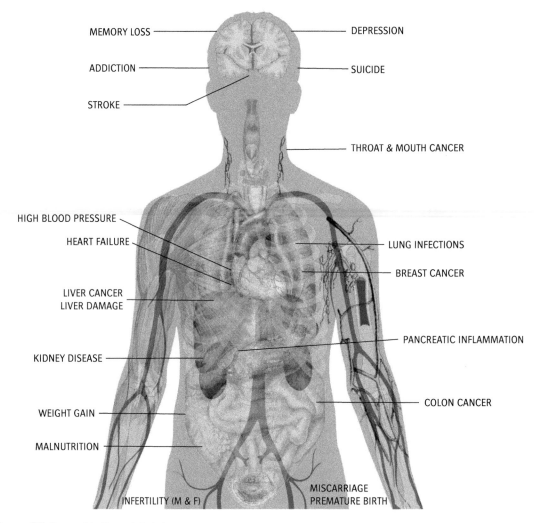

Figure 22.4 Harmful effects of alcohol.

Reproduced courtesy of Nathan Grills. This image is not covered by the Creative Common licence terms of this publication. For permission to reuse please contact the rights holder.

- More than seven million people die from the effects of tobacco each year and more than eighty per cent of smokers live in LMICs.[17]
- Around half of the world's billion smokers can be expected to die prematurely from smoking unless they quit.[18]
- Despite their diversity, *all* tobacco products are dangerous.
- Lung cancer is the second leading cause of death from tobacco and seventy-one per cent of lung cancers are due to smoking.[19]
- Tobacco is a leading preventable cause of heart disease and stroke.
- Tobacco has over 250 harmful chemicals in each cigarette and harms nearly every organ of the body.[20]

Why do people still smoke given how toxic tobacco smoke is? It might be that people lack awareness. More likely it is because tobacco in any form is highly addictive, and those who use it need help to stop. Figure 22.5 can be used in a participatory exercise that highlights the harmful effects of tobacco. Begin with an outline drawing of a body and ask participants to draw a line to any part of the body that is affected by tobacco, and discuss how it is affected.

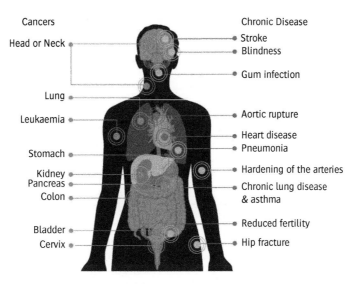

Cancers
Head or Neck

Lung
Leukaemia

Stomach
Kidney
Pancreas
Colon

Bladder
Cervix

Chronic Disease
Stroke
Blindness

Gum infection

Aortic rupture

Heart disease
Pneumonia

Hardening of the arteries

Chronic lung disease
& asthma

Reduced fertility

Hip fracture

Figure 22.5 The damage that smoking does to the body.

Healthy diet

Poor diet leads to intermediate risk factors such as high BP, obesity and diabetes (see Figure 22.1). NCDs such as stroke, heart attack, diabetes, and some cancers can all be traced back to poor diet. The key messages about diet are (see also Figure 22.6):

- *Eat five servings of fruit and vegetables (about 400 grams) per day.* This will provide the required fibre, vitamins, and anti-oxidant nutrients to help reduce the risk of cancer. In many communities it is impossible to either grow or buy this number of different fruit and vegetables for our meals. However, the greater the number and the wider the range, the better.[21]

- *Eat wholegrain cereals (whole-wheat, brown rice), legumes and nuts.* These provide (a) soluble fibre, which lowers cholesterol and reduces heart attack and stroke risk, and (b) insoluble fibre, to keep the gut healthy and reduce the risk of bowel cancer.[22]

- *Limit fats and oils.* Fatty foods are concentrated sources of energy and make it more difficult to maintain a healthy weight. Saturated fats also increase 'bad' cholesterol in the blood and increase the risk of heart disease. Saturated fats are found in dairy foods (butter, cheese, cream and whole milk), fatty meat, lard, hard margarine, coconut oil, and red palm oil. For cooking, choose vegetable oils, especially sunflower, olive, rapeseed, or safflower.

- *Limit sugar intake, especially sodas, colas and other sweet drinks.* Sugary foods and sodas are concentrated sources of energy and contribute to becoming overweight. Sodas contain large amounts of sugar.

- *Reduce salt intake.* High salt intake increases the risk of high BP, which contributes to heart disease and stroke. Hidden salt is in processed food such as cheese, meat, packet and canned soups, stock cubes, snacks, and ready-to-eat meals. Avoid adding salt at the table, and aim to gradually decrease the amount of salt added to cooking.

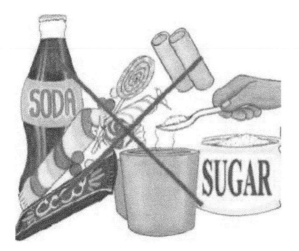

Figure 22.6 Foods to avoid.

What we need to prepare

Scope the burden of disease and context

We should start by asking what the main burden of disease is in our country, our district, and our community. For the big picture, we can refer to the Global Health Estimates published by the WHO.[4] The Ministry of Health and the District Medical Officer may have useful information, as may other local Civil Society Organisations (CSOs), government services, hospitals, clinics, and local practitioners. Our PA or community survey (see Chapter 6 and Figure 22.7) may have already given us the main information.

Next, we should consider what contributing factors could be present in our community. For example, obesity is a status symbol in many African countries.

Tap into existing resources

There are many resources that exist locally, and it is important to seek these first before going elsewhere. Local resources may include:

1. *The community*: it will provide resources and viewpoints that represent the local understanding of issues and problems (see Chapter 6).
2. *Schools*: We can discover what health teaching already occurs, and where in the curriculum there is overlap with preventing NCDs (e.g. cooking classes, life skills).
3. *Secondary and tertiary centres*: Document and develop referral pathways.
4. *Churches and religious institutions*: Find out if they are open to helping. The WHO outlines the effectiveness of NCD lifestyle interventions when conducted in religious settings.[12]

In addition to the excellent resources listed at the end of this chapter, other CSOs may well share materials available for preventing and responding to NCDs in the community.

Plan the programme

- Forward planning is important to ensure that what we do is based on evidence and will actually work, instead of approaching the situation from an opportunistic point of view, or just doing what is easiest.
- In addition to a three-to-five-year logframe and yearly work plan, additional checks will help plan a successful programme.

- Involving the community, including local and religious leaders and congregational members, is important as they can, and should, determine their priorities in dealing with NCDs.
- Discuss plans with the local government and work with them if possible.
- Invite other programmes working to address NCDs to review the plan, which can generate useful feedback, and strengthen links.

  If we ask how can we design our programme so that it integrates with and benefits your work, the opportunities for mutual sharing of knowledge (and possibly resources) increase. Discussing plans with the local government may encourage opportunities to work with them as well.
- Establish a workable and pragmatic timeframe.

  NCD programmes by definition are long term and need to be increasingly understood, managed, and owned by the community, in association with government services. There is no place for CSOs that appear, run a programme for one or two years, then depart.

Prepare health promotion materials

We can get materials from various outside sources or, better still, our local community or local school can develop health promotion materials. This approach will ensure:

1. The materials convey the message in a right way;
2. That graphic, direct messages are not unnecessarily offensive;
3. Learning happens as the materials are developed;
4. Local leaders are engaged in the process.

Integrate with existing community programmes

Rather than starting a new programme, we could add NCDs to our existing community health programme, or work alongside another existing programme with capacity and willingness to tackle NCDs. We should involve *existing* local workers such as community health workers (CHWs) or equivalent. According to Beaglehole and colleagues, primary healthcare is ideally placed to find cases, start and monitor treatment, promote health, and teach prevention, and non-physician clinicians (NPCs) will have an increasing role, which will include CHWs.[23] Therefore, we need to train CHWs and NPCs to:

- Identify those at high risk of NCDs (e.g. using the screening tool in the next section);
- Refer high-risk individuals for medical assessment and treatment;
- Follow up patients regularly, to check treatment adherence;
- Look for signs that the NCDs might be progressing (e.g. diabetic wounds, ulcers) and refer; and,
- Hold training sessions (especially for those at high risk) on avoiding NCD risk factors.[24]

A community health programme in India began to focus on tobacco as the leading risk factor for NCDs in the community. They designated CHWs as tobacco control advocates (TCAs). This is an additional role for CHWs, who are ideally placed to convey tobacco control messages (see Figure 22.8).

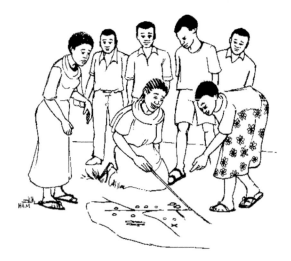

Figure 22.7 Understanding a participatory appraisal (PA).

Reproduced courtesy of Centers for Disease Control and Prevention. Available at http://www.cdc.gov/vitalsigns/tobaccouse/smoking/infographic.html. This image is distributed under the terms of the Creative Commons Attribution Non-Commercial 4.0 International licence (CC-BY-NC), a copy of which is available at http://creativecommons.org/licenses/by-nc/4.0/.

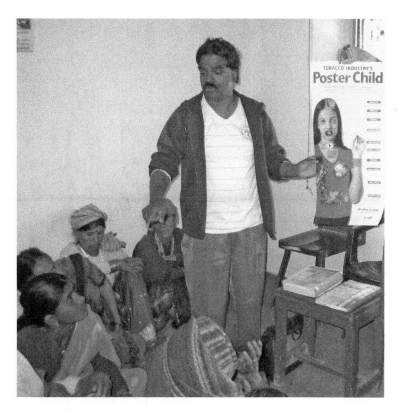

Figure 22.8 A community health worker teaching about risk factors.

Reproduced courtesy of Nathan Grills. This image is distributed under the terms of the Creative Commons Attribution Non-Commercial 4.0 International licence (CC-BY-NC), a copy of which is available at http://creativecommons.org/licenses/by-nc/4.0/.

What we need to do

This section details five components of an effective NCD response at the community level. These may run together, in sequence, or in whichever way suits the community and the programme's resources. Additionally, the actions we take should also address the social determinants (upstream causes) that increase the risk of NCDs (see Figure 22.1).

Screening

Screening is simply checking for early stages of disease or unhealthy habits. This means we can intervene at an early stage before much damage is done by an NCD. Screening can either be an opportunistic screening, where it is integrated with routine check-ups and other healthcare actions or via a screening programme (mass or selective). A screening programme provides an opportunity to screen an entire village or subgroup (age, school), which can be a good way to start an NCD programme. The programme needs to be carefully planned or it can harm the project and the people being screened (see Figure 22.9). When planning a screening programme, we must be sure to:

1. Clearly identify the problem.
2. Ensure that there is evidence for the effectiveness of the screening tool.
3. Create the awareness in the community regarding the importance of screening.
4. Get permission and support from the people and the village leaders.
5. Prepare equipment: BP cuff, height and weight measures, glucometer to measure blood glucose, etc.
6. Ensure that follow-up is available, affordable, and effective.

Adult Screening Sheet

Date:_____

Name _____   Age:_____   Gender: M /F

Questions

		Yes ☑	No ☑
1	Do you smoke?		
2	Does anyone from your house smoke?		
3	Does anyone from your family (father/mother/sister/brother) have diabetes?		
4	Do you have any of the following: (increased thirst, increased urination, unexplained weight loss, sores that don't heal)		
5	Do you get less than 30min exercise a day?		
6	Do you regularly drink more than 1 alcoholic drink per day		

Examination

A. **HEIGHT & WEIGHT FOR BODY MASS INDEX**

Weight (Kg):_____ Height (m)_____

BMI $\dfrac{\text{Weight (kg)}}{\text{Height}^2\ (\text{m}^2)}$:

Underweight = BMI less than 8.5
Normal weight = BMI 18.5 – 24.9
Overweight = BMI 25-29.9
Obesity = BMI 30 or greater

B. **BLOOD PRESSURE & PULSE**

	Record Value	Normal ·	Pre hypertension	Hypertension
Systolic	_____mm/hg	Less than 120	120-139	140 or greater
Diastolic	_____mm/hg	Less than 80	80-89	90 or greater
Pulse	_____beats/minute	60-100	Less than 60 may be normal for athletes	

C. **BLOOD GLUCOSE (RANDOM)**

	Record Value	Normal	Pre diabetes	Diabetes
Random blood sugar	_____mmol/ L	Less than 7.1	7.1 - 11.0	11.0 or greater

Refer   Yes / No (refer if high BMI, hypertension, symptoms of diabetes)
_____
_____
_____

Figure 22.9 A screening record that includes a health education message.

The following subsections provide guidance on aspects of screening in the community setting.

Short survey

We can make our own screening survey but we should use standard questions to ask about alcohol and tobacco use, salt/sugar/fat intake, physical activity level, and symptoms of diabetes (e.g. weight loss, sores, urination, thirst, family history). The exact questions differ between areas and communities. For example, in the mountains of North India we removed physical activity, as people averaged two to three hours of physical activity a day. This question was replaced with one about mouth ulcers, given there is high incidence of mouth cancer due to tobacco chewing.

BMI measurement

Where possible, height and weight measurement should be without shoes, coats, and heavy outer clothing. When recording height measurements, a good vocal cue might be, 'Look straight ahead, keep your heels flat on the floor, and stand with your back against the board, stand as straight as you can, like a soldier'.[25] Box 22.1 shows the formula for determining adult BMI, as well as adult BMI ranges. The formula is the same for children and adults but the normal ranges are different. For children, use a specific BMI-for-age chart or calculator.

Blood pressure

CHWs and others can learn how to take BP readings (see Figure 22.10). This needs to be part of a carefully drawn-up plan with detailed training.

- If >140/90 mmHg ➔ give lifestyle advice and refer for repeat measurement and possible medical treatment.

> Box 22.1 **BMI formula and adult ranges**
>
> *BMI Formula for metric*: weight (kg)/[height (m)]^2
> *BMI Formula for imperial*: Formula: weight (lb)/[height (in)]^2 x 703
>
> - below 18.5 indicates underweight.
> - 18.5–24.9 is normal.
> - 25–29.9 is overweight.
> - 30 and above is obese.

- If pulse is irregular or >100 bpm ➔ refer for ECG and review.[26]

Random blood glucose testing

A random non-fasting blood sugar level is a helpful and convenient point-of-care test to measure blood glucose levels. Kits are easily available. The WHO provides information and guidance on measuring blood glucose.[27] The following levels indicate that further testing and/or intervention may be necessary:

- Random non-fasting blood sugar level >200 mg/dL (11.1 mmol/L) suggests diabetes and needs further assessment, including a fasting blood glucose level or HbA1c.
- Fasting blood sugar level of >125 mg/dL (7 mmol/L) on more than one occasion indicates diabetes.[28]
- Fasting blood sugar level of 100–125 mg/dL (5.6–6.9 mmol/L) indicates pre-diabetes and needs follow-up testing/referral.

If any of the measurements above are abnormal, then we should refer for further assessment including a fasting blood glucose level or HbA1c. If HbA1c is available, the parameters are:

- Diabetes: >48 mmol/mol or >6.5 per cent; or
- Pre-diabetes: 39–46 mmol/mol or 5.7–6.4 per cent.

While a urine dipstick for sugar is helpful if the above tests are not available, it misses many people with diabetes.

Next steps

Brief verbal health education can be effective. Consider prescribing a lifestyle modification such as walking for 30 minutes five times a week. Distribution of handouts on how lifestyle changes (diet, exercise, stopping smoking) may help to prevent problems. Finally, follow up any people you have referred for further testing and treatment.

Promoting healthy behaviours

Health promotion is the process of enabling people to take control over their health and improve it. Our NCD programme aims to enable people to increase their physical activity, have a healthy diet (less sugar, fat, salt, and alcohol), and stop smoking.

However, promoting healthy behaviour involves looking beyond the individual. The Ottawa Charter in Health Promotion reminds us of the many complex

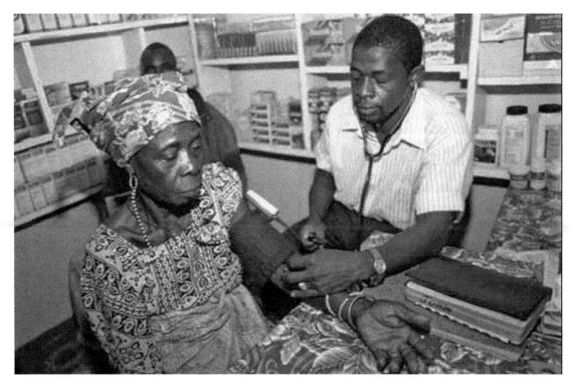

Figure 22.10 Blood pressure reading.

influences on behaviour,[29] and that health promotion activities should try to make healthy choices easier. We can use the Ottawa framework to help us address the 'upstream factors' that affect individual health behaviour (see Table 22.2).

Educating for healthy behaviour

Health education activities will be central to our NCD programme. Health education is especially effective where current knowledge levels about risks to health are low. Making people aware of a clear link between behaviour and illness can enable helpful changes (see 'Health Education Program for Developing Communities' in 'Further reading and resources' at the end of this chapter).

We can incorporate health education into existing programmes across various contexts. For programmes that are clinic-based, we can link our programme with the clinic (see Chapter 13), and provide information in the waiting room (e.g. a DVD playing) and registration (e.g. give pamphlets). We can encourage local practitioners to refer patients to us when they are ready and

willing for health education. This helps to reorientate health services towards prevention.

For community-based programmes, a useful way to promote NCD awareness and to strengthen community action is via local festivals (see Figure 22.11). The festival may also act to recruit at-risk people for targeted courses and programmes.

> **Quit-to-win community event**
> At a community festival in North India we offered US$25 to three volunteers to stop smoking and abstain from smoking for six months. That would be equal to one life saved if they continue as non-smokers. Such 'quit-to-win' programmes can be effective and those who quit can in turn become community 'quit champions' in their communities and lead others to stop smoking. Following the event, at least four other people stopped smoking.

School-based programmes are often very successful. Children learn rapidly, and we can work with teachers to incorporate NCD health education into the curriculum. Additionally, we can form health

Table 22.2 **Ottawa Charter for Health Promotion framework**

Ottawa Charter Action	Definition	Brainstorm interventions for ... (e.g. smoking)
Develop personal skills	Personal development through providing information, education for health, and enhancing life skills.	E.g. Health education about dangers.
Strengthen community action	Facilitate community involvement in setting priorities, making decisions, planning strategies, and implementing.	E.g. Public event on quitting. Get church involved.
Creating supportive environments	Creating a space where people can work, rest, and play in safety. Make healthy choices easy.	E.g. Make no-smoking zones.
Re-orientation of health care services	Facilities to focus on prevention, health promotion, and integrate with primary and community health.	E.g. Establish quit clinic at hospital.
Building healthy public policy	Advocate for legislation, regulations, rules, incentives, and disincentives.	E.g. Advocate for enforcement of local anti-smoking laws.

clubs to spread messages around NCD risk factors. We can also encourage the school to use child-to-child methodology.[30]

Finally, faith-based settings can be excellent for health promotion. Studies have shown that religious beliefs impact on health habits, especially when faith leaders are convinced of the value of healthy lifestyles, and can model them and teach about them. For example, in one west African city the head of the cathedral realized that many in the congregation were unhealthy and overweight. Arrangements were made for BP checks to be carried out after the evening worship, as an entry point into a wider NCD programme in the city.

Assisting behavioural change

Our NCD programme should include various activities to help people build personal skills for behaviour change. Below are some ideas, but the numerous resources available will also be helpful:

- *Group courses and classes*. We can run tobacco cessation courses, Alcoholics Anonymous (AA) groups, and, if we have skilled and experienced staff, group courses for other unhealthy behaviours.
- *Individual counselling*. Health workers can be taught to use the '5 A's' approach, for all risk factors: *A*sk about habit, *A*dvise on dangers, *A*ssess the level of use, *A*ssist them to change, *A*rrange additional help.

- *Share important aids and tools*. Aids and tools such as the '4 Ds' (*D*o something else, *D*rink water, *D*elay, *D*eep breathe) are available at various websites.[31]
- *Facilitate special health clubs*. Exercise clubs can encourage group exercise. It is known that people who exercise with friends are more willing to stick to an exercise programme than those who exercise alone.
- *Healthy eating programmes*. Develop tailor-made programmes for healthy eating.

Tips for success in education

- Engage at multiple points with the same message: at school, on street hoardings, at community events, at public meetings.
- Recruit champions for healthy behaviours from the community, or even nationally. Sports and film stars are especially helpful.
- Consider what engages the community. If it is cricket or football, use them as examples (Figure 22.11).
- Focus on what people care about, such as their appearance, their children, current livelihood, etc. They might not care much about a disease that might occur in ten years' time.
- Be positive. Avoid just discussing a list of harms. Instead, use positive terms such as money saving, having more energy, feeling younger.

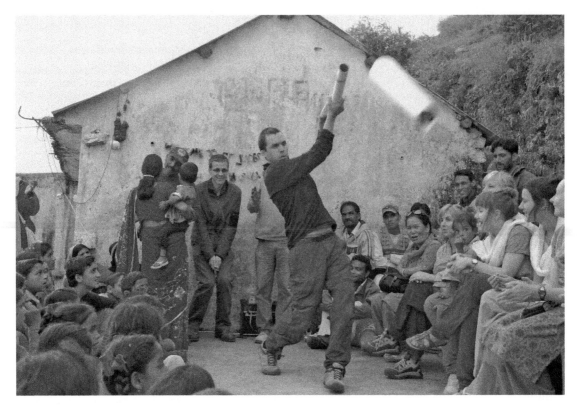

Figure 22.11 A health play undertaken at a community festival.

For more ideas on how to creatively get messages across, see 'Creative ways of communicating health messages' from Tearfund's *Footsteps*.[32]

Advocacy

Advocacy is an important aspect of the Ottawa framework and can help make healthy choices the easy choices.

Advocate for regulation

In controlling tobacco, the most effective high-level actions include raising taxes, regulating advertising, and banning smoking in public areas. Village health committees, women's groups, or others can exert pressure to help bring these about. The use of Avaaz (https://secure.avaaz.org/en/) and other online advocacy programmes is proving effective in some places. For example, one NGO programme raised awareness about laws on sales and advertising of tobacco. An influential village person noticed illegal advertising in his village and in partnership with the village committee asked the vendors to remove it.

Advocate for better services

We can advocate for improved access to NCD care, reliability of supplies, and affordability. While community-based health centres may have limited ability to provide these, members can still become effective advocates for these services to be provided.

Advocate for children

NCD damage starts at a young age. Children are particularly vulnerable to starting smoking (highly addictive) and initiating other risky behaviours. Advocacy to protect children is important, and usually has widespread community support. Measures might include:

● Limiting access, e.g. banning tobacco sales near schools and banning liquor sales to children.

● Opposing alcohol and tobacco advertising near schools.

● Ensuring junk foods are not available within or near schools.

- Advocating for safe places for play and physical activity.

Disease-specific treatments and interventions

Although specific therapy for NCDs is often expensive and the initial diagnosis and treatment needs to be done by doctors or other skilled professionals, there is a huge role for community health programmes. With training and supervision, CHWs can identify, refer, and follow up cases in the community and ensure medication is taken regularly using a DOT (Directly Observed Treatment) approach, either themselves or by training family members.

Cardiovascular disease (high BP, stroke, heart conditions)

Uncontrolled hypertension is the leading risk factor for death worldwide.[33] CHWs can monitor anyone who has a high BP reading. If they repeatedly have high readings the CHW can counsel them on behaviour change (e.g. exercise, weight reduction, salt intake, smoking and/or alcohol) and refer as the person may need to start medication.

For people on medication, CHWs can monitor their BP and remind them to take tablets as prescribed every day (since high BP is usually a lifelong condition), and use a DOT approach until habits are well established by individuals within their families.

Regular use of low-dose aspirin (75–150mg) can be given to people with certain risk factors like previous heart attacks, stroke, or high BP. When there are signs of a heart attack, 300mg of aspirin can be given.[33]

Cancer

Addressing the PATH risk factors (page 389) is important for preventing cancers. Additionally, certain immunizations can be highly effective in preventing cancer and we should promote them within our community. Hepatitis B immunization can prevent seventy per cent of liver cancer and is usually part of the childhood immunization programme (see Chapter 15). The use of HPV immunization is strongly recommended and is effective in preventing cervical cancer.

It should be noted that cancer screening programmes probably have low benefit at the community level in resource-poor areas. However, this depends on the incidence of specific cancers and any national programmes that may be in place. Mammography is thought to have value from the age of 45 and up, but only in areas where there is a high incidence of breast cancer and where screening is possible, affordable, and accurate.

Respiratory disease (asthma, chronic bronchitis, emphysema (COPD))

In all settings, we must stress that *all* tobacco use, including passive smoking, endangers health. We must also work to reduce indoor smoke pollution, especially from cooking fires.

Asthma is increasingly common and dangerous but the use of inhalers can save lives and help affected children to live normal lives. Inhalers are especially important in urban areas with high pollution levels, which can often cause or exacerbate asthma. One especially dangerous period for asthma sufferers is after celebrations when huge numbers of fireworks increase air pollution to dangerous levels, e.g. in Delhi during Diwali or New Year. It is important to recognize and refer serious infectious exacerbations of chronic lung disease.

Diabetes

Identifying diabetes cases is a basic part of any NCD programme following which certain community-based interventions can be very effective. Firstly, controlling blood sugar level and BP is essential in patients with diabetes.[34] Dietary control and, in most cases, weight loss is crucial to control blood sugar and BP. If these behaviour modifications are not enough to stabilize blood sugar levels, then medication may be needed. Tablets are usually the first type of medication to use; metformin is typically the first line drug and can be organized at the primary care level. When tablets are insufficient to control blood sugar, insulin injections may be needed and excellent resources are available for insulin use in community programmes.

Importantly, diabetes patients need regular monitoring for common problems associated with diabetes including:

Regular eye tests are needed to check the retina for damage. Eye tests can determine if the patient has any changes in vision, such as blurred eyesight or a sudden decline in vision;

Regular examination of the feet is also important, as patients with diabetes often develop foot ulcers or numb feet. We must look for any swollen areas, cuts, or sores, and treat these immediately. Patients must be encouraged to wash and dry their feet daily, as well as to wear well-fitting and comfortable shoes.

Evaluate and monitor the NCD programme

Finally, an essential part of our work is to constantly monitor our programme. We should not see it as a test to pass, but as an opportunity to learn from what has happened, and to improve what we are doing.

Because NCDs are so complex and broad, it is difficult to lay down any hard and fast indicators. Each programme will need to choose the most effective qualitative and quantitative indicators for their own context. Example objectives against which the programme could be evaluated might include:

- All adults over the age of 35 are screened for common NCD risk factors once every three years.
- Prevention messages are promoted in three different ways each year.
- A community health awareness festival is undertaken each year.
- The community is supportive, provide space for, and assist with screening camps.
- Each person with diabetes and high BP receives a monitoring visit every two months and is checked for complications.
- Fifty per cent of people with diabetes have adequate blood glucose control (determined by HbA1C <5.7), within three years, seventy-five per cent within five years.
- Fifty per cent of those with high BP have their BP controlled (<140/90) within six months, seventy-five per cent within one year.
- All those found with symptoms and/or signs of cancer are referred for assessment and treatment.
- The prevalence of tobacco use falls by ten per cent each year.

Further reading and resources

Carter I. *Healthy Eating: A PILLARS Guide*. Teddington: Tearfund; 2003. Available from: http://learn.tearfund.org/~/media/files/tilz/publications/pillars/english/pillars_healthy_eating_e.pdf

Health Education Program for Developing Communities. 2016. Available from: www.hepfdc.info

Lancet Commissions: Dementia prevention, intervention and care. *Lancet*. 2017; 390: 2673–734.

STEPS Surveillance Manual. Geneva: World Health Organization; 2017. Available from: http://www.who.int/chp/steps/manual/en/

Time to deliver: report of the WHO independent High Level Commission on NCDs. *Lancet*. 2018; 392: 245–52.

Tearfund. Non-communicable diseases. *Footsteps*. 2012; 87. Available from: http://tilz.tearfund.org/~/media/Files/TILZ/Publications/Footsteps/Footsteps_81-90/87/FS87.pdf

Websites

Alcoholics Anonymous. http://www.aa.org

Chatterjee S, Khunti K, Davies MJ. Type 2 diabetes. *The Lancet*. 2017; 389 (10085): 2239–51.

Global Burden of Disease resources. http://vizhub.healthdata.org/gbd-compare/

Global CHE network. https://www.chenetwork.org/

Hesperian Health Guides. http://www.hesperian.org/

International Diabetes Federation. http://www.idf.org

Samarasekera U, Horton R. Women's cancers: Shining a light on a neglected health inequity. *The Lancet*. 2017; 389 (10071): 771–3.

The Tobacco Atlas. http://www.tobaccoatlas.org/

References

1. World Health Organization. *Factsheet—Non-communicable diseases*. Geneva: World Health Organization; Updated 2017. Available from: http://www.who.int/mediacentre/factsheets/fs355/en/

2. World Health Organization. *Global status report on non-communicable diseases*. Geneva: World Health Organization; 2011.

3. Balbus J, Barouki R, Birnbaum LS, Etzel RA, Glubkman PD, Sir, Grandjean P, et al. Early-life prevention of non-communicable diseases. *The Lancet*. 2013; 381 (9860): 3–4.

4. World Health Organization. *Global Health Estimates, Projections of mortality and causes of death, 2015 and 2030*. Geneva: World Health Organization; 2012. Available from: http://www.who.int/healthinfo/global_burden_disease/projections/en/

5. Political declaration of the high-level meeting of the General Assembly on the prevention and control of non-communicable diseases. United Nations General Assembly, A/res/66/2, 24 January 2012.

6. World Health Organization. Sixty-fifth world health assembly. 2012; 21–26 May. Geneva, Switzerland. Available from: http://apps.who.int/gb/DGNP/pdf_files/A65_REC1-en.pdf

7. Gaziano T, Abrahams-Gessel S, Denman CA, Mendoza Montano C, Khanam M, Puoane T, et al. An assessment of community health workers' ability to screen for cardiovascular disease risk with a simple, non-invasive risk assessment instrument in Bangladesh, Guatemala, Mexico, and South Africa: An observational study. *The Lancet Global Health*. 2015; 3 (9): 556–63.

8. *Global Burden of Disease Study 2017. The Lancet*. 388 (10053). Available at: http://thelancet.com/gbd/2017

9. Das P, Horton R. Rethinking our approach to physical activity. *The Lancet*. 2012; 380 (9838): 189–90.

10. Lee I-M, Shiroma E, Lobelo F, Puska P, Blair SN, Katzmarzyk PT. Impact of physical inactivity on the world's major non-communicable diseases. *The Lancet*. 2012; 380 (9838): 219–29.

11. World Health Organization. *Global recommendations on physical activity for health*. Geneva: World Health Organization;

2010. Available from: http://apps.who.int/iris/bitstream/10665/44399/1/9789241599979_eng.pdf

12. Anderson J. *Interventions on diet and physical activity: What works: summary report*. Geneva: World Health Organization; 2009. Available from: http://www.who.int/dietphysicalactivity/summary-report-09.pdf

13. World Health Organization. *Global health risks: Mortality and burden of disease attributable to selected major risks*. Geneva: World Health Organization; 2009.

14. The World Health Organization. *Public hearing on harmful use of alcohol*. Geneva: World Health Organization; 2009.

15. The World Health Organization. *WHO report on the global tobacco epidemic*. Geneva: World Health Organization; 2008.

16. U.S. Department of Health and Human Services. *The health consequences of smoking—50 years of progress: A report of the Surgeon General*. Atlanta, GA: U.S. Department of Health and Human Services; 2014. Available from: https://www.surgeongeneral.gov/library/reports/50-years-of-progress/full-report.pdf

17. World Health Organization. *Factsheet—Tobacco*. Geneva: World Health Organization; 2017. Available from: http://www.who.int/mediacentre/factsheets/fs339/en/

18. Britton J. Death, disease and tobacco. *The Lancet*. 2017; 389 (10082): 861–2.

19. World Health Organization. *WHO global report: Mortality attributable to tobacco*. Geneva: World Health Organization; 2012.

20. US National Cancer Institute. *Harms of cigarette smoking and health benefits of quitting*. Available from: https://www.cancer.gov/about-cancer/causes-prevention/risk/tobacco/cessation-fact-sheet

21. Aune D, Giovannucci E, Boffetta P, Fadnes LT, Keum N, Norat T, et al. Fruit and vegetable intake and the risk of cardiovascular disease, total cancer and all-cause mortality: A systematic review and dose-response meta-analysis of prospective studies. *International Journal of Epidemiology*. 2017; 46 (3): 1029–56.

22. World Health Organization. *Diet, nutrition and the prevention of chronic diseases: Report of the joint WHO/FAO expert consultation*. WHO Technical Report Series, No. 916. Geneva: World Health Organization; 2003. Available from: http://www.who.int/dietphysicalactivity/publications/trs916/en/

23. Beaglehole R, Epping-Jordan J, Patel V, Chopra M, Ebrahim S, Kidd M, Haines A. Improving the prevention and management of chronic disease in low-income and middle-income countries: A priority for primary health care. *The Lancet*. 2008; 372(9642): 940–9.

24. Farzadfar F, Murray C, Gakidou E, Bossert T, Namdaritabar H, Alikhani S, et al. Effectiveness of diabetes and hypertension management by rural primary health-care workers (Behvarz workers) in Iran: A nationally representative observational study. *The Lancet*. 2011; 379 (9810): 47–54.

25. World Health Organization. *STEPS Surveillance Manual*, Part 3, Section 5: Taking Physical Measurements. Geneva: World Health Organization; 2017. Available from: http://www.who.int/chp/steps/Part3_Section5.pdf?ua=1

26. *Atrial fibrillation and stroke: unrecognised and undertreated. The Lancet*. 2016; 388 (10046): 731.

27. The World Health Organization. *STEPS Surveillance Manual*, Part 3, Section 6: Taking Biochemical Measurements. Geneva: World Health Organization; 2017. Available from: http://www.who.int/chp/steps/Part3_Section6.pdf?ua=1

28. Mayo Clinic. *Tests and diagnosis or diabetes*. 2012; Available from: http://www.mayoclinic.com/health/diabetes/DS01121/DSECTION=tests-and-diagnosis

29. World Health Organization. First international conference on health promotion, Ottawa. *The Ottawa Charter for Health Promotion*. Geneva: World Health Organization. 1986. Available from: http://www.who.int/healthpromotion/conferences/previous/ottawa/en/

30. Child-to-Child Trust and The World Health Organization. *Children for health: Children as partners in health promotion*. London: Macmillan; 2005.

31. QUIT Resource centre. Available from: www.quit.org.au/resource-centre/

32. Tearfund. Non-communicable diseases. *Footsteps*. 2012; 87. Available from: http://tilz.tearfund.org/~/media/Files/TILZ/Publications/Footsteps/Footsteps_81-90/87/FS87.pdf

33. World Health Organization. *A global brief on hypertension: Silent killer, global public health crisis*. Geneva: World Health Organization; 2013. Available from: http://apps.who.int/iris/bitstream/10665/79059/1/WHO_DCO_WHD_2013.2_eng.pdf?ua=1 PAGE 20

34. Ray K, Seshasai S, Wijesuriya S, Sivakumaran R, Nethercott S, Preiss D, et al. Effect of intensive control of glucose on cardiovascular outcomes and death in patients with diabetes mellitus: A meta-analysis of randomised controlled trials. *The Lancet*. 2009; 373 (9677): 1765–72.

CHAPTER 23

Disability and community-based rehabilitation

Nathan Grills and Jubin Varghese

What we need to know

Defining disability?

At long last, disability is being recognized as a common, important condition that can affect anyone. The Paralympic Games have helped to draw the world's attention to disability with both its challenges and its immense hopes.

The UN General Assembly adopted the United Nations Convention on the Rights of Persons with Disabilities (UNCRPD). Persons with disabilities is a general term used to refer to those 'people living with a disability' of any kind. We avoid using the term 'the disabled' or 'disabled people' as they are people first and foremost. The UNCRPD defined disability as 'the interaction between persons with impairments and attitudinal and environmental barriers that hinder their full and effective participation in society on an equal basis with others.'[1] For many people, that important definition takes a bit of understanding. We hope this chapter will help to bring some clarity.

Facts about disability in today's world:

- Ten to fifteen per cent of the world's population live with a disability.

- Persons with disabilities constitute the world's largest minority.

- Eighty per cent of persons with disabilities live in developing countries.

- Twenty per cent of the world's poorest people are disabled.

- In 62 countries, there are no rehabilitation services to help persons with disabilities.

- Between 51–53 per cent of Persons with disabilities cannot afford healthcare.

- Children with disabilities are much less likely to attend school than those without disability.

- Persons with disabilities tend to experience higher unemployment and have lower earnings than those without disabilities.[1,2,3]

The UNCRPD emphasizes the importance of 'mainstreaming disability issues as an integral part of relevant strategies of sustainable development'. This means that disability is a crucial health need that our community health programmes must incorporate.[1]

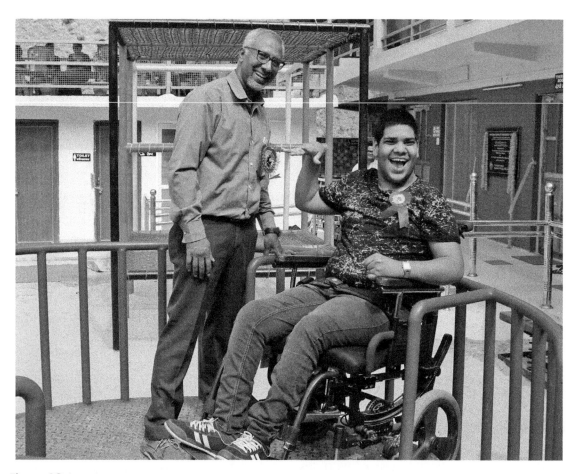

Figure 23.1 Our community health programs must include people with disability.

What is community-based rehabilitation (CBR)?

CBR is a strategy that focuses on providing equal opportunities to persons with disabilities so they can participate in community life.[4] In doing this, CBR enhances quality of life. When CBR was first developed in the 1980s, it centred on providing access to community-level health and therapy. CBR has since evolved to address access to education, employment, and social services. To achieve such changes, we must engage at multiple levels with the following groups:

- Persons with disabilities and their families;
- The local community and their leaders;
- Government departments and health services; and
- Educational and employment institutions.

Any CBR-inspired programme should be based on the principles outlined in the UNCRPD:[1]

- Respect for inherent dignity and individual autonomy.
- Non-discrimination.
- Full and effective participation and inclusion in society.
- Respect for difference and acceptance of persons with disabilities as part of human diversity and humanity.
- Equality of opportunity.
- Accessibility.
- Equality between men and women.
- Respect for the evolving capacities of children with disabilities and respect for the right of children with disabilities to preserve their identity.

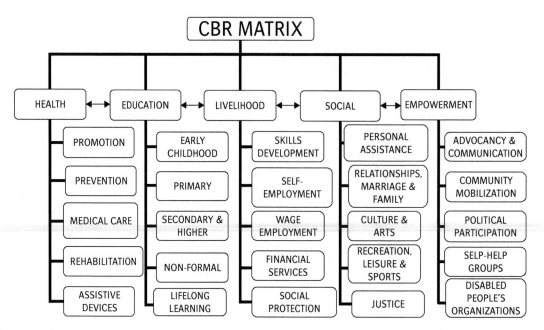

Figure 23.2 Community-based rehabilitation matrix.

Components of CBR

CBR involves a variety of approaches to disability. Therefore, the World Health Organization (WHO) has developed a CBR framework, or matrix, that includes the various components of an effective CBR programme. These are health, education, livelihood, social, and empowerment. Each component has five key elements (see Figure 23.2).

Although our CBR programme might not cover all these components, the matrix helps us consider the inter-related aspects of disability. We should work closely with other programmes and government services to ensure that all components are being addressed in a community.

Why CBR?

• It helps to make rehabilitation services more available.

The WHO estimates that 30 million people in Africa, Asia, and Latin America require approximately 180,000 rehabilitation professionals. In the absence of professionals, however, we can meet many of the needs of persons with disabilities locally without referral to specialized, expensive services. For example, we can train local CBR volunteers to provide support and basic therapy. Additionally, we can advocate for local health services to actively include persons with disabilities.

• It promotes culturally appropriate services.

Local people understand the cultural context and are able to challenge stereotypes in a non-threatening manner.

• It brings value to community life.

By enabling communities to respond to persons with disabilities in their midst, CBR promotes acceptance of all, allows everyone to contribute to society, and helps communities to become more sensitive and interdependent.

• It puts into practice the CBR 'philosophy of care'.

Many disability services follow a purely medical approach to disability, i.e. people are viewed in terms

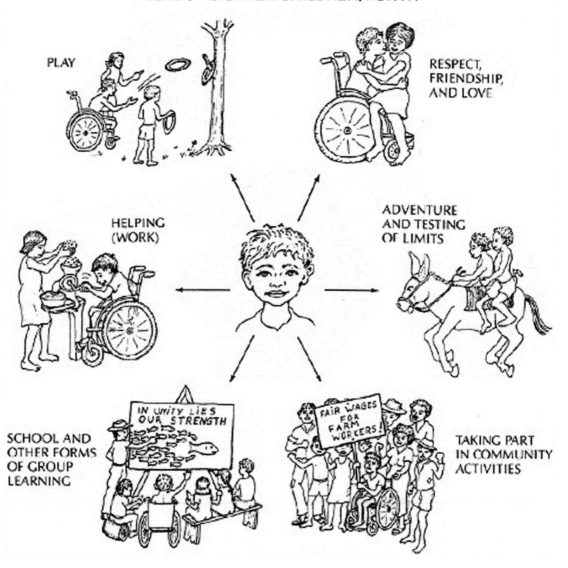

Figure 23.3 Needs of a child with disability.

of their impairment or difficulty, whereas CBR has a holistic approach that sees a person in their social context and treats persons with disabilities with full dignity (see Figure 23.3). CBR brings about a paradigm shift whereby persons with disabilities are seen as more than just their impairment. It is important to note that CBR is not the only approach to provision of disability services. For example, centre-based disability programmes are another valid approach and can work in conjunction with CBR. However, they tend to require more resources and expertise.

What we need to prepare

Assess the situation

We need first to identify persons with disabilities, and then do some analysis to understand their actual situation.

- Disability screening survey.

Initially, we can undertake a simple community survey to identify persons with disabilities. We can define the type and severity of disabilities present. We can outline the various barriers experienced including social, physical, political, geographical, but above all, attitudinal. The survey findings will indicate where to focus, what disabilities to address, and the life situations of persons with disabilities.

- Assessment of functioning.

An important part of this survey involves assessing function. Table 23.1 below sets this out.

- Participatory appraisal (PA).

We will need to 'triangulate' data (i.e. check data from two or more sources) using different PA tools (see Chapter 6). We need to decide who to involve in order that the findings represent the entire community (see Figure 23.4). Persons with disabilities should be fully involved in making an appraisal, which should include:

- Considering physical accessibility of venues and providing transport if needed.
- Additional support to facilitate participation by individuals with special needs, e.g. sign language for the hearing impaired.
- Helping those with difficulty in reading and writing by:
  a. Keeping written exercises to a minimum.
  b. Keeping written points short, clear, and reinforced with a verbal explanation.
  c. Using pictures and illustrations as much as possible.
  d. Helping illiterate participants with any reading and writing tasks.
- Regularly checking participants' understanding.
- Fostering participation by people with hearing difficulties through:
  a. Seeking family assistance.
  b. Speaking loudly and clearly (but not shouting).
  c. Inviting those with hearing difficulties to sit at the front.

Table 23.1 **Assessment of functioning**

Questions	Some difficulty	Lots of difficulty	Unable to do it at all	Comments/ remarks
Does anyone in your family have difficulty seeing, even if wearing glasses?				
Does anyone in your family have difficulty hearing, even if using a hearing aid?				
Does anyone in your family have difficulty* walking or climbing steps?				
Does anyone in your family have difficulty* remembering or concentrating?				
Does anyone in your family have difficulty* with self-care, such as washing all over or dressing?				
Using your language, does anyone in your family have difficulty* communicating (e.g. understanding or being understood by others)?				

* Difficulty that is abnormal for their age if <5 years.

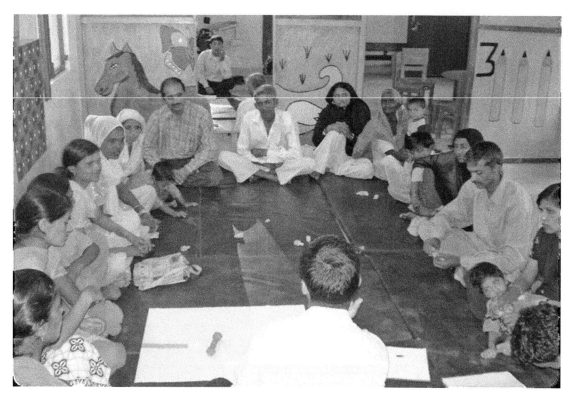

Figure 23.4 A participatory appraisal group.

Reproduced courtesy of Herbertpur Hospital. This image is distributed under the terms of the Creative Commons Attribution Non-Commercial 4.0 International licence (CC-BY-NC), a copy of which is available at http://creativecommons.org/licenses/by-nc/4.0/.

Connect people together

The CBR matrix is multi-dimensional; clearly no one programme can provide all aspects. So CBR requires the involvement of a wide variety of people and organizations (stakeholders): relevant government departments, community leaders, religious institutions, health and educational facilities, civil society organizations (CSOs), and others. A key foundation for successfully working towards CBR is to develop collaborative links with these stakeholders. This helps to gain widespread support for CBR, facilitates referrals, and encourages sharing of resources. We also need to create momentum within the community and to spark creative discussions about making CBR as effective as possible.

Another crucial step is connecting with the community. There are numerous ways to do this, e.g. creating forums with community leaders, persons with disabilities, and their families. This keeps disability on the agenda while preparing the community for the CBR programme.

Select CBR workers

CBR workers should be selected from the community for the reasons described in Chapter 8. They may be the existing CHW, the parent of a person with disabilities, or a respected community member. A number of CBR workers should be persons with disabilities themselves. A mixture of male and female CBR workers will help work across the pillars of the CBR matrix. The role of the CBR worker is to undertake basic therapy, support inclusive education, advocate for those with disability, raise the community's awareness about disability, and assist persons with disabilities to link with other NGOs and services.

Once identified, CBR workers need to be trained, perhaps through external courses, or a specific training course could be developed nearby. Their training will need to be supplemented later by refresher days.

What we need to do

Each CBR programme looks different, because it is guided by its particular situation. All planning will be shaped by findings of the survey, PA, and analysis, in which the community will be fully involved. However, all CBR programmes, whichever CBR component they focus on, tend to involve six steps:

1. Screening and assessment.
2. Maximizing function.
3. Parent support groups and disabled peoples' organizations (DPOs).
4. Advocacy.
5. Mainstream inclusion.
6. Programme monitoring and evaluation.

Screening and assessment

Screening is a simple way of identifying disabilities in people as early as possible (see Figure 23.5). We can then follow up each individual, make further assessments, and refer as needed. The earlier we do this, the better, as it helps maximize the ability of the person with disability to function and to prevent secondary complications. Screening children with disabilities can be done within our community, e.g. at our clinic or within our immunization programme. Schools are another place where children are often screened for learning, hearing, or visual difficulties.

Screening requires a clear plan with defined follow-up and referral paths:

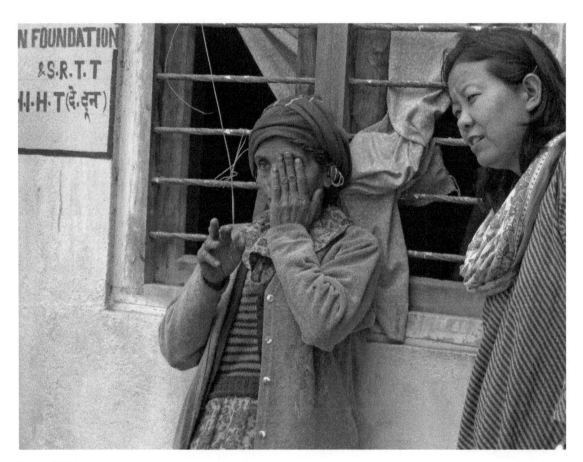

Figure 23.5 Screening for disability.

Screening tools are often designed in English before being translated into local languages. While the forms get translated and back-translated, the words used in the forms may be rarely used in regular conversations. Colloquial expressions must be captured in the forms. Equally important is learning to ask questions in a non-threatening, non-harmful manner. For example, in rural North India, questions asked on family history of neuropsychiatric illnesses can be quite sensitive as the mother already bears the blame for the child's disability. While the paternal history is often ignored, the maternal history is dissected, which can result in further blame on the mother.

- Obtain permission to conduct the screening.
- Conduct an awareness programme in the community about the screening camp/clinics.
- Develop screening tools[5] that are concise, simple, culturally appropriate, and in the local language (see Box 23.1).
- Train CBR team members how to identify those requiring further assessment, and how to record them accurately.

Assessments are undertaken at intervals and are useful to:

- confirm the diagnosis;
- decide on therapy goals;
- draw up plans to help the person with disability to become independent in daily activities like feeding, grooming, etc.;
- decide on assistive devices that may be required;
- decide on home modifications that may be needed;
- set learning goals with an aim to integrate into mainstream schools;
- identify skills and interests which could lead on to vocations or careers; and
- set goals for vocational training and independence.

There will be people identified during screening who require further assessment, and the CBR team can conduct this themselves or refer individuals to an appropriate service.

After confirming the diagnosis and drawing up the management plan, the CBR worker helps with further actions that need to be taken and if required, arranges further assessments. Additionally, the CBR worker can provide emotional and spiritual support to families who are coming to terms with the disability.

Maximizing function

Enabling a disabled person to maximize their function is an important first step. But it is also an entry point to other parts of the CBR matrix (Figure 23.2), such as health education. 'Assistive technologies' are key opportunities for realizing people's rights, and for promoting access and empowerment.[6] The WHO is leading a movement to make an essential list of assistive products that should be made available to persons with disabilities. However, disabilities are diverse, and the range of physical therapy and means of prevention are disability-specific and too detailed to list here.

Eye health

If eye problems are identified by screening, the CBR programme can try to link with a visiting ophthalmologist–simple interventions like cataract operations and providing glasses can have a dramatic impact. There are other useful actions that can also be taken, including eye hygiene, eye safety, control of blood sugar in diabetes, and vitamin A supplementation (an important factor in preventing blindness in many countries, especially south Asia;[7] see Chapter 14). Simple messages such as encouraging hand and face washing can be very effective in helping to prevent trachoma, and routine eye checks as part of CBR programme can pick up problems at an early stage when they are still preventable.[8]

For ideas on helping children with visual impairment to develop all their capabilities, see the *Community Eye Health Journal*[8] and *Helping Children Who Are Blind*.[9]

Orthopaedic disabilities

It may be helpful to link a person with disabilities to a hospital or orthopaedic surgeon. However, most persons with disabilities have learned to live with their disability, and surgical operations occasionally worsen function. Persons with disabilities need to have the information, ability, and opportunity to decide whether to access orthopaedic interventions (Figure 23.6).

Orthopaedic aids and appliances can be very helpful, though often they are expensive. In contexts where the cost for such aids and appliances is too high, we can develop skills within the community to help meet the need. For example, we could organize a prosthetic and orthotic workshop for a local carpenter so they can copy

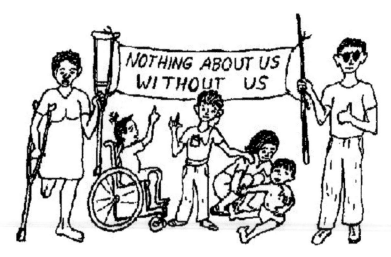

Figure 23.6 Nothing about us without us.

some model aids and appliances. A physiotherapist can also train CBR workers and volunteers in how to do basic therapy. For more suggestions of ways to make innovative aids and equipment, interested readers are referred to David Werner's *Nothing about us without us: Developing innovative technologies for, by and with disabled persons.*[10]

Something of key importance for injury reduction is to educate communities in road safety. Road trauma can be addressed by promoting seatbelt use, helmet use, an understanding of basic road safety, vehicle maintenance, and helping the community to understand it is completely unacceptable (and illegal) to ride bicycles, or to operate *any* vehicle, when under the influence of alcohol or drugs.

Hearing and speech impairment

It is often difficult to find expert assessment and surgical treatment despite deafness being common in many developing countries. Therefore, prevention is key. Children are very susceptible to otitis media and deafness, when they are subject to tobacco smoke and household smoke from cooking fires. Smoking, especially around children, should be strongly discouraged.

Speech therapists are often hard to find. But with a little training, CBR workers can develop useful skills to help children communicate better.

Helping Children Who Are Deaf[11] (Figure 23.7) is full of suggestions for parents and other caregivers about building language and communication skills through signing and other approaches.

Developmental delay/intellectual disability

If identified early, the CBR worker can address both developmental delay and intellectual disability by:

- Co-ordinating action that needs to be taken;
- Making regular home visits to review progress and promoting skills such as writing, drawing, or speech lessons;
- Training parents to include teaching and development activities into everyday interaction; and
- Constantly working to overcome stigma from the family and communities.

Where possible, an occupational therapist or special education teacher could be invited to train CBR volunteers in basic assessments and interventions. A number of small changes to an environment can make a huge difference for persons with disabilities. For example, a hand rail and a simple modified chair that fits over a squat toilet can allow independent toileting, build self-esteem, and simplify home life.

Follow-up

Even if our programme is fortunate enough to have some specialist inputs, the specialists may not be able to provide follow-up. Again, CBR workers can be taught to follow up after operations (with dressings, hygiene, etc.) and to continue with basic therapy. Follow-up visits from the trained CBR volunteer can be useful in many ways, helping persons with disabilities maximize their physical function, increase their self-sufficiency, and

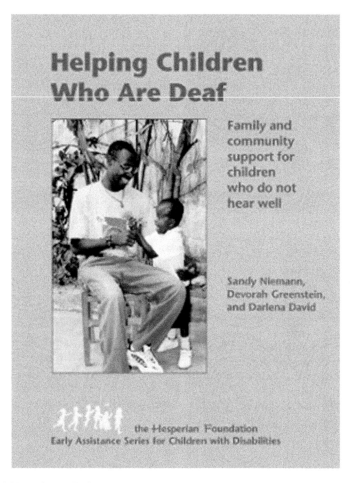

Figure 23.7 Helping children who are deaf.

bring greater understanding and acceptance of disability to the community.

Parent support groups and disabled peoples' organizations (DPOs)

Working with persons with disabilities and their families, we learn quite quickly that we do not share their unique joys, griefs, and struggles. Families of persons with disabilities often seek out others with similar problems for mutual support and to learn from each other.[12] A CBR programme should foster these links and to help Persons with disabilities and their families find a safe meeting environment.

The composition of support groups varies. A disabled peoples' organization (DPO) is run by people with disabilities to identify and address the problems they face. DPOs may be formal and registered as societies, or they may be informal self-help groups (SHGs). These informal DPOs may focus on local issues and advocacy at the local level. Alternatively, a registered DPO may focus on regional activities and be involved in advocacy at a district, state, or national level[12] (see Box 23.2).

SHGs and DPOs are important because people with disabilities are often hidden in the community. These groups provide opportunities for persons with disabilities to interact with each other and with the wider community (Figure 23.8). Persons with disabilities become more independent and learn skills to make decisions about their lives.

Box 23.2 **An example of a DPO**

Persons with disabilities in Sahaspur, India, started meeting as an informal group five years ago. They primarily met to work on getting entitlements like disability certificates and pensions. However, as they met regularly and listened to each other's stories, they began looking beyond their own needs.

They heard about a young man with spinal cord injury who had unmet medical needs and who was being looked after by an elderly mother. The group visited the young man and then approached the Chief Minister to apply for funds for his treatment. They raised money from among themselves to support the elderly mother.

For Road Safety week, the group stopped motorcyclists without helmets who were travelling on one of the main roads near their villages, and gave them roses and information about wearing helmets.

Once a DPO becomes registered, it has greater access to speak out in district- and state-level forums. The Sahaspur DPO has been instrumental in the district in disability-inclusive disaster risk reduction.

For health programmes, the process of starting a parents' support group or DPO is similar to the process of starting any SHG:

- Formation when the members begin to come together;
- Development of vision and focus;
- Group strengthening with capacity building;
- Monitoring; and
- Registering as a society (if the group chooses to do so).

Advocacy

Advocacy can bring about important change at community level—especially ensuring that persons with disabilities have access to entitlements and rights—and influence state, national or international policy.

One key aim in advocacy is teaching persons with disabilities about their rights, and empowering them to stand up for these rights. We need to support the individual, DPO, or parent support group to work with local leadership to remove the barriers that stop persons with disabilities achieving their potential. These include social, physical, and attitudinal barriers (Box 23.3).

Advocacy is in large part about helping the marginalized to access services to which they are entitled, but which bureaucratic, unfair systems or degrading attitudes in the community stop them from receiving. The services are often those that our programme cannot provide, so we need to help persons with disabilities to access both mainstream and specialist services. Some services like rehabilitation are disability specific, but other needs can be met by mainstream services that already exist.

CBR staff need to keep informed about relevant government schemes and other entitlements and make this information available to persons with disabilities, parent groups, and DPOs. We need to find out:

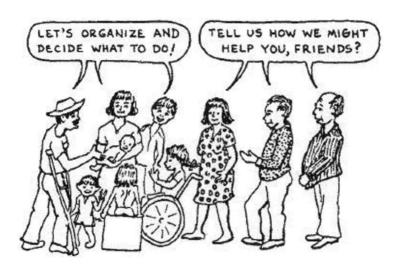

Figure 23.8 Forming a disabled people's organization (DPO).

> Box 23.3 **Case study**
>
> Chebi, a girl with cerebral palsy from Zambia, was refused entry into school by the local teacher. The CBR programme mobilized the local parents' group to approach the village leadership. They asked the teacher to admit the child as required under law, and their request was granted. The CBR programme also helped Malika to acquire a special seat to sit on at school.

- The name of the scheme;
- The relevant government department;
- Who is eligible;
- Documents needing to be completed to access the scheme;
- Copies of the forms that need to be filled; and
- Ideas on what to do if there is no action.

Mainstream inclusion

The previous four activities are largely *disability-specific* activities. But there is also a concept known as the Twin Track Approach[13] (see Figure 23.9) that is *disability inclusive*. This approach is central to a community approach to disability. It requires our CBR programme to work in conjunction with other mainstream development activities to enable the inclusion of persons with disabilities. 'Mainstreaming' disability could entail inviting persons with disabilities to join existing self-help groups, such as literacy groups and youth groups, helping persons with disabilities access schemes that alleviate poverty (e.g. employment schemes, housing schemes, water schemes), or enlisting persons with disabilities in the decision-making process through participation in the relevant community bodies.

Our CBR programme, along with the parent support groups and disabled peoples' groups, should make it a priority to create awareness of disability inclusion, and advocate for changes in attitude and practice within communities. Both arms of the Twin Track Approach ultimately increase the rights and opportunities of persons with disabilities. A key guide for this approach is called 'Inclusion made easy'[14] (see also Figure 23.9, Box 23.4).

Programme monitoring and evaluation (M&E)

As in any other community programme, M&E is essential. We should not see this as a test to pass, but as an opportunity to learn and improve our programme. One approach we can use is to appoint an evaluator or an evaluation team, comprising the following:

- An expert in CBR who has evaluated other CBR programmes, and who can share ideas from other successful programmes. *Ideally* this person should also have local experience, so their insights, feedback, and ideas are appropriate, and relevant to the culture and context.
- A representative from the government.
- Persons with disabilities and their families.

Indicators that could be utilized in the evaluation will vary according to the exact CBR focus, but could include:

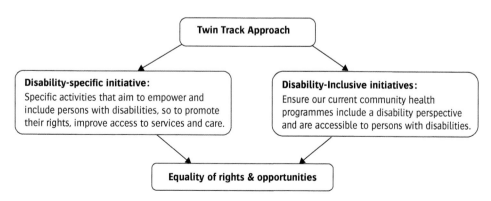

Figure 23.9 The Twin Track Approach.

Box 23.4 Case study

Maelika is a young woman with disability and she is the eldest of six. Following her father's death, it fell to her to be a co-provider for her family. Finding a job was difficult. A volunteer with a local CBR programme encouraged her to ask the village decision-making body for help. The committee helped Maelika obtain a disability pension card, and gain employment as a local preschool worker. The salary and disability pension now allow her to support her family financially. Maelika has started motivating others with disability by sharing her story and highlighting that they also have a right to employment under the UN Charter. Today, Maelika is a channel of transformation for persons with disabilities in her community (see Figure 23.10).

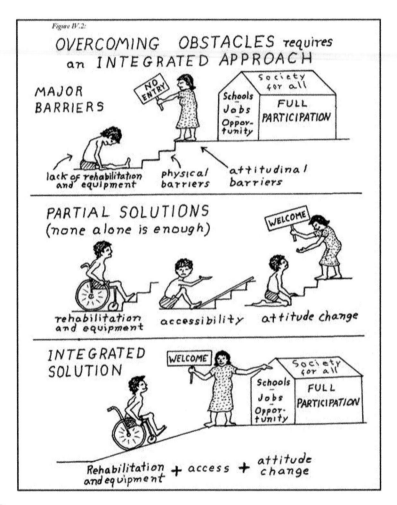

Figure 23.10 Overcoming obstacles by working together.

- Involvement of people with disability in each aspect of the CBR programme;
- Number of children with disability attending school;
- Health status of those with disability;
- Inclusion of persons with disabilities in public consultations and village decision making;
- Persons with disabilities and their employment status;
- Number of persons with disabilities who are involved in a DPO (or similar); and
- Community attitudes towards those with disability.

After the M&E produces an evaluation report and recommendations, we should organize a review meeting with the programme staff and other key stakeholders (donor, local partners, and managers) to plan the way forward. A rough structure could be inspired by the SWOTAC approach:

- *Strengths*: celebrate the successes.
- *Weakness*: discuss areas where improvement is needed.
- *Opportunities*: discuss potential ways forward.
- *Threats*: consider barriers to progress and/or to implementing action.
- *Action plan*: build new actions into the existing or next programme plan (or logframe).
- *Celebrate*: place emphasis on noting the successes, to encourage and thank both our staff and the community, and to build stronger links with the community we are serving.

Through all these elements of CBR programme planning and staffing, persons with disabilities will receive services, be included in programmes, and become empowered in such a way that their disability will no longer prevent them from living a meaningful and valuable life.

Further reading and resources

Elwan A. *Poverty and disability: A survey of the literature.* Social protection discussion paper series, No. 9932. New York: The World Bank; 1999. Available from: http://siteresources.worldbank.org/DISABILITY/Resources/280658-1172608138489/PovertyDisabElwan.pdf

Morris A, Sharma G, Sonpal D. *Working towards inclusion: experiences with disability and PRA. Participatory Learning and Action.* 2005; 25: 5–11. Available from: http://pubs.iied.org/pdfs/G02138.pdf

Tearfund. People with Disabilities. *Footsteps.* 2001; *49*. Available from: http://tilz.tearfund.org/Publications/Footsteps+41-50/Footsteps+49/

Werner D. *Disabled village children.* Berkeley, CA: Hesperian Foundation; 1987.

World Health Organization. *Community-based rehabilitation guidelines.* 2010. Available from: http://www.who.int/disabilities/cbr/guidelines/en/index.html

World Health Organization. *Disability and health factsheet.* WHO Media Centre, 2016. Available from: http://www.who.int/mediacentre/factsheets/fs352/en/index.html

References

1. United Nations. *Convention on the Rights of Persons with Disabilities.* 2006. Available from: http://www.un.org/disabilities/convention/conventionfull.shtml
2. United Nations Department of Economic and Social Affairs. World's largest minority needs to be included in the MDGs. *DESA news* [online]. 2010; 14 (12). Available from: http://www.un.org/en/development/desa/newsletter/desanews/feature/2010/12/index.html
3. World Health Organization. *World disability report.* 2011. Available from: http://www.who.int/disabilities/world_report/2011/en/
4. World Health Organization. *Community-based rehabilitation.* 2015. Available from: http://www.who.int/disabilities/cbr/en/
5. Werner D. Guide for identifying disabilities. In: *Disabled Village Children.* Berkeley, CA: Hesperian Foundation; 1987. p. 51–8.
6. Khasnabis C, Mirza Z, et al. Opening the GATE to inclusion for people with disabilities. *The Lancet.* 2015; 386 (10010): 2229–30.
7. World Health Organization. *Guideline: Vitamin A supplementation in infants and children 6–59 months of age.* 2011. Available from: http://whqlibdoc.who.int/publications/2011/9789241501767_eng.pdf
8. Mactaggart I. Working with communities to improve their eye health. *Community Eye Health Journal* [online]. 2015; 88 (27). Available from: http://www.cehjournal.org/working-with-communities-to-improve-their-eye-health/
9. Niemann S, Jacob N. *Helping children who are blind: Family and community support for children with vision problems.* Berkeley, CA: Hesperian Foundation; 2000.
10. Werner D. *Nothing about us without us: Developing innovative technologies for, by and with disabled persons.* Palo Alto, CA: Healthwrights; 1997.
11. Niemann S, Greenstein D, David D. *Helping children who are deaf: Family and community support for children who do not hear well.* Berkeley, CA: Hesperian Foundation; 2004.
12. Young R, Reeve M, Grills N. The functions of disabled people's organisations (DPOs) in low and middle-income countries: A literature review. *Disability, CPR and Inclusive Development (DCID).* 2016; 27 (3): 45–71.
13. CBM International. *CBM and the Twin Track Approach to disability and development.* 2008. Available from: http://www.cbm.org/article/downloads/53994/Twin-Track_Paper_final_version_October2008.pdf
14. CBM International. *Inclusion made easy.* 2012. Available from: http://www.cbm.org/article/downloads/78851/CBM_Inclusion_Made_Easy_-_complete_guide.pdf

CHAPTER 24

Setting up community mental health (CMH) programmes

Julian Eaton

What we need to know

Why mental health is important for well-being and community development

The expression 'there is no health without mental health' refers to the close connections between physical and mental health. Until recently, health services have generally just included physical health. Finally, however, more people now realize the huge importance of mental health.

The Sustainable Development Goals (SDGs) state that:

By 2030, [we should] promote mental health and well-being and strengthen the prevention and treatment of substance abuse, including narcotic drug abuse and harmful use of alcohol.

The field of 'global mental health' can be described as the science and practice of improving care based on evidence and equity around the globe. It often focuses on parts of the world where mental health is most neglected.

It is increasingly clear that mental illnesses are very common. They not only cause individual disability, but

have a negative impact on community development. Mental illness traps people in poverty. Poverty also increases people's risk of mental illness, forming a vicious cycle that makes community development more challenging. Many mental illnesses affect people from a young age, can last throughout their lives, and can affect those years where they would normally be working and earning a living for themselves and their family (Figure 24.1).

Happily, growing evidence shows that many conditions respond well to treatment, which reduces disability, increases quality of life, and can be achieved in a cost-effective way. This means that it is increasingly possible to improve mental health as an essential part of overall health and well-being, which in turn helps to promote community development.

Despite this, in many low-income countries, only around 15 per cent of people receive the mental health care they need. This unacceptable treatment gap slows global development, prevents some people from participating in community life, and may even cause exclusion. There is increasing research demonstrating the neglect of mental health globally. Growing advocacy and action by people affected by mental distress

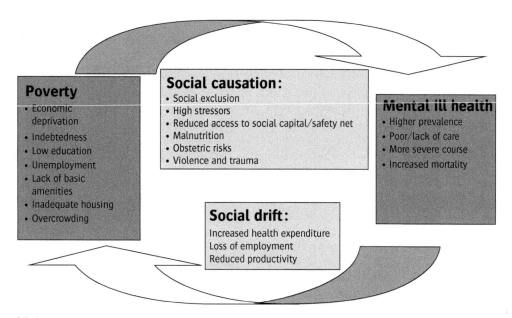

Figure 24.1 Mental ill health and poverty form a vicious cycle, each reinforcing the other negatively.

has led to a movement for coordinated action for mental health and scale-up of mental health services, especially in low and middle-income countries (LMICs, Box 24.1).[1]

The role of culture and the history of approaches to mental health care

Mental illness occurs in all societies, and usually at similar rates. But the way that it is understood and explained varies greatly across cultures. Often, because of changes in behaviour and thinking, it is thought to have a spiritual cause. Traditional healers and religious healers remain the first port of call for many people who become mentally ill in Africa, Asia, and Latin America. As health care workers we may wish to follow bio-medical approaches to treatment and care, but we need to recognize these spiritual dimensions and work with traditional healers if we want to develop an effective mental health programme.

The practice of medical psychiatry was introduced to many parts of the world during the colonial period. From the early 1900s this was usually through building asylums, often which were the then-accepted model of mental health care. But few effective medical treatments for severe mental illness were available until the 1950s.

The 1960s saw a dramatic shift away from institutions, and by the 1980s, there was a strong consensus in favour of community-based mental health care. In richer countries, this move away towards care in the community has become the norm. But apart from a few notable exceptions, like the Aro Village System in Abeokuta in Nigeria in the 1950s, this process has not happened enough in many LMICs, resulting in huge treatment gaps. The institutional focus of mental health services often leads to abuses of human rights both in institutions, and in communities. People with severe mental illness can end up in prisons, chained, or locked up.

In some countries, asylums have become modern specialist centres, connected with university hospitals, but these few centres, and the small number of professionals, cannot begin to meet the needs of the many people needing access to care. Ideally, mental health services should be integrated into the publicly provided health care system, and should be geographically accessible. Integration of physical and mental services can increase access to care and ensure that people with combined physical and mental health problems can be seen at one location, which helps to reduce the stigma of mental illness. This integration is also effective at community level. For example, community health workers (CHWs) can raise awareness about mental health, recognize cases, provide care, and refer when needed, alongside their other tasks.

Box 24.1 **What do we mean by mental health and mental illness? Some notes on terminology**

Good mental health is when somebody feels good about themselves, can cope with the stresses of life, and can meet their normal day-to-day responsibilities. When someone is mentally healthy, they can maintain good relationships with those around them and effectively contribute to society.

Policies, programmes, and research that address mental health in poor settings usually include common problems like insomnia, mild depression, and anxiety, as well as severe and disabling conditions like severe depression, schizophrenia, and bipolar affective disorder. Although the way that people understand and experience mental illness, and seek care, varies according to culture, the illnesses seen across the world share many similarities, and treatment, if given appropriately, can benefit people from any country.

Due to the similarities in pathways to care, stigmatizing attitudes of society, and treatment needs, epilepsy (a neurological condition) and dementia have generally been addressed under the same programmes as mental illnesses. Similarly, problems associated with alcohol and substance use have also been included in the same programmes and packages of care. This grouping is often called *Mental, Neurological and Substance Use Disorders (MNS)*, and is the term used by the WHO and others.

While childhood mental illness is an important part of this field, generally, *intellectual disability* (usually due to permanent brain injury before or around the time of birth) does not share many of the characteristics of mental illness, and services are focused on education rather than medical treatment (though some individuals may have both problems, and programmes may address both issues).

The term that people living with disability by social and psychological consequences of mental illness have come to use at an international level is *psychosocial disability* (reinforced by the use of this term in the UN Convention on the Rights of Persons with Disability). This recognizes the enormous impact on quality of life that the experience of discrimination and rejection has for many. This discrimination can be institutionalized, with arbitrary imprisonment, chaining, and social exclusion often being enacted in a way it is not for other people.

Mental health is something we all have, to some degree, whereas people might or might not have a *mental illness*. In fact, while all of us might experience mental distress sometimes (e.g. when we lose a loved one), we do not consider this to be mental illness unless a person stops being able to function well in their home relationships, work life, or social role.

It is possible to do many things that promote individual and Community Mental Health (CMH), and there is an important role for people and communities outside formalized care in promoting resilience, even in stressful circumstances. Mental health programmes ideally include preventive and promotional aspects, as well as addressing negative social attitudes.

Essential elements of a community mental health (CMH) programme

This section outlines the *types of intervention* needed in programmes, as well as considering the way *they are organized*, to meet the mental health needs of community members. Box 24.2 It suggests some ways we can bring about improvements in health systems. These are widely relevant for any government-run mental health services, for private health care providers, and for local-level approaches through civil society organizations (CSOs). These groups can all play a role in meeting the needs of people with mental health problems (Figure 24.2).

The effects of mental illness can be seen in every aspect of people's lives: mental, psychological, and social.

Medical: mental illnesses have a major impact on physical health. For example, children with epilepsy are at risk from falling into fires and water, and people with schizophrenia die on average 15 years younger than their peers. In addition, where there is a need for medication, there is a risk of side-effects.

Psychological: as well as coping with the typical symptoms of mental illness such as low mood, unusual thoughts, or hallucinations, people often experience stigma and exclusion from social activities.

Social: family relationships, education, employment, human rights, interaction with the justice system, spiritual life, and involvement in religious and cultural pursuits can all be profoundly affected by mental illness.

We have to consider all these factors together, because a purely medical approach will be incomplete.

> ### Box 24.2 Principles of health system reform to improve mental health care
>
> - Services need to be locally accessible and, ideally, integrated into the general health care system, which is less stigmatizing and allows for better continuation of care and management of comorbidity.
> - Clinical care should be offered by general health professionals as well as mid-level mental health professionals (e.g. mental health nurses, psychologists).
> - This 'task sharing' approach implies a systematic shift in roles towards less-senior health staff in locations outside of large metropolitan cities having greater responsibility for frontline treatment.
> - Psychiatrists and other senior professionals should engage in public health/system planning, and in training and supervision of other clinicians, as well as their traditional clinical role.
> - Critically, other aspects of the health system need to be strengthened to ensure proper integration of quality mental health care, such as ensuring an adequate supply of medication, and the inclusion of mental health statistics in the routine health information management systems.
> - Given the low priority that mental health usually has in the system, it is necessary to create strong management structures and to ensure ongoing advocacy, support, and resources for reformed systems.

In addition, we must put ourselves into the shoes of someone with a mental health problem. What do they see as a successful outcome: reducing symptoms or also having an improvement in their social life? This approach, which encourages people to identify their own priorities, is called the 'recovery approach'. This approach in mental health is equivalent to the concept of communities owning their own futures, a key emphasis in community-based health care.

All these approaches to care work much better if they link as much as possible to the communities where people live, and take place within communities. For

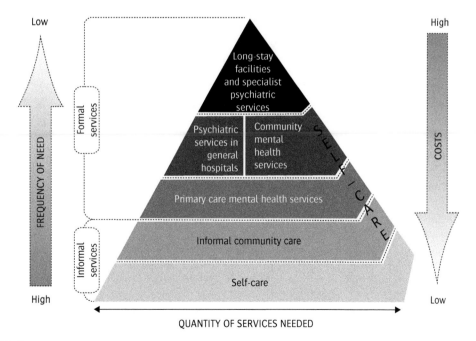

Figure 24.2 The ideal service mix, focusing more on locally accessible services. In many countries, this pyramid is inverted, with almost all funds used at the specialist level.

example, CHWs can address underlying issues which affect mental health, e.g. excessive alcohol or drug use, violence against women, child abuse, high levels of unemployment. In some cases, health workers need to visit patients at home when they cannot (or do not) seek care at a clinic. Good links between communities and services at all levels allows the health team to identify, care, treat, and follow up patients to prevent relapse.

Community members themselves are the best people to provide initial support for anyone who is distressed, has a mental illness, or requires support. Being a supportive family member or a good friend is important for helping people with mild or short-term mental distress. It is also useful for family and community members to work alongside professional care where there is more serious illness. There are many ways that health programmes can recognize and support the essential role of families and informal carers of people with mental illnesses. For example, programmes can teach them skills, inform them about their relative's illness, and even protect the mental health of the carers themselves (see Box 24.3).

Finally, each of us has the capacity for self-help. With guidance and practice, we can improve our own mental health, become more resilient to stress, and aid our own recovery from mental illness. Some practical examples of self-help include getting adequate sleep, building positive relationships, having a good work-life balance, taking regular exercise, and avoiding alcohol or drug abuse.

Medical Care

It is essential in a mental health programme to be able to provide medical care since many of the most severe mental illnesses, e.g. schizophrenia or severe depression, as well as epilepsy cannot be effectively treated without appropriate medication. If a person is very unwell, psychological and social interventions may only be effective once symptoms have been stabilized. There is now good evidence for effectiveness of medical and psychological interventions in low-income settings, as well as guidelines on how packages of care can be effectively delivered.[4] Many guidelines specifically include community-based approaches.

It is often possible to use local medical services to provide this care on a referral basis. In some cases, it may be necessary to advocate for and support the local services to establish mental health care if it is absent. This has the advantage of creating local health resources for the wider community, and can simplify the requirements for a new programme, as medical licensing and provision of medication can be complicated and has legal requirements.

Additionally, as a Community Mental Health programme will be limited to outpatient services, good connections with more specialized services will be essential for the occasional patient, even if they are far away. Such services may be able to offer supervision, training, advice, or guidance on other aspects of programme

---

Box 24.3 **Case study 1: Supporting caregivers, and people with their own mental health needs**

In low- and middle-income countries, family caregivers are the most important source of support for a family member with mental distress. Burans is a partnership project between the Emmanuel Hospital Association and the Arukah Network in Uttarakhand, India.[3] The Burans programme initially focused on providing information and support to people with mental distress and facilitating access to care. It quickly became apparent, however, that caregivers were critical in supporting their family members in all aspects of rehabilitation and recovery, and therefore needed to be formally included in the programme.

In collaboration with caregivers, Burans developed a programme component where community health workers facilitate the formation of caregiver support groups of between seven and ten caregivers living in a neighbourhood. These support groups meet weekly or fortnightly and follow a nine-week facilitated programme which builds caregiver knowledge and skills. It covers topics such as how to increase affected family members' engagement in self-care and household responsibilities, strategies to build and support positive new behaviours, and how to support their relative with getting the most out of talking therapy and medicines that have been prescribed. The modules also address ways caregivers can identify their own mental distress and keep themselves well. Caregivers describe this programme as very helpful and, for some, the changes have been transformational for both themselves and other family members. Formal evaluation of the programme is ongoing.

management, e.g. medication availability, evaluation and research.[5]

If no local primary mental health care or psychiatric services can be found, it is necessary to establish an independent service with suitably qualified staff, e.g. psychiatric nurses trained in prescribing, a primary care doctor, a psychiatrist. Such staff may well need update training on best practice and there are excellent resources available using the WHO mhGAP training.[2] Standard treatment guidelines or protocols are a good way of maintaining quality, consistency, and safety, and may include referral guidance as in a stepped care approach. If clinical staff are relatively junior or inexperienced, it is important that sufficient supervision is in place.

In order for any health care service to work well, we need to ensure that medicines are available and affordable, that good records are kept, and that patients can be referred when necessary. The WHO recommends the use of high-quality generic medicines (see Chapter 11). There is little added benefit in using branded drugs, and their high prices make them unaffordable in low-income settings (Table 24.1). Fortunately, a wider range of useful generic medicines is now available.

Psychological care

While some conditions require medical treatment, many respond better to psychological (talking) therapies. Even those people who do need medication may well benefit from psychological therapies as well, so we need to make this available. There are three main ways in which talking therapies can be used.

1. *Counselling skills* and *good communication* are needed by any health team members who are dealing with patients, carers, and community members.

Treating people with respect, good listening skills, and being able to communicate messages and ideas well make a huge difference in how well people respond to care. Good communication can help to make an accurate diagnosis, as well as increase the likelihood of people returning for follow-up care. In addition, learning these skills helps community members to offer peer support to relatives and friends.

2. Advice and education (*psycho-education*) is an important part of any programme.

Alongside any medical or psychological treatment, there are some essential messages for the patient and carer on how to improve their health. For example:

- preventing relapse (how to avoid falling ill again);

Table 24.1 **A typical standard drugs list.**

Drug	Form
Anti-Psychotic drugs	
Chlorpromazine	100 mg Tabs
Haloperidol	5 mg Tabs and 5 mg Injection
Risperidone	1–2 mg Tabs
Olanzapine	5 mg Tabs
Anti-Depressant drugs	
Amitriptyline	25 mg Tabs
Fluoxetine	20 mg Tabs
Anti-Epileptic drugs	
Carbamazepine	200 mg Tabs
Phenobarbital	30 mg Tabs
Phenytoin	50 mg Tabs
Sodium Valproate	100 mg Tabs
Injectable Depot Anti-psychotic drugs	
Fluphenazine Decanoate	25 mg Injection
Others	
Benzhexol (anticholinergic (side-effect) drug)	5 mg Tabs
Lorazepam (benzodiazepine)	1 mg Tabs

This table only shows available drugs and forms/dosages and is not a prescribing guide. Please ensure national guidelines are carefully followed.

- how to take medication safely and manage side effects;
- what to do in an emergency;
- how to avoid causes of stress or triggers for epileptic seizures;
- how to care for a family member with dementia; and
- how to manage difficult behaviour.

These messages would normally be given routinely during appointments or community visits, possibly with appropriate literature to reinforce them.

3. Specific therapies should be used when there is evidence to support them.

For example, specific therapies have been shown to work well for panic attacks, anxiety, obsessive compulsive disorders, and depression. However, it can be difficult to find suitably qualified staff and to organize ways

> ### Box 24.4 **Case Study 2: Care for post-natal depression in Pakistan**
>
> In low-income countries, perinatal depression affects one in five women, and is associated with infant malnutrition, and lasting effects on both physical and psychological health. A team at the Human Development Research Foundation in Pakistan decided to adapt a proven treatment for depression for the local setting.[6] The Thinking Healthy Programme (THP) aimed to reduce perinatal depression in low socio-economic settings and improve health outcomes in children through using an adaptation of cognitive behaviour therapy (CBT) delivered by CHWs.
>
> In partnership with primary care clinics, CHWs supported mothers from pregnancy to one year after birth. Participants received 16 sessions of the evidence-based approach that combined talking therapy with activities to improve maternal well-being, ways in which mother and children related, and social support for mothers.
>
> The intervention cost was under US$10 per woman per year, and led to recovery in three out of four women treated in a randomized controlled research trial. There were also significantly better health outcomes for their children. The THP is now available as a WHO manual.[7]

of delivering these therapies. This will often mean that people will first need referral before they can access these treatments.

Some basic techniques can be taught to non-specialist HCWs or even to community members, e.g. problem solving and relaxation techniques. There is also evidence that some specific techniques can be effectively used by community workers (see Box 24.4). A number of effective 'low-intensity' scalable interventions, often delivered to groups, are now becoming available. These can address a wide range of problems and therefore do not depend on an exact diagnosis.

Social care

Those with mental health problems will often value support to help get back to a more normal social life, e.g. employment, marriage, etc. It is important that these aspects of people's lives are part of our CMH programme. This is usually best done by members of the health team liaising with others involved with the same people (such as community-based workers).

Examples of things we can do:

- Visit schools to advocate for a child to be re-admitted after her epileptic seizures no longer occur because of treatment. This may include educating the teachers and students that epilepsy is not contagious and teaching them the basics of how to manage an epileptic seizure if it occurs.
- Work with a family to encourage them to take their family member with schizophrenia for treatment, rather than chaining them in the village.
- Persuade the police to recognize that a person's mental illness played a role in behaviour that resulted

in arrest, thus making sure they are treated, rather than imprisoned.

Although all people should receive education, support, and advice at clinic visits, carers who are particularly struggling may need extra home visits, e.g. a family with an elderly relative with dementia whose behaviour is difficult to manage. In addition, we must pay attention to the high risk of human rights or other abuse, and where this is found, take appropriate action. There are now some helpful tools to help ensure our programmes are respectful of human rights.[8]

Community-based rehabilitation (CBR, see Box 24.5 and Chapter 23) is a particularly effective model for ensuring all relevant aspects of patients' needs are considered.[9] It focuses on social inclusion and empowerment, but also ensures that there is relevant access to medical care, education, livelihood assistance, and other support where necessary. Many CBR programmes will have field workers with training and experience in this comprehensive approach. Where this is the case, disability associated with mental ill health is not very different from any other.

Extended role of the community health worker

Especially important is the work of CHWs who are well placed to know the day-to-day challenges and needs of those in their community.

For the work of CHWs to be safe and effective in the support of those with mental health issues, we need to clearly define their role and the resources needing to back them up. They also require careful training, supervision, and teaching about how and when to refer patients if their needs become too great to cope with.

The CHW's role might include:

- *Medical aspects*:
  - identifying and referring people with mental health needs, and helping them to access appropriate services;
  - planning their treatment with them, and considering what to do if the illness gets worse;
  - educating people and their families about the illness and how to stay well, including the importance of taking medication as prescribed; and
  - following up clients at risk of relapse, especially when they miss clinic appointments.

- *Psychological aspects*:
  - developing long-term trusting relationships with families, and providing basic counselling and messages about maintaining good mental health; and
  - if properly trained, provide psychological treatments such as problem management, or behavioural activation therapy.

- *Social aspects*:
  - addressing social issues that worsen mental health, e.g. gender-based violence or family conflict;
  - community awareness-raising about mental health and human rights;
  - setting up self-help groups (SHGs) or ensuring that people with mental health problems are included in other community groups; and

  - making sure that people with mental illnesses or psychosocial disabilities benefit from the same rights as other people, e.g. social welfare benefits, education, employment.

In some countries, CHWs are already being given a more extended role, including diagnosis and initiating or following up medical treatment. There is huge potential in this as CHWs become an increasingly important part of health systems; however, there is an important need to establish clear guidelines for treatment and adequate support mechanisms. Even if this is formally the case, it is often necessary to ensure training and skills are up to date, and support is available, e.g. supervision and medication supply. Senior health workers like nurses and doctors should also consider psychological and social aspects of care when formulating treatment plans.

Important tasks at community level

There are a number of activities we can do at a community level to improve mental health and reduce the risk of mental illness. Specific evidence-based ways we can promote mental health and prevent illness include:[10]

- Help to change community attitudes.

Many negative beliefs and myths reinforce the stigma and discrimination experienced by people with mental health problems. By improving attitudes, we can promote better inclusion into community life. CHWs can be effective in changing negative attitudes, but there is good evidence that people who have experienced mental health problems themselves are the most effective

---

Box 24.5 Case Study 3: Integration of mental health into community-based rehabilitation (CBR)

In the Upper East Region of northern Ghana, the Presbyterian community-based rehabilitation (CBR) programme in Sandema recognized that the large population of people with mental illness and epilepsy were not accessing care. Many experienced stigma and discrimination and there were high rates of abuse, including by some traditional healers. The only medical treatment was too far for most people to reach, and even there, medication was expensive and the relapse rate was high.

The programme therefore decided to integrate support for people with mental conditions into the CBR programme. They trained the fieldworkers to raise awareness in communities, and to recognize mental health problems. Self-help groups (SHGs) of people with psychosocial disabilities were established with the aim of providing mutual support, and enabling people to re-integrate in the community, both socially and economically. Initially, they invited a psychiatric nurse to visit occasionally, but later the SHGs advocated with local political and health leaders to open a mental health clinic in the local primary care centre, and to make affordable medication available. Now they access care near their community, and have a powerful collective voice.

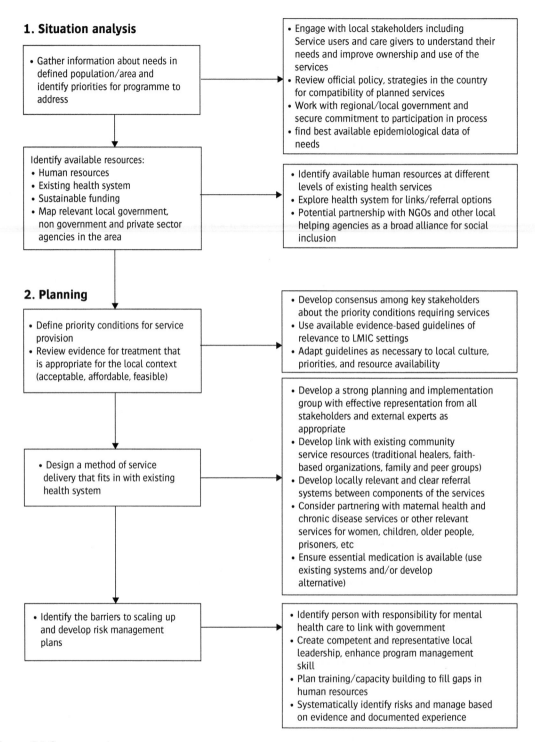

1. Situation analysis

- Gather information about needs in defined population/area and identify priorities for programme to address

- Engage with local stakeholders including Service users and care givers to understand their needs and improve ownership and use of the services
- Review official policy, strategies in the country for compatibility of planned services
- Work with regional/local government and secure commitment to participation in process
- find best available epidemiological data of needs

Identify available resources:
- Human resources
- Existing health system
- Sustainable funding
- Map relevant local government, non government and private sector agencies in the area

- Identify available human resources at different levels of existing health services
- Explore health system for links/referral options
- Potential partnership with NGOs and other local helping agencies as a broad alliance for social inclusion

2. Planning

- Define priority conditions for service provision
- Review evidence for treatment that is appropriate for the local context (acceptable, affordable, feasible)

- Develop consensus among key stakeholders about the priority conditions requiring services
- Use available evidence-based guidelines of relevance to LMIC settings
- Adapt guidelines as necessary to local culture, priorities, and resource availability

- Design a method of service delivery that fits in with existing health system

- Develop a strong planning and implementation group with effective representation from all stakeholders and external experts as appropriate
- Develop link with existing community service resources (traditional healers, faith-based organizations, family and peer groups)
- Develop locally relevant and clear referral systems between components of the services
- Consider partnering with maternal health and chronic disease services or other relevant services for women, children, older people, prisoners, etc
- Ensure essential medication is available (use existing systems and/or develop alternative)

- Identify the barriers to scaling up and develop risk management plans

- Identify person with responsibility for mental health care to link with government
- Create competent and representative local leadership, enhance program management skill
- Plan training/capacity building to fill gaps in human resources
- Systematically identify risks and manage based on evidence and documented experience

Figure 24.3 Steps in developing community mental health programmes.

Source: data from Eaton, J. et al. Scaling up services for mental health in low- and middle-income countries. The Lancet. 378(9802), 1592-1603. Copyright © Elsevier 2011. This image is distributed under the terms of the Creative Commons Attribution Non-Commercial 4.0 International licence (CC-BY-NC), a copy of which is available at http://creativecommons.org/licenses/by-nc/4.0/

3. Implementation

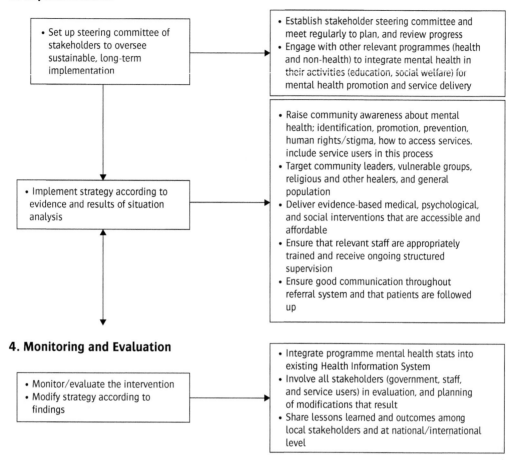

Figure 24.3 Continued

change-makers. Awareness campaigns in mass media, or using posters and leaflets or public talks, are a valuable way of correcting wrong attitudes, and informing people about new or existing services available in the area, and also that treatment can be effective when it continues to be taken regularly.

The most important thing is to show that people with mental illnesses can participate in all aspects of community life. This can be done by, for example, inviting them to participate in activities like livelihood programmes or community celebrations, and to join disability rights organizations and community groups. Language can often reflect and reinforce negative attitudes, and it is a good idea to examine whether language used to describe

mental illness is unintentionally insulting. Even a programme name that is inclusive and implies that mental health problems are common and can be experienced by anyone, can reduce stigma, e.g. Programme for Stress Reduction.

● Reduce suicide rates.

Suicide is a common cause of death in many places, and rates increase in highly stressful environments. Rates can be lowered by reducing access to the means of suicide (e.g. reducing access to guns, or locking pesticides in a central store) and by reducing stress (e.g. lowering student workload, allowing students to retake exams quickly if they fail). Two other things are known to help: encouraging people to talk about how they feel so they can seek help, and encouraging the media to reduce coverage about the methods that people use in suicide.

- School-based life skills education.

Helping students to think about their emotional well-being, and teaching them to cope with problems constructively is known to improve long-term mental health.

- Early life interventions.

The environment that infants experience has a long-term effect on both their mental and physical well-being. We can identify and support mothers who are depressed or struggling to cope (see Box 24.4). We can help mothers to interact with their children in supportive ways. Similarly, when parents of children who have behavioural and emotional problems can learn skills for adjusting behaviour, family relationships and child mental health both improve.

- Reduce alcohol use.

We can ask people about their alcohol use and give simple advice. This should include explaining about dangerous levels and practical ways to drink less. Reducing access to alcohol, including raising prices and reducing advertisements, is also known to be effective.

Empowering service users

People with mental health problems are often a very marginalized group. Those who are most people living with disability, e.g. those diagnosed with schizophrenia, have often been given little choice about their own lives; in many places this is still the case.

Self-help peer groups can provide support and encouragement, and even work together on livelihoods, i.e. ways in which both income and self-confidence can be generated. They can form the basis for advocacy. These groups can allow members to share their preferences about how they live in their communities—something always denied to them. For too long, those with mental illness and other disabilities have been deprived of any choice about how they are treated. We need to challenge the idea that people with disabilities cannot make decisions about their own treatment or understand and give consent for medicines and other support (Box 24.5).

Ensuring that care is continuous and integrated

Many mental illnesses are long-term (chronic) conditions that tend to vary in severity over time (relapsing and remitting). For these problems, continuity of care is especially important. This is best ensured by providing review, follow-up, and access to medication as close to patients' homes as possible.

Keeping the costs of medication down is also essential, as most people in poorer countries pay for their own medicines. Care for long-term conditions can be especially difficult for families to afford. Ways of reducing medication costs include rational prescribing (see Chapter 11), using generic rather than branded versions, and using government pharmacies where they are cheaper.

With any chronic condition, but particularly with severe mental illness, regular follow-up care is vital. It must be made as easy as possible, but there also needs to be a system for recognizing when a patient has not attended for follow-up appointments, and contacting them to find out why. Apart from the cost and inconvenience, it is common for people to abandon treatment once they start to feel better.

An important factor that leads to patients stopping medicines is unpleasant side effects of medicine. The cure may feel worse than the problem. It is important that team members in a CMH programme are familiar with the common side effects, know which ones require more urgent action, and have helpful strategies to help patients persist with taking medicines (see *Where there is no psychiatrist* in 'Further reading and resources').

In some situations, patients can be followed up in outpatient clinics, as many will need to attend regularly, perhaps every month. In reality, however, there may be only one or two practising psychiatrists in the whole district or country. Additionally, the expense and inconvenience of travelling to the clinic can make it almost impossible for patients to attend.

Therefore, health care centres clearly should be as close and accessible to communities as possible. When clinicians visit communities and patients in their own homes, they can better understand the difficulties and constraints people face, and the reasons why some clients do not attend the health centre. This leads to the growing idea that mental health services and chronic non-communicable diseases should be integrated to make the best use of resources; it also shows the value of the holistic primary health care approach. If people with mental distress primarily get care through general services, they are not stigmatized. We need to help patients to have a 'single record' that all those caring for the patient are able to see. This can be done through use of a family folder system (see Chapter 13).

What we need to do

Assess the situation

Health programmes must respond to the needs of the community, but as discussed in previous chapters, we must also ensure that the community understands its own assets and abilities. There are more details on how we do this in Chapters 2 and 6.

When it comes to mental health needs, we need to analyse the situation carefully in some detail. Firstly, we must discover the type and the extent of mental health needs in the community, which are often hidden. Secondly, we must assess those resources that are available in the community, or within its reach given support and training. Table 24.2 gives some guidance and more detail.

There may be a variety of organizations in a community with a role to play in mental health. These include government services, CSOs, disabled persons' organizations (DPOs), advocacy organizations, and groups working in other sectors, e.g. education. All these stakeholders should be involved in the analysis and planning. This brings a greater understanding of the situation, but it also helps them to contribute and to own the change process. Full participation also allows co-ordination of efforts and avoids confusion and duplication.

We therefore need to set up a steering group or action team that represents a wide variety of people. This gives greater buy-in and makes integration of the programme activities into the wider system more likely.

Plan with all groups involved

The situation analysis is likely to highlight a wide range of needs, and we will need to decide on priorities, bearing in mind the available people and resources. It is also helpful carefully to consider barriers that may make it harder to implement our plans, i.e. perform a risk analysis. Having done this, a programme of activities can be developed to address these priorities.

We should include the following:

- Understanding what services need to be delivered at each level of a health system, e.g. community, health post, referral centre, and evaluating tasks that each member of the team might be able to do. See Chapter 1 on the important topic of task shifting.
- Preventing mental illness and promoting good mental health are always top objectives.

Table 24.2 Information to consider as part of situation analysis.[11]

Context	Population demographics. Health indicators. Social indicators
Need for care	Prevalence of different conditions. Current proportion of people accessing care. Risk factors for mental illness in the target area.
Policy and legislation	Political support. Mental health policy and plans. Mental health legislation.
Human resources	Personnel at different grades and locations • availability for programme/ costs.
Health system infrastructure	Administrative structures for health. Services providing mental health care • at different levels of system. • public and private, NGO. • in specialist and general health care.
Health information system	Indicators that should be collected by services for health system, and to measure expected impact.
Community	Local beliefs about mental illness • cause, treatment and stigma. • community and family support. • discrimination and abuse. Traditional care availability and its use.
Other sectors	Availability of welfare, livelihood support, special education, access to rights, justice system.
Key stakeholders	Health system leaders, mental health professionals, potential service users, community and traditional leaders

- Using local resources and partnerships to increase our impact and efficiency.
- Integrating mental health into wider health and social care as far as possible. This means avoiding a separate, vertical programme (or silo) that suggests mental health is in some way unique, which can reinforce stigma.

Plans must be realistic, practical, and need to include funding, human resources, management, supervision, and monitoring and evaluation (M&E).[12] Plans need to be structured in a clear way with timelines, clear allocation of duties, and the people responsible for those duties named. Having these practical details in place makes it easier to keep the whole programme accountable. If a plan is agreed by all partners in advance, it is more likely to succeed. Getting support from as many stakeholders as possible at this stage is likely to reap rewards during the implementation phase.

Implement the programme

Implementation will need competent staff and good leadership. We may need to enhance skills, provide leadership, coaching, and learn from good practice elsewhere. We need to ensure there is continuing professional development and build the capacity of the whole team. Ideally, this would also involve staff in services outside the programme, e.g. PHC nurses and doctors who might be the first point of contact for patients, social workers, etc. Also, we must not forget pathways to care, e.g. traditional healers and religious leaders.

Good guidelines for implementation and training materials now exist for different grades of worker, e.g. under the WHO's excellent mhGAP programme (see 'Further reading and resources').

There are three other issues we need to prioritize:

1. Sustainability.

This is a key issue from the start. We need to integrate CMH care into existing structures as much as possible. Although we may have a strong team running the programme, management structures for mental health at national and district levels are often very weak and require support and encouragement in order to back up local services. This requires communities and teams to lobby policy makers and others to include mental, neurological, and substance use disorders into health systems.

2. Vulnerable groups.

We must pay special attention to any group that has higher mental health needs, e.g. single women head of households, women after delivery, socially excluded groups, and as capacity allows, migrants, displaced persons, and prisoners. This can be done by deliberately looking for them and seeking to understand their specific needs. Sometimes we will discover them when we are doing our initial survey, or they may come to light when CHWs become more involved in the community. We should consider partnering with others who have particular skills, e.g. in child and maternal health, chronic diseases, HIV, neglected tropical diseases (NTDs), services for older people, and prisoners. Other chapters in this book give more information on these groups.

3. Advocacy.

People who have experienced mental illness can become powerful advocates for change, especially when working as part of a team (for a similar approach advised by programmes working with HIV, see Chapter 20). Our health programme must foster a strong voice for advocacy by empowering service user organizations. We also need to follow human and civil rights approaches and help people claim the services and benefits that should be provided by government (see Box 24.5).

Monitoring and evaluation (M&E)

Any health programme requires regular oversight and adaptation to make it work well. Routine and systematic monitoring of a programme is essential to keep activities aligned to its original objectives. Periodic evaluation, taking into account information that has been routinely collected, allows for assessment of progress and responding to any problems identified. Such M&E is also used to keep programmes and services accountable to those who are funding work. An important addition to this is giving a voice to those who are using services, and taking their feedback seriously.

The process of M&E of programmes should begin during the initial design of the programme, so that its expected impact is clear, and can be used as a guide for M&E.

Examples of useful information to measure are:

- Basic service use statistics.

Numbers of men, women, boys, and girls who use the service, e.g. every month, plus a list of their diagnoses. Providing this information to government health authorities allows them to measure coverage of mental health services and shows the importance of the programme.

- Service quality.

Whether the staff are delivering the care in a way that helps patients to get better. This can be done by observation, checking knowledge gained after training, and by asking patients if they are satisfied with their care. This can be made 'semi-quantitative' by them numbering questions from 1 to 5, 5 being the best.

- Resource availability.

Whether all the key resources are in place, e.g. if medication is available, whether the right staff are in place all the time, and whether quiet and confidential rooms are available to see patients.

- Mental health outcomes.

There are useful questionnaire tools that can be used to identify people with mental illness, e.g. SRQ 20, PHQ9, GHQ12 (see http://researchonline.lshtm.ac.uk/7829/), and to measure the extent of disability, e.g. WHO DAS 2.0 (see http://www.who.int/classifications/icf/more_whodas/en/).

Using specific and validated tools is important to measure outcomes and impacts of programmes.

Not only will M&E help focus on providing for the needs identified in the community, but it will also allow lessons learned to guide others, as work in this neglected area of health and development is scaled up elsewhere.

Further reading and resources

Bhugra D, Tasman A, Pathare S, Priebe S, Smith S, Torous J, et al. The WPA-*Lancet Psychiatry* Commission on the future of psychiatry. *The Lancet Psychiatry*. 2017; 4 (10): 775–818.

CBM Community Mental Health Implementation Guidelines. Available from: https://www.cbm.org/article/downloads/54741/CBM_Community_Mental_Health__CMH__-_Implementation_Guidelines.pdf

Lancet Commission on Global Mental Health and Sustainable Development, 2018. Available from: www.globalmentalhealthcommission.org

The Lancet Global Mental Health Series; 2007 and 2011. Available from: http://www.thelancet.com/series/global-mental-health and http://www.thelancet.com/series/global-mental-health-2011

Mental Health Innovations Network. Available from: http://www.mhinnovation.net

Movement for Global Mental Health. Available from: http://www.globalmentalhealth.org

Patel V. *Where there is no psychiatrist*. London: RCPsych Publications; 2018.

World Health Organization. WHO Mental Health Gap Action Programme (mhGAP). Available from: http://www.who.int/mental_health/mhgap/en/

References

1. Lancet Global Mental Health Group. Scale up services for mental disorders: A call for action. *The Lancet*. 2007; 370 (9594): 1241–52.

2. World Health Organization. *Mental Health Gap Action Programme (mhGAP): Scaling up care for mental, neurological and substance abuse disorders*. Geneva: World Health Organization; 2008.

3. Emmanuel Hospital Association. *Nae Umeed (New Hope)—strengthening community based caregiving*. 2017. Available from: http://projectburans.wixsite.com/burans

4. Patel V, Thornicroft G. Packages of care for mental, neurological, and substance use disorders in low- and middle-income countries. *Public Library of Science Medicine Series*. 2009; 6 (10): e1000160.

5. Thornicroft G, Tansella M. Balancing community-based, and hospital-based mental health care. *World Psychiatry*. 2002; 1 (2): 84–90.

6. Rahman A, Malik A, Sikander S, Roberts C, Creed F. Cognitive behaviour therapy-based intervention by community health workers for mothers with depression and their infants in rural Pakistan: A cluster-randomised controlled trial. *The Lancet*. 2008; 372 (9642): 902–9.

7. World Health Organization. *Thinking healthy: A manual for psychological management of perinatal depression*. 2015. Available from: http://www.who.int/mental_health/maternal-child/thinking_healthy/en/

8. World Health Organization. *WHO QualityRights guidance and training tools*. 2014. Available from: http://www.who.int/mental_health/policy/quality_rights/guidance_training_tools/en/

9. Cohen A, Eaton J, Radtke B, George C, Manuel V, De Silva M, et al. Three models of community mental health services in low-income countries. *International Journal of Mental Health Systems*. 2011; 5 (3). DOI: 10.1186/1752-4458-5-3

10. Patel V, Chisholm D, Dua T, Laxminarayan R, Medina-Mora ME, editors. *Mental, Neurological, and Substance Use Disorders*. Disease Control Priorities, Volume 4. Washington, DC: The World Bank; 2015.

11. PRIME. *Situation Analysis Tool*. 2014. Available from: http://www.prime.uct.ac.za/research/160-prime-s-situational-analysis-tool

12. Basic Needs. *Community mental health practice: Seven essential features for scaling up in low- and middle-income countries*. Bangalore: Basic Needs; 2009.

CHAPTER 25

Helping communities to manage disaster risk

Joel Hafvenstein and Jonathan Stone

In the communities where we work and live, we want to see people able to choose the best future for themselves. We want them to thrive in spite of uncertainty, conflict, natural hazards, and changing climates. Sudden shocks and long-term stresses (hazards) often mean that this is not their reality. External threats can prevent communities from enjoying their rights, capabilities, and freedoms. As populations grow and the climate changes, the number of people affected by disaster is rising and will probably continue to do so.[1]

We need to build resilience into our community health programmes (CHPs) and support the community in understanding and managing their disaster risk. Health workers know that 'prevention is better than cure'; in the same way, helping communities become resilient is more effective than relying on emergency relief after a disaster happens.

We must be aware not only of what type of hazard the community currently faces, but also whether that frequency is increasing and whether new hazards are likely to develop. Climate change, e.g. less predictable growing seasons for crops, greater likelihood of flooding, is an increasing area of concern.

What we need to know

Managing disaster risk

It is easy for people anywhere to feel helpless against natural disasters—to think of them as 'acts of God' or 'acts of nature'—and that they are completely beyond our control. To change this mindset, it is important to distinguish between hazards and disasters. A hazard is an extreme, disruptive event that is often beyond human control. A disaster is the impact of a hazard on vulnerable people.

For example, cyclones or earthquakes are hazards. For a hazard to cause a disaster, there needs to be

---

Box 25.1 Game for disaster management training

(Useful supplies: a cardboard box, a rope, a motorcycle helmet, a first aid kit)

1. Loop the rope around a volunteer, and point out that they are now 'tied up,' unable to move.
2. Hold the box high over their head and explain that it represents a heavy weight. This volunteer is now living with the risk that at any time the weight will fall and injure their head. Ask what can be done to prevent or reduce the disaster of the falling box hitting the volunteer.

Your group may come up with ideas like the following:

- Untie the volunteer, so they can move out from under from the box (note that if the box falls with no one underneath, it is still a hazard, but not a disaster).
- Have someone else watch the box, and shout a warning when it is starting to fall, so the volunteer can dodge.
- Protect their head from the box, by building a shelter or having them wear a helmet at all times (you can illustrate this with a real motorcycle helmet).
- Have a strong person ready to catch the box when it falls.
- Be prepared to provide first aid immediately after the box falls, to limit the long-term injury from the disaster (you can illustrate this with a real first aid kit).

These ways to prevent the falling box 'disaster' are similar to the key ways that we can address real disasters: moving to a less exposed area (e.g. building houses above flood level); establishing early warning systems; disaster mitigation (i.e. acting to reduce the impact of future hazards); and preparing for emergency response.

The key message is that even when we cannot directly affect the *hazard*, there are still many ways to mitigate the *disaster*.

---

vulnerability—the susceptibility of individuals, communities, or systems to the impacts of hazards. Mobilized communities have the potential to reduce this vulnerability, starting by making full use of existing community capacities, in other words, their own knowledge, strengths, and resources. By reducing people's vulnerabilities and strengthening these capacities, communities can manage disaster risk significantly. For example, imagine an earthquake occurring in a city where every building has been built to a quake-resistant design, so no structures are seriously damaged and no one is seriously injured.

The game described in Box 25.1 is an entertaining way to illustrate this distinction and to start people thinking of ways to manage disaster risk.

The essential nature of community-level action

Often, we think that disasters are too big a problem for local communities to deal with, so we shift responsibility to governments or other outside support agencies such as international non-governmental organizations (INGOs), the United Nations (UN), and civil society organization (CSOs). However, disaster risk management can start locally and then be integrated with wider efforts.[2]

This is easier said than done, unless disasters are so frequent that communities learn the value of owning a response. When disasters are rare in any given location, it can be difficult to demonstrate the need for preparedness. Communities must decide whether they should put their time and resources into preparing for a disaster that may never happen or into livelihoods, health, education, or dealing with conflict. There are also false understandings of risk. For example, one colleague told the author, 'We've just had a big earthquake. We don't need to worry about another one for 100 years'. Thus, it is helpful if risk reduction is seen as an integral part of community-based health care, rather than a separate programme.

Why must disaster risk management be based in the community?

1. **Many disaster risk management activities are only effective if owned by the community.**

The community knows more than any outside group about its own vulnerabilities. However, a community may not always recognize its own capabilities to cope with disasters unless we can raise awareness and help it to use these effectively. For example, in floods or

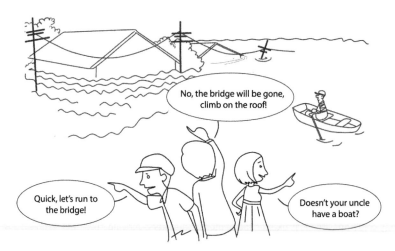

Figure 25.1 Everyone needs to know the evacuation plan.

cyclones, rapid evacuation to a safe place is vital to save lives. But an evacuation plan needs to be understood and rehearsed by the whole community—otherwise people will not know what to do when the disaster happens, and the most vulnerable (the sick or people living with disability) may be forgotten (Figure 25.1).

All across the world, unequal social structures leave women and girls more vulnerable to disasters than men and boys. Outsiders can only help to a limited extent to change the practices and restrictions that put women at greater risk. It largely needs to be done by the community themselves championing inclusion.

2. **Communities are best placed to deliver 'first response' in an emergency.**

Community volunteer teams who have been trained and equipped for evacuation, emergency rescue, and first aid can save many lives in the hours before external help arrives. They know best who is vulnerable and in need of help.

3. **The international system of emergency response has major and growing gaps.**

Globally, there is evidence that the number, severity, and economic impact of some types of disaster—particularly floods and storms—is increasing.[3] Humanitarian relief funding has been inadequate in many disasters, and there is little sign of that gap shrinking. Moreover, while the international humanitarian system and most government disaster agencies are set up to assist after large-scale disasters, many communities are affected as much or more by smaller disasters: local floods, fires and landslides that recur, often annually. These 'everyday disasters' may seem to cause relatively limited damage, but their frequency and cumulative effect can trap people in poverty—sometimes even more so than major disasters. And these smaller, less dramatic situations rarely inspire government or international response, and are often left out of official disaster statistics.[4]

Types of hazard

In our communities we need to understand two things. The first is what types of hazard are most likely to occur. The second is what community vulnerabilities might turn those hazards into disasters (Table 25.1).

Depending on the type of hazards we face, a community will emphasize different aspects of disaster reduction. For example, in rapid onset disasters for examples with tsunamis (tidal waves), it is especially important to have timely early warning systems and a community contingency plan that everyone knows and has practised. We need to note the difference in response needed for large-scale disasters affecting a wide area, and small-scale disasters that affect only the community and surroundings. We also need to be aware of the likelihood and frequency of any disaster.[5]

Table 25.1 **Key categories of disaster**

Type	Description	Hazard examples	Vulnerability examples
Sudden-onset	Sudden shocks caused by extreme natural phenomena. They strike with little or no warning and do immediate harm to human populations, activities, and economic systems. The frequency and severity of many weather-related disasters (including some epidemic diseases) is changing due to climate change.	• Cyclones • Wildfires • Floods • Storm surges • Avalanches • Earthquakes • Tsunamis • Volcanoes • Pest outbreaks • Epidemics	• Ineffective early warning system. • Houses built in highly exposed areas (e.g. steep hill slopes, unprotected coast). • No community contingency plan (e.g. for evacuation or rescue). • Weak house construction. • Most people lack necessary skills (e.g. swimming) or knowledge of what to do in disaster (e.g. 'drop, cover, hold on' in quake). • Poorly planned development.
Slow onset	Disruptive changes which cause people's livelihoods to slowly decline to a point where they will struggle to survive. Usually due to climatic extremes, but made worse by ecological, social, economic, or political conditions.	• Drought • Famine • Salinization • Water-logging • Desertification • Environmental degradation	• No knowledge of drought-resistant crop varieties. • Lack of access to irrigated land or healthy pasture. • Lack of drainage channels. • Weak institutions for natural resource management.
Human-made	Emergency situations whose principal, direct causes are identifiably human actions, deliberate or otherwise. Sometimes separated into 'conflict-related' and 'industrial/ technological' categories.	• War • Conflict-related displacement • Village or urban fires • Severe pollution • Nuclear accidents	• Lack of information/warning about actions of warring parties. • Local livelihoods rely on easily plundered assets (e.g. livestock). • Lack of organized fire brigades. • Poorly regulated industry (e.g. oil drilling, chemical plants). • Imbalanced power structures.

What we need to do

Set up a disaster response team (DRT)

Raising individuals' awareness, although important, is not enough to manage disasters. The community must organize itself and take collective action to address vulnerabilities. If there is willingness to do this, our programme can help facilitate the process.

Any community that experiences regular, unpredictable, or serious hazards needs a carefully chosen, trained DRT (Figure 25.2). They will be responsible for many of the actions described in this chapter. DRTs should include one or more CHWs, women, students, and a person living with disability. Teachers and others with responsibility in the community should also be part of this group.

There is no reason to create a new committee if an existing group, such as a village health committee can take on the role, but it must have a proven track record of completing projects.

Understand community hazards and capacity

We need to talk with the community to identify and understand the main hazards. The DRT can assess the community's disaster risk using the participatory tools described in Chapter 6, such as a timeline (Figure 25.3). Ask questions such as:

• How often does this hazard occur?
• How severe is it in a "normal" year and a bad year?

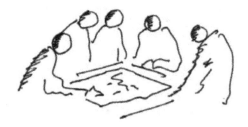

Figure 25.2 Form a disaster response team.

- What area does it usually affect?
- How long does it last?
- How much warning do you have?
- Have you observed any changes over time in the hazard, e.g. in its frequency or severity?
- What are the usual *impacts* of the hazard (i.e. the disaster) on this community?

It is crucial to reflect on and make use of the community's capacities, i.e. the strengths, abilities, and skills that make them resilient to disaster. If some people in the community were less affected by the disaster, what helped them? What else can we think of that might avert disaster? The community can often make more use of their capacities. For example, a mosque loudspeaker or church bells could send an early warning of a hazard. Community members who know how to swim, put out fires, or build hazard-resistant housing may be able to teach others.

Lead risk-reduction activities

Once the community group understands community vulnerabilities, it can start acting on reducing them and increasing capacities for managing disaster. A community risk reduction plan should be based on the community's own capacities, not just as an appeal for outside aid. One aspect of risk reduction is building design. As discussed in Chapter 13, community clinics should be built simply, using local materials and building styles, but advice should be sought from a qualified person on hazard resistance. For further information on this, consult Build Change.[6]

Plan practically for disasters

The DRT should develop a contingency plan spelling out the actions that the community will take immediately before, during, and after a disaster. A good contingency plan should include the following.

Warning systems

Early warning systems do not always result in action, often because the level of hazard is difficult to predict

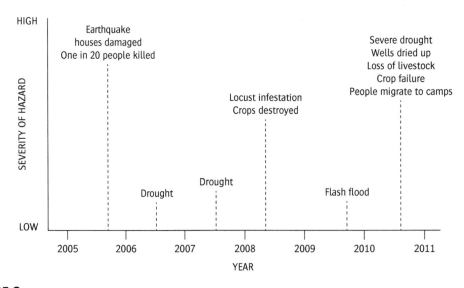

Figure 25.3 A sample timeline of community hazards.

or because people are unwilling to take action 'in vain'.[7] If official early warning is available, e.g. through radio, measures can be taken to make sure it reaches all community members. For every hazard type, the local warning system will be different and have different levels of effectiveness and reliability.[8] For cyclones and hurricanes in resource poor areas, handheld megaphones or signal flags are widely used. With hazards like flash floods, church bells, mosque loudspeakers, and mobile phones can all be used to raise the alarm.

For example, in Bangladesh, trained community leaders used mobile phones and flags to disseminate warnings from the national flood centre. The floods in 2007 and 2008 were successfully forecast ten days ahead and action was taken to evacuate and protect livelihoods. For every $1 spent on the project, about $40 were saved; on average the amount saved per household was between four and five hundred dollars.[9]

With drought, conditions deteriorate slowly, but many drought-prone areas have a government or meteorological department warning system. Farmers often have their own traditional ways of forecasting drought, e.g. interpreting insect behaviour, wind directions, tree flowering patterns. It is important not to disregard these methods.

Evacuation centres

The DRT should work with the community to designate a building as an emergency shelter and ensure it is safe, clean, and equipped with a safe drinking water supply, emergency lighting, a first aid kit, and men's and women's toilets. Women, girls, and vulnerable adults must be able to use their designated toilets without any shame or risk.

Care for the most vulnerable

The plan should include specific plans to assist the evacuation of highly vulnerable people, the elderly, the long-term sick, or those living with disability. We must also make provision (in some societies) for widows and women whose husbands are away.

Links with government

Many governments have a plan and resources allocated to help communities cope with disaster. Wherever possible, the community's contingency plan should relate to local and national government plans. Equally, the community group can ensure that the government plan actually reflects community needs. They should also maintain a communication system that is likely to work in a disaster to guarantee links between the community and the government and outside actors.

Practice/drill

Any contingency plan needs to be rehearsed in simulation in order to identify any practical problems and embed it in the memories of all community members. In addition, the CHP should have its own contingency plans, considering the following:

● Access/transport.

Will people be able to reach the clinic in the event of a disaster? If transport in and out of the community is affected, what will that mean, e.g. for the CHWs' supply chain? For referrals? We may need emergency stockpiles of essential medicines.

● Communications.

How will we communicate with the outside world following a disaster, e.g. to report emergency needs? Remember that mobile networks may be damaged by disasters or needed by official disaster responders.

● Shelter.

We should have a plan for use of the building and its surrounding area in a disaster, keeping in mind that emergency medical needs will probably increase.

● Identify who is most vulnerable.

In an emergency, knowing who is likely to need help is essential. The CHW will already be working with many of them—mothers and children, the chronically ill, persons with disabilities, and people from marginalized groups and castes.

● Plan casualty management.

Depending on the type and severity of the disaster, the CHW's first aid skills may not be sufficient, or she may be injured. Thus, it is important to train and equip a community volunteer first aid team to support the CHW in emergencies. First aid kits with an adequate supply of wound dressings must be kept in a secure location and reserved for times of disaster.

● Prepare for the public health impacts of disaster.

For example:

1. Disasters often affect water sources and sanitation, increasing water-borne diseases like cholera and typhoid.

   ● A CHP should have a contingency plan for highly infectious diseases, in particular cholera, whenever there is any chance this may occur.

2. Floods and storms may affect the number of mosquitoes causing dengue fever, malaria, etc.

   • The DRT should be aware of the signs of epidemic diseases and give early warning to the health authorities.

3. Might people from other disaster-affected areas take refuge in our programme area?

   • If so, what would this mean for the programme, and for public health needs?

4. Disasters can increase HIV transmission via an increase in violence and/or transactional sex.

   • The danger of physical and sexual abuse including rape may be increased.

5. When the food supply is affected, child malnutrition is likely to rise.

6. Households may lose health-related assets such as smokeless stoves, mosquito nets, and water storage units.

The DRT along with CHWs should be ready to raise community awareness of these post-disaster health risks, and scale up their normal public health work as necessary to address them.

7. Be prepared to keep working without support.

After a disaster, as mentioned in Chapter 8, CHWs may have to operate without contact with programme leaders or supervisors for some time. CHWs should be trained with this possibility in mind.

Deliver disaster safety messages

As part of their public health information role, the DRT and CHW need to communicate key messages about personal and household safety for each type of disaster.

Key safety messages: earthquake

1. Before the quake:

   • Identify 'safe' places.

Identify or create safe places in each room of your home, workplace or school where you can Drop, Cover, and Hold On in a quake. A safe place will be away from windows that can shatter or tall furniture that could fall on you. It could be under a sturdy table, or against an interior wall.

   • Prepare your home.

It is important to have an emergency exit or 'fire exit' as a quake may block the main door and can also cause fires. Place all furniture at the sides of your room and store any heavy objects such as sewing machines low to the ground. Shut and (if possible) lock high-up cupboards at night. Keep footwear and a torch (flashlight) by your bed.

2. During the quake:

   • Drop, Cover, Hold On (Figure 25.4).

This simple formula is usually the best way to avoid injury in a quake. 'Drop' means drop down to the floor. 'Cover' means protect your head and neck with your arms or padding, e.g. a school-bag or cushion. Try to get under a table if possible. 'Hold On' means hold something secure, like a large, bulky piece of furniture that will not fall on you. If there is no such furniture, sit on the floor next to an interior wall. Never go onto stairs during an earthquake!

If you are in bed when the quake begins, stay there, curl up, and hold on, protecting your head with a pillow or blanket if possible. If you are outside when the shaking starts, find a clear area (away from trees, buildings, power lines, etc.) and drop to the ground. Stay there until the shaking stops.

3. After the quake:

   • Local dangers.

If there is any danger of gas leaks, do not light a flame or turn on an electric switch or appliance. Be aware of broken glass and other sharp debris. Look for damage in your home. Try to put out any small fires.

   • The danger is not over when the shaking stops.

An earthquake is often followed by strong *aftershocks* (Figure 25.5). Once the ground has stopped shaking, if

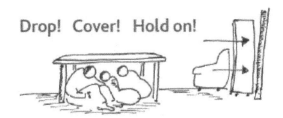

Figure 25.4 What to do in an earthquake.

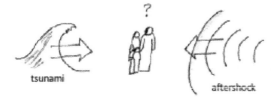

Figure 25.5 After the earthquake …

the building you are in has been damaged, leave calmly and carefully. Stay out of damaged buildings. Each time you feel an aftershock, follow the earthquake rule: Drop, Cover, Hold On.

A quake has related secondary hazards, e.g. landslides, fires, or tsunami (enormous waves triggered by the earthquake). If you are living near the coast, move to high ground *immediately* in case there is a tsunami. Keep alert for any public messages about a tsunami.[10]

Key safety messages: flood

1. Before the flood:

Identify an area which is high enough to be safe from flooding, and a safe evacuation route. Practise evacuating along this route.

2. During the flood:

Move to high ground as soon as you receive warning of rising water. Watch out for any power lines on the ground that could electrocute you. Only walk through water if it is not moving.

People who cannot swim may need a buoyancy aid; locally available options might include a cluster of sealed plastic containers, bunches of coconuts, or banana tree trunks. Do not swim out to rescue people in fast-moving water unless you are secured by a rope to a tree or a group of rescuers.

3. After the flood: water safety.

The DRT should remind community members that flood waters are likely to be contaminated with sewage (Figure 25.6). All exposed food should be thrown away to prevent the spread of disease.

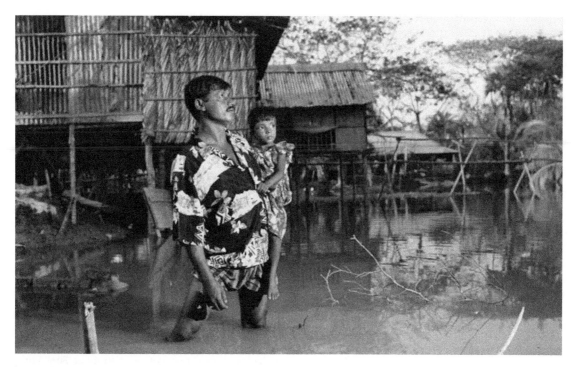

Figure 25.6 Rafiqsa Shikari and his family faced flooding after a cyclone or hurricane in Bangladesh.

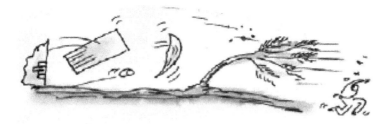

Figure 25.7 The Open Field System.

Key safety messages: cyclones or hurricanes

1. Before the cyclone:

    *   Identify emergency shelter.

There needs to be a designated safe place where families can shelter for the duration of the storm (Figure 25.7). This should be on high ground, with plenty of room to accommodate people. In some countries, government, the Red Cross, Red Cresent and CSOs have built strong cyclone shelters which are raised off the ground on pillars. More commonly, schools, clinics, religious buildings, government offices, or grain stores are used. They need to be cleared and prepared before the storm arrives. If no emergency shelter exists then preparation of the shelter should be the responsibility of the DRT (or a trained volunteer team). Practise evacuating to the shelter.

    *   Get to safe shelter.

When people hear early warning of a cyclone, they need to evacuate with their family as practised. Plan to quickly evacuate the elderly, those with disabilities, pregnant mothers, those with long-term sickness, and young children with support from community volunteers.

2. During and after the cyclone: landslides.

Heavy rainfall during a cyclone often causes landslides. In 1998, landslides associated with Hurricane Mitch killed 18,000 people across four countries. Landslides are often most destructive in urban areas, where shortage of land has forced people to build on steep, unstable slopes. During a storm, stay alert and listen for unusual sounds that might indicate moving debris, such as trees cracking or rocks falling. A trickle of flowing or falling mud or debris may precede larger landslides.

Landslide warning signs include leaning posts or trees, soil cracks, changes in natural water flow and disruption to piped water supply. If you are near a stream or channel, be alert for any sudden increase or decrease in water flow and for a change from clear to muddy water. These indicate landslide activity upstream, so be prepared to move quickly. Don't delay—save yourself, not your belongings.

Key safety messages: fire

House fires are especially common in slum communities with unsafe or illegal electricity connections, or in flammable homes with interior cooking.

1. Before the fire:

    *   Prepare your home.

You should have an emergency exit or 'fire exit' in case the main door is blocked by fire/smoke. Keep combustible materials as far from your cooking area as possible. Keep at least one means of extinguishing fires (e.g. fire blanket, water pot, sand bucket) in the kitchen and any other fire risk areas.

    *   Precautions/Prevention.

Teach children about fire safety, and not to play with burning objects. Cooking and smoking cigarettes are two major causes of house fires. Be prepared to extinguish cooking fires quickly. If you smoke, always extinguish cigarettes in a cup or tray; never smoke in bed. Ideally, don't smoke at all

2. During the fire:

    *   Putting it out.

Most big fires start small; they need air and heat to spread. If you see a small fire, put it out immediately by throwing earth, sand, or water onto the fire, or by covering it with a blanket or towel to cut off air. Also shout 'Fire!' immediately to alert others and summon help.

    *   Stop, Drop, Roll.

If clothing catches on fire, *stop* running, *drop* to the ground, and *roll* around until the fire is extinguished.

* Avoid smoke.

Most deaths in fires result from people breathing in smoke. If you are in a smoky room, crouch down low (where there is less smoke), cover your face with a wet cloth, and crawl to the nearest exit.

These messages should not just be delivered verbally. The DRT should help people *practise* disaster safety through household and community drills, allowing space for local solutions.

Co-ordinate and support teams of volunteers

Depending on the context, the DRT may need to organize the following volunteer teams.

Early warning team

These volunteers may be responsible for warning specific vulnerable groups, e.g. the elderly or persons with disabilities.

First aid/rescue team

The first aid/rescue team is responsible for rescuing people who have been trapped or injured by a disaster. The team members should have physical strength for moving debris and materials, carrying bodies, using rescue equipment (e.g. ropes, ladders, digging tools), or using boats or canoes. They should also have up-to-date first aid training—the CHP should be able to provide this.

Food distribution team

If food aid needs to be brought in from outside, volunteers are needed to handle this food and organize daily distribution. These volunteers should be able to record basic information, such as family details, and to manage food stocks. This team may also have to organize food for people who are ill or who cannot come to a distribution centre. In major disasters they will need to act with strength and fairness when large numbers of people are desperate to access supplies.

Shelter and toilets team

When people are displaced by a disaster, these volunteers will help them to construct temporary shelter. They should monitor the shelters to make sure they are effective in bad weather and make changes accordingly. They will also manage sanitation, e.g. building temporary latrines, digging and managing trench toilets or defaecation fields. The latter is a controlled version of the 'open field system' described in Chapter 21, in which the field is divided into strips with fixed boundaries and only one strip is used at any one time—or shallow trench toilets which are filled in as they are used (see Figure 25.8). NB: The safety and dignity of women and children is an *essential* consideration in choosing any sanitation solution, especially in emergencies.

Counselling team

These volunteers provide emotional and spiritual support through listening, counselling, and (as appropriate) praying with those who are suffering from bereavement. Ideally, they should be able to recognize those more seriously traumatized and at risk of post-traumatic stress disorder (PTSD) and know referral options.

Report on post-disaster needs and ensure they are met

The DRT will be responsible for ensuring that information about post-disaster needs is gathered and reported to government and other appropriate relief providers. Immediate needs for information include:

* estimates of deaths;
* injuries and urgent health needs, physical and mental;
* damage (to houses, water/sanitation, infrastructure); and
* the number of people without adequate water, food and shelter.

The DRT will work with the volunteer groups and any external aid providers to coordinate the process of meeting the whole community's basic needs for water, food, shelter, sanitation, and medical care. This will require special care for the most vulnerable. It should monitor progress of the response and seek additional resources where needed.

Sustain disaster preparedness

We have already discussed the need for a DRT to lead the process of disaster reduction by planning and mobilizing collective action. However, DRTs can easily lose momentum, especially if disasters are infrequent. After an initial burst of activity, they may have little to do and may question their own value. Their training will need updating when members are replaced by new ones, or there are major changes. Often, they will need some basic equipment, e.g. life jackets, radios, SAT

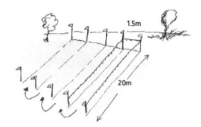

Figure 25.8 An 'open field' system.

Reproduced with permission from Bill Crooks and Tearfund. Disasters and the local church. Copyright © 2011 Bill Crooks/Tearfund. Available at http://learn. tearfund.org/~/media/files/tilz/churches/disasters_and_the_local_church/ disasters_and_church_web.pdf?la=en. This image is distributed under the terms of the Creative Commons Attribution Non-Commercial 4.0 International licence (CC-BY-NC), a copy of which is available at http://creativecommons.org/ licenses/by-nc/4.0/

phones, and even phone credit. Sustaining a DRT to re-main prepared needs to be considered carefully (Box 25.2). The following are ongoing roles of a DRT.

Representing the community on disaster issues

The DMT should be the voice of the community on dis-aster planning and response to local and national gov-ernment, other communities, CSOs, and other actors. This communications and public relations aspect of the work is increasingly valuable. It enables other people,

organizations, and communities to be able to learn from them, as well as helping to build their own profile. Reviewing the community response to a disaster is a key task and unless local and small scale will need to be done as part of a wider monitoring group.

Community updates

As hazards, vulnerabilities, and capacities change, the group will be responsible for updating community risk assessments and any disaster plans. It will also be respon-sible for making sure the whole community is aware of any important new plans.

Further reading and resources

Coppola D. Natural hazards, unnatural disasters: The economics of effective prevention. Washington, DC: World Bank; 2011. Available at: https://www.gfdrr.org/sites/gfdrr/files/publica-tion/NHUD-Report_Full.pdf

Crooks W, Mouradian J. *Disasters and the local church: Guidelines for church leaders in disaster-prone areas.* Teddington: Tearfund; 2011. Available at: http://tilz.tearfund.org/~/media/Files/ TILZ/Churches/Disasters_and_the_local_church/Disasters_ and_church_web.pdf?la=en

Joint Statement: Scaling Up the Community-Based Health Workforce for Emergencies. Global Health Workforce Alliance, UNICEF, UNHCR, WHO, IFRC. 2011. Available at: http://www.searo. who.int/srilanka/documents/community_care_in_emergen-cies.pdf?ua=1

Lavell A, Maskrey A. The future of disaster risk management. *Environmental Hazards*. 2014; 13 (4): 26–80.

Mattsson E. *Improved seismic-resistant design of adobe houses in vulnerable areas in Peru*. BSc [dissertation]. Uppsala, Sweden: Uppsala University; 2015. Available from: https://uu.diva-portal.org/smash/get/diva2:853417/FULLTEXT02.pdf

UNISDR. *Global Assessment Report (GAR) on Disaster Risk Reduction*. 2011. Available from: https://www.preventionweb.net/english/hyogo/gar/2011/en/home/index.html

References

1. Centre for Research on the Epidemiology of Disasters. *The Human Cost of Natural Disasters 2015: A global perspective*. 2015. Available from: http://reliefweb.int/sites/reliefweb.int/files/resources/PAND_report.pdf

2. Hansford R. *Roots 9—Reducing Risk of Disaster in our Communities*. 2011. Tearfund. Available from: http://tilz.tearfund.org/~/media/Files/TILZ/Publications/ROOTS/English/Disaster/ROOTS_9_Reducing_risk_of_disaster.pdf

3. EMDAT, *The International Disaster Database*. Available from: http://www.emdat.be

4. Global Network of Civil Society Organisations for Disaster Reduction. *Views from the Frontline: Findings from VFL 2013 and recommendations for a post-2015 disaster risk reduction framework to strengthen the resilience of communities to all hazards*. 2013. Available from: http://gndr.org/images/newsite/documents/VFL2013/vfl2013%20reports/GNFULL_13_ENGLISH_FINAL.pdf

5. Abarquez I, Murshed Z. *Community based disaster risk management: Field practitioners' handbook*. Pathumthani: Asian Disaster Preparedness Center, 2004. Available from: http://www.adpc.net/igo/category/ID428/doc/2014-xCSf7I-ADPC-12handbk.pdf

6. Build Change. 2015. Available from: http://www.buildchange.org/

7. Coughlan de Perez E, van den Hurk B, van Aalst MK, Amuron I, Bamanya D, Hauser T, et al. Action-based flood forecasting for triggering humanitarian action. *Hydrology and Earth System Science*. 2016; 20: 3549–60.

8. Ibrahim M, Kruczkiewicz A. *Learning from experience: A review of early warning systems*. Milton Keynes: World Vision; 2016. Available from: http://www.wvi.org/sites/default/files/WV_EWEA_Doc_FINAL_Web.pdf

9. UNISDR Scientific and Technical Advisory Group. *Using science for disaster risk reduction: report of the ISDR scientific and technical advisory group, 2013: Case Study 3*. Available from: http://www.unisdr.org/we/inform/publications/32609

10. Earthquake Country Alliance. *Staying safe where the earth shakes*. Available from: http://www.earthquakecountry.org/downloads/StayingSafeWhereTheEarthShakes_StatewideEdition.pdf

Use of information and communication technologies (ICT) in community health programmes

Smisha Agarwal and Trinity Zan

What we need to know

Background and growth of information and communication technologies (ICT)

Over the last decade, there has been a huge increase in the number of mobile phone users around the world. Even in the remotest areas, it is becoming easier to connect, and in most cities, even in slum areas, mobile phone use is the norm. In addition to mobile phones, other digital devices, e.g. tablets and laptops, have become increasingly available, making it possible to reach resource-poor communities with health care information and services.

The use of mobile phones and other wireless devices to deliver health services and information is referred to as 'mHealth'. The term 'digital health' usually refers to the use of both wired devices for the delivery of health care, such as computers and laptops, and also to mobile devices such as mobile phones. These two terms are sometimes used interchangeably, but this chapter uses the term 'mHealth'.

There are two points worth making at this stage. First, we need to realize that setting up mHealth and other forms of ICT requires time, ingenuity, and connection between a wide variety of people in the development and rollout of the service. Before beginning the implementation process, we need to be sure that our programme has both the need and the capacity.

Second, we must not allow the demands of the technology (or of the developers) to make us 'unlearn' important community development principles. One definition of development is 'a process through which people gain greater control over the circumstances of their lives'. Will any digital service we set up contribute to this or undermine it?

Types of mHealth programmes

In practice, mHealth involves the use of digital devices for a wide variety of issues. Mobile phones (including SMS technology) may be used as a tool to reach the

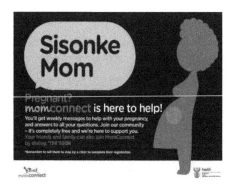

Figure 26.1 Mobile Academy delivers audio training for health workers delivered by a fictitious character, Dr. Anita.

Reproduced courtesy of Mobile Academy and BBC Media Action. This image is distributed under the terms of the Creative Commons Attribution Non-Commercial 4.0 International licence (CC-BY-NC), a copy of which is available at http://creativecommons.org/licenses/by-nc/4.0/

community with important health information, to support health care workers (HCWs) in providing better care, or to help strengthen the health system. Figures 26.1 and 26.2 illustrate some specific examples.

mHealth programmes for clients

Digital tools such as mobile phones are useful for community members to receive health information, or to communicate with healthcare workers and with other members of the community.

There are several examples of mHealth programmes that provide important healthcare information. Two examples are The Mobile Alliance for Maternal Health Action (MAMA) in Bangladesh,[1] and MomConnect in South Africa.[2] A key element of both these national programmes is to send text messages with important nutritional and health information to pregnant women and new mothers. In addition, these programmes use behavioural change approaches to influence families' 'health-seeking behaviour' for essential antenatal and postnatal services (Figure 26.2).

Another programme, Mobile for Reproductive Health (m4RH), developed text messages on family planning methods that can be accessed by mobile phone users in Kenya and Tanzania. To access information about different types of contraceptives, users can opt-in to the

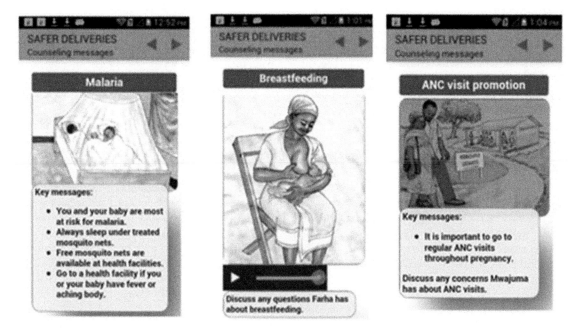

Screenshots from D- Tree International's counselling section of the mobile application

Figure 26.2 Screenshots from D-Tree International's counselling section of the mobile application.

Reproduced courtesy of D-tree International. This image is distributed under the terms of the Creative Commons Attribution Non-Commercial 4.0 International licence (CC-BY-NC), a copy of which is available at http://creativecommons.org/licenses/by-nc/4.0/

service by sending a text 'm4RH' to a short-code telephone number to receive an SMS with a menu of options. m4RH has been implemented in Afghanistan, Kenya, Tanzania, Rwanda and Uganda and has been adapted to reach young people.[3]

ChatSalud in Nicaragua works similarly to m4RH but has broader scope—in addition to family planning information, it covers topics such as safer sexual practices, sexually transmitted infections/HIV, and pregnancy-related care.[4]

mHealth programmes for healthcare providers

Often community health workers (CHWs) or facility-based health workers may not have all the training, experience, or support they need to provide quality services to the community. Mobile phones can be used to provide training in new technical areas, as well as to assist HCWs in providing routine diagnosis and treatment. For example, in several states in India, Accredited Social Health Activists (ASHAs) have access to a programme called Mobile Academy—an audio training health course on preventative health behaviours (Figure 26.1). ASHAs can access this in a series of eleven chapters and quizzes on their mobile phones through simple voice calls. They can take the course free-of-cost by dialling a mobile number through any mobile handset. The course is delivered by a fictitious, engaging female character called 'Dr Anita.' Lessons can be completed at the ASHAs' own pace. They receive a pass or fail score and a certificate of completion at the end of the course.[5]

There are also valuable tools that support screening, diagnosis and treatment which can be put on mobile phones or tablets to help guide HCWs. For example, in Malawi, the Integrated Community Case Management (iCCM) application uses mobile checklists and information to help the assessment of children with symptoms such as diarrhoea, fever, cough, and rapid breathing. Health surveillance assistants (HSAs) use this mobile tool to capture information about the child on a mobile form, including symptoms and danger signs. The mobile application then guides the HSA to ask a series of questions that helps to reach a diagnosis and treatment.[6] Similar systems to strengthen iCCM are being tested in Mozambique and Uganda.

Other uses of mHealth for healthcare providers include using a mobile phone to consult with other colleagues or supervisors about how to manage medical complications, notifying higher-level health facilities about patients needing referral, and playing short videos displayed on phones or tablets to educate members of the community.[7]

mHealth for systems strengthening

mHealth interventions provide ways not just to support CHWs but also to connect them to health care facilities, and to improve the quality of care by streamlining how services are delivered. For example, mobile phones may be used to collect data about clients for specific services, and to register a birth or death (i.e. tracking vital events in real time) and to follow up on these events, as appropriate (see Chapter 8). Instead of the traditional paper registers, CHWs can use their mobile phones or tablets to record information about pregnant women or immunizations received by children. This data, if collected digitally, can then be used to develop automated reminders for CHWs to follow-up on their clients in a timely manner.

Real-time recording of data in a digital format reduce the delays by reporting data from the community to the district health team. Here, the information can be used for planning health services. It can also alert the district health team to important disease outbreaks with minimum delay, which is immensely important in case of epidemics, for example, cholera, and Ebola.

One successful example of an mHealth programme to strengthen health systems is the cStock programme in Malawi.[8] HSAs use their phones to send a monthly SMS to the system about the level of essential medicines they have in stock. This combined data from HSAs helps the district health team to know more accurately about current drug stocks, calculate resupply quantities needed for each HSA, and send them a message about when the medicines will become available at the health facility to ensure sufficient stocks are available or will need to be sent out. This reduces the dreaded situation when essential medicines are not available as patients need them, and also prevents the HSA from making unnecessary trips to restock at short notice.

Another example is mHero, a two-way mobile communication system that uses text messaging to connect Ministries of Health and HCWs; mHero was developed in 2014 by Intrahealth International and UNICEF to respond to the Ebola outbreak in Liberia. Using mHero, messages can be sent to HCWs in a crisis. Crucial information about health facilities and availability of essential medicines and services can then be reported to the Ministry. In the initial stages of the Ebola crisis, mHero was widely used to communicate with HCWs around the country and to coordinate the availability of workers and services in health facilities that were on the frontline of treating affected patients.[9]

Do mHealth interventions actually work?

Currently, there is no clear overall evidence on the efficacy of mHealth interventions as research on its wide range of uses is still in its early stages. There are many anecdotes, opinions, and stories that add support to the value of this technology. One area that has been reviewed is mHealth's value in the wider uptake of breastfeeding. Sending mothers informative text messages increases the number of women who start breastfeeding and still breastfeed at six months. Another study suggests that using text messages increases the use of antenatal services and skilled attendants at the time of birth (see Chapter 17). However, to date the use of messaging to improve the uptake of reproductive

healthcare is still inconclusive. Based on available evidence, the World Health Organization, is in the process of developing guidelines to support development of digital strategies to advance healthcare (https://www.who.int/reproductivehealth/topics/mhealth/digital-health-interventions/en/).

mHealth should not be thought of as an intervention in itself. Rather, it should be considered as a valuable tool to increase the effectiveness of healthcare, and to overcome barriers in delivering services to difficult-to-reach communities. Regardless, we must always keep costs in mind. There are large initial infrastructure costs in setting up an mHealth programme and this can be much greater than using traditional methods. However, if our programme is able to reach a larger number of people, costs will reduce and our coverage will improve. Therefore, if using a digital tool can help us overcome barriers to making health services more effective, then it is worth exploring.

Box 26.1 **Important definitions and basic concepts**

Beta-testing: Testing the technical aspects of an mHealth programme in pilot version, before implementation, provides an opportunity to identify and address any technology-related problems.

Communication channels:
- *SMS* (Short Messaging Service) allow users to send and receive text messages on their mobile phones.
- *USSD* (Unstructured Supplementary Service Data) is similar to SMS, but may be thought of more like a chat session which allows two-way exchange, and ends when the communication ends. USSD is the mechanism used in many countries to check and to top-up airtime.
- *Multimedia messaging service (MMS)* is a messaging service that allows the transfer of text messages, pictures, voice, video or all four. To exchange multimedia messages, users must have a phone that is running over a GPRS or a 3G network.
- *Interactive Voice Response* or *IVR* allows the clients to communicate with an automated pre-recorded human voice. The voice may share important information or guide the client to respond either with voice or using the mobile keypad. IVR may be valuable for programmes operating in areas with limited literacy, but its costs should be compared to those of other communication channels.
- *General Packet Radio Service (GPRS) or 3G*: Technologies that allow transfer of data through

mobile phone networks. GPRS and 3G refer to the strength of the signal for transferring data, browsing websites, watching videos etc.
- *Interoperability*: How and whether two technical systems can work together and exchange data, i.e. 'talk to each other'. If community programmes want to share digital data or send reports to a health facility, donor, or government health system, it is important that the systems are interoperable.
- *Open-source software*: Software or computer programme code that can be publicly accessed and modified by programmers other than those who developed it. In contrast, proprietary software can only be used by the team that created it, and requires a special license (and possibly a fee) if others want to modify it for their use.
- *Mobile money*: Refers to a cash management service available on a mobile phone that can be used to transfer money between users. M-Pesa, widely used in Kenya and Tanzania, is an example of a mobile money service.
- *Short codes*: Special telephone numbers, shorter than a full telephone number, that can be used to send messages. Short codes are easier to read and remember, and can therefore be used by programmes aiming to communicate with clients through messaging.

Some basic concepts

To develop mHealth programmes, we need to work with programme managers, those working in public health, engineers, and computer programmers. This means we first need to understand some basic concepts and terms used in mHealth (Box 26.1).

Understand the context

Before we design and implement an mHealth service, we need to answer two key questions:

1. Is a digital solution the most appropriate for the problem we are trying to solve?
2. Is it realistic to think that a digital solution will work in our setting?

mHealth may seem attractive, but it is not always the best solution. Sometimes, a simple, old-fashioned solution is the most effective and efficient answer to a problem. To help us decide whether digital technology is the best solution, we must first be very clear about the problem we are trying to solve. Then we need to brainstorm different potential solutions, and list the advantages and disadvantages of each. For example, for each option we need to ask:

- How much time do we estimate it will take (it may be longer than we think)?
- How many and what types of resources will we need?
- Do we think this is likely to be the most effective solution to the problem or barrier we have defined?

- Which option is most inclusive of community members?
- Which solution do we, as a team, tend to think will bring the greatest benefit?

If, after doing this, we believe that a digital technology may be appropriate, then we will need to look in more detail at our context.

How are people using existing technology?

First, we need to know if the people we expect to use mHealth actually own digital/mobile devices, and that they know how to use them (Box 26.2). For example, if we are considering developing an app on a mobile phone that would help CHWs to screen children for common childhood illnesses, then we need to know whether CHWs own smartphones, or a feature phone without a touch screen, or at least have easy access to a mobile phone, e.g. a husband's or older child's. However, sharing a phone can be very sensitive and all those involved would need to be entirely happy to do this. The same would go for another valuable use of mHealth: developing a service to enrol pregnant women in our community to receive text messages about how to be healthy during pregnancy.

Box 26.2 **Questions to help understand the community and context**

- Who owns or uses a digital device (mobile phone, tablet, computer) in the community? Men only? Women? Is there a difference between men and women regarding phone ownership or shared use of phones? Young people? Health workers (at facilities or CHWs)?
- How do people use their phones, tablets, and computers? Do they make and receive calls only? Do they send and receive text messages? Do they visit websites? Do they listen to music or watch videos? Do they use WhatsApp or similar?
- Is there generally good mobile phone reception in the community?

- Is there Internet connectivity in the community (via fibreoptic cable or phone lines)?
- How quick, easy, or near is it to access the Internet?
- Do health facilities have digital devices (computers, tablets, mobile phones) for use by the health workers?
- How do people charge their digital devices?
- How much do people pay per month to use their digital devices (for phone credit/airtime)? Who pays for this? Does cost affect how people use their phones (e.g. they will call people but hang up before the person picks up, in order not incur charges (sometimes called a 'flash')?

Literacy levels are an important consideration when designing digital services. For example, a programme that sends text messages to mothers, or an app that helps a health worker screen a client for TB will require the user to be literate. Some services, however, do not require this, e.g. a call-in phone number with IVR messages about various health issues.

We also need to consider how people do, or do not, use and value digital devices in their everyday lives, as this can influence how we design a programme. Most will consider it a status symbol, meaning in any programme where we donate smartphones to health workers, e.g. to CHWs, we would need to be careful about what other community members might think and whether it could create tension within the community.

What kind of infrastructure is in place to support technology?

We will also need to discover any structural challenges that would make implementing our digital health solution difficult. Some important questions to ask include:

- Is there good mobile phone reception?
- Is there 3G connectivity that enables going online via mobile phones?
- How reliable and strong is current Internet connectivity, e.g. is it possible to watch a YouTube video without interruptions?
- How long does it take for a website to load fully?
- Do most people have access to electricity to charge digital devices, e.g. at health facilities?

Are other people or organizations already doing something similar in our community?

In addition to these questions and issues, we need to know if there are any similar initiatives more widely underway in the country, region, or district. If so, we may be able to adapt what already exists, or talk to people who can offer us helpful tips and back-up. We may believe that we are pioneering the use of digital services in our health programmes, but it is likely that others will be doing this soon; we should collaborate as much as possible.

How can we get information to answer these questions, and more?

We can talk directly to different community members, either individually or in small groups. But we also need to know more specifically if anyone else is using (or has used) mHealth in our country or district; if so, we should connect with them.

To help us find out, we can search online for mHealth 'communities of practice' or technical working groups in our area. We can also visit online project repositories, e.g. mHealth Knowledge,[10] and we can reach out to digital health listservs.[11] It is also important that we are well informed about whether our country has an existing digital health policy or strategy that would guide the development and implementation of our mHealth service. For example, there may be specific policies regarding how we must protect clients' personal data or where it should be stored. Connecting with relevant decision makers who know these answers might also open connections to local technology firms or other potential partners who could be involved with our work.

Ok, we think a digital tool will work—what next?

Once we understand whether an mHealth intervention is appropriate for our area, we can then start thinking about the steps we need to take. This is not very different from planning any other health intervention. We need to define clear goals, how the digital services will be able to reach people, and what resources are needed for this to happen. Using planning tools such as a logframe (see Chapter 7) can help us clarify the programme goals and objectives.

The digital component of the intervention also requires a number of specific steps to help us develop the correct technology, partnerships, and testing needed in the context of our programme.

Technology decisions

We should think of an mHealth intervention as an addition to an existing health programme in order to target a specific health challenge or need. First, we must make a number of decisions about what exactly this mHealth intervention will look like (Box 26.3).

The two key questions are:

1. Cost: we must calculate the cost of the programme, both for initial development and maintaining the technology.
2. Ease of use: at each step of planning, we must keep the end users in mind and ensure we develop a system that people will find useful and easy to use.

We must also determine the types of mobile phones that will be employed for the programme. Here are some questions to help us make this decision during our planning stages:

- What kind of functions do our end users already use on their phones?

- *Core functions*: What are the core technology functions that are needed for the programme (Enter and send data? Automatically send content to people? Provide a menu of options)? What is the user expected to do with the technology?
- *Communication type*: What kind of communication format will be used? Examples include SMS, IVR, MMS. Is this one-way communication where information is being sent to the user, or two-way communication where the user can also respond to the system?
- *Access*: How will the users access the programme? Does an app have to be downloaded on their phones? How will that be accomplished? Can users self-register to the programme? If so, what kind of outreach is needed?

- *Frequency*: How often will the user engage with the system? For example, if this is a text messaging service, how frequently will the messages be sent to the user?
- *Language*: In what language will the programme be available?
- *Data use*: If the system is collecting data, how would we like to access the data? Examples include in the form of spreadsheets or as a dashboard which can be accessed online. If a dashboard is needed, we would need to identify the specific indicators that we would like to see on the dashboard.
- *Security*: If the system is storing data, what are the requirements, if any, for data security and back-up?

- What is the ideal screen size needed to perform the functions?
- What other functions are needed on the phone (local language capability, multimedia, Internet connectivity, compatibility with other platforms, etc.)?
- What is the length of the mobile battery life?
- Is the mobile device available locally?
- Do we have local programmers and technical support available for the maintenance of the phones?

If we only need call or messaging functions, we may be able to use the most basic mobile phones widely used in many countries. Alternately, for more advanced functions, we will need feature phones and smartphones/android phones, which are rapidly becoming more available and affordable. Feature phones are typically low-cost basic phones with Internet access but lacking the advanced functions of a smartphone. Smartphones are able to download a variety of applications and have a touchscreen interface and functions similar to that of a computer. If a large screen size is needed, we may use tablets instead of mobile phones.

Partnerships

Before considering partnerships in our mHealth development it is vital that those involved in the technology side must have a real understanding of the global health issues and community needs that we are addressing. It can be time consuming and frustrating if programmes are developed that are out of synch with our programme and its current needs. We also need to check again whether more traditional ways of working will bring better outcomes and community connection.

It will help greatly if we have tech-savvy people on our team, and also in the community. Developing an mHealth programme can be a good way of bringing greater connection with the community. Greater numbers of 'millennials' are interested, gifted, and informed about digital services. This means that for a relatively simple digital intervention, we, along with community members, may consider developing the technological component ourselves. For example, routine digital data collection surveys can easily be programmed by non-technologically minded people using open-source software such as Open Data Kit (ODK). Similarly, a programme that sends informational messages to clients could be programmed using TextIt (https://textit.in) or similar software.

However, in most cases, planning an mHealth intervention will require partnering with an organization that provides technology support. A technology partner can also help us to understand what the development and maintenance costs are likely to be. Technology partners will require a brief of our specific requirements. In order to provide a brief, we need a clear understanding of the mHealth services we are planning, as the technology partner typically estimates their costs based on hours of programming required. We should not hesitate to ask questions to clarify technical and engineering terms (see Box 26.4). Also, we must ensure that the technology partner understands how we intend the health intervention to work and who are the main users.

We also need other types of partnership. Depending on the kind of service we are planning, we may need a more formal partnership with local government stakeholders, such as health facility staff. Local NGOs or universities may already have some or all of the appropriate

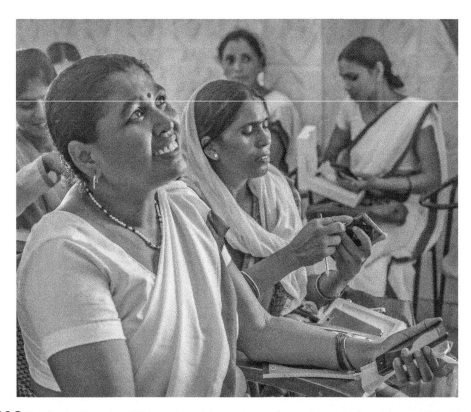

Figure 26.3 Frontline health workers (FLWs) receive training on the use of smartphones and the mSehat mobile health platform in rural Uttar Pradesh, India.

content we need. We may consider consulting local decision makers (such as governors, community leaders, teachers, etc) on the most appropriate and relevant design for the cultures we are working with. If we get this wrong, it can lead to delays, increased costs, and frustration.

Content development and testing

The first point: colleting information. In the early stages of designing an mHealth service, we collect information to help us decide whether we should use digital technology to address a particular health problem. As part of that process, we compile the profile of the individuals who will use the technology—whether they can read and write (and in what languages), how they normally use mobile phones or computers, and what devices they own. This also will help us to decide on the most appropriate type of technology to use—IVR, SMS, video, etc.

The second point: developing content. A key step is developing the content that our mHealth service will provide to an individual, either directly to patients, or in the form of a tool or guide for a health worker. To do

this we need to find out what information will be most important or useful, and how can we efficiently develop accurate information.

To address the first point, we can look at research and information on the specific topic we have chosen. For example, if we are hoping to improve community members' knowledge of HIV, there will be written and online sources of the information. These may include documented levels of awareness, common rumours and misconceptions, and gaps in knowledge in our country or area. We could also consider doing our own research with members of our community—through focus group discussions, in-depth interviews, or key-informant interviews, to gather more specific information that will help us develop the content (see Chapter 6).

To address the second point, it is always good to start with what already exists. We may have identified similar services in another part of the country and are able to use that content and adapt it to our needs. We should also look further afield to other sources of content, including existing health norms, guidelines, tools, and training

> ### Box 26.4 **Questions for technology partners**
>
> - What is their prior experience with a project of our type and size? Do they have previous experience working in our country/district setting?
> - Will an open-source software or a custom-developed/proprietary software be used? More information about types of software can be found here: https://www.k4health.org/sites/default/files/table_4.1_ict_toolkit.pdf
> - How many people can use the system at the same time? What is the total capacity of the system?
> - What kind of hardware does the programme need to operate? Hardware could include modems, types of phones, and SIM cards.
> - What kind of training and support services are provided after the initial development cycle is completed?
> - What is the annual maintenance and licensing fee? How will it change over time?
> - How often are the data backed-up?
> - How is data privacy maintained? Does it follow any local regulations?
> - Can the system integrate with other health information systems?

materials that other groups may have developed. When it comes to developing and reviewing content, we need to include a variety of individuals, including healthcare providers, intended end users, programme managers, and local leaders. This variety will expose us to a wide range of ideas and increase the numbers of people who feel engaged with the service and will be more likely to use it. Many groups create an advisory committee or technical working group for this purpose.

Content and usability testing

Once we have drafted the content, we need to organize end-user testing to determine if it is fit for purpose, that they understand it, and how it can be improved. We can do this on a small scale with anywhere between 5–15 people who are of the same profile as those who will use the service. For example, if we want to offer information about child nutrition and growth monitoring to parents, then we should identify parents of young children to review our content. If we have developed content for a series of short training films for HCWs who provide TB testing and services, then we should find a sample of those same providers to review our content. The content should be reviewed in the order that it will appear. A facilitator or interviewer should ask the group what they understand each message to mean, whether anything is confusing, and whether they would suggest any changes (Box 26.5).

Sometimes programmes choose to test the content with the users before it has been programmed into the technology, and sometimes they test it as part of the technology. The latter is called usability testing (Box 26.6). It focuses on making sure that the individual understands how to use the device itself, how to navigate through the content, how to get from one place to another, how to start and stop the service, etc. It is

another opportunity to get feedback on what the end user likes and does not like, in both the content and in the technology. For example, it helps us to see if there are specific technological problems (things that don't work as intended). We should test the content and the use of the technology at least twice. This helps us to make improvements based on feedback, and ultimately to make a better service that more people will use (Figure 26.4).

Implementing the programme

If we have followed the steps so far, then we have built a strong foundation to begin implementing our mHealth programme. We have investigated what information and tools people need, how they currently use technology, and what capacity and skills they may require to use our service. We have established partnerships with institutions and individuals who can help us design and implement the service. We have developed and tested the content and the technology to make sure that it works and that those who are supposed to use it understand how to use it.

To prepare for implementation, we must now put into place the skills, structures, and systems to support our service.

Putting together a management team

While it may sound obvious, it is essential to have a management team in place to oversee the implementation of the mHealth programme. The team may vary in size, depending on the needs of the specific mHealth programme. The team should usually include those with specific skills and understanding in training, managing partnerships, collecting and analysing data, technology, budgeting, and finance. The team will need to develop a plan for how the members communicate

---

Box 26.5 **Case study: Content testing**

After m4RH was developed and tested in Kenya and Tanzania, it was adapted and expanded for young people between 10 and 24 years of age in Rwanda. The team took the content that was already developed in those two countries and used it as the foundation for the new work in Rwanda. Using local sources of sexual and reproductive health information and input from local stakeholders on specific needs of adolescents, they developed the new content for young people. This included information on sex, pregnancy, gender-based violence, HIV, and STIs. After local stakeholders reviewed the content and suggested changes, the team conducted focus group discussions (FGDs) with young people, parents, and caregivers, as well as with influential community leaders. These FGDs helped to determine what was acceptable to the different audiences, to make it relevant to and trustworthy to young people, and to decide on the best format for messages. Ten FGDs were conducted with 15–24-year-old males and females stratified into same-gender groups of 15–17-year-olds and 18–24-year-olds. Four FGDs were conducted with adults (parents, educators, local leaders). After more revisions were incorporated, the content was programmed into the technology (in this case, USSD and SMS) and the team conducted usability testing.

Excerpt from FGD guide to test m4RH content with youth in Rwanda (This is included to show how essential it is to use the right wording in any information we provide, especially if it's in digital format)

Interviewer reads: 'Puberty' messages provide information on puberty, female bodies, male bodies, changes in emotions, and sexual decision-making. Here some examples *(Hand out slips of paper with messages written on them)*. Please read the messages.

Ingingo z'ingenzi (Puberty menu)

1. What do you understand Ingingo z'ingenzi to mean?
2. Is there a better way to say this word? *(PROBE: What language do young people use to describe this idea?)*

Message 1: Ubwangavn n' ubugimbi (Puberty)

1. What do you understand Ubwangavn n' ubugimbi to mean?
2. Is there a better way to say this word? *(PROBE: What language do young people use to describe this idea?)*

Message 2: Imibiri y'abakobwa n'imyororokere (Girls' Bodies)

1. What do you understand Imibiri y'abakobwa n'imyororokere to mean?
2. Is there a better way to say this word? (PROBE: What language do young people use to describe this idea?)

---

with each other and with others outside the team, what they will communicate about (including data collected through monitoring and evaluation), and at what frequency.

Training users on how to use the programme

This applies mainly to mHealth programmes that will be used by HCWs, managers, and administrators as part of their daily routine. As discussed, this will vary, depending on whether it is a tool on their mobile phone to help them screen children for pneumonia or an app that allows them to enter client data and automatically generate follow-up appointments sent via SMS. This training must give an overall understanding of the service and its purpose, any special requirements about client privacy or protection of personal data, and a plan for how and when to report any malfunction in the system. For services that are targeted at individual community members, training on how to use the service must also include making sure as many community members as possible know about the service and use it.

Training those individuals who will supervise and give support to users

As with any newly acquired skill, we will need to provide those using the mHealth programme with frequent support. They will need guidance on how to use it most effectively, how to solve problems and support to build their confidence. Therefore, we will need to provide training and orientation to supervisors. Supervisors and users should receive the same basic training, but supervisors should also learn how to assess the technology competence of the healthcare workers and others using the service. They must know appropriate ways of giving useful feedback on how well they are doing and on any special issues that may arise.

> ### Box 26.6 **Excerpt from m4RH usability testing guide to test technology and content with youth in Rwanda**
>
> *Interviewer says:* Thank you very much for consenting to participate in this programme today. This interview will be broken up into several sections including questions regarding the m4RH programme menus and messages. As you go through the system, I will ask you questions. Remember, there are no right or wrong answers to these questions and we are interested in both your positive and negative opinions. Do you have any questions before we begin?
>
> 1. Main menu (Level 0) (10)
>   a. Please text the word 'm4RH' to 6474.
>   b. Please read the message that you received out loud.
>   c. Please reply with the number of the language you want.
>   d. Please read the message that you received out.
>   *Note: If the participant has chosen English, ask him/her to restart and choose Kinyarwanda.*
>   *Amount of time passed while participant read the introduction screen_____*
>
> 2. Based on the response you received what can you do? What would you do if you wanted information about 'puberty'? What would you do if you wanted information about 'sex and pregnancy'?
>
> 3. Topic Menus (Level 1) (10)
>   Please choose one of the first three options.
>   a. Did you receive another menu of choices? Please look at it now and read the menu out loud.
>   b. Based on the response you received what can you do?
>   c. If you accidentally selected this information (e.g. replied with the wrong code) or if you wished to receive additional or other information, what would you do?
>
> 4. Messages (Level 2) (10)
>   Please look at the text messages you received.
>   a. How many messages did you receive?
>   b. Were they in the correct order?
>   c. Please read the messages you received out loud.
>   *Note: Please note if the participant had trouble reading the message*
>   *How easy or difficult was it for participant to read the text messages? Easy, Okay, Difficult*
>   d. Is this the information you expected to receive? [If no, what information did you expect to receive?]
>   e. What did you think of the length of the message? [PROBE was it too long, too short, or just right?]
>   f. Was it new information? Was the information useful? Do you trust the information?
>   g. What would you do if you wanted information about another topic?

Encouraging responsibility and maintaining interest

In some cases, we may decide to actually provide phones or tablets to health workers or community members to use as part of our mHealth programme. Many programmes around the world have done this, including the one million health worker programme (Chapter 8). Inevitably, there have been cases of people losing or stealing phones or misusing them for personal purposes (rather than strictly for work). If we decide to provide phones or tablets, we should draw up a simple contract for the recipient to sign that outlines expectations for proper use, or any penalties for recurrent misuse (e.g. reimbursing all or part of the cost of the device in case of loss). This helps people to take greater responsibility when they receive the smartphone or other hardware. One other problem commonly occurs. A new piece of technology can be very exciting

at first, but users lose interest as time passes, unless it is clearly relevant to their needs. A clear statement about the correct and ongoing use of the device should also be included. Supervisors can point users to the contract when this and other problems arise.

Making sure people know about the new mHealth service

Part of our planning and preparation is making sure people are aware of our mHealth service. We should have already included a variety of people in our previous discussions, plans and training, such as local leaders, health workers, programme managers and, community members. However, for an mHealth service that will be used by the wider community and beyond, we need to think about how they will hear about it. We can promote or advertise the service in many ways—on radio, using posters

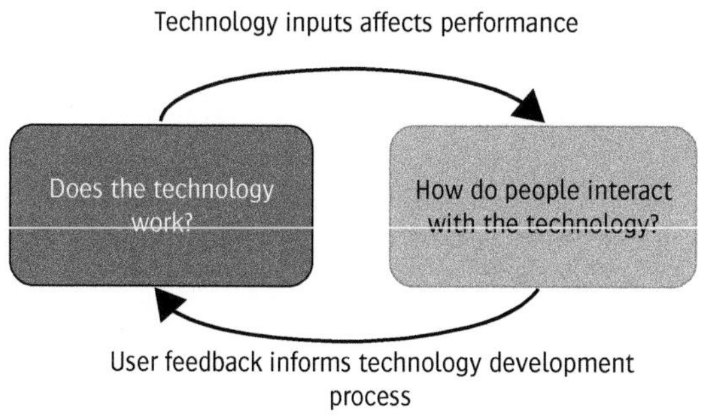

Technology inputs affects performance

User feedback informs technology development
process

Figure 26.4 People and technology.

or flyers, or through community talks or household visits. HCWs including CHWs can inform the community about the service in the health clinic or in people's homes.

Doing a trial-run before full-scale implementation

It is essential to schedule a thorough trial-run, prior to full-scale implementation. This is called 'beta-testing.' Although we have already tested the technology once or twice, this provides another opportunity to see how the technology operates on a slightly larger scale in the real-world setting, and to work out any kinks. It is a way to minimize the risk of big, unexpected problems arising

later (Figure 26.4; Box 26.7). Once we have conducted a trial-run, we are ready to fully launch our mHealth service, to support and monitor its use and effectiveness, and to make on-going improvements as necessary.

Monitoring mHealth programmes

mHealth programmes need to be continuously monitored to make sure they are working as intended and reaching our target communities. We can use traditional principles of monitoring and evaluations described in Chapter 9. mHealth programmes also have technical components that need to be assessed as easily as possible. For example, most mHealth programmes have some level of automated data collection, usually referred to as 'backend data', so a programme that sends informational text messages to users will automatically collect information, such as what day and time the message was sent (i.e. timestamp), to which clients the information was sent, and whether the message was received and opened. By using this information, it becomes possible to monitor, over time, the number of individuals that the programme has successfully reached.

It is easy to become overwhelmed by the large amount of data that mHealth systems can produce, especially if we do not have experienced data analysts on our team. From the start, we need to determine the indicators that are of most interest. We then need to discuss with the technology partner how to capture and analyse this data. Usually the technology partner will provide

---

Box 26.7 **Further tips for successful implementation**

1. Build around the existing workflow patterns and the felt needs of health workers.
   a. Build solutions to real problems faced by health workers.
   b. Time is precious—avoid adding unnecessary new tasks that take more time.
   c. Data collected should be useful to the collector as well as the manager.
2. Minimize recurrent costs by ensuring technology is used for designed functions and not inappropriately overused.
   a. Do not rely on distant experts.
   b. Create point-of-care applications and 'tech fixers' that provide answers directly and quickly by those trained in the community. Delays are frustrating for all.

c. Build on existing programmes instead of replacing them.
3. Ensure phone applications function the same way a mobile phone app usually functions.
4. Thoroughly test any new application or device before release.
   a. After release, do 'post-marketing surveillance' of their use in the field.
   b. Avoid adding in apps for leisure purposes that can be distracting.

data on a regular (weekly, monthly, etc.) basis, or provide us access to a dashboard that allows us download the information in a spreadsheet (such as MS Excel), or simply view our data onscreen.

Choice of indicators is especially important. For example, in areas where mobile network reception is poor, we will need to monitor whether the messages sent to the clients are actually being received. If the programme intends CHWs to have mutual links with community members about specific health issues, data will be generated each time a community member asks a question, receives an answer, or offers information. We should identify, as a team, which services are most important for us to monitor, and define the most appropriate indicators.

Further reading and resources

Källander K, Tibenderana JK, Agpogheneta OJ, Strachan DL, Hill Z, ten Asbroek AHA, et al. Mobile health (mHealth) approaches and lessons for increased performance and retention of community health workers in low-and middle-income countries: A review. *Journal of Medical Internet Research*. 2013; 15 (1): e17. DOI: 10.2196/jmir.2130

Labrique AB, Vasudevan L, Kochi E, Fabricant R, Mehl G. mHealth innovations as health system strengthening tools: 12 common applications and a visual framework. *Global Health: Science and Practice*. 2013; 1 (2): 1–12.

Mitchell M, Hedt-Gauthier BL, Msellemu D, Nkaka M, Lesh N. Using electronic technology to improve clinical care–results from a before-after cluster trial to evaluate assessment and classification of sick children according to Integrated Management of Childhood Illness (IMCI) protocol in Tanzania. *BMC Medical Informatics and Decision Making*. 2013; 13 (95). DOI: 10.1186/1472-6947-13-95

World Health Organization. Monitoring and evaluating digital health interventions: a practical guide to conducting research and assessment. 2016. Available from: http://apps.who.int/iris/bitstream/10665/252183/1/9789241511766-eng.pdf

Useful weblinks

Global Digital Health Network website: https://www.mhealthworkinggroup.org/

Hesperian Foundation, http://www.hesperian.org produces apps and a wide variety of valuable online resources for use at community level

International Telecommunication Union. National eHealth Strategy Toolkit. Available from: http://www.itu.int/pub/D-STR-E_HEALTH.05-2012

mHealth Assessment and Planning for Scale (MAPS) Toolkit: http://who.int/reproductivehealth/topics/mhealth/maps-toolkit/en/

mHealth Evidence: https://www.mhealthevidence.org/

mHealth Knowledge: http://mhealthknowledge.org/

mHealth Planning Guide: https://www.k4health.org/toolkits/mhealth-planning-guide

Principles for Digital Development: http://digitalprinciples.org/

References

1. UN Foundation. *What we do: Mobile Alliance for Maternal Action (MAMA)*. 2013. Available from: http://www.unfoundation.org/what-we-do/issues/global-health/mobile-health-for-development/mama.html

2. Department of Health, Republic of South Africa. *Momconnect briefing*. Available from: http://www.health.gov.za/index.php/mom-connect

3. FHI 360. *Mobile 4 Reproductive Health Toolkit*, 2016. Available from: https://www.fhi360.org/sites/default/files/media/documents/resource-m4rh-toolkit.pdf

4. Ippoliti NB, L'Engle K. Meet us on the phone: Mobile phone programs for adolescent sexual and reproductive health in low-to-middle income countries. *Reproductive Health*. 2017; 14:11. DOI: 10.1186/s12978-016-0276-z

5. Chamberlain S. A mobile guide toward better health: How Mobile Kunji is improving birth outcomes in Bihar, India. *Innovations: Technology, Governance, Globalization*. 2014; 9 (3–4): 47–56. Available from: http://mitpressjournals.org/userimages/ContentEditor/1415302178306/INNOVATIONS_DIGITAL-INCLUSION.pdf

6. D Tree International. *Tella Matias uses mobile app to save lives in Malawi*. 2016. Available from: http://www.d-tree.org/success-story-tella-matias-uses-mobile-app-save-lives-malawi/

7. D Tree International. *Safer deliveries*. Available from: http://www.d-tree.org/saving-lives/womens-lives/safer-deliveries

8. mHealth cStock. *Supply Chains 4 Community Case Management*. Available from: http://sc4ccm.jsi.com/emerging-lessons/cstock/

9. Mhero. Available from: http://www.mhero.org/

10. MHealth Knowledge. Available from: http://mhealthknowledge.org/

11. Global Digital Health Network Listserv (formerly the mHealth Working Group). Available from: http://www.mhealthknowledge.org/resources/global-digital-health-network-listserv-formerly-mhealth-working-group

CHAPTER 27

Community-level responses to domestic violence and abuse

Peter Grant and Amanda Marshall

This chapter looks at issues of violence and abuse at the community level, and outlines some responses, both immediate and longer-term. Violence can take many forms and has many causes, which on a wider scale is often through ethnic, economic, and political conflicts. This chapter focuses mainly on domestic abuse usually by men against women. Violence and abuse result from a breakdown of relationships and the abuse of power. Reconciliation needs to address these basic issues and focus on restoring relationships.

In the words of former UN Secretary General Ban Ki-moon, 'There is one universal truth, applicable to all countries, cultures and communities: violence against women is never acceptable, never excusable, never tolerable.'[1] And yet one in three women worldwide will suffer violence during her lifetime. Violence against women occurs in every nation and community in the world (Figure 27.1).

What we need to know

Definitions and incidence of violence and abuse

The United Nations has a complex but full definition of violence against women as 'any act of gender-based violence that results in, or is likely to result in, physical, sexual, or psychological harm or suffering to women,

including threats of such acts, coercion, or arbitrary deprivation of liberty, whether occurring in public or in private life.'[2]

Violence against women and girls (VAWG) shows itself in four main ways: physical, sexual, emotional, and economic abuse. The most universal ways in which these are shown include domestic and intimate partner

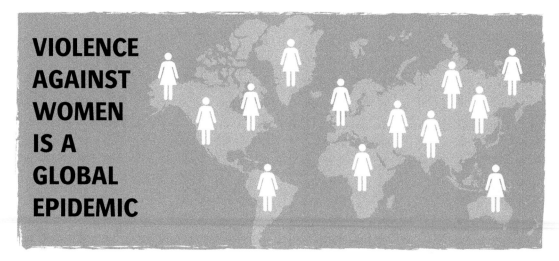

Figure 27.1 Violence against women is a global experience.
Reproduced courtesy of Restored Relationships, https://www.restoredrelationships.org/. This image is distributed under the terms of the Creative Commons Attribution Non-Commercial 4.0 International licence (CC-BY-NC), a copy of which is available at http://creativecommons.org/licenses/by-nc/4.0/

violence, non-partner sexual violence (including rape in warfare), sexual trafficking, bullying, and sexual harassment.

Other widespread forms worldwide include harmful practices, such as female genital mutilation/cutting (FGM/C) and child, early, and forced marriage (CEFM). Less-documented forms include crimes committed in the name of 'honour': femicide, prenatal sex selection, female infanticide, elder abuse, dowry-related violence, bride kidnapping, and acid-throwing.

Women and girls are at risk of multiple forms of violence throughout their lives. In some countries up to 70 per cent of women have experienced physical and/or sexual violence in their lifetime from an intimate partner.[3] Further, virtually all women are affected by the *possibility* of violence and *threats* to their emotional and physical well-being.[4]

Domestic abuse

Phumzile Mlambo Ngcuka, the current (2017) Executive Director of UN Women, has stated 'All countries worry me because of the universality of violence against women. The fact that 75% of violence against women is domestic violence is the issue. The home is the unsafest place for a woman to be.'[5]

Domestic abuse is characterized by controlling and coercive behaviour. *Controlling behaviour* is designed to make a person feel inadequate and/or dependent by regulating their everyday actions, isolating them from others' support and depriving them of the means of

independence, resistance, and escape. In addition, the perpetrator often exploits the victim's personal resources for themselves. *Coercive behaviour* is an act or a pattern of assaults, threats, humiliation, intimidation, or other abuse used to harm, punish, or frighten the victim.

Domestic abuse is a repeated pattern of behaviour. It happens in all kinds of relationships, both heterosexual and same sex. It can happen between people who are dating, have children together, are partnered or married to each other, when people live together or separately, and even after the relationship or marriage has ended. Domestic abuse is largely founded on gender inequality and discrimination against women. At its heart is the abuse of power over another individual.

Domestic abuse can happen to anyone regardless of age, race, disability, sexuality, class, or income

- Women are particularly vulnerable to abuse when pregnant or seeking to leave a relationship.
- Older people and disabled people can be particularly vulnerable to domestic abuse.
- Children experience domestic abuse in many ways, including through directly intervening to protect one of their parents, being forced to join the adult abuser, and hearing and witnessing violent attacks and brutality.
- Coercive and controlling behaviour in a domestic situation is usually exerted over the whole family so any children suffer as well as the adult victim.

The impact and consequences of abuse can be devastating and lifelong. Women may suffer the horrific consequences of abuse such as broken bones, lifelong health issues, diminished roles in public and private life, and loss of earning power. It also leads to loss of relationships with friends and family, loss of self-confidence, and to psychological trauma which is often life long. In the worst cases, violence against women results in the loss of life itself.

Sexual violence

Sexual violence affects an estimated one in five women globally. The impact and consequences of an intimate violation of the body can result in extensive physical and psychological trauma, along with unwanted pregnancies. Sexual violence in conflict has been long recognized as a tactic of war. In the Democratic Republic of Congo (DRC) an average of 36 women and girls are raped every day. It is estimated that 200,000 women have been raped in the DRC since the conflict began.[6] During the genocide in Rwanda in 1994 it is estimated that around 250,000 women were raped.[7]

Female genital mutilation

Female genital mutilation is one of the most widespread and severe forms of sexual violence:

It is estimated that at least 200 million women and girls currently live with the consequences of FGM. Carried out on females of various ages, from newborns to women about to be married, FGM is prevalent in 28 countries in Africa, alongside some communities in the Middle East and Asia, as well as within certain ethnic groups in Central and South America. However, FGM is not a phenomenon that is limited to the above-mentioned geographical regions. Increasingly, other countries are faced with the challenge of FGM within diasporas in Europe, the USA, Canada, Australia and New Zealand.[8]

One of the main challenges of the current worldwide campaign against FGM is the trend of medicalization. Medicalized FGM has been defined by the World Health Organization (WHO) as FGM carried out by a member of any category of *health care provider*, regardless of the setting in which the procedure takes place.

Global action on VAWG

In recent years, there has been increased global commitment to addressing VAWG, and greater international co-ordination. Recently, efforts to tackle VAWG have been given greater emphasis by two important global statements. The first is the inclusion of commitments on VAWG in the Sustainable Development Goals (SDGs). SDG 5 commits signatory states to achieve gender equality and empower all women and girls. It includes these specific targets:

- Eliminate all forms of violence against all women and girls in the public and private spheres, including trafficking and sexual and other types of exploitation.
- Eliminate all harmful practices, such as child, early, and forced marriage and female genital mutilation.

The second global statement is the 57th session of the Commission on the Status of Women (CSW57) in 2013 for which 'the elimination and prevention of all forms of violence against women and girls' was the priority theme. CSW57 called on member states to take measures to tackle VAWG.[9]

Current research summary

According to Lori Heise's widely accepted ecological model, violence is caused by many factors that interact at various levels of the 'social ecology', not only the level of the individual, but also the household, community, and society.[10] The likelihood that a man will become abusive, that a woman will be abused, or that one community will have a higher rate of violence than another depends on many factors that interact at different levels. Social ecology includes the life histories and personalities that men and women bring to their relationships, as well as the context of their everyday lives. The ecology also includes social norms and structural factors: outside factors such as religious institutions and ideology, the way economic power is distributed between men and women, and factors such as laws and policies to prevent and punish violence. Often these are not implemented because many legal systems reinforce gender inequalities.

Some factors are nearly always associated with VAWG, while others are more specific to the context. Factors that are commonly present and increase the risk of VAWG[11] include:

- For domestic abuse:
  - exposure to violence in childhood
  - presence of community norms that support wife or partner abuse; and
  - binge drinking, harmful notions of masculinity and rigid gender roles.
- For non-partner sexual violence, the factors are:
  - adverse childhood experiences;
  - personality disorders;
  - peer influences; and

- delinquency and ideals of masculinity that emphasize heterosexual performance and control of women.

VAWG has many negative consequences for women and girls, and more widely. VAWG is a major cause of ill health among women and girls. Its impact can be seen in death and disability caused by injuries, exposure to sexually transmitted infections (STIs), increased physical and mental illness, and alcohol abuse. VAWG may also result in unwanted pregnancy and abortions and low birth weight among infants. Violence and the fear of violence severely limit women's ability to escape poverty, and their potential contributions to social and economic development.[12]

Overall research concludes that interventions covering a number of areas are more effective than single-component ones in preventing VAWG. For example, media campaigns were more effective when combined with targeted outreach efforts and training workshops at local level. Livelihood programmes alone were less effective than those which included gender training.[13]

What we need to do

Involve men

Men are the main, but not the only, perpetrators of all forms of violence and abuse. But only a minority of men are perpetrators. Men must take responsibility in approaches to ending violence and abuse at community level. It is their actions that need to change if violence is to be halted. In their roles as faith and community leaders, it is also often men who have to take the lead in responding to violence.

In recent years, there has been a greater emphasis on working with men and boys to address violence against women. The reasons and ways of doing this have evolved over time, and have faced criticism from some. In 2014, an academic article in *The Lancet* discussed how interventions that help prevent abuse have developed from simply treating men as perpetrators of VAWG to approaches that seek to transform the relations, social norms, and systems that sustain gender inequality and violence.[14] The authors recommend that future interventions should emphasize work with both men and boys and women and girls to change social norms on gender relations. Also, it recommends that programme design should bear in mind the differences between men and women.

Evidence suggests that it is important to work with men and boys and that interventions working with both men and women are more effective than single-sex interventions. It also showed that helping to transform ideas of gender is more effective than simply working through attitude and behaviour change.[15] Similarly, guidance published by the UK's Department for International Development suggests that programmes targeting men and boys are effective at tackling VAWG only when they explicitly focus on transforming unequal power relations between women and men, including promoting alternative notions of masculinity.

A report by the UK's Gender and Development Network[16] (GADN) describes how faith organizations and faith leaders can have a strong impact, both positive and negative, on how VAWG is perceived within local communities. It also explains how CSOs are placing greater emphasis on including people of faith to help end violence. The GADN states that this is particularly important with the current rise of religious fundamentalisms. It cites research by the Association for Women's Rights in Development, which has found that women's rights activists frequently mention that VAWG increases with religious fundamentalism.

Community-level justice and reconciliation

Many countries do not have functioning legal systems that deal effectively with violence and abuse at community level. This means that communities need to set up systems that hold perpetrators of violence to account so that they have to face the consequences.

Most perpetrators are men, which reflects the sense of male privilege and entitlement that are so prevalent in our societies. This is seen, for example, within churches or other religious bodies. Church and other faith leaders, spouses, and prominent lay members have been found to be perpetrators of abuse. More recently, sport and, in particular, football clubs have been centres of abuse. Corporations, political parties, and the film industry are increasingly being discovered as centres of serious and often hidden abuse, which have given rise to worldwide movements such as the #MeToo Movement (https://metoomvmt.org).

It is vital that all organizations and institutions within society consider how they may be condoning domestic and sexual abuse and what they can do to prevent it.

Being accountable and knowing that there are serious consequences are important ways of reducing abuse. Seeing change in perpetrators is a long-term process. There are some programmes which aim to change some of the underlying attitudes and beliefs that drive domestic abuse, but they are very expensive and unlikely to be a realistic option for most communities.

NB: It is also important to remember that homophobic abuse is widespread and that male rape is significant, particularly in armed conflict.[17]

Debunking myths

Many people have conceptions and attitudes about domestic abuse that are incorrect. It is important for us to challenge these myths. Helping people to learn new and more enlightened attitudes is also needed if communities are to address violence effectively, without stigmatizing victims. The next sections describe some common myths about domestic abuse.

Myth 1: It happens to certain types of people

Many people assume that domestic abuse happens to people from certain socio-economic, religious, or cultural backgrounds. This is not the case. Although domestic abuse and violence may be more common in certain contexts, it can happen to anyone at any time.

Myth 2: It happens because of …

Domestic abuse is complex, and is not easily explained by a single theory. We may think that abuse happens because of alcohol misuse, unemployment, being abused as a child, mental or physical ill health, or other environmental factors. Although these may be contributory factors, abuse basically happens because an abusive person chooses to behave in that way. Often perpetrators use the list above to give reasons and excuses for their behaviour.

Myth 3: A victim can cause a perpetrator to become abusive

Often an abusive person will tell a victim 'you made me do it'. A victim is never responsible if a perpetrator chooses to behave in an abusive and controlling way.

Myth 4: A victim can fully understand what is happening to them

When someone is in a relationship where they are subject to abuse, they will often feel very confused about what is happening. They are sometimes not even sure that what they are experiencing is abuse or not.

Myth 5: A victim can choose to leave; if they don't, they are choosing to stay

People ask why victims continue to stay in a situation where they are suffering abuse. They assume that it is easy to leave and to escape their situation and start a new life. This is not the case on either an emotional or a practical level. A perpetrator will work to ensure that the victim feels that they cannot cope on their own—that leaving is a dangerous or impossible thing to do. Practically, it may be financially impossible to leave the situation, particularly when there are children. It may be safer to stay than to leave.

Myth 6: Domestic abuse is about anger

Domestic abuse is a choice to act in a controlling way. It is not primarily about being angry, but often does include anger or fake anger.

Myth 7: Domestic abuse doesn't happen in our community

Domestic abuse happens in every community. With one in three women affected, it is extremely likely that there will be those in our locality who have been affected by domestic abuse.

Sexual violence and rape also carry powerful myths around sex, temptation, and location. Myths abound, resulting in attitudes like 'what did she expect wearing that?', 'what was she doing there at that time of night?', and 'he is a man and he needs sex'. Rape is about power and abuse of power and control, and using sex as a tool of that power for the destruction of the woman. Statistics show that most rape is committed by a person the woman knows, dispelling the myth that strangers are the main danger.

Understand specific forms of abuse

In addressing VAWG at community level we also need to mention specific forms of abuse that are dependent on culture. These include honour crimes, honour killings, forced marriage, female genital mutilation, abuse of children and women related to alleged possession by evil spirits, or dowry problems. In all these contexts, the need to protect the victim is the main priority, irrespective of the cultural context in which the domestic violence occurs. Some of the forms of abuse mentioned here are frequently found in the context of a variety of religions and educational backgrounds. Leaders often justify them as a way to assert patriarchal power and control. Often the violence is carried out by members of the same extended family, with the collusion of others in the community.

Honour-based violence (HBV)

HBV is defined as 'a collection of practices, which are used to control behaviour within families or other social groups in order to protect perceived cultural and religious beliefs and/or honour'.[18] Such violence often occurs when perpetrators perceive that a relative has shamed the family or community by breaking an 'honour code'. The honour code is set at the discretion of male relatives. Women who do not abide by the code are punished for bringing shame on the family. Practices seen to justify HBV may include an intimate relationship outside of marriage; rejecting a forced marriage; becoming pregnant outside marriage; interfaith relationships; seeking divorce, and inappropriate dress or make-up.

Women and girls are the most common victims of HBV. However, males can also be victims. Examples include when a relationship is thought to be inappropriate because it is, or may be perceived as, same-sex, or when a present or future partner has a disability. HBV is not only perpetrated by men. Sometimes female relatives will support, incite, or assist. It is also not unusual for younger relatives to be selected to undertake the abuse, as a way to protect senior members of the family, or as a way of showing them the consequences if they ever dishonour the family name.

Crimes committed in the name of 'honour' might include:

- domestic abuse;
- threats of violence;
- physical assault;
- sexual or psychological abuse;
- forced marriage; or
- being held or taken somewhere forcibly.

Forced marriage

A forced marriage is one where either, or both, people in the marriage do not (or in cases of people with learning disabilities, cannot) consent to it. There is a clear distinction between a forced marriage and an arranged marriage. In arranged marriages, the families of both spouses take a leading role in arranging the marriage, but the choice of whether or not to accept the arrangement still remains with the couple involved.

However, in forced marriages, one or both spouses are coerced into it. The pressure put on people to marry against their will can be physical: threats, actual physical violence, and sexual violence. It can also be emotional and psychological, e.g. when someone is made to feel they are bringing shame on their family. Financial abuse such as taking away wages or refusing to give money also happens. Vulnerable adults who lack the capacity to consent to marriage may not be directly coerced—it is just made to happen.

When we come across a case of forced marriages, we should not dismiss it as a simple domestic issue. For many people, seeking help is a last resort, meaning that all disclosures of forced marriage should be taken seriously.

Female genital mutilation (FGM/C)

Sometimes referred to as female circumcision or cutting, (FGM/C) refers to procedures that intentionally alter or cause injury to the female genital organs for non-medical reasons. FGM/C affects between 100 and 140 million girls worldwide with another three million girls estimated to be at risk of FGM.[19]

School-aged girls living in cities or studying in other countries may be taken back to their home villages so that FGM/C can be carried out during the school holidays. This allows them time to 'heal' before they return to school. FGM/C does not just affect children and adolescents. It is also carried out on adults.

Case histories and personal accounts indicate that FGM/C is an extremely traumatic experience for girls and women that stays with them for the rest of their lives. For boys, group circumcision in some cultures may involve coercion and abuse.

Where harmful traditional practices such as child marriage and FGM/C are widely practised, they are social norms which both men and women support. Anyone departing from the norm may be condemned, harassed, or ostracised. FGM/C is a deep-rooted social practice that is entrenched in the culture, with origins going back thousands of years.[20] It is even believed that it is in the girl's best interests, because uncut girls cannot marry and will be stigmatized or even thrown out of the community. A systematic review of FGM/C interventions in Africa found that the main factors that supported FGM/C were tradition, religion, and the need to reduce a woman's sexual desire.[21] FGM/C is not required by any religion, but religion may sometimes become one driver of the practice, e.g. in some areas it is incorrectly believed to be a requirement of Islam.

Child- or adolescent-to-parent abuse

This type of abuse is likely to be a *pattern of behaviour*. This can include physical violence from a child or adolescent towards a parent, or other abusive behaviours, such as damage to property, emotional abuse, and economic/financial abuse. These forms of abuse can occur together or separately.

Abusive behaviours can include, but are not limited to humiliating language and threats, belittling a parent, damaging property, stealing from a parent, and displaying heightened sexualized behaviours to shock parents. Patterns of coercive control are often seen. Some families experience episodes of explosive physical violence from their adolescents, with periods of fewer controlling, abusive behaviours. We also need to understand the pattern of behaviour in the family as a whole. For example, siblings may also be abused or abusive. There may be past or current domestic abuse between the parents of the young person.

Domestic abuse is notoriously difficult to identify. This can become even harder if the abuse is child- or adolescent-to-parent abuse. Like other forms of domestic abuse, it is very likely to be under-reported. Many affected families may be facing multiple issues such as substance use, mental health issues, and domestic violence. Many families may not recognize that they need support for this issue and may feel unable to ask for help due to stigma and shame. Other issues include a lack of awareness of existing support (e.g. family support groups); parents not seeing themselves as legitimate recipients of support; lack of knowledge on drugs, alcohol, and their effects; an 'it'll never happen to us' mind-set; and a lack of consensus on the best course of action within couples.

We need to recognize the effects that this form of abuse may have on both the parent and the young person. Only then can we establish trust and support for both. It is important that a young person using abusive behaviour against a parent receives a response that also safeguards them.

Elder abuse

Elder abuse is a hidden, and often ignored, problem in society. It is the mistreatment of an older person, and both older men and women can be at risk. People can be abused in different ways, including physical, psychological, financial, sexual, and spiritual abuse. Neglect is common, including inappropriate use of medication. The abuse can occur anywhere: someone's own home; a carer's home; day care; residential care; a nursing home or hospital. The abuser is usually well-known to the person being abused. They may be a partner, son, or daughter; a friend or neighbour; a paid or volunteer care worker; a health or social worker, or other professional. Older people may also be abused by a person they care for.

There is a variety of reasons why abuse occurs. Abuse may range from a spontaneous act of frustration to systematic premeditated assaults on an older person. At home, a common cause is a carer feeling unable to provide the level of care required. There is also the frustration of caring 24 hours a day, often without a break, for an older person who needs extensive care, e.g. those with dementia or other chronic problems.

Teenage-related abuse

This type of abuse occurs in the age group of those between 16 and 24 years of age, and those in this group are at quite high risk of domestic abuse. Domestic abuse is still a 'hidden' issue in society; it is even more so for teenagers. This is made worse by the fact that adolescents can be more accepting of, and dismissive about, this form of behaviour than adults. It is important to remember that cases involving those under 18 years of age may include a mix of domestic abuse, sexual abuse, child sexual exploitation, and street gang-related sexual and other violence. Sexification, pornification, and grooming largely through social media and mobile phones, e.g. 'sexting', are extremely widespread.

These experiences may have both immediate and long-term effects on young people. One feature of teenage-related abuse which can be unique and challenging is the difficulty in finding support. Simply because of their age, many young people are unable to access the same levels of support as over 18s. There may be also safeguarding factors to consider when working with young perpetrators of violence, as they may be subject to abuse themselves.

Raise awareness at community level for prevention, and 'do no harm'

As individuals and organizations, we can play a key role in preventing domestic abuse. We can raise awareness and challenge attitudes and behaviours that create a culture in which domestic abuse is tolerated or accepted. There are many opportunities to do this through community organizations, faith groups, and by working with groups of adults and young people. One particular opportunity to raise these issues is in marriage preparation courses, which can be useful in many cultures.

Other ways we can work specifically to raise awareness of abuse

- Run school-based programmes where children and adolescents learn the norms of behaviour; these can be powerful entry points for interventions.
- Health services are an ideal place to identify and start to address the violence that women and girls suffer at home. In many contexts, health services are the first port of call for women who have experienced VAWG. Health care settings allow women and children to talk about experiences and receive a safe, supportive response. Communities can make leaflets and books available and there are helpful websites which highlight the nature of abuse and ways of giving advice. It is good practice for us to discuss issues openly.
- Raise awareness powerfully through the arts, such as theatre and poetry, tapping into research about what works well.
- Families and communities can model positive, healthy relationships that break cultural stereotypes and treat women with dignity and respect. They can be bold in standing against a culture that diminishes women, and challenge others when women are treated abusively (see Box 27.1).

There are also group-based approaches which are known to work. These include:

- Relationship-level interventions working with males and females (NB: commonly-used couple counselling and anger management approaches tend not to be effective in dealing with domestic abuse).
- Group-based microfinance combined with training on gender.
- Working with communities to change social norms.
- Protection orders, shelters and parenting programmes.

Finally, routine screening of women for experience of violence in health facilities is not helpful for prevention, nor is arrest in cases of domestic violence, although this may be necessary for the protection of the women and children affected.

Be informed and aware of the legal position and of local services

When involved in abuse situations, we must have a basic knowledge of the rights of those affected by violence and the legal situation in the country where we are working. We should link into available local services where these are available. Organizations, such as those providing services for women affected by violence, often need practical support within agreed guidelines. For example, practical items are needed for safe houses, since women have often left home with very little clothing or other essentials.

Box 27.1 **An example from Burkina Faso**

Modelling healthy relationships can be a powerful witness to the local community as a church in Vipalgo village, Burkina Faso discovered. They taught a marriage course and invited couples from the church to take part. The marriage course ran over several weeks with couples putting into practice what they had learned each week. Neighbours started to notice changes happening in the households. One couple said that their neighbours began to visit on a regular basis and chat and observe how the couple were interacting with one another. The biggest change came when, completely against the local culture, the husband moved into the same house as his wife and children. In that particular culture, the husbands usually had a separate home in order that they could sleep well and not be bothered by the children in the night. The subtle changes, and this big change, saw neighbours, friends, and others in the village come to the local church and ask the pastor if they could join the course. They had witnessed the positive improvements in the relationships of the couples attending the marriage course and wanted it for themselves.

Respond appropriately to victims and survivors

Many different models and methods have been used to tackle VAWG. These include finding ways to prevent and respond to abuse, working across different government, social, and civil society sectors, and being guided by the best ways of addressing different forms of violence, according to the best evidence.

Examples of ways we can respond appropriately to victims and survivors include:

- Psychosocial counselling, through trained providers
- Special programmes for perpetrators
- Physical response such as shelters, specialised gender units in police stations, safe homes
- Responses based on legal and justice approaches
- Population-based prevention such as awareness-raising campaigns, social marketing approaches and group education

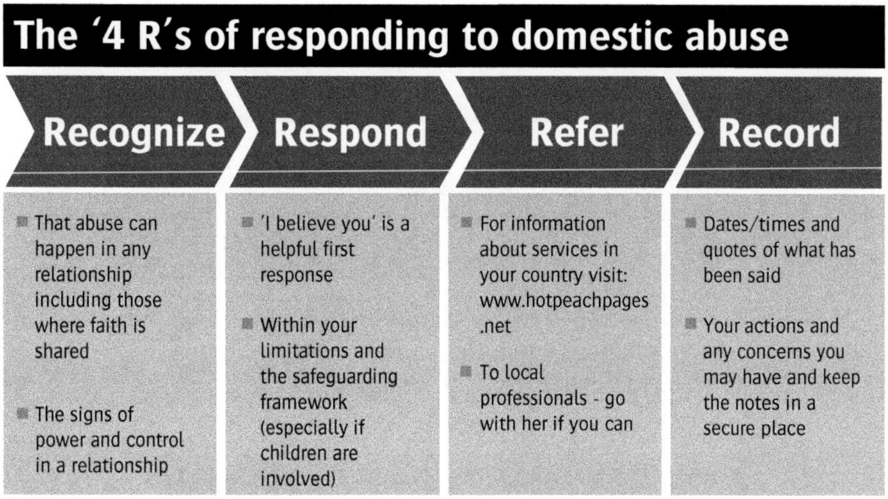

The '4 R's of responding to domestic abuse

Recognize	Respond	Refer	Record
▪ That abuse can happen in any relationship including those where faith is shared ▪ The signs of power and control in a relationship	▪ 'I believe you' is a helpful first response ▪ Within your limitations and the safeguarding framework (especially if children are involved)	▪ For information about services in your country visit: www.hotpeachpages .net ▪ To local professionals - go with her if you can	▪ Dates/times and quotes of what has been said ▪ Your actions and any concerns you may have and keep the notes in a secure place

Figure 27.2 The 4Rs: Recognise, respond, refer, record.

Reproduced with permission from Church of England. 2011. Responding well to domestic abuse. Available at: https://www.restoredrelationships.org/. This image is distributed under the terms of the Creative Commons Attribution Non-Commercial 4.0 International licence (CC-BY-NC), a copy of which is available at http://creativecommons.org/licenses/by-nc/4.0/

- Group-based training or workshops for prevention of VAWG, including empowerment training for women and girls, school or community workshops to promote changes in social norms and in behaviours that encourage VAWG
- Responses to reduce poverty and improve livelihoods

Good frameworks for looking at response are given in Figures 27.2 and 27.3:

We can also look at the 5Ps:

- *Prevention*—education, awareness, cultural change.
- *Protection*—law, policing.
- *Provision*—rape crisis, refuges, counselling, and support.
- *Prosecution*—implementing the law, community-level justice.
- *Partnership*—working with others locally and nationally who have expertise.

It is difficult to draw up a simple list to identify if domestic abuse is happening, because abuse can occur on many levels and in many ways. Also, both victims and perpetrators can behave and respond in a range of different ways. We can use the following list for guidance but it is not exhaustive:

- Unexplained bruises/injuries, providing excuses for the injuries, e.g. an accidental fall;
- Signs of feeling suicidal;
- Becoming unusually quiet or withdrawn;
- Panic attacks;
- Frequent absences from work or other commitments;
- Wearing clothes that conceal, even on warm days;
- Stopping talking about her/his partner;
- Unusually anxious or rushes away;
- Never appearing alone in public but always accompanied by their partner;
- Becoming more isolated, possibly moving away from home, withdrawing from friends and family;
- Children—being 'clingy', tired, and lethargic, having behavioural difficulties, and struggling in social settings and at school.

We must always consider safety of children and victims, as well as our own. For example, telephone calls, written information about domestic abuse support services, texts, e-mails, photographs and accessing relevant websites all create potential risks when these are discovered.

If a victim discloses abuse, we should consider that most survivors want to be asked. If we are able to broach the subject, our offer of help could be the first step in enabling them to seek help. For example, we could ask: 'How are things at home?' and if it becomes appropriate, 'Is anyone hurting you?' If these types of conversation do happen, try wherever possible to talk in a safe, private place where there will be no interruption, or arrange to talk again; someone in distress may start talking anywhere.

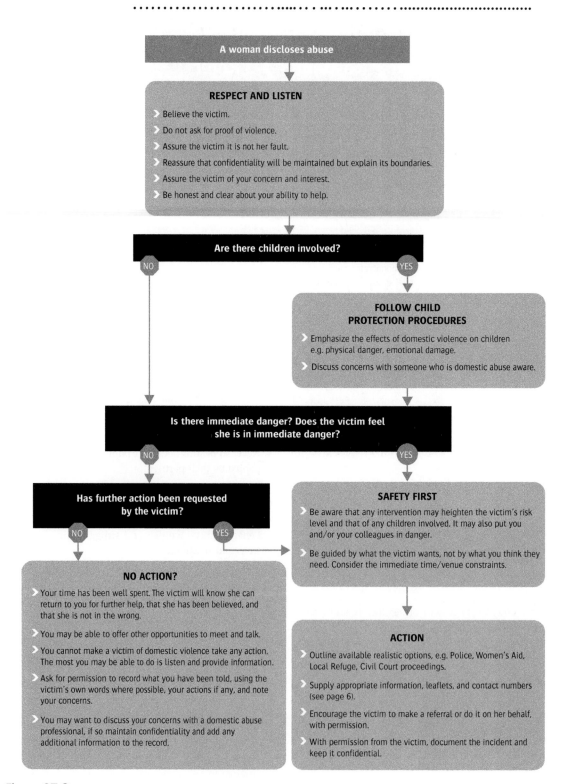

Figure 27.3 Responding appropriately to victims and survivors.

> ### Box 27.2 **Examples of effective responses**
>
> - HEAL Africa in DRC have promoted community education for changing traditional law and practices, setting up a safe house, and linking to local police and lawyers.
> - Campaigns, including One Man Can in South Africa and First Man Standing in the UK, have engaged men in speaking out against violence against women.
> - A church in the UK has linked to a local refuge and provided care packages, plus help with moving on and into housing, repairing fences, cupboards, painting, and other moving-in practicalities.
> - Vigilance in Burkina Faso have provided youth relationship education and Christian AIDS Taskforce in Zimbabwe have provided relationship and gender education.

We must also try to make it clear that complete confidentiality cannot be guaranteed, depending on the nature of what is disclosed. While we might respect an individual's right to confidentiality, disclosure may happen, e.g. if someone is being hurt and a criminal offence has been committed, if someone is in danger, or when children are involved.

Finally, take plenty of time to listen and believe what is being said. If someone thinks they are not being believed, they may be discouraged from speaking again.

Responding to the disclosure

- Do be sensitive to people's backgrounds and cultures, checking our own as well as their understanding of how the cultural issues affect them. Ask them about the attitude of their families and what support they can expect.
- Do affirm the strength and courage it takes to have survived the abuse, and even more to talk about it.
- Do express concern for their safety and discuss it, e.g. do they have somewhere to stay? Help them to develop a safety and exit plan
- Do ask about the children, e.g. are they abused or witnesses to abuse? If so, we may need to persuade them to report it or to allow us to do so. We have no option but to do so if a child is at risk.
- Do encourage them to focus on their own needs—something they may not have been able to do since the abuse began, but which is critical in helping them to change their situation.
- Do reassure them that, whatever the circumstances, abuse is not justified and not their fault.

- Do ask them what they want from us or any support team or organization we belong to.
- Do offer help which is in response to their needs and preferences and which lets them keep in control.
- Do give information about where to get specialist help, particularly help that is available locally.
- Do encourage them to seek professional help even if they do not want to leave the situation where abuse is taking place.

We should be sure to perform careful record-keeping and follow-up when speaking with a victim of abuse. We must check if it is all right to contact them at home before doing so. Ask them what their preferred means of contact is and confirm that this is safe. Always keep information confidential and never pass on an address without consent (unless it is a child protection issue).

When we confer with the victim, we must make a brief objective note of date, facts, and context of what has been said, including exact words but keep any opinions separate. This should be kept in strict confidence. We can share the incident with someone who is qualified and can support or give help as we think through the issues and action.

Finally, we must review the safety and risk issues in relation to the perpetrator. When victims are leaving a controlling abuser, they often have to leave with nothing and have access to very limited financial support. We should consider how our organization or (where relevant) our church or faith community can provide practical support to survivors.

Engage men, community leaders, and faith groups

Men

Thankfully there are many men who choose not to abuse and are good fathers, husbands, and partners. But often these men do not speak up or challenge violence and abuse when it is seen or heard. There are several recent campaigns that engage such men in the response to violence against women. These include the White Ribbon Campaign, initially in Canada and now worldwide, Sonke Gender Justice's (Box 27.2) 'One Man Can' and Restored's 'First Man Standing'. These campaigns encourage men to respect all women, challenge other men's attitudes and actions towards women, and join in the cause with women to end violence against women.[22] The UN recently re-launched 'He for She',[23] a solidarity movement for gender equality, which includes ending violence against women.

Violence against women is not a 'women's issue' but a human issue, and men need to stand alongside women in addressing it. In some ways, we could argue that it is a men's issue, since it is men's attitudes and actions that must change if violence is to end. Men need to listen to women who can contribute and advise on courses of action. It is vital for women and men to work together to bring violence against women to an end. All men need to reflect as husbands, fathers, work colleagues, consumers, and in all their other roles on what it means to respect women. Men who have changed their attitudes, strengthened their relationships, intervened to stop violence, and brought these issues into their work and personal lives can have a huge impact (Box 27.3) on those who have yet to do so.

The roots of violence against women lie in the abuse of power and in gender inequality. In turn, these depend on our understanding of masculinity and femininity, and what it means to be a man or woman in the twenty-first century. We need to emphasize understandings of masculinity that recognize the diversity of men and allow space for women to exercise leadership and fulfil their potential.

Men and boys can also be victims of domestic and sexual violence. The frequency and severity of domestic violence against men is lower than that against women. The issues, however, of stigma and secrecy apply as much, if not more, to men. All survivors of violence need to be recognized and supported. We need to emphasize that a person's identity is not destroyed by what they may have experienced and that the responsibility for the violence always lies with the perpetrator and not the victim.

Community leaders

Community leaders play a key role in setting standards of acceptable behaviour and implementing community-level justice. It is ideal, but not always possible, for community leaders to attend basic awareness training on domestic abuse and safeguarding. We can encourage local organizations to have procedures in place against domestic abuse, and a quick referral system, e.g. by phone, so that women who are abused know who to contact and that they will be listened to in safety.

Adopting a charter related to domestic abuse is another way a community-level organization can address the issue of abuse in general, with the charter being prominently displayed or distributed in the organization or faith community. This signifies that the organization is aware of the issue of domestic abuse and is prepared to take action. For victims and survivors, it signals that the organization is a safe place, and for perpetrators that there is zero tolerance of domestic violence. This charter needs to come out of a formally adopted policy and procedure on domestic abuse, so that everyone knows what to do and who to contact when a person discloses abuse.

Tackling domestic abuse should not be seen as an optional add-on for community health programmes. It is a key issue in all communities and needs to be understood and actioned in ways which work best in each context.

Faith groups

The first action that faith groups can take is to acknowledge the reality that domestic abuse happens in their communities, too. This acknowledgement can then lead into discussions and solutions offered by faith communities depending on their own context and resources. One church has devoted whole services to the issue of abuse and produced a liturgy[24] to address domestic abuse. Using theology and sermons to challenge abuse can be incredibly helpful to a victim and a survivor. It can challenge perpetrators of abuse who may well be sitting in the place of worship. Being clear that all violence against women is wrong and must stop helps to break the myth that abuse cannot, and does not, happen in religious communities.

Pursue justice, reconciliation, and hold perpetrators to account

We have noted that violence and abuse affect one in three women worldwide. Very few men, however, are prosecuted or held to account for these actions. The first priority for achieving justice is to challenge perpetrators of violence and to end the culture of impunity that protects men from the consequences for their actions. This requires not only watertight laws but also commitment from politicians and institutions to ensure that they are applied. It also means a shift in culture so that such violence is no longer tolerated. We all have a role to play in making that happen.

Perpetrators are very good at hiding their behaviour. Behaviour traits of perpetrators can include (although the list is not exhaustive):

- presenting themselves confidently;
- focusing on themselves with little empathy for their partner;
- assertively claiming victim status;
- finding no fault in themselves;
- making unfounded accusations;
- putting partner down and portraying partner often as unreasonable or unstable;
- never considering the children's experiences;
- making disparaging remarks about their partner in public;
- using their wedding vows as leverage to keep their partner tied to them—'you promised …';
- expressing suspicion about legitimate activities of partner;
- restricting access to partner's family and friends;
- recruiting others to back them up against their partner;
- using inappropriate humour;
- trying to engender pity in order to manipulate and recruit colluders;
- exhibiting unpredictable, changeable behaviour in order to keep control;
- using religious texts to justify behaviour.

Everyone has an important role in challenging inappropriate behaviour. This can, however, lead to increased risks for both the victim and the person who challenges the perpetrator. This needs to be done in a careful and sensitive way—one that does not place a victim at increased risk (Box 27.4). Factors which help us may include:

- Ensuring that the victim is the highest priority in terms of safety and well-being, and that any action is victim centred;
- If meeting the perpetrator, ensuring that the meeting is in a public place, and that there are others in the meeting;
- Maintaining an awareness of the danger that the perpetrator may pose to any person offering help or support, including the need for personal safety;
- Sharing concerns with a properly trained professional and ensuring that a clear plan is made for the perpetrator;
- Co-operating and working with an appropriate formal authority, ensuring that information concerning

> ### Box 27.4 **Perpetrator programmes**
>
> The attitudes that underpin domestic abuse are often deeply-rooted and difficult to change. Some success has been achieved through Domestic Violence Intervention Programmes for perpetrators. These are extended (often six to nine months) group-based sessions which challenge the attitudes and behaviours of perpetrators. Parallel groups are organized for their partners to ensure that they are held to account. Attendance at a perpetrator programme is often mandated by a court but it is possible in some parts of the world for men to self-refer to such programmes.

the victim is only given to them and not to the perpetrator.

Actions to avoid in responding to perpetrators include:

- Never colluding with, excusing, or minimizing their behaviour.
- Never trying to investigate. Only those professionally trained should discuss any issues formally with them.
- Never giving the perpetrator any information about the victim, particularly their whereabouts. This could cost the victim their life.

Reconciliation

Violence often hides a deeper problem. If wrong attitudes, the abuse of power, and broken relationships are at the root of violence, then reconciliation must involve restored relationships. If underlying attitudes and the relationship are not addressed, then violence could more easily break out again in the future. In cases of domestic violence, the safety and welfare of those affected by violence is the first priority. A change of heart by a perpetrator of violence must be clearly seen over an extended period by a change in attitudes and actions linked to accountability and true change of heart and practice. We must deal with the underlying causes of the problem as well as the symptoms, if change is to be sustainable. Restoring relationships can also avoid conflict on other issues in the future.

Dealing with specific forms of abuse

This section examines responses to honour-based violence, forced marriage, and children abusing adults.

How and when we make these responses will depend a great deal on the context. Ideally, we should be working with community members, and CSOs to take the lead in these sensitive areas. If we come as outsiders, it is usually inappropriate and unsafe to take action directly, both for ourselves and for victims.

Responding to a disclosure of actual or potential 'honour-based' violence

Do:

- Recognize and respect their wishes.
- See them immediately in a secure and private place where the conversation cannot be overheard.
- See them on their own—even if they attend with others.
- Establish a way of contacting them discreetly in the future.
- Obtain full details.
- Consider the need for immediate protection and placement away from the family.
- Seek advice as soon as possible, from a trained specialist who has knowledge of forced marriage.

Do not:

- Send the person away.
- Approach members of her family or the community unless the person expressly wishes it and the risks have been carefully assessed.
- Attempt to be a mediator.

We may only have one chance to speak to a potential victim. If the victim is allowed to walk out of the door without support, that one chance might be lost.

Responding to a disclosure of actual or potential forced marriage

Do:

- Recognize and respect their wishes.
- See them immediately in a secure and private place where the conversation cannot be overheard.
- See them on their own—even if they attend with others.
- Establish a way of contacting them discreetly in the future.
- Obtain full details.
- Consider the need for immediate protection and placement away from the family.

- Seek advice as soon as possible, from a trained specialist who has knowledge of forced marriage.

Do not:

- Send the person away.
- Approach members of her family or the community unless the person expressly wishes it and the risks have been assessed.
- Attempt to be a mediator.

Forced marriage cases can involve a variety of complex and sensitive issues that should be handled by a child protection or adult protection specialist.

Responding to disclosure of child-to-adult abuse

Do:

- Remember this is domestic abuse and the general domestic abuse considerations outlined still apply.
- Consider whether other children are at risk in the house. If so, you will also need to treat this as child abuse.

Do not:

- Assume that this is a parenting issue—the parent is the victim in this situation.
- Joke or make light of the situation.
- Underestimate how difficult it is for the parent to report the incident and for the young person to accept responsibility.
- Wait until something more serious happens before taking action.

Acknowledgement

Acknowledgement is given to 'Responding well to domestic abuse,' Church of England (March 2017) from which text has been used with permission.

References and further reading

1. Commission on the Status of Women in New York. UN Secretary-General Ban Ki-moon. 2008. Available from: http://www.un.org/press/en/2008/sgsm11437.doc.htm
2. Declaration on the Elimination of Violence against Women. United Nations General Assembly, Resolution 48/104,1993. Available from: http://www.un.org/documents/ga/res/48/a48r104.htm
3. UNWomen. *Facts and figures: Ending violence against women.* Updated February 2016. Available from: http://www.

unwomen.org/en/what-we-do/ending-violence-against-women/facts-and-figures

4. Turning Promises into Progress. Report. Gender and Development Network, Gender Action for Peace and Security, UK SRHR Network, London, March 2015. Section 2. Available from: http://gadnetwork.org/gadn-resources/turning-promises-into-progress

5. Dugan E. Phumzile Mlambo-Ngcuka: Home can be the unsafest place for women. *The Independent*. 26 April 2015. Available from: http://www.independent.co.uk/news/people/phumzile-mlambongcuka-home-can-be-the-unsafest-place-for-women-10204379.html

6. Violence against women in Eastern Democratic Republic of Congo: Whose responsibility? Whose complicity? Brussels: International Trade Union Confederation; 2011.Available from: https://www.ituc-csi.org/IMG/pdf/ituc_violence_rdc_eng_lr.pdf.pdf

7. United Nations. *Background information on sexual violence used as a tool of war*. 2013. Available from: http://www.un.org/en/preventgenocide/rwanda/about/bgsexualviolence.shtml

8. Robertson L, Szaraz M. The Medicalisation of FGM. *28 Too Many*. 2016; 1–37. Available from: http://www.28toomany.org/media/uploads/report_final_version.pdf

9. UN Women. Commission on the Status of Women 57th session. 2013. Available from: http://www.unwomen.org/en/csw/previous-sessions/csw57-2013

10. Heise LL. *What works to prevent partner violence? An evidence overview*. London: STRIVE; 2011. Available from: http://strive.lshtm.ac.uk/resources/what-works-prevent-partner-violence-evidence-overview

11. Fulu E, Heise LL. *Evidence reviews. Paper 1: State of the field of research on violence against women and girls*. Pretoria: What Works; 2015.

12. Arango DJ, Morton M, Gennari F, Kiplesund S, Ellsberg M. *Interventions to prevent or reduce violence against women and girls: A systematic review of reviews*. Washington, DC: World Bank; 2014.

13. Fulu E, Kerr-Wilson A, Lang J. *Effectiveness of interventions to prevent violence against women and girls: A summary of the evidence*. Pretoria: Medical Research Council; 2014.

14. Jewkes R, Flood M, Lang J. From work with men and boys to changes of social norms and reduction of inequities in gender relations: A conceptual shift in prevention of violence against women and girls. *The Lancet*. 2015; 385 (9977): 1580–9.

15. Fulu E, Kerr-Wilson A. Evidence reviews. Paper 2: Interventions to prevent violence against women and girls. Pretoria: What Works; 2015.

16. Gender & Development Network. Turning Promises into Progress: Gender Equality and Rights for Women and Girls—Lessons Learnt and Actions Needed. London: Action Aid; 2015.

17. Sivakumaran S. Sexual violence against men in armed conflict. *European Journal of International Law*. 2007; 18 (2): 253–76.

18. *Honour-based violence and forced marriage*. Crown Prosecution Service; Legal guidance, Domestic abuse. Revised: 28 June 2018. Available from: http://www.cps.gov.uk/legal/h_to_k/honour_based_violence_and_forced_marriage/

19. World Health Organization. *Female genital mutilation (FGM)*. 2017. http://www.who.int/reproductivehealth/topics/fgm/prevalence/en/

20. FGM Unit. *Female genital mutilation: The case for a national action plan*. Great Britain House of Commons Home Affairs Committee. London: 2014.

21. Berg RC, Denison E. *Interventions to reduce the prevalence of female genital mutilation/cutting in African countries*. London: 3ie; 2013.

22. First Man Standing. Restored. Available from: http://www.restoredrelationships.org/firstmanstanding/pledge/

23. UN Women. He For She. 2014. Available from: http://www.heforshe.org/

24. Restored Relationships. *Ending domestic abuse: A pack for churches*. Teddington: Restored; 2011. Available from: http://www.restoredrelationships.org/resources/info/51/

CHAPTER 28

Community palliative and home-based care

Mhoira Leng

Palliative care is a key, neglected area of care in community settings. This is partly because other causes are seen to be more important, such as maternal and child health, and also because, until recently, fewer people survived to an age when palliative care might be needed. It is a difficult, challenging subject to deal with at community level without good training and availability of the best medication. This chapter looks at a wide range of issues affecting communities. It overlaps with, and is sometimes referred to as, home-based care (Figure 28.1).

With correct training and good community management, most palliative care can be provided at community level by competent, informed care teams, with clear pathways for care, which might include the hospital. In resource-poor settings, empowering the person and family with knowledge and skills to care and cope is paramount. This, supported by a caring community, can bring to the surface the potential for care present in every person and family, resulting in effective palliative care.[1] Therefore, this chapter includes rather more detail on medication than many chapters, as it is such a key part of effective care.

What we need to know

Defining palliative care

The World Health Organization (WHO) defines palliative care as 'an approach that improves the quality of life (QoL) of patients and their families facing problems associated with life-threatening illness, through the prevention and relief of suffering by means of early identification and impeccable assessment and treatment of pain and other problems, physical, psychosocial and spiritual.'[2]

Interestingly, this is the only WHO definition in which the word 'spiritual' occurs. This illustrates how, for the great majority of those living in low- and middle-income countries, spiritual issues and religious customs related to death and dying are of high importance.

Palliative care helps people and families live with chronic illness. It relieves pain and suffering, improves QoL and maintains dignity. Hospice or supportive care are terms that are used in some settings, but usually

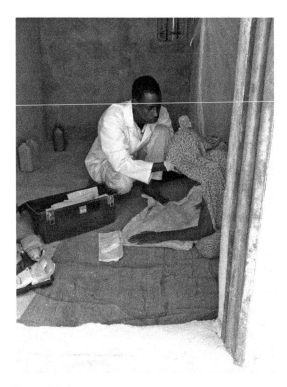

Figure 28.1 Palliative care nurse supports wound care at home in Mauritania.

Reproduced courtesy of Dr David Fearon. This image is distributed under the terms of the Creative Commons Attribution Non-Commercial 4.0 International licence (CC-BY-NC), a copy of which is available at http://creativecommons.org/licenses/by-nc/4.0/

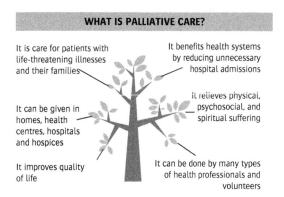

Figure 28.2 What is palliative care?

Reproduced with permission from World Health Organization. Infographics on Palliative Care. Available at http://www.who.int/ncds/management/palliative-care/pc-infographics/en/. This image is distributed under the terms of the Creative Commons Attribution Non-Commercial 4.0 International licence (CC-BY-NC), a copy of which is available at http://creativecommons.org/licenses/by-nc/4.0/

mean the same as palliative care, although hospice care refers to facility-based, rather than community-based, care (Figure 28.2).

Who requires palliative care, and when?

Palliative care should be available for all people who are living with chronic and life-limiting illness, regardless of the type of disease, the stage of that disease, the age of the person, or the setting where they are living. We need to think about the different settings in which we live and work. Some of us will see people living with communicable diseases such as HIV/AIDS or multidrug-resistant tuberculosis (MDR-TB). We may see children living with cerebral palsy caused by problems at birth or by infections such as malaria. We may also see children, including neonates, with a congenital illness or another chronic illness. Overall, we see increasing numbers of people living with non-communicable diseases (NCDs),

e.g. cardiovascular disease, cancer, chronic lung diseases, diabetes, and mental health problems.

We know that the number of people living with these diseases is growing across the world, especially in low- and middle-income settings. We also know that as people grow older,[3] they may have several chronic illnesses, e.g. AIDS plus cardiovascular disease, diabetes plus hypertension, or stroke disease plus dementia. This is multiple disease or multimorbidity and may include up to five chronic illnesses. This means we should focus primarily on the person and their needs, not the disease(s). The WHO estimates that over 40 million people are in need of palliative care, likely to be an underestimate and to increase rapidly in the future.

The best model showing when to start palliative care is shown in Figure 28.3 It should be an approach that starts as soon as we know there is a chronic, life-limiting illness and should be delivered alongside treatment options, e.g. antiretroviral therapy for HIV/AIDS, chemotherapy for cancer. Care is focused on the sick person but also includes the family and carers, offers support during the dying phase, and continues after a death has happened to support the loss and adjustment of those who are bereaved.

It has been suggested that we combine this palliative care approach to include health promotion, as many people, especially in low- and middle-income settings and rural communities, delay coming to health care workers (HCWs) until their illness is very advanced. Some people may never see a doctor, far less a specialist, and will often not have a clear diagnosis.

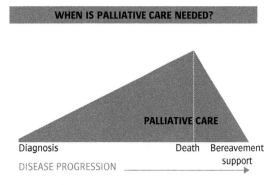

Figure 28.3 When is palliative care needed?

Reproduced with permission from World Health Organization. Infographics on Palliative Care. Available at http://www.who.int/ncds/management/palliative-care/pc-infographics/en/. This image is distributed under the terms of the Creative Commons Attribution Non-Commercial 4.0 International licence (CC-BY-NC), a copy of which is available at http://creativecommons.org/licenses/by-nc/4.0/

Global palliative care

Recognition and development

To integrate evidence-based, cost-effective and equitable palliative care services in the continuum of care, across all levels, with emphasis on primary care, community and home-based care, and universal coverage schemes.

World Health Assembly, *Strengthening of palliative care as a component of comprehensive care throughout the life course,* Doc. 67/19. June 2014

In 2014, the World Health Assembly approved a resolution for palliative care with an emphasis on providing care without gaps and including community settings.[4] The resolution also emphasizes the need to integrate training for palliative care in all the relevant curriculums, ensure access to essential medicines, and adjust health policy towards implementing palliative care. This approach is important because palliative care does not fit into one single area of health care, but touches many disciplines. Palliative care is recognized under the human right to health, and failure to provide pain relief has been reported as crossing the boundary to mistreatment, which, in some cases, risks being tantamount to torture.[5]

Palliative care has been developing rapidly in the past 50 years. It has been successfully integrated into a few health care systems, e.g. the UK and Australia (more than 90 per cent integration), but services are only available in less than half the countries in the world and often only to a very small proportion of the population (Figure 28.4).

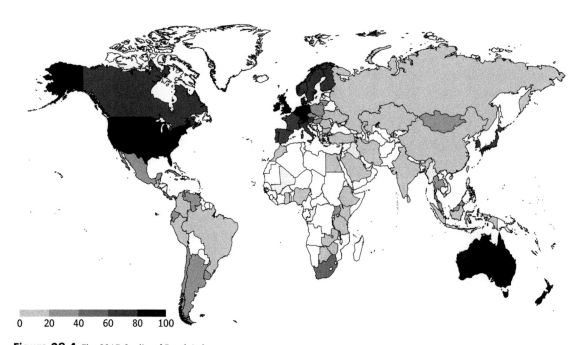

Figure 28.4 The 2015 Quality of Death Index.

Reproduced courtesy of The Economist Intelligence Unit Limited. This image is distributed under the terms of the Creative Commons Attribution Non-Commercial 4.0 International licence (CC-BY-NC), a copy of which is available at http://creativecommons.org/licenses/by-nc/4.0/.

Palliative care as a component of Universal Health Coverage

> Universal health coverage (UHC) means that all people and communities can use the promotive, preventive, curative, rehabilitative and palliative health services they need, of sufficient quality to be effective, while also ensuring that the use of these services does not expose the user to financial hardship.
>
> World Health Organization, 2015.

We know that ensuring everyone has access to health is an equality-based, compassionate approach but it also makes economic sense. Universal health coverage focuses on the patient journey and ensures access to health care without financial hardship. People living with chronic illness and facing the end of their lives face huge financial burdens due to the costs of the health care. They may waste their scarce resources seeking treatments that do not help. They may try seeking traditional options such as herbalists, or sell possessions and land to travel for more conventional treatments.

Lack of information may result in people being unable to make the best choices for themselves and their families. Families seek to 'do all they can,' mistakenly thinking this means accessing expensive hospital treatments. This can mean people do not get the choice of where to die, which, for many people, is in their own home or community setting, and not in a hospital or health facility. It is of concern that this lack of choice and family pressures in higher and middle-income countries is leading to a rapid increase in people dying in intensive care units. Early palliative care can reduce unnecessary hospital admissions and support choice. However, this is only possible if those needing palliative care are identified early in the community or primary care setting, e.g. by a community health worker.

Palliative care offers an opportunity to influence health systems not only to provide better palliative care but to encourage and develop a values-based and person-centred approach to health. The skills we learn include core values such as holistic care, professionalism, effective communication, ethics and patient-centred care. The strengthening of our communities and health systems will promote resilient, compassionate, healthy societies. Our goal is to see palliative care integrated across health systems to ensure people have the care they need and deserve, starting at community and primary health care level (Figure 28.5).

Barriers and gaps to providing palliative care

> 'Cancer is killing us. Pain is killing me because for several days I have been unable to find injectable morphine in any place. Please Mr. Secretary of Health, do not make us suffer any more ... '
>
> Unidentified woman with cervical cancer,
> *El Pais*, Columbia, 12 September 2008

We know that most palliative and home-based care needs are not being met. We also know that pain relief is not available in most of the world; in particular, strong pain-killers such as opioids (morphine and its derivatives) are difficult to access. This causes untold and needless suffering. The WHO has guidelines on the organization of palliative care services, essential medicines, and pain control.[6]

Often there is a failure to identify those needing palliative and home-based care, which prevents interventions from being offered early. Those people most

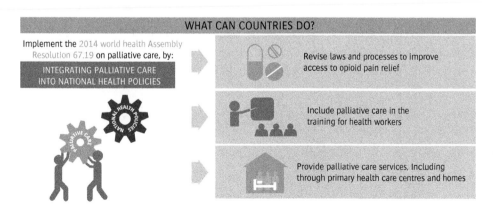

Figure 28.5 What can countries do?

WHAT ARE THE GAPS?

86%	83%	98%
of people who need palliative care do not receive it	of the world's population lack access to pain relief	of children needing palliative care live in low- and middle income countries

Figure 28.6 What are the gaps?

Reproduced with permission from World Health Organization. Infographics on Palliative Care. Available at http://www.who.int/ncds/management/palliative-care/pc-infographics/en/. This image is distributed under the terms of the Creative Commons Attribution Non-Commercial 4.0 International licence (CC-BY-NC), a copy of which is available at http://creativecommons.org/licenses/by-nc/4.0/

lacking palliative care are the vulnerable and marginalized without a strong voice. We need to identify them in our communities. They are often children, women, the poor, those with mental health problems, those affected by stigma or whose lifestyle choices are different, those in prison, and refugees fleeing natural disaster, oppression, and conflict.

More often than not it is simply those who are nearing the end of their lives, requiring regular care but no longer able to earn money or support themselves. How we care for the vulnerable in our communities is one of the most important indicators of a thriving, compassionate society (Figure 28.6).

There are many reasons and barriers to explain this massive inequality in the provision of palliative care which include (Figure 28.7):

- A lack of awareness and understanding among the public, policymakers, and HCWs and many myths relating to the use of opioids as strong pain-relieving medicines. This leads to poor training added to the overall scarcity of health workers.

- Social and cultural barriers. Some cultures contain strong beliefs about the causes of illness, including curses and blame.

- An emphasis on a medical model of health can lead to a 'death denying' culture with the myth that palliative care is only appropriate in the final weeks of life, or for specific diseases such as cancer or HIV/AIDS.

- A concern that opting for palliative care means 'giving up' or may shorten life.

In reality, there is good evidence that relief of suffering and a focus on QoL improves satisfaction for the patient, family, and HCW, allows for better decision-making, allows personal and family priorities to be respected, and should be started early alongside treatment options. Palliative care is 'adding life to days not just days to life' (Figure 28.7).

Delivering palliative care

Good palliative care is possible with limited resources

Palliative care is best delivered by a team approach that is person-centred, empowering to communities, and interdisciplinary. This team may include some or all of these professionals: a nurse, doctor, social worker, nutritionist, psychologist. The team can also contain trained volunteers who are crucial in community settings alongside empowered families.

Palliative care is largely based on attitudes, skills, and values. Expensive technology is not needed for good care, and the list of essential medicines is short and largely inexpensive. In practice, palliative care is even more important when people have few resources and may be unable to access medical treatments. Innovative models of palliative care show how families and communities can be empowered and mobilized to be the mainstay of palliative care and support (Figure 28.8).

WHAT ARE THE BARRIERS?

Poor public awareness or how palliative care can help	Cultural and social barriers, such as beliefs about pain and dying	Insufficient skills and capacities of health workers	Overly restrictive regulations for opioid pain relief

Figure 28.7 What are the barriers?

Reproduced with permission from World Health Organization. Infographics on Palliative Care. Available at http://www.who.int/ncds/management/palliative-care/pc-infographics/en/. This image is distributed under the terms of the Creative Commons Attribution Non-Commercial 4.0 International licence (CC-BY-NC), a copy of which is available at http://creativecommons.org/licenses/by-nc/4.0/

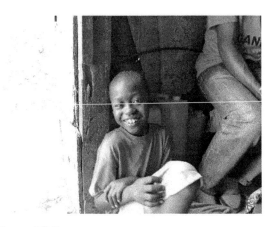

Figure 28.8 Patient in urban slum Kampala.

Reproduced courtesy of Dr Mhoira Leng. This image is distributed under the terms of the Creative Commons Attribution Non-Commercial 4.0 International licence (CC-BY-NC), a copy of which is available at http://creativecommons.org/licenses/by-nc/4.0/

This community cohesion is a rich resource in community settings. Palliative care can be integrated into every level of the health care system, including trained volunteers, thus making it available in the most rural settings and in urban slums. In addition to providing care and support, the community has a role in raising awareness and ensuring that end-of-life issues are recognized and supported by district and national health systems. In some countries, there are national awareness programmes in the media, schools, and community groups.

Technology is increasingly being used to support palliative care, e.g. using mobile devices to support data transfer, access medications, or facilitate specialist advice and support. E-learning and e-medicine are now becoming available in low-resource settings.

Models of palliative care

There are different delivery models of palliative care across the world (Box 28.1). The principles are the same

---

Box 28.1 **How have others set up community PC initiatives?**

There are many examples of good practice in low- and middle-income countries that help us work out a model for our community. Here are a number of examples:

1. Kerala, India: Whole communities have been engaged in identifying those who have palliative care needs, with large numbers of volunteers trained to take the lead. Health care teams work closely with the volunteers to ensure care is given as close to home as possible but also ensure that patients with complex problems can be referred. These networks have also made essential medicines, e.g. oral morphine, available in the home setting, and Kerala now has a state policy and roll-out programme for palliative care. In addition, a mental health organization, MEHAC, provides community-based support established via a project identifying, supporting, and building networks for those with chronic mental health needs.

2. Uganda: The lead was given by a partnership between an NGO, Hospice Africa Uganda, and the Medical Officer of Health to improve access to oral morphine by allowing trained nurses and clinical officers to prescribe. Recent research has showed the effectiveness of this approach. There are also community outreach teams, mobile palliative care services, and training programmes at all levels, including a degree in palliative care.

3. Rwanda: A new cadre of community worker with six months' training has been established—the *home-based care practitioner*. They help to identify and manage people living with chronic disease, including palliative care needs.

4. Tanzania: A district hospital in Muheza helped to develop a network of trained community workers, but also worked with leaders at the community level to increase awareness of palliative care.

5. Delhi, India: An amazing network of services based in communities across the city provides outreach domiciliary support for palliative care. They also have a helpline, day-care facilities, and provision of essential medicines including oral morphine. These networks are present in some slum communities.

6. Bangalore India: The Bangalore Baptist Hospital offers an integrated model, and pioneered guidelines to empower families to use the subcutaneous route at home to give morphine and other medication when the person is unable to take oral medication. This is also being promoted in the Christian Medical Association of India network of hospitals.

7. Northern Uganda: In the refugee camps, a trained palliative care nurse has worked with the national palliative care team at Makerere University to develop focal points for palliative care in some health centres serving refugees who have fled the conflict in South Sudan.

but we need to think how best to apply these principles in our own settings. We can think of palliative care provision in three levels.

1. Level 1 or a basic palliative care approach.

Patients and families have relatively simple needs, which can be met by health and social care workers, including volunteers and CHWs, provided they are given basic training.

2. Level 2 or intermediate.

Patients and families have more intricate needs, which can be met by health and social care workers who deal with chronic disease and have had some additional training. This level may include primary care, community health, gynaecology, medical and surgical specialties, and paediatrics. When trained, such people may act as focal points for palliative care, and be able to supervise the care in level 1.

3. Specialist or level 3.

Patients and families have complex problems and these can met by HCWs with specialist training using a multidisciplinary approach. Specialist teams also offer the training, mentorship, and support for all levels of palliative care.

Communication: the key skill in palliative care

Experienced palliative care practitioners use their communication skills with the same skill that surgeons use their scalpels. As a surgeon learns to operate, we can learn, practise, and refine our methods of communication. We should take any occasion to learn this in action, e.g. by shadowing a respected palliative care team or observing an experienced and sensitive listener. We can also find excellent video demonstrations on the Internet (Box 28.2).

Communication is not limited to giving information—it is a two-way process. It involves receiving, giving, and being present (accompanying). We communicate through verbal and non-verbal methods, whether we are aware of it or not. Verbal tools include:

- Open questions that allow the patient to describe what is important to them.
- Clarification, which demonstrates that we are following the story and are interested in what is being said.
- Repetition and summarizing what the patient said, often useful at the end of the consultation to verify

> ### Box 28.2 **An uncomfortable challenge**
>
> One effective way of improving our communication skills is to video our consultations. We just need a simple video-enabled camera or phone and a willing patient. After the consultation, we can watch ourselves and reflect upon our words and actions following the guidelines provided. Our mentors may be interested in watching and providing feedback. Remember to:
>
> - Ask permission from the patient.
> - Start with some simple consultations.
> - Protect the patients' data: do not share or publish it.
> - Delete all copies after learning.
>
> Reproduced with permission from Makerere University and Mulago Hospital. Palliative Care Guidelines 2012. Copyright © 2011 Makerere University. This box is distributed under the terms of the Creative Commons Attribution Non Commercial 4.0 International licence (CC-BY-NC), a copy of which is available at http://creativecommons.org/licenses/by-nc/4.0/

that we have understood correctly before agreeing a management plan.

As we try to choose appropriate words in our verbal communication, we also have to choose the components of our non-verbal communication. We should become aware of our:

- Eye contact.
- Body posture, such as sitting forward.
- Behaviours, such as head nodding.
- Not being distracted by mobile phones.

In this way we show that we are actively listening to the patient. This makes the patient feel more confident and supported, and we are rewarded with a more in-depth history and better rapport.

Giving bad news

All new HCWs are nervous about giving bad news at the beginning. It is correct to approach this subject with seriousness and respect. However, we should not make the mistake of thinking that this information belongs to us; it rightly belongs to the patient. It needs to be delivered in a gentle and appropriate manner. There is a range of consequences from the level of bad news. We can gain experience through employing the following suggestions in simpler situations before approaching more complicated, life-changing, news. A tool to help us is the SPIKES protocol:[7]

● *Set up.*

Know the family, patient, and the information. Invite the patient to bring a family member. Consider some of the potential resulting questions beforehand.

● *Perception.*

Try to assess what the patient already knows. We often find the patient knows much more than we expected.

● *Invitation.*

What do they want to know? Not everyone wants all their medical information. Some prefer not to know, for their own reasons.

● *Knowledge and information.*

Give a 'warning shot': say you have some serious news. Give information in short, clear segments in a gentle manner. Evaluate the response as you speak. It may be appropriate to spread the information over several conversations.

● *Emotions.*

Empathize. Sometimes reflecting a person's feelings helps them open up, with phrases such as 'I know this must be difficult for you'. Allow people to express their feelings.

● *Strategy and summary.*

Clearly outline what happens next, e.g. a follow-up appointment or visit. Not knowing what is happening or

---

> **Box 28.3 Prognosis**
>
> Special consideration is required prior to giving information on prognosis. In resource-rich contexts, a prognosis is dependent upon multiple factors, including staging of illness, comorbidity, and locally available treatments. It is often not accurate. This is more complicated in resource-limited contexts. It is advisable that we refrain from providing a specific prognosis. We may refer to local specialists, if available.
>
> Reproduced with permission from Makerere University and Mulago Hospital. Palliative Care Guidelines 2012. Copyright © 2011 Makerere University. This box is distributed under the terms of the Creative Commons Attribution Non Commercial 4.0 International licence (CC-BY-NC), a copy of which is available at http://creativecommons.org/licenses/by-nc/4.0/

---

believing you are being talked about can be discouraging and disempowering for a patient (Box 28.3).

QoL is a subjective experience. We each ascertain different values to different components of our lives. These values may change over time and in response to events like illness. It is not for us to decide another's priorities. It is our job to explore their priorities and try our best to help patients maintain their priorities as long as possible. For example, an 80-year man fears pain, and is willing to accept any treatment to prevent pain. In respecting these wishes, we may manage his symptoms differently than for a 30-year old lady whose main desire is to remain fully alert for as long as possible in order to help care for her family.

What we need to do

Assess the need for palliative care

It is practically impossible for one individual to provide all the components of good palliative care; meeting the physical, emotional, spiritual, and social needs of the patient, and, in addition, the needs of the family. Therefore, we need to empower others to meet these needs, ideally forming a multidisciplinary team within a wider network of enthusiastic individuals or associations. Time spent finding partners is a worthwhile investment, as the complex challenges of providing palliative care become apparent (Figure 28.9).

Early on we need to assess palliative care needs in the community (see Chapter 6 for ways of doing this), concentrating on health concerns in the community that link to palliative care, and the need for home-based care.

We can also ask:

● What is the extent of palliative care needs?
● Who is currently caring for palliative patients in the community?
● How are these patients treated?
● In what ways does the community come together to help?

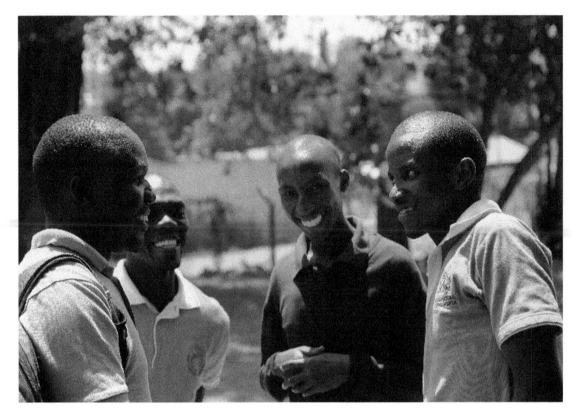

Figure 28.9 Trained volunteers supporting palliative care.

Reproduced courtesy of Dr Mhoira Leng. This image is distributed under the terms of the Creative Commons Attribution Non-Commercial 4.0 International licence (CC-BY-NC), a copy of which is available at http://creativecommons.org/licenses/by-nc/4.0/

- Are CHWs involved in home-based care?
- What are the cultural views about death?
- What do the local faith communities have to say about pain control and the inevitability of death?

Access the necessary medication, including pain relief

At least 70 per cent of patients with cancer or AIDS have pain and therefore access to palliative care medications is crucial. Unfortunately, there are barriers to access in many settings, especially for opioid pain relief (i.e. morphine or its derivatives). We should discover what medications are available in our country and region. It is worthwhile knowing how we can access them *before* we are faced with a patient in severe pain. There may be supplies in the capital city and it is sensible to establish links with cancer services and tertiary hospitals, either to access medications or as a point for referral. We should always connect with government and use any supplies they may provide and work co-operatively together.

Although effective palliative care is not possible without access to pain-relieving medications, it is important to remember that palliative care is far more than just pain relief. It is, of course, difficult to provide emotional, social, and spiritual care while severe pain remains a problem and we should always work to find a way to have pain relief, including oral morphine, available. It can be argued that those in pain have an even greater need to be accompanied and supported, but early identification and thorough assessment of pain lays the foundation for other aspects of care. Examples include positioning of the patient, massage, or the use of additional medications, e.g. corticosteroids for headaches secondary to raised intracranial pressure, or tricyclic antidepressants for neuropathic pain.

Offer holistic care

When we have identified someone living with a chronic, life-limiting illness who has palliative care needs, we need to assess the whole situation before offering care for the whole person. Although this section separates the different dimensions—physical, psychological, social, and spiritual—these are all overlapping and interacting. If someone is in severe physical pain, they will feel anxious and depressed and if they are not able to work, they may be unable to care for their children and lose hope for the future. This is known as 'total' pain.

Our approach should be stepwise:

1. Assess, listen, re-assess with examination and investigations.

2. Agree a problem list highlighting the patient's priorities.

3. Identify and treat any reversible problems, e.g. a urinary catheter for retention.

4. Discuss and inform patients and family.

5. Agree a care plan including holistic care and any relevant prescription or referral.

6. Review and reassess.

Figure 28.10 shows a helpful list of essential practices for palliative care that can help us.

Identify, evaluate, diagnose, treat, apply solution measures for:	Identify, evaluate, provide support, apply solution measures and refer when necessary for:
Physical care needs	
■ Pain (all types)	■ Fatigue
■ Respiratory problems (dyspnoea, cough)	■ Anorexia
■ Gastrointestinal problems (constipation, nausea, vomiting, dry mouth, mucositis, diarrhoea)	■ Anaemia
	■ Drowsiness or sedation
■ Delirium	■ Sweating
■ Wounds, ulcers, skin rash and skin lesions	
■ Insomnia	
Psychological/emotional/spiritual care needs	
■ Psychological distress	■ Spiritual needs and existential distress
■ Anxiety	■ Depression
■ Suffering of family or caregivers	■ Bereavement support for family/caregivers

Consider and manage:
Care planning and coordination
■ Identify support and resources available; develop and implement care plan based on patient's needs
■ Provide crae in the last weeks/days of life
■ Facilitate the availabilityand access to medications (especially opioids)
■ Identify the psychosocial/spiritual needs of professionals providing care (including self)
Communication issues
■ Communicate with patient, family and caregivers about diagnosis, treatment, symptoms and their management, and issues relating to care in the last days/weeks of life
■ Identify and set priorities with patient and family/caregivers
■ Provide information and guidance to patients and caregivers according to available resources

Source: Adapted from IAHPC (5).

Figure 28.10 IAHPC Essential Practices List 2012.

Physical care needs

Pain assessment

There is no laboratory test for pain. We need to ask the patient to describe their pain and actively listen to what is said. Our aim is to quickly and safely control the pain so that the patient can carry on with their life. To do this, we assess, treat, and reassess.

We can use the SOCRATES tool to help with assessing pain, but we should remember there may be more than one pain (Box 28.4). Use a body chart to help identify the site. Use a tool like the hand scale to help measure the severity and the effectiveness of treatment.

In children or non-verbal adults, we may need to use behavioural markers, e.g. body posture, loss of appetite, crying, withdrawal, or physiological markers such as raised pulse and sweating. If the child is older, we can use a tool like the faces scale for them to identify the picture that most looks like their experience of pain (Figure 28.11).

Managing chronic pain using the WHO approach

The WHO uses four principles to manage chronic pain:

1. By the ladder.
2. By the clock.
3. By the mouth.

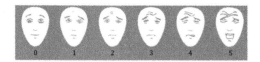

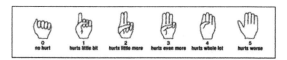

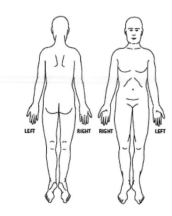

Figure 28.11 These body charts and hand scales.

Reproduced courtesy of Dr Mhoira Leng. This image is distributed under the terms of the Creative Commons Attribution Non-Commercial 4.0 International licence (CC-BY-NC), a copy of which is available at http://creativecommons.org/licenses/by-nc/4.0/

4. By the individual.

The WHO pain ladder guides our prescribing (Figure 28.12). It uses simple analgesics or painkillers and then moves to stronger analgesics called opioids or medications related to morphine.

We start at step one with a non-opioid, e.g. paracetamol, establishing a pattern of giving pain medications at regular intervals, preferably by the mouth if possible. A breakthrough or rescue dose of medications is prescribed for when pain is severe and occurring between the regular dosing of analgesia. We re-assess the pain at regular intervals. We move up the ladder when the pain does not respond sufficiently to the medication. The prescription of strong opioids is restricted to trained and registered prescribers and depends on local and national regulations. If we are unable to prescribe, we can find out where it is available locally. When prescribing opioids, we should always also prescribe a laxative, as opioids cause constipation.

For children, a two-step approach is recommended and in many parts of the world this is also used for adults (Figure 28.13).

Box 28.4 **SOCRATES**

Site: Where is the pain? Where are the different pains?
Onset: When and how did it start?
Character: How is it described, e.g. sharp, dull, stabbing?
Radiation: Does the pain move and how is the movement described?
Associations: Is there a relationship between the pain and other symptoms?
Time course: How is it changing over time?
Exacerbating or relieving factors: What makes the pain worse? What helps the pain?
Severity: How bad is the pain?

Reproduced with permission from Makerere University and Mulago Hospital. Palliative Care Guidelines 2012. Copyright © 2011 Makerere University. This box is distributed under the terms of the Creative Commons Attribution Non Commercial 4.0 International licence (CC-BY-NC), a copy of which is available at http://creativecommons.org/licenses/by-nc/4.0/

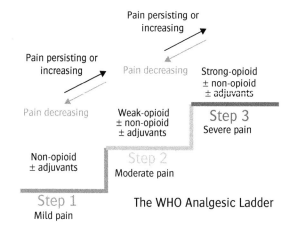

Figure 28.12 The WHO Analgesic Ladder.

Adjuvant medications for certain causes or types of pain

Adjuvant medications are not pain medications, but work with pain medications to help certain causes or types of pain. They should only be used in combination for managing pain.

- Inflammation and swelling.

Tumours can cause pressure on surrounding tissues causing pain. Steroids are used to reduce the swelling: Dexamethasone 16mg a day for suspected

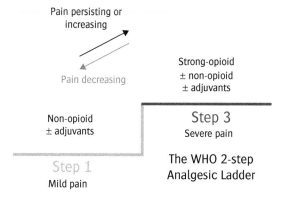

Figure 28.13 The WHO 2-step Analgesic Ladder.

spinal cord compression or raised intracranial compression, and 8mg a day for other swelling related symptoms. This is often a short-term management to get symptoms under control and consider further management. Remember to review, as long-term steroids have serious side effects.

- Nerve pain.

Pain due to nerve damage is often described by the patient as a burning, shooting, or electric shock. It can be severe so that even light touch causes severe discomfort. Treatment options include tricyclic depressants (amitriptyline 12.5–25mg at night) or epileptic medications (clonazepam 0.5–1mg at night or sodium valproate 200mg twice a day)

- Skeletal muscle spasms.

These often occur in patients confined to bed and in those with neurological or musculoskeletal problems. Diazepam 5mg at night, titrated up to 20mg.

- Abdominal cramps and smooth muscle spasm.

Check the patient is not constipated first but consider hyoscine butylbromide (Buscopan) 20mg four times a day (Figure 28.14 and Figure 28.15).

Respiratory problems

Breathing difficulties can be extremely distressing. As we stay calm, we can reassure the patient and the family, and try to explore their fears. General measures include changing position, helping the patient to slow their breathing down, and encouraging breathing with their diaphragm as well as helping to maximize their activity while conserving energy. This can mean finding alternative ways of doing things, such as sitting for washing or cooking but avoiding total inactivity if possible (Figure 28.16).

Cough

A cough can disrupt normal life and lead to exhaustion for the patient and the family. It affects communication, reduces oral intake, and can disturb the sleep of everyone in the household. Cough can be caused by the disease process, its treatment, or it may be unrelated. Treatable causes include chest infection, TB, asthma, chronic obstructive pulmonary disease, pleural effusion, sinusitis, and reflux disease. These should be treated as appropriate.

To manage the cough symptom, we can consider:

- Cough suppressants: codeine (15 to 30mg every four hours) and morphine (2.5–5mg every four hours).
- Nebulized saline 0.9%.

Step	Analgesics	Comments	Adjuvants
Step 1 (non-opioid)	Paracetamol 1g 6 hourly or Diclofenac 50mg 8 hourly	• Continue with step 1 analgesic when moving on to step 2 and 3	• Amitriptyline 12.5-25mg nocte for neuropathic pain (can be increased to 50-75mg if tolerated)
Step 2 (Weak opioid)	Morphine 2.5-5mg 4 hourly during the day with a double dose at night or Codeine Phosphate 30-60mg 6 hourly or Tramadol 50-100mg 6 hourly	• Low dose morphine is considered a step 2 analgesic and is recommended first line if available as it is cheaper than codeine or tradamol • Discontinue step 2 analgesics when starting step 3	• Clonazepam 0.5-1mg nocte for neuropathic pain second line • Dexamethasone 4-8mg od for swelling/oedema e.g. liver capsular stretch • Hyoscine Butylbromide (buscopan) 20mg qds for smooth muscle spasm • Diazepam 5-20mg nocte for painful skeletal muscle spasm
Step 3 (Strong Opioid)	Morphine 7.5-10mg 4 hourly during the day with a double dose at night Increase the dose as required to control the patient's pain	• The elderly and/or those with renal impairment may require a dose adjustmet • (For children see separate guideline)	

Figure 28.14 Steps 1–3.

Step	Analgesics	Comments	Adjuvants
Step 1 (non-opioid)	**Infants from 1 to 3 months** • Paracetamol 10mg/kg every 4-6hrs max 4 doses/day **Children from 3 months to 12 years** • Paracetamol 10-15mg/kg every 4-6hrs max 4 dosed/day, max 1g at a time • Ibuprofen 5-10mg/kg every 6-8 hours	• Aspirin is rarely used in children	• Amitriptyline - children from 2-12 years, 0.2-0.5mg/kg (max 25mg) at night - increase if needed to max 1mg/kg twice a day • Carbamazepine - 5-20mg/kg day in 2 or 3 divided doses, increase gradually to avoid side effects. • Diazepam (used for associated anxiety)
Step 2 (Weak opioid)	**Infants from 1 to 3 months** • Oral morphine - 0.08-0.2mg/kg every 4 hrs **Children from 2 to 12 years** • Oral morphine 0.2-0.4mg/kg every 4hrs **Children from 2 to 12 years** • Oral morphine 0.2-0.5mg/kg every 4hrs	• **Titration:** After a starting dose, the dosage should be adjusted to the level that is effective with a maximum dosage increase of 50% per 24 hours.	• 1-6 years: 2-10mg/day in 2-3 divided doses • 6-14 years: 2-10mg/day in 2-3 divided doses • Hyoscine Butylbromide • 1month - 2 years: 0.5mg/kg po 8hrly • 2-5 years: 5mg po 8 hrly • 6-12 years: 5mg po 8 hrly • Prednisone - 1.2mg/kg/day

Figure 28.15 Steps 1–2.

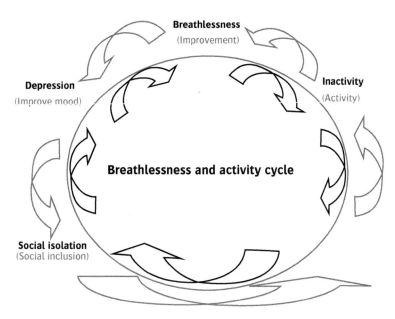

Figure 28.16 Breathlessness and activity cycle.

- Corticosteroids: oral dexamethasone (8mg once a day) or inhaled steroids (use the formulation available locally for asthma).

Breathlessness

Breath is the essence of life and we should acknowledge that breathlessness feels like life is being withheld from us. Identified causes should be treated as appropriate. Try the simple methods in Box 28.5. There is good evidence that stimulating the facial nerve can ease the sensation of breathlessness; the simplest is to use a handheld or table fan and blow air across the face. We can also use medications to help breathlessness (Box 28.6). The mainstays are low-dose oral morphine and benzodiazepines. If we have access to short-acting medications such as lorazepam 0.5 to 1mg, this can be very useful for panic attacks and the oral preparation can be used sublingually and is useful in the community. In general, oxygen is not helpful and has many limitations, although it provides a strong placebo effect. Try to use fans as described.

Gastrointestinal problems

Constipation

Constipation is very common in palliative care. Early advice and prescribing can prevent many difficult cases. Remember that even when oral intake is greatly reduced,

---

> ### Box 28.5 **Breathing techniques**
>
> 1. Diaphragmatic breathing; place one hand on your abdomen and one on your chest. Now breathe in and try to make sure the hand on your abdomen moves more than the one on your chest. Repeat for 10–20 minutes three times a day while lying supine. This can help build respiratory muscle strength and improve the depth of breathing.
> 2. Pursed lips; breathe in through your nose and out through your mouth with lips pursed as if you are blowing out a candle. This can be helpful when breathing rates are increasing.
> 3. Square breathing; breathe in for four seconds, then hold for four seconds. Breathe out for four seconds, and then hold for four seconds. This can be helpful when breathing rates are increasing.
>

> ### Box 28.6 **Medications to help breathlessness**
>
> - Low dose morphine e.g. 2.5–5mg po every four hours can improve symptoms of breathlessness (if already on morphine for pain control, increase the dose by 20 per cent and advise on taking break-through doses as required).
> - Diazepam 2.5–5mg po up to tds. This can be very helpful when the breathlessness is associated with significant anxiety or panic attacks.
> - Consider oxygen if hypoxic (however there is no evidence to support the use of palliative oxygen in patients with normal oxygen saturations).
> - Regular nebulized saline 0.9% may be helpful for patients with sticky bronchial secretions.
>
> Reproduced with permission from Makerere University and Mulago Hospital. Palliative Care Guidelines 2012. Copyright © 2011 Makerere University. This box is distributed under the terms of the Creative Commons Attribution Non Commercial 4.0 International licence (CC-BY-NC), a copy of which is available at http://creativecommons.org/licenses/by-nc/4.0/

there should be at least a small bowel motion every couple of days. Patients can feel very unwell if they become severely constipated, suffering nausea, vomiting, abdominal bloating, and cramping pain. Causes include medication, low oral intake, poor mobility, as well as problems in the bowel itself. Firstly, assess whether there is bowel obstruction, which is characterized by large-volume vomiting with no flatus being passed. Sometimes an abdominal X-ray helps us diagnose this. If this is a possibility, consider referral for surgery if suitable and such facilities are available. If there are no signs of obstruction, encourage oral fluids and increased intake of fibre-rich foods, e.g. fruit and vegetables. Rectal examination can help to identify very solid stools or a ballooned empty rectum which may mean the constipation is higher up. Usually we need both oral and rectal measures. Rectal measures which may be available include glycerol or bisacodyl suppositories or enemas. Oral options should include a stimulant such as bisacodyl (5–10mg) or Senna tablets (1–2 tabs), both taken at night as well as a softener such as liquid paraffin (10–20ml) or sodium docusate (50–300mg/day). Speak to the community as there may cheap effective local remedies, such as dried and ground paw paw (papaya) seeds, which act as a fibre laxative.

Nausea and vomiting

Nausea and vomiting are distressing symptoms and are a common problem. We should think carefully about the cause by taking a careful history and as usual identify any reversible causes. Our medications should be given specific to the cause, as different causes respond to different treatments. Table 28.1 may appear daunting, but it is important to approach nausea and vomiting with careful consideration.

Confusion

Delirium

Delirium is confusion usually associated with a drop in conscious level. It is important to diagnose early and consider the treatable causes. Relatively simple problems can result in delirium in palliative patients, such as urinary tract infection. It is unlikely that the patient presenting with delirium can describe the cause. We should listen to relatives as they are often best placed to identify early changes in cognition and behaviour. Many causes can be tackled quickly and cheaply with limited resources. We should not forget to check things like impaired hearing and sight, which can make symptoms worse. The two commonest causes are new medications and infection. We need to warn relatives that delirium can last several weeks, even when a reversible cause has been successfully managed. Our approach should include:

- Any new medications? Is the patient taking the right doses of established medications? Has anything changed that might lead to medication toxicity?
- Signs of infection. We should thoroughly examine the patient, thinking of local infections such as malaria or meningitis; we should dipstick urine.
- Think about blood sugar. Both high *and* low blood sugar can cause delirium.
- Assess for urinary retention. If in doubt, pass a catheter. Sometimes the blockage is higher up and results in kidney failure, but this is often irreversible.
- Look for dehydration, especially if there are problems with drinking.
- Always assess for constipation as it is often overlooked, and it is best to prevent or manage it as early as possible.
- Think of organ failure, specifically liver and renal. May require blood tests.
- Has the patient been dependent on any substance, e.g. alcohol?

Sometimes confusion and agitation are part of the end-of-life scenario and we should prepare family and ensure symptoms are well controlled.

We care for the patient providing a quiet, calm environment with a member of the family present. Talking to the patient in a calming manner can help the patient, the

Table 28.1 **Treatment of nausea and vomiting**

Cause	Clinical picture	Treatment	Remember to ...
Metabolic upset or side effect to medications.	Persistent nausea unrelieved by vomiting.	Haloperidol (500 micrograms to 1.5mg opd) Metoclopramide (10mg tds to qds)	Stop the offending medication. Check blood if appropriate to look for renal failure, liver failure, and or high calcium.
Slowing or stopping of the gastrointestinal system.	Vomiting is more of a problem than nausea. Patient feels relieved after vomiting, which is often of a large volume.	Metoclopramide (10 to 20mg qds)	Rule out obstruction in patients potentially suitable for surgery.
Intracranial problems such as tumours and meningitis.	Associated with headache and worse with movement	Cyclizine (25 to 50mg orally tds) Dexamethasone 8-26 mg opd	Consider whether there is any infection needing treatment.
Stomach and oesophagus irritation.	Nausea worse with eating. Reflux symptoms.	Ranitidine 150mg bd Omeprazole 20mg bd	Consider if there is peptic ulcer disease that needs further treatment.

opd=once daily; bd=twice daily; tds=thrice daily; qds=four times daily

family, and ourselves. Restraints are unnecessary and best avoided, as they will worsen the agitation. Medications are best avoided as they can exacerbate the problem, but sometimes we need to use a short-term intervention to control severe agitation. Try using haloperidol titrated from 0.5mg up to 3mg three times a day as required until they are settled. This can be given either orally or subcutaneously. If unavailable, chlorpromazine is an effective alternative. Benzodiazepines are not a replacement as they do not help cognition, although they can reduce anxiety and a small evening dose may be appropriate.

Dementia

In dementia, the onset of confusion and impaired thinking is slower than delirium and usually associated with an underlying cause, e.g. stroke. Worldwide, the most common form is Alzheimer's, followed by vascular causes. With dementia, consciousness is less affected, compared with delirium, unless there is an additional cause of confusion, e.g. infection or side-effects of medications.

One of the most distressing things for the person and family affected by dementia is the progressive, prolonged nature of the illness and the loss of communication and even recognition of loved ones, alongside physical deterioration. Open and sensitive communication is very important as well as helping plan for the future, e.g. how to manage legal and financial issues. As far as possible, support the person to maximize their function and help them feel involved and safe. Avoid sedating medications as this can make symptoms worse. Short-term memory is most impaired, but long-term memory may be intact so consider music, stories, and spiritual practices that can create a calm, familiar environment and aid communication. Dementia is also associated with physical problems so very good assessment, symptom control, and management of problems, including hearing and sight, is needed instead of simply attributing every problem to brain failure.

Skin problems

There are three major categories to consider.

Skin infections

Cancers, both primary and secondary, can cause large fungating wounds, which are embarrassing to the patient and family and can have an offensive smell. The impact is not just the physical problems but also the loss of self-esteem, disordered body image, social exclusion, and hopelessness. In many low- and middle-income settings people come with very extensive, advanced disease, especially with breast and cervical cancers. We should:

- Reassure the patient and involve the family in the care provided.
- Consider whether any referrals are needed for surgical or oncological treatment.
- Avoid abrasive products, e.g. betadine or hydrogen peroxide, which cause further trauma.

- Clean the wound using a salt solution (1 litre boiled and cooled water to 2 teaspoons of salt).
- Dress with clean gauze or local cotton. Initially change the dressings daily, or more frequently if there is a large discharge. Newspaper can be layered in the dressings if there is a lot of leakage. After cleaning, Vaseline gauze can be used if available.
- Maggots can be manually removed with forceps. A cloth soaked in turpentine, held close to the wound, can help draw the maggots out of the wound to be removed manually. We should remember that maggots are more offensive for the patient than for us, especially in the genital or head and neck regions.
- Offensive smells can be treated with crushed, uncoated metronidazole tablets. This is sprinkled onto the wound just before the new dressings. In some settings we will have metronidazole gel which is easy to use but expensive. For deep fungating wounds in head and neck cancers, nebulized parenteral metronidazole has been effective.

Problems from posture and poor skin health

These are mainly pressure sores and other wounds that fail to heal. Skin breakages can be managed as described. There are several simple ways to prevent pressure sores:

- Clean bedding on a foam mattress
- Encouraging changes of position every two hours, including sitting up or moving around if possible.
- Using pillows, or rubber gloves filled with water, to relieve pressure, e.g. next to a healing pressure sore, or to reduce friction between knees. Some communities have used resources like rubberized canvas to make a simple water bed that can be filled at the bedside.
- Look after the skin. Keep clean and well moisturised using petroleum jelly or barrier creams.
- Make sure than any measures include regular change of position.

'Is my wound getting better?'

We should take our time changing dressings. Patients and families often use this time to ask the care giver whether the wound will get better. If handled appropriately, this can be a helpful gateway to a deeper conversation about the illness and prognosis. Responding with a question, such as 'What do you think?' can provide illuminating answers. It is not necessary to have the full discussion while changing the dressing. We can acknowledge the importance of the question and bring it up later at a suitable moment.

Insomnia

Most people are affected by insomnia at some point in their lives, although transient insomnia is not usually a major problem. It becomes a problem when it is chronic, potentially leading to mood disorders, irritability, and a lack of motivation and energy. There is often a combination of physical and psychological causes. Physical causes include pain, caffeine intake, and urinary problems. Psychological causes include stress, anxiety, and depression.

We can advise and prescribe for the physical causes and try to offer a safe space in which concerns and challenges can be discussed. We may not have all the answers, but this is not the objective of listening. Having someone to talk with, outside of the family, is often what the patient wants and needs.

Relaxation techniques can be taught and tried with no need for expensive materials or medications. Techniques include:

- Protection of the sleep environment. Keep the bedroom quiet, dark, and cool if possible. Avoid unnecessary stimulation in the evening, such as television or late visitors.
- Meditation or prayer may be part of the culture or can be learned. This may include visualizing a peaceful place or experience.
- Focusing on breathing and then progressively contracting then relaxing muscles can be a useful practice.

Medications such as hypnotics can play a role, but should be used sparingly.

Social and legal issues

When we look at the needs of patients and families especially in low- and middle-income settings, social issues are a common, significant source of distress. For many this is financial when the illness has led to high medical costs or loss of income. Even travelling for clinic appointments can be a huge drain. People may also want to complete a task like paying for school fees or arranging a child's wedding. As discussed, palliative care can be a tool for alleviating poverty as we help people to have the best information and make the best choices. Setting clear and realistic goals together is a key part of palliative care (Figure 28.17).

Living with chronic illness leads to many different losses. People may lose their role as the bread-winner or decision maker in the family. They may struggle

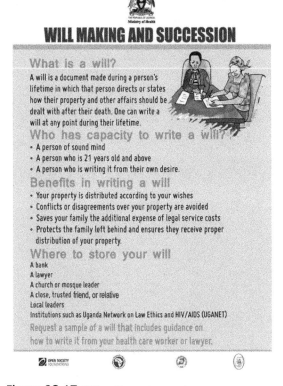

Figure 28.17 Will making and succession.

with stigma, isolation from work and friends, loss of self-esteem, and disordered body image. This may impact on relationships in many ways, including sexuality, and it is important to create safe environments for these difficult issues to be discussed and then support offered.

One area that is often neglected is legal issues. Making a will might ensure that the patient's wishes regarding property or resources are known and respected. This may reduce family conflict and ensure non-family members are included and vulnerable people are protected. It may help a patient to think through and communicate their wishes. It may also allow closure in the knowledge that they have provided for their dependants. Some teams have training in paralegal skills and can signpost to more formal legal advice. However, some people feel it is almost inviting death or 'putting on a curse' to plan for end-of-life care or make a will.

Psychological, emotional, and spiritual care needs

Many HCWs, even in resource-rich settings, are intimidated by the psychological and spiritual needs of patients and avoid this subject. Patients and families are often much more comfortable discussing these issues than their health worker, especially in resource-poor situations.

One helpful suggestion is to approach this subject as a learner, rather than a teacher. This starts with a genuine interest in the other person as a person, not just as a patient. This goes a long way to opening up the channels of communication about things that are important to the person and their family.

We value the contribution of professionally trained counsellors, psychologists, and pastoral care workers, although access to these services is limited. The support we can provide, as non-specialists, is often well received, especially when we follow the advice in the communication section earlier in the chapter.

Teamwork is crucial to good psychological and spiritual care. Our team should include members of the local community, including from religious faith groups. Team training will be helpful for us all in this domain (Figure 28.18).

Psychological distress

The impact of a life-limiting illness is traumatic for the patient and their family and requires significant adjustment. These periods of adjustment can lead to anxiety and difficulty coping and manifest as psychological distress. This is more common in situations of unrelieved physical suffering, poor communication, challenging social circumstances, and unanswered questions. We

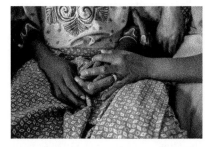

Figure 28.18 Palliative care hand-in-hand with patients.

should explore past experiences and current concerns, such as,

- Relationship difficulties—in the family and in the community.
- Worries—about how to provide food or support family, about employment.
- Views of others—how is their illness viewed by their neighbours, fear of contagion or taboo.
- Fears—about the future, about pain, about dying.
- Anger—about the illness or the treatment.

We can ask open questions about worries and fears and how they are coping. Sometimes these periods of adjustment lead to more significant symptoms of anxiety and depressed mood and we may need to offer medication (such as antidepressants or anxiolytics) alongside support. We will not, nor is it possible to, have all the answers. Listening is our choice of therapeutic tool.

Spiritual distress

Spiritual distress is perhaps the area we most avoid as HCWs. Even the concept of spiritual pain can be difficult to explore with patients and their carers. It is helpful to think of our spiritual needs as relationship or connection with God, relationship and connection with others, and our sense of purpose, meaning, and hope. Culture, beliefs, values, and relationships all make a big contribution to our spiritual context. Many of us express our spirituality through a faith-based framework but it is useful to think of spirituality in a broader sense (Figure 28.19).

So, when we are exploring these issues, we may ask questions like 'when you face difficult times, what gives you strength and hope?' 'do you feel at peace?' 'what lessons in life do you want to pass on to others?' 'are there relationships where you need to forgive or be forgiven?' and 'do you have a faith that supports you?' Discussion about spiritual issues can be a healing experience, allowing patients to reflect on their lives, find meaning and purpose, and even explore issues that they have not addressed before. Serious illness can make us review our priorities and be a time of spiritual growth.

Faith leaders have an important role to play but may benefit from training in palliative care; in particular, to avoid the tendency to connect physical wellness with God's blessing and burden the patient with an extra load of guilt.

As many of us have experienced in our own lives, it can be stressful and tiring to look after ill family

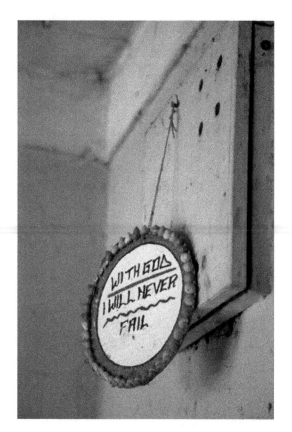

Figure 28.19 Spiritual care reminder in patient's home.

Reproduced courtesy of Dr Mhoira Leng. This image is distributed under the terms of the Creative Commons Attribution Non-Commercial 4.0 International licence (CC-BY-NC), a copy of which is available at http://creativecommons.org/licenses/by-nc/4.0/

members. This stress is multiplied in resource-poor situations where the family have limited control over their situation. They may have little confidence in the local health care structures, but have no alternative. In certain contexts, families may have a range of doubts as they face a life-limiting illness. They question whether this illness was an 'illness of doctors' and that perhaps they should have consulted a traditional healer earlier.

This fluctuating process will continue from the moment of first symptoms until after death. Conflicting advice from friends and other family members may worsen the situation as the family try to do their best within cultural expectations. There may be shame associated with certain illnesses leading to hiding ill relatives from the community, even from health workers. Warning signs of stress include fatigue, poor concentration, neglect of duties, feelings of helplessness, and anxiety.

Planning for end-of-life care

Our good intentions of preparing the patient and the family for death can lead to a temptation to predict the moment of death. We are frequently wrong. We can cause harm through the creation of unhelpful expectations. The capacity to accurately predict the moment of death is not required for good-quality palliative care. We may even find that the idea of timetabling death is contrary to our adopted culture, which may consider the timings of life and death as exclusively under the control of a supreme being. Our attempts at predicting the future may be offensive or laughable to them. We should encourage realistic, culturally appropriate expectations of the timing of death. As we look back over the course of the illness with the patient and family, most will make their own presumptions about the potential timings. Our job is to guide, prepare, and accompany. We maintain the objective of providing good QoL until the moment of death and into the period of bereavement.

It is important, however, that when the patient is actively dying, we can identify, support the family, and make the dying process as comfortable as possible through ongoing symptom assessment and control. Signs of nearing death include:

- Changes in breathing.
- Decreased consciousness.
- Skin colour and temperature changes as the peripheries shut down.

Suggestions for the family:

- Continuing to speak with the patient helps both the family and patient as their hearing may be intact until late stages, even if they seem to be barely conscious.
- Use a wet cloth to moisten the mouth and petroleum jelly to protect the lips. Avoid food or drink when conscious level is low, as this may lead to aspiration. This is distressing to the patient and to the family due to the increased gurgling sounds in the chest.
- Turn the patient every two hours to prevent pressure sores.
- Explain how noisy respiratory secretions may be distressing to the patient and show them how simple repositioning can help.
- Encourage them to follow their usual customs, for example reading holy literature or inviting a religious leader to visit.

Suggestions for the care team:

- Good symptom control should continue and plan for the common symptoms and consider planning access to these medication in advance. Some community services train families to give medications and others have end-of-life care packs.
- Many regular medications can be stopped, such as diabetic and hypertensive medications.
- Necessary medications may be administered through alternative routes, with rectal, nasogastric, sublingual, and subcutaneous routes being useful if the patient is unable to swallow. Try to avoid using IV lines but if repeated injections are anticipated a butterfly needle can be inserted and used as a route for regular injections.

Good end-of-life care which allows patients and families to make the best choices for them in their context may include stopping futile or unnecessary treatments (Figure 28.20). Excellent symptom control, including the use of medications that may have some sedative effects, may be helpful if there is agitation. It is important to emphasize that this is good medical practice with the aim of a dignified end to life in the place of choice. This should not be confused with euthanasia, which is the deliberate ending of a person's life and is illegal in most settings.

Bereavement care

Palliative care focuses also on the family and therefore support should continue after a person has died. The community may be best able to offer culturally appropriate support. However, it is worth remembering that some people may need additional help. Risk factors include those with a very dependent relationship, a distant relationship, previous mental health issues, multiple losses, sudden death or lack of time to adjust and make choices, poor symptom control at the end of life, and lack of support systems.

We should encourage people to understand grief is a normal reaction and to express how they are feeling. Active listening, presence, and reassurance can be very important. Most people will rebuild their lives and we can support them in this, recognizing this can take many months. People do not so much get over grief but rather integrate this experience. They move on to a new phase of living.

Support for the care team

Palliative care is a rewarding and needed service. It keeps us close to our own mortality, the mortality of those around us, and our personal journeys with grief. For all of us involved in this intensity of care, which includes

Symptom	Enternal Route	Subcutaneous Route
	Morphine 5 – 7.5 mg 4hrly	Morphine 2.5 – 5 mg 4hrly
Pain		
Morphine dose will depend on the patient, clinical problem and previous opioid use. If the patient is already taking opioids 1/6th of 24 hour oral dose can be given orally when needed or 1/2th of the 24hour oral dose can be given SC when needed.		
Anxiety or Agitation	Diazepam 5-10mg od titrated to tds, Lorazepam 0.5 to 2mg SL	Midazolam 2 to 5mg SC
Excessive bronchial secretions		Hyoscine butylbromide 20mg or Hyoscine hybrobromide 0.4mg od titrated to tds
Anti-secretory medication should be given when symptoms first occur and will be less helpful if given later.		
Issues of Hydration and Nutrition	• Patients should eat and drink as they wish and take sips of water as long as they are able. • Families should be educated that it is normal for patients to lose their appetite, sense of thirst and stop feeding towards the end of life. They should not feed	

Figure 28.20 Symptom control.

family members, we must not neglect our own emotional, spiritual, physical, and social needs. Burnout is common owing to chronic physical, emotional, and/or spiritual exhaustion. It is associated with feelings of being ineffective, cynical, and defeated. In health care settings, common features include wanting to withdraw from clinical practice and depersonalization. In other words, patients are no longer equal human beings, but rather we think of them as diagnoses, problems, or disruptions to our busy, important schedules. Other signs include tiredness, poor concentration and mistakes, anger, avoidance of patients and colleagues, becoming argumentative, and making frequent complaints (Figure 28.21).

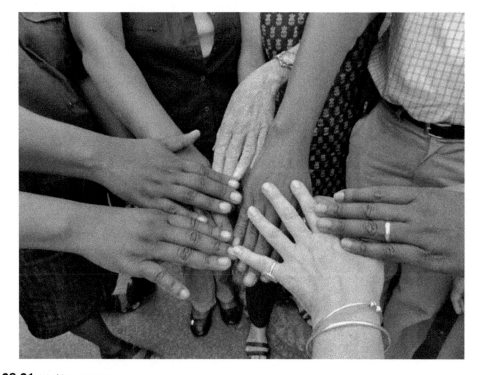

Figure 28.21 Working as a team.

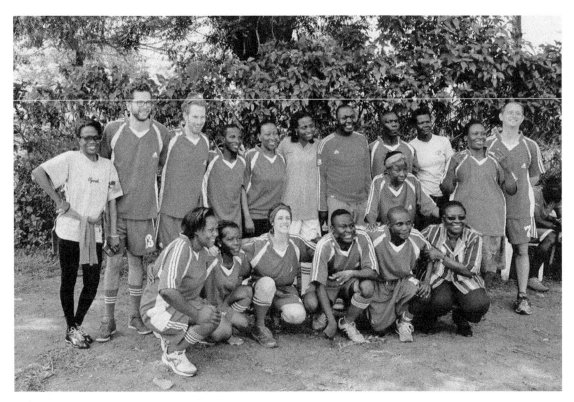

Figure 28.22 Participating in World Hospice and Palliative Care Day.

Reproduced courtesy of Dr Mhoira Leng. This image is distributed under the terms of the Creative Commons Attribution Non-Commercial 4.0 International licence (CC-BY-NC), a copy of which is available at http://creativecommons.org/licenses/by-nc/4.0/

Burnout, like most symptoms, is easier to prevent than to treat. A healthy work–life balance is important (Figure 28.22). Suggestions on avoiding burnout in ourselves and colleagues include:

- Accountability structures.

We should all have at least one mentor, to whom we are accountable, and one mentee, whom we hold accountable. It can be beneficial if these are from outside of our teams. These relationships help us to avoid burnout in ourselves and others.

- Ongoing training improves competencies and confidence.
- Regular work meetings with colleagues.

These meetings can provide a forum in which we can discuss and reflect upon challenging, and deceased, patients. Significant Event Analysis can be a useful tool to aid reflection following memorable events, both positive and negative.

- Regular time off work, including fun activities and enjoying other hobbies or interests.
- Non-work activities, e.g. social gatherings with colleagues, sport and exercise at least three times a week.

Further reading and resources

International Collaborative for Best Care for the Dying Person. *Supporting care in the last days or hours of life.* Liverpool: Marie Cure Palliative Care Institute Liverpool; 2014. Available from: http://www.palliativzentrum.kssg.ch/content/dam/dokument_library/container_palliativzentrum/palliativzentrum/Dokumente/International%20Model%20Document%20ICP.pdf.ocFile/International%20Model%20Document%20ICP.pdf

Lancet Commission Report: alleviating the access abyss in palliative care and pain relief – an imperative of Universal Health Coverage. *Lancet.* 2018; 391: 1391–454.

de Lima L, Bennett MI, Murray SA, Hudson P, Doyle D, Bruera E, et al. International Association for Hospice and Palliative Care (IAHPC) List of Essential Practices in Palliative Care. *Journal of Pain and Palliative Care Pharmacotherapy.* 2012; 26 (2): 118–22.

Available from: https://hospicecare.com/resources/palliative-care-essentials/iahpc-list-of-essential-practices-in-palliative-care/

World Health Organization. *Planning and implementing palliative care services*. 2016. Available from: http://www.who.int/ncds/management/palliative-care/palliative_care_services/en/

World Health Organization. *Reference guide for the development of a national health financing strategy*. 2015. Available from: http://www.who.int/health_finacninf/en/

Websites

African Palliative Care Association. Available from: https://www.africanpalliativecare.org/

Cairdeas International Palliative Care Trust. Available from: http://www.cairdeas.org.uk/

Indian Association for Palliative Care. Available from: http://palliativecare.in/

International Children's Palliative Care Network. Available from: http://www.icpcn.org/

International Hospice and Palliative Care Association. Available from: http://hospicecare.com/

Pallium India. Available from: http://palliumindia.org/

World Hospice and Palliative Care Alliance. Available from: http://www.thewhpca.org/

Useful textbooks available online

Amery J. *A Really Practical Handbook of Children's Care*. Lulu Publishing; 2016. Free download. Available from: https://itunes.apple.com/gb/book/a-really-practical-handbook-of-childrens-palliative-care/id1110435299?mt=11

Bates J. *Inspiring hope: Helping churches to care for the sick*. Available from: https://www.emms.org/about-emms/publications/inspiring-hope-palliative-care-handbook/.Registration required.

Downing J, Atieno M, Debere S, Mwangi-Powell F, Ddungu H, Kiyange F, editors. *Beating pain*. Kampala: African Palliative Care Association; 2010. Available from: http://www.icpcn.org/wp-content/uploads/2017/08/Beating-Pain-APCA-Handbook.pdf

Downing J, Atieno M, Debere S, Mwangi-Powell F, Kiyange F, editors. *Handbook of palliative care*. Kampala: African Palliative

Care Association; 2010. Available from: http://apps.who.int/medicinedocs/documents/s19115en/s19115en.pdf

Worldwide Hospice Palliative Care Alliance. *Palliative care toolkit and training manual*. Available from: http://www.thewhpca.org/resources/palliative-care-toolkit

Photographs (all taken by Dr Mhoira Leng with permission)

Child in urban slum, Uganda.
Palliative care volunteers, Uganda.
Supporting at home, Uganda.
With God I will never fail; on wall of patient's home, Uganda.
Hands together, Zambia.
Uganda MPCU team taking part in World Palliative Care day football tournament, Uganda.

References

1. Sallnow L, Richardson H, Murray SA, Kellehear A. The impact of a new public health approach to end-of-life care: A systematic review. *Palliative Medicine*. 2016; 30 (3): 200–11.
2. World Health Organization. *Palliative Care*. 2017. Available from: http://www.who.int/ncds/management/palliative-care/introduction/en/
3. Beard JR, Officer A, Araujo de Carvalho I, Sadana R, Pot AM, Michel J-P, et al. The World Report on ageing and health: A policy framework for healthy ageing. *The Lancet*. 2016; 387 (10033): 2145–54.
4. United Nations. *Strengthening of palliative care as a component of comprehensive care throughout the life course*, Doc. 67/19. 67th World Health Assembly. 2014. Available from: http://apps.who.int/gb/ebwha/pdf_files/WHA67/A67_R19-en.pdf
5. Human Rights Watch. *Access to pain treatment as a human right*. 2009. Available from: https://www.hrw.org/
6. World Health Organization. *Planning and implementing palliative care services*. 2016. Available from: http://www.who.int/ncds/management/palliative-care/palliative_care_services/en/
7. Baile W, Buckman R, Lenzi R, Glober G, Beale EA, Kudelka AP. SPIKES-A six-step protocol for delivering bad news: Application to the patient with cancer. *Oncologist*. 2000; 5 (4): 302–11

APPENDIX A

Supplies needed by a small health centre

Each project will need to draw up a list specific to its needs. Here are items that are likely to be needed by most clinics.

Medical equipment

Ambubag
Ampoule file
Aural forceps
Blood pressure machine
Clinical thermometers
Crutches adult/child
Dental forceps/gum retractor/syringes/needles
Dressing tray
Ear syringe
Eye bath
Eye-testing lenses and charts
First aid equipment
Foetal stethoscope
Forceps, various
Gallipots
Haemoglobinometer
Hair clippers
Height measurer
Jugs
Kidney bowls
Medicine measurers/pill counters
Microscope

Nasal hook for foreign bodies
Nasal speculum
Needle holders
Ophthalmoscope/spare batteries, bulbs
Otoscope/spare batteries, bulbs/speculums
Patella hammer
Plaster knife/shears
Portable suction
Probe
Scalpels
Scissors
Sigmoidoscope/proctoscope
Splinter forceps
Splints
Stethoscope
Tape measure
Tourniquets
Trolley
Tuning forks
Vacuum extractor
Vaginal speculums
Weighing scales adult/child

Renewable medical supplies

Adhesive tape
Aprons
Bandages, various, including crepe/triangular
Bottles, etc., for dispensing
Butterfly needles
Child feeding tubes
Cotton wool
Delivery kits
Dressings, various
Elastic (crepe) bandages
Episiotomy set
Family planning supplies, including IUDs
Gauze bandages
Gauze compresses
Gloves (rubber), large, small/maternity, and non-latex
HIV test kit
Intravenous giving sets and cannulas/butterfly sets
Insect repellent containing DEET
Labels for dispensing
Laboratory supplies
Lancets for malaria tests
Lubricant, e.g. KY jelly
Malaria rapid diagnostic tests
Mediswabs

Micropore (non-allergenic) tape
Midwives' kit
Mosquito nets, impregnated
Nailbrush
Needles, gauges 26, 22,18
Paraffin gauze dressings
PVC sheeting
Safety box (sharps containers)
Safety pins
Soap and soap dishes
Spoons, plastic
Steri-strips for small wound closure
Sugar/salt/spoon for demonstrating ORS
Suturing materials
Swabs and swab sticks
Syringes, 2 ml, 5 ml, 10 ml
Tongue depressors
Tweezers
Umbilical cord clamp/tie
Urinary catheters, varying sizes/spigot
Urinary dipsticks
Urine drainage bag
Vaccine vial monitors
Water buckets and dippers

General equipment

Autoclave/sterilizer/pressure cooker with needle and syringe rack, drums/autoclave tape, labels, wrapping cloths
Batteries
Basins
Bedpans and urinals
Blankets, pillows, etc.
Brooms, dustpans, scrubbing brush, etc.
Buckets
Candles
Chairs/benches
Clock (timer)
Cold boxes
Computer, software and accessories
Examination couches (foldable)
Fuel
Generator/cable
Kettle
Keys/locks
Lamps/lanterns

Matches
Mobile phones
Money box
Refrigerator (with temperature monitor)
Screen (privacy)
Storage cupboards
Stove
Stretcher
Tables
Teaching aids, e.g. flashcards, drama props, videos
Tool and repair kit
Torch/kerosene lantern
Tray (plastic)
Trolley (cart for dressing/dispensing)
PC, Video/DVD player, and other ICT equipment
Water filter with replacement 'candles'
Whiteboard/chalkboard and coloured crayons

Records, registers, etc.

Books (medical)
Calculator
Cash books, ledger, etc.
CHW notebooks/diaries
Clinic Essential Drug list
Digital recording equipment
Family folders
Folders and files
Patient numbers (cardboard)
Petty cash container

Prescription pads
Record cards (including self-retained), tally sheets, report forms, etc.
Referral letters
Registers (strong)
Rubber stamps/ink pads
Standing orders/treatment protocols
Stationery, including paper, pens, drawing pins, paper clips, etc.
Stock cards/order forms

APPENDIX B

Community health resources

Please note that many resources are mentioned at the end of each chapter. Here, we have compiled a list of some more general and international sources. Each reader and each country will have its own, and our apologies for any you may feel have not been mentioned.

Africa Christian Health Associations Platform.

Website: http://africachap.org/en/

In its Constitution ACHAP defines its mission as 'inspired by Christ's healing ministry. ACHAP supports Church related health associations and organizations to work and advocate for health for all in Africa, guided by equity, justice and human dignity'. The website gives information on and links to the many Associations in sub-Saharan countries

Aga Khan Development Network.

Website: http://www.akdn.org/

AKDN aims to transform health care systems by training thousands of nurses, midwives, and doctors. It operates community health projects, often in conjunction with rural development programmes, in some of the poorest and remote areas

Arukah Network for Global Community Health (previously Community Health Global Network, CHGN).

Email: team@arukahnetwork.org

Website: http://www.arukahnetwork.org

This is a networking and training organization that aims to link, share information, and strengthen community based health programmes.

Names, addresses and emails change frequently but were correct at the time of publishing. If you have trouble finding the organisation search on line e.g., through Google.

Teaching Aids at Low Cost (TALC) (now commonly known as Health Books International) PO Box 49, St Albans, Herts, AL1 4AX, UK.

Tel: +44 (0) 1727 853869.

Fax: +44 (0) 1727 846852.

Email: info@talcuk.org

Website: http://www.talcuk.org

It is helpful to be on TALC's free mailing list.

Voluntary Health Association of India,

B 40 Qutab Institutional Area, South of IIT, New Delhi, 110 016, India.

Email: vhai@vsnl.com and vhai@sify.com

Website: http://www.vhai.org

VHAI publishes journals, e.g. *Health for the Millions* and health educational materials in regional languages. It runs training programmes and acts as resource and advisory centre on all forms of community-based health care. It has associated branches in each state of India. Its website is worth accessing by all programmes working in South Asia and beyond.

General International Development Resources

British Overseas NGOs for Development (BOND)

Regent's Wharf, 8 All Saints Street, London N1 9RL, UK

Email: bond@bond.org.uk

Website: http://www.bond.org.uk

A membership organization valuable for information and networking.

Centers for Disease Control and Prevention (CDC).

Website: https://www.cdc.gov

Based in the United States, CDC and their publications and website are an excellent resource for worldwide global health information.

Footsteps Magazine

Tearfund, Resources Department, 100 Church Road, Teddington TW11 8QE, UK.

Fax: +44 (0) 1746 764594.

Email: enquiries@tearfund.org.uk

Website: http://learn.tearfund.org/ from which current and back copies can be downloaded

A free international newsletter on practical aspects of health and development. Published four times per year in English, French, Spanish, Portuguese and other languages. This is highly recommended for all programmes

Hesperian Health Guides (Hesperian Foundation)

1919 Addison Street #304, Berkeley, CA 94704, USA.

Email: hesperian@hesperian.org

Website: http:// www.hesperian.org

Outstanding books, health information and newsletters and health wikis and illustrations. Original publishers of Where There is No Doctor. We recommend every programme to be in touch with Hesperian and make use of their resources and their website

Nossal Institute for Global Health

University of Melbourne, Australia

Website: http://mspgh.unimelb.edu.au/centres-institutes/nossal-institute-for-global-health

Their mission is to support improvements in health of vulnerable communities in partnership, through research, education and inclusive development practice

Oxfam Publishing

Oxfam House, John Smith Drive, Cowley, Oxford OX4 2JY UK

Email for orders: policyandpractice@oxfam.org.uk

Website: http://policy-practice.oxfam.org.uk/?cid=rdt_policyandpractice.

Oxfam also has regional offices in many countries. It advises about community health, development, and funding and publishes a variety of useful books and manuals, including valuable country profiles.

Pan-American Health Organization (PAHO)

525 23rd Street, NW, Washington DC, 20037, USA.

Website: http:/www.paho.org.

A major health resource centre for the Americas.

The Panos Institute

9 White Lion Street, London N1 9PD, UK.

Email: info@panos.org.uk

Website: www.panos.org.uk.

This institute specializes in information and communications for sustainable development.

Practical Action Publishing (previously known as Intermediate Technology).

Website: http://www.practical action.org or https://practicalactionpublishing.org

Email: publishing@practicalaction.org.uk.

Publishes many books and also has a comprehensive book catalogue covering all aspects of health, development and technology.

Swiss Resource Centre and Consultancies for Development (SKAT) (Includes both SKAT Consulting and SKAT Foundation)

Vadianstrasse 42, CH-9000 St Gallen, Switzerland.

Email: info@skat.ch.

Website: http://www.skat.ch.

Produces lists of publications in various languages on development, appropriate technology, water and sanitation. Also a quarterly newsletter.

World Health Organization (WHO)

Marketing and Dissemination, CH-1211 Geneva 27, Switzerland

Website: www.who.int/publications with details of how to order, and information about all WHO publications.

Also on their website is a vast range of health information, which, with careful searching, will give information about many aspects of community-based health care. Most chapters in this book have links to particular areas on their website for more information on their specific programmes. The WHO is the definitive United Nations agency that advises governments worldwide on all aspects of health care. It publishes a large number of books, journals, reports, and other resources. Details of their regional offices can be obtained from their website.

Specific community health topics

Child Health Care

Centre for International Child Health

Imperial College London, Section of Paediatrics, Division of Infectious Diseases, Department of Medicine, 2nd Floor Wright Fleming Building, Room 232, St Mary's Campus, London, W2 1PG

Tel: +44 (0) 20 7594 8839

Email: cich@imperial.ac.uk

Website: https://www.imperial.ac.uk/centre-for-international-child-health

Facilitating research partnerships and educational activities for global child health.

Child-to-Child

Institute of Education, 20 Bedford Way, London WC1H OAL, UK.

Tel: +44 (0) 207 612 6649

Fax: +44 (0) 207 612 6645

Website: http://www.child-to-child.org.

Child-to-Child publishes a whole range of resource books, readers and activity sheets to enable children to teach other children and family members, or for schemes who include children as partners in health and development. Many of these materials are also available from TALC.

Save the Children UK and Save the Children International

Website: http://www.savethechildren.org.uk.and https://www.savethechildren.net

This large international organization dedicated to bringing lasting benefits to children is committed to the principles of community-based health care. It helps to set up long-term health and development programmes worldwide. It publishes a wide range of books on all aspects of children, including conflict, emergencies, development, and food security.

UCL Institute of Child Health

30 Guilford Street, London WC1N 1EH

Webiste: http://www.ucl.ac.uk/ich

The mission of the UCL Great Ormond Street Institute of Child Health is to: 'improve the health and well-being of children, and the adults they will become, through world-class research, education and public engagement'.

UNICEF (United Nations Children's Fund)

UNICEF House, 3 UN Plaza, New York 10017, USA.

Website: http://www.unicef.org/publications.

Advises governments and agencies on programmes for children. Provides a large range of resource materials, journals, and books. Their regional offices will provide advice on all aspects of child health care, and they also publish regional journals. The *State of the World's Children* is a major report published yearly.

Eye Health

International Centre for Eye Health

London School of Hygiene and Tropical Medicine, Keppel Street, London WC1E 7HT UK

Email: icehorg@iceh.org.uk.

Website: http://www.iceh.lshtm.ac.uk.

Advises and publishes information on all aspects of eye care, including prevention of blindness.

Health Technology

Tropical Health Technology

Website: http://www.tht.ndirect.co.uk

THT has its prime focus in laboratory services and associated information and technology.

Mental Health

Developing Mental Health

PRIME, Beckett House, Mitre Way, Battle, East Sussex, TN33 0AS UK

Website: http://www.developingmentalhealth.org.

A key resource for community mental health care, a subject of growing importance.

Primary Health Care

African Medical Research Foundation (AMREF)

HQ Langata Road, PO Box 00506, 27961 Nairobi, Kenya

Email: info@amrefhq.org.

Kenyan office email: info@amrefke.org

Website: http://www.amref.org (Offices in various other countries.)

Publishes books, journals, and other literature. Runs training courses and seminars. Acts as a comprehensive advisory centre on primary health care.

Medical supplies and equipment for primary health care: A practical resource for procurement and management. Kaur M, Hall S. Coulsdon: ECHO International; 2001.

Available from: http://apps.who.int/medicinedocs/documents/s20282en/s20282en.pdf

Provides a detailed suggestions for equipping a primary health care centre.

MAP International

2200 Glynco Parkway, Brunswick, Georgia 31525-6800 USA.

Email: map@map.org.

Website: http://www.map.org.

A resource and information consultancy on community health development with offices through-out the world. MAP also supplies essential drugs and medical equipment for primary health care programmes and runs training courses.

Sexual Health & Family Planning

International Planned Parenthood Federation (IPPF)

4 Newhams Row, London SE1 3UZ, UK

Tel + 44 (0) 939 8200.

Email: info@ippf.org.

Website: http://www.ippf.org.

Advises and publishes information on all aspects of family planning and child spacing.

Water and Sanitation

Global Handwashing Partnership

Website: http://www.globalhandwashing.org

Provides training, research summaries and education resources on handwashing and its impact on international health.

Water, Engineering and Development Centre (WEDC)

Loughborough University, Loughborough, Leics LE11 3TU, UK.

Email: wedc@lboro.ac.uk.

Website: http://wedc.lboro.ac.uk

A resource centre and consultancy on all aspects of water supplies and sanitation.

Journals with community health emphasis

Bulletin of the World Health Organization
Available from: http://www.who.int/bulletin/en/

The Christian Journal for Global Health
Available from: http://journal.cjgh.org/index.php/cjgh

An open access, peer reviewed journal on global health, it provides faith-inspired approaches to promoting global health and offers innovative solutions to many of the most vexing health challenges. Published monthly and containing many articles of interest and relevance, it includes evidence-based and thoughtful discussion and facilitates broad-based and holistic learning and sharing within an academic framework. Areas covered include community and public health, health care services, and mission and health.

Community Eye Health Journal
Available from: https://www.cehjournal.org

A publication of the London School of Hygiene and Tropical Medicine sent free to over 22,000 health care providers worldwide, mainly in low and middle-income countries, providing up-to-date and relevant information to eye care workers of all levels in the countries where the burden of eye disease and blindness is greatest.

Family and Community Health Journal
Available from: http://journals.lww.com/familyandcommunityhealth/pages/default.aspx

This journal publishes rigorous scholarly work from multiple disciplines using qualitative, quantitative, and mixed methods to highlight the full spectrum of family and community-focused research undertaken to reduce health disparities and to achieve health equity.

International Journal of Community Medicine and Public Health (IJCMPH)
Available from: http://www.ijcmph.com/index.php/ijcmp

An open access, international, monthly, peer-reviewed journal publishes articles of authors from India and abroad with special emphasis on original research findings that are relevant for developing country perspectives including India.

Journal of Community Health
Available from: https://link.springer.com/journal/10900

A publication for health promotion and disease prevention, coverage includes preventive medicine, new forms of health manpower, analysis of environmental factors, delivery of health care services, and the study of health maintenance and health insurance programmes.

The Lancet Global Health
Available from: https://www.journals.elsevier.com/the-lancet-global-health/.

This exciting journal is dedicated to publishing high-quality original research, commentary, correspondence, and blogs on the following subjects as they pertain to low- and middle-income countries: reproductive, maternal, neonatal, and child health; adolescent health; infectious diseases, including neglected tropical diseases; non-communicable diseases; mental health; the global health workforce; health systems; health policy; and public health.

The Lancet medical journal plublished weekly is the leading worldwide journal dedicated to global and planetary health in addition to publishing high-level research on a wide range of key heath topics

Tropical Doctor

The Royal Society of Medicine Press Ltd, 1 Wimpole Street, London W1G OAE, UK

Tel: +44 (0) 207 290 2928

Fax: +44 (0) 207 290 2929

Email: rsmjournals@rsm.ac.uk.

Available from: http://journals.sagepub.com/home/tdo

A useful journal for doctors and nurses working in community health programmes and rural hospitals.

Note:

Names, addresses and emails change frequently but were correct at the time of publishing. If you have trouble finding the organisation search on line e.g., through Google.

APPENDIX C

Using the family folder system

This is a template which can be helpful if you are using the Family Folder System described in Chapter 6 to which you will need to refer to understand the boxes below. It is deliberately designed to be very simple.

Each programme will need to make its adaptation to the sections on family conditions, and in particular to relevant diseases in the programme area, as well as the most important immunizations and types of family planning used in your context.

FAMILY FOLDER FORM

Name of head of family	Occupation	Folder number	Date of survey
Village/town/colony	District	Region	State/Province
Religion	Languages	Type of family (nuclear/joint)	

HOUSEHOLD CHARACTERISTICS

Type of house	Electrical supply	Lighting	Cooking fuel used
Ventilation	Latrine type	Waste disposal system	Handwashing facility
Drinking water source	Malaria prevention measures	Animals and housing	Transport/mobility
Communication devices and media	Significant nutritional patterns	Health education status	Income/socioeconomic Status

DETAILS OF FAMILY'S CONDITIONS

		1	2	3	4	5	6	7	8	9	10	11	12	13	14
Remarks															
Education	Sch. Lit.														
	Adult lit.														
Addiction	Tobacco														
	Alcohol														
Family planning	Elig for fp														
	If pregnant														
	Coil														
	O/c pill														
	Vas														
	Tub														
Immunization	Tet tox														
	Measles														
	Polio														
	Dpt														
	Bcg														
Diseases and conditions	Nutritn (<5)														
	Other														
	Disability														
	Tb														
Family profile	Relation to others														
	Relation to Head														
	Sex														
	DOB														
	Name														
	Number	1	2	3	4	5	6	7	8	9	10	11	12	13	14

VITAL EVENTS SINCE SURVEY

Births

Name	Sex	Father's name	DOB

Deaths

Name	Age	Cause	Date of death

Migration

Name	Sex	Date of mig.	Relation to head	In/ out	Reason

FELT PROBLEMS—What are the main problems affecting your family?

1.

2.

3.

USE OF EXISTING SERVICES—Who and where does the family attend when sick? And how distant?

1.

2.

3.

Index